100270

HEALTHIER LIVING

1770

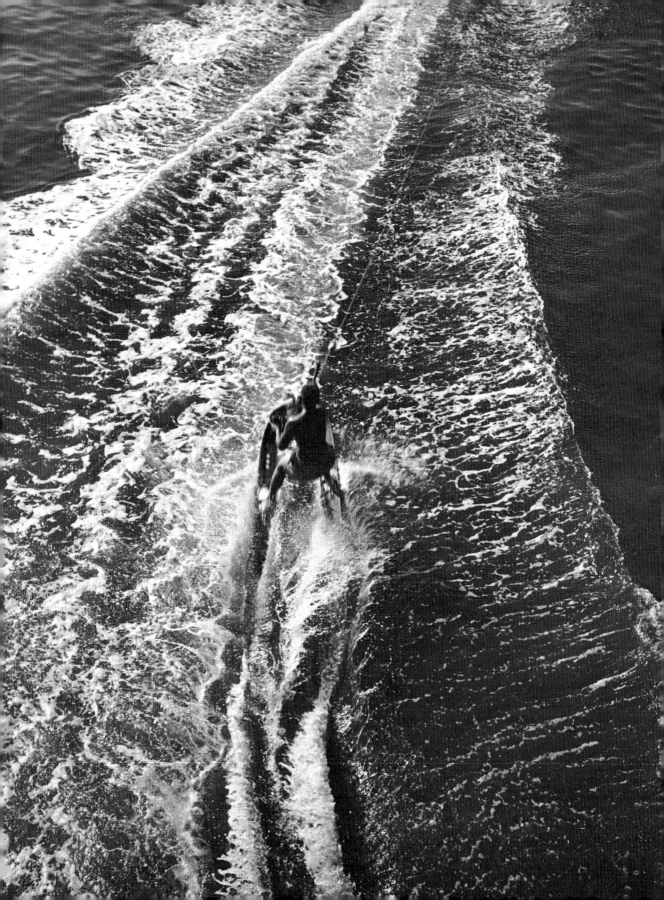

HEALTHIER LIVING

A College Text with Readings in Personal and Environmental Health

THIRD EDITION

JUSTUS J. SCHIFFERES, Ph.D.

Director, Health Education Council; Formerly: Medical
Editor, National Foundation for Infantile Paralysis;
Associate in Hygiene, Columbia College; Instructor in
Health Education, Teachers College, Columbia University

With a Foreword by
WILLIAM HAMMOND, M.D.
Editor of the New York State Journal of Medicine

JOHN WILEY & SONS, INC.
New York · London · Sydney · Toronto

TO MY FAMILY
Cecile, Stephen, Sande

A Health Education Council Book

Books by Justus J. Schifferes include

Essentials of Healthier Living
Third Edition

Healthier Living
Second Edition

Library of Congress Catalogue Card Number: 76-96957

SBN 471 75945 7

Printed in the United States of America

10 9 8 7 6 5 4 3 2 1

PREFACE

THE PURPOSE OF THIS NEW BOOK IS TO PROVIDE A COMPREHENSIVE, SCIENTIFIC, up-to-date textual foundation *with selected readings* for a thorough college course in health education.

There have been five precursors: the original edition, 1954; a revised edition, 1965; and three briefer editions (*Essentials of Healthier Living*), 1960, 1963, and 1967. While this new edition has a wealth of new and updated material, it still retains the editorial features that prompted the adoption of the earlier versions in some 250 colleges and universities in the United States.

This book is divided into five major parts, which may also be regarded as major concepts in modern health education. They are: (1) mental health, (2) personal health, (3) family living, (4) health hazards, and (5) environmental health. A detailed view of the different topics in each of these parts can be gleaned from the Table of Contents or by leafing through the book. The wealth of material here will make it possible for instructors to assign some parts for careful study and others for outside reading.

Readings

What is chiefly new in this edition is the inclusion of carefully selected readings from a wide variety of sources. These reading materials are not otherwise readily at hand—either for the student nor in many cases for the instructor.

The readings cluster about a few major, and frequently controversial, subjects—drug abuse, perspectives in sexuality, and environmental health. These readings add breadth and depth to the classroom considerations of these subjects.

A book of readings alone—and there are such books—usually lacks continuity and perspective with reference to the whole field of subject matter to be covered. A textbook without readings often suffers from lack of timeliness and a narrowness in point of view. This book, including both text and readings, has only one author but it also has over 30 other contributors, each with a specific and personal point of view on an important topic. This volume may be considered as *two books in one;* text and readings.

Highlights of New Material

Another feature of this book is a newly written chapter on *drugs and drug abuse,* a critical subject on many campuses. It is often the duty of health educators to convey specific and timely information on this subject to college students.

Considerable new material has been added on the following topics:

Birth control, a subject that can no longer be avoided in realistic health education courses.

Personality development, a discussion of theories of personality other than that of Sigmund Freud (Adler, Jung, et al).

The psychology of obesity, an important factor to be taken into account when dieting to lose weight.

Two new exercise hobbies, jogging and "aerobics," that have gained considerable acceptance.

Numbers of people in the health professions, a new tally.

Motorcycle accidents, an increasingly serious addition to the annual toll of motor vehicle accidents.

Sleep, a discussion of new experiments utilizing REM (rapid eye movements).

A Philosophy of Health Education

The fundamental principles on which this book is written are time-tested. If I may be permitted to quote a few sentences from the preface to the original edition of this work, I willingly repeat:

"This is a book on health, not disease. It stands on the premise that promotion of health, for which you may read happiness, is something different from and beyond the prevention of disease, though not completely divorced from it.

"This book is written on the principle that all learning is one learning. It draws on history, literature, anthropology, sociology, psychiatry, psychology, child development, and a host of other academic disciplines, including [English poetry]. . . .

"I see the aim of modern health education as that of inspiring a course of human conduct illumined by an understanding of the structure and function of the human body. . . . But bodily function is modified and controlled by the human mind and emotions, and it takes place within a social framework. I have given fuller consideration, therefore, to the social factors that play upon mind and body and thus account for bodily function or malfunction (disease). I can sum this up in one polysyllabic phrase: namely, a multidisciplinary approach to sociopsychosomatic medicine."

This book seeks to stimulate, motivate, and inspire readers to wise health behavior, based on well-marshaled scientific facts and well-considered attitudes. Hence, it does not preach. On many important but unresolved health issues, it frankly presents pro-and-con opinions, drawn from recent authoritative sources. I trust the reader, who is and must be treated as an adult, to come to intelligent, personal—and therefore meaningful—decisions in his health conduct. On such crucial matters of student interest as eating, drinking, driving, dieting, smoking, family living, drugs, and the like, I have sought to present information that would evoke intelligent personal decisions; but I have tried to avoid telling readers exactly what they should or should not do.

Teaching Aids

No textbook can take the place of good teaching—although a well-prepared textbook can make good teaching easier. A number of teaching aids have been "built in" to this book, for example, the Summary Review Questions at the end of each chapter. Special attention may be called to the "sense or nonsense" questions for starting a classroom discussion.

The various appendices offer further *teaching aids*. Newly added to this edition is a *glossary*. Other appendices include "A Short Reference Catalog of Common Human Ailments," a "Calorie Counter of Common Human Foods," and "First Aid—Condensed and Illustrated."

Illustrations

Many new and striking illustrations have been added to this book. Illustrations play a functional role; for example, they summarize most of the anatomy and physiology that is presented here. The full-color "transvision" insert offers a unique opportunity to "see through" the human body. Charts and graphs carry much solid statistical information not elsewhere repeated. Up-to-date photographs make an impact that words alone cannot convey.

Acknowledgements

A textbook as comprehensive as this must draw its facts from many sources. These have been duly credited in earlier editions, in instructor's manuals, in footnotes and in Appendix E, "Chapter References and Bibliography."

Every book is a cooperative enterprise. I wish to acknowledge and express my grateful appreciation to many individuals and organizations whose cooperation made this book possible. They are mentioned by name in a formal acknowledgements section, which is Appendix F, page 563.

An acknowledgement that I must give in this preface is to Charlotte Shelby, whose depth-editing, keen sensibility, and devotion to the details of making this a first-rate textbook can hardly be overestimated.

I have been encouraged in the preparation of this book by the hope that its carefully chosen subject matter—including the new readings—its scientific orientation, and its literary style might guide some students along the path to healthier living.

Justus J. Schifferes, Ph.D.

Livingston, New Jersey
January 1970

FOREWORD

THIS NEW BOOK, LIKE SO MANY OF ITS AUTHOR'S EARLIER WORKS, CONTAINS a great store of up-to-date health and medical information. An informed opinion and a rational point of view pervade the work. While written primarily for the college student, this book might well serve a parallel need for intelligent adults of any age.

I have known Dr. Schifferes both as a health educator and a medical writer, a valued Fellow of the American Medical Writers Association and the American Public Health Association. He has gone far toward mastering that most difficult art of communication—namely, science writing for the general and student publics. The facts herein presented on the human body in health and disease are developed in the best tradition of the art.

We are all—college students included—subjected to a barrage of misinformation, half truths, and sensationalism about health matters. This misinformation is widely scattered by the faultless technique and efficiency of the various modern media of mass communication. Books like this one are necessary to set the matter straight. Of this particular book it may be said that it does the job forthrightly and with all essential detail.

Throughout the book Dr. Schifferes stresses the recognition of the third component involved in "healthier living." Social wellbeing, he emphasizes, goes along with physical and mental wellbeing in achieving reasonable health goals. We have long been aware of this fact but are just now beginning to apply it. As the author pertinently concludes, "The physical health and survival of the human race are inextricably interwoven with its mental health and moral vision."

There is valuable material here on physical and emotional fitness with a sensible and workable program for attaining and maintaining balance in these important spheres. It must be recognized that poor health still is an important cause of college drop-outs and that emotional disturbance ranks highest among the reasons.

The section of the book which discusses sexual drive and family life is noteworthy. Without preachment, these highly sensitive areas of life are clearly explained and put in proper perspective.

While this book has been designed as a college textbook, and offers a wealth of teaching opportunities at this level, it should also prove valuable to anyone called upon to counsel young adults in relation to their physical or emotional health.

Health education in the modern world has not one but many faces. Its locale ranges from the physician's office, through schools and colleges and various voluntary health agencies, to the depth of jungles. That is why it is good to see in this book an outline of the functions of the World Health Organization and a generous presentation of the factors involved in the area of environmental health at home and abroad.

It is the function of health education to impart information, change attitudes, and induce behavior in the direction of healthier living. When a physician gives advice and writes a prescription for an individual patient, he is in effect a health educator as well as a therapist. Through his advice and the information he imparts, often limited by the time factor, the physician seeks to induce healthier behavior on the part of his patient. Unfortunately, with the exception perhaps of pediatrics, people rarely seek his advice until they are ill. He has relatively little opportunity to practice preventive medicine. This gap can be largely closed by the efforts of the professional health educator, who may be doing his work under the auspices of school, college, public health department, or voluntary health agency.

Formal health education in the college or university has special responsibility. Here, usually, is the last chance to provide young people with an organized course in the wide variety of subjects that comprise modern health education. On this score I can do no better than quote the statements of Alexander G. Ruthven, then president of the University of Michigan, on the occasion of the Third National Conference on Health in Colleges:

"Health is one of the cardinal principles of education. . . . I submit as a basic and enduring reality of life that knowledge of present, accepted, scientific facts is a determining factor in the protection and promotion of health and should be made part of the equipment of every student. . . . A curriculum should include basic courses in personal and community health, family health and mental health. . . . Since we cannot hope to give our students all of the knowledge they will need for the rest of their lives, relative values should be considered, and some of the less important offerings sacrificed for more adequate instruction in the science of keeping well."

This text, the third edition of *Healthier Living,* contributes wisely and thoroughly to the acknowledged goals of modern health education.

William Hammond, M.D.

Editor, New York State Journal of Medicine;
Fellow, American College of Physicians;
Past President, American Medical Writers Association

CONTENTS

INTRODUCTION

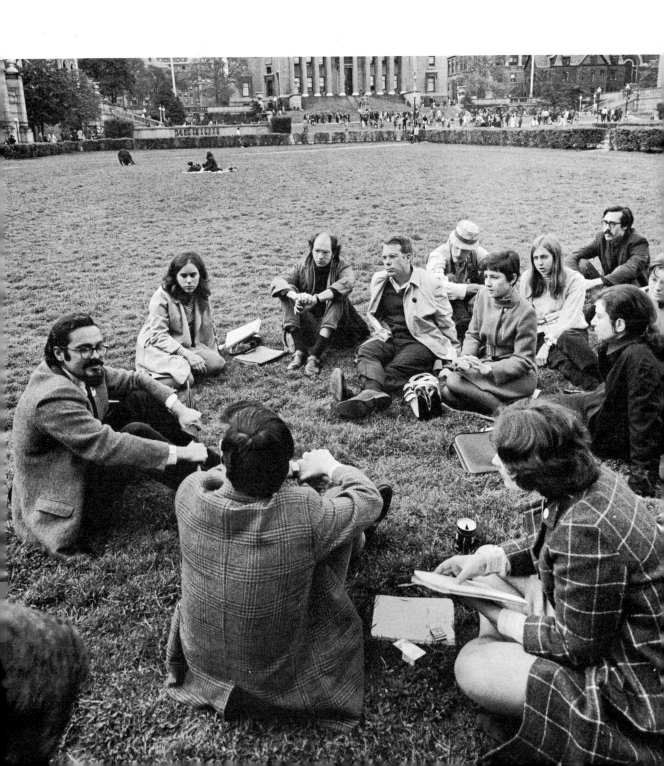

OVERLEAF
College life brings with it new ideas, new people, new books, new living quarters, and new problems. (Photograph by Zimbel-MONKMEYER)

1

HEALTH IN
THE COLLEGE COMMUNITY

Health is a state of complete physical, mental, and social
well-being and not merely the absence of disease or infirmity.
Statement of the World Health Organization

HEALTH, AS DESCRIBED ABOVE, IS A GOAL toward which anyone and everyone in the world can aspire, but relatively few reach. Health, although a personal possession, depends on the existence of sound and well-rounded community health resources. In a healthy state we do not live with or to ourselves alone. As a crude example, your face might be pocked instead of smooth if there were no public health mechanism for vaccination against smallpox.

Health and disease are not complete opposites; the individual and the community harbor degrees of each. Many people, despite pain and disability, maintain a cheerful and healthy attitude toward life. Even very sick people retain a great number of normal bodily functions. On the other hand, rigorous clinical examination of some of the apparently healthiest specimens of mankind may detect incipient weaknesses or flaws—a tendency toward high (or low) blood pressure, a slightly oversensitive digestive tract, or a fear of closed places (claustrophobia) for example. It should be especially noted that the overdeveloped, heavily muscled strong man and the pancake-thin, self starved beauty are in no better health than less conspicuous men and women.

We move toward health as we move away from disease, and vice-versa. Indeed that is why we have chosen to title this book "Healthier Living." Health is relative.

It is even possible to express this partly sick, partly well concept as it applies to communities in a mathematical formula, worked out by epidemiologist Dr. John Gordon of Harvard, as follows:

$$\frac{D}{H + D} + \frac{H}{H + D} = 1$$

where D represents the number of people in the community (or mathematical universe) who are sick, or more diseased than healthy, at a given time; and H the number who are healthy, or at least on the healthier side of the ledger. This formula is particularly valuable for ascertaining how ravaged a given community may be by an epidemic of an infectious disease.

Community health is the sum and extension of the personal health of each and all individual members of the community. But personal health is also the function of the operative health resources of the community: its pure water supply, enforcement of sanitary regulations, availability of doctors, nurses, hospitals, and hundreds of other things. It is not easy to be a well person in a sick community.

3

Community is a word of many images. A community of human beings might be as small as a single household or as large as a nation. It might be as geographically pat as a township, village, city, county, or state; or as scattered and diverse as a racial or religious group, or people of specific national origin within another country. The essence of community is *community of interest*.

Health in the College Community

We can speak, therefore, of a college community; primarily students and faculty, but also including, when you think of it, parents of students, alumni, custodial employees, and many others. It is also possible to define, outline, and attack specific college health problems. Indeed the American College Health Association and its individual members associated with college health services have been doing this pointedly for a number of decades. Great progress has been made, for example, in the management of infectious mononucleosis, a common campus disorder popularly called "student's disease." Medical schools and colleges, of course, are the lifeblood of the scientific and clinical research upon which depends further conquest over disease. Some colleges and universities, of which Ohio State is a prime example, are spearheads of health promotion and health education within the larger geographic communities they serve.

Healthwise a college, *alma mater,* owes several obligations to its students and faculty—notably adequate health service facilities, usually known as the college or student health service, and opportunities for health education at an adult level. Between 15 and 20% of the colleges in the United States do not fulfill these obligations. But you who have this book in hand have at least embarked upon a course of adult health education, and will find yourselves miles beyond the old-fashioned rules of hygiene learned in grammar school: "Brush your teeth, wash your hands, move your bowels."

What will be required of you is a genuine appreciation of the human body; the cultivation

of attitudes toward life, which result in more personally and socially satisfying behavior; a more sophisticated understanding of the physiological and psychological relationships between the sexes; a more exact knowledge of the reciprocal relationship between personal and community health, and how the one enhances the other.

Health Education: Roots and Goals

While the scientific facts that you learn in an adult course in health education should be of lifetime value to you, much of the information will also have an immediate usefulness and may help you to stay in college. For your academic success you should recognize that there is a physiology as well as a psychology of learning. That great nineteenth-century educator, Horace Mann, asserted: "No person is qualified to have care of children a single day who is ignorant of the leading principles of physiology." What you learn and, conversely, what you can teach will be dependent in important measure on the state of your health and to some extent on your physical fitness for life and learning. The human mind and body are all of one piece. One can obviously be too tired to study; but it is also possible to be too undernourished to learn, too weak to pay attention, or too anxious to think.

Health education has deep-set roots that can be traced back to the ancient Greeks, who believed that about half a young man's, or a young woman's, educational experience should be related to physical development. The ancient Romans echoed this opinion in their famous axiom, "A sound mind in a sound body" (*"Mens sana in corpore sano"*). In the twentieth century we see it reflected and reborn in campaigns and demands for "physical fitness," of which we shall say a great deal more in Chapter 7.

Your mental acuity and stamina are unquestionably influenced by your physical condition, your personal or physical fitness measured in long or short spans. The purpose of your instruction in the whole field of health and physical education is to keep you on your feet—not flat on your back—on your toes—alert to the intellectual challenges around you—and alive in every sense of the word to the opportunities that arise as a part of or as the result of your college adventure.

Healthier Living

Healthier living takes no magical formulas and does not proceed by well-worn slogans, such as "Eat a good breakfast." "Sleep eight hours every night." "Wash your hair every week." It requires a sound, scientific but not overdetailed background of human anatomy, physiology, and hygiene; and the simple determination to take sensible actions and precautions in health matters —without pushing yourself to extremes or questioning every move you make. Healthier living should be more comfortable living, happier living. Indeed it turns out that the same factors which make for happier everyday living also make for longer life. Good health is a means to an end, not a goal in itself.

A considerable number of young men and women are forced to leave college every year "for health reasons." Many might have been, and still could be, spared this unfortunate step through better health education, more intelligent concern for their health, or better collegiate facilities for taking care of their problems. More than a century ago, in 1856, an alert and concerned college president, William A. Stearns of Amherst, spoke out critically: "The breaking down of the health of students, especially in the spring of the year, which is exceedingly common, involving the necessity of leaving college in many instances, and crippling the energies and destroying the prospects of not a few who remain, is in my opinion wholly unnecessary if proper measures could be taken to prevent it."

There has been more than a century of progress on campuses around the world toward taking "proper measures" to safeguard and improve the health of students. You can undoubtedly find an excellent health service in your own institution. No substitute has been found, however, for the student's own intelligent care and concern for

his or her own personal health. The subtle line between legitimate and abnormal concern for one's health (hypochondria) is one that every well-educated man or woman must learn to draw and walk; and they are fortunate who draw the line early in their undergraduate days.

Why Students Leave College ("Dropouts")

You who are studying from this textbook as an assignment in a regularly organized college course are successfully matriculated college students. You must, however, face up to the fact that half the students who enter college do not finish. At least 50% drop out before they get their degrees. In the freshman year alone nearly half the class (25% of the overall total of dropouts) leaves school or fails to return!

This should not be viewed as alarmist warnings. Anyone who genuinely wants to complete his or her college career and is not irreparably handicapped can usually manage to do so. Temporary dropout and some delay in completing degree requirements are occasionally advisable and helpful.

Why do so many students leave college? If we consider mental or emotional health, as we should, along with the more familiar category of physical health (it is hard to separate the two!), poor health is probably the principal reason for college drop-outs. Lack of intelligence is rarely a reason for leaving college—once you are admitted. Indeed more than one-third of those who drop out of college are in the highest intellectual brackets; approximately one-fifth are making excellent academic records.

In examining the following list of reasons for college dropouts, two facts should be kept in mind: almost every condition enumerated can be either (1) ameliorated or (2) corrected.

Money. Financial difficulty is often given as the reason for leaving college permanently or temporarily. However, it will be frequently found that there are previously undiscovered loan or scholarship resources available. What may come as a shock to some students, who have up to that time been liberally supported by their families, is accepted as an obvious fact of life by many others; namely, that they must finally begin to help support themselves financially, and wholly or partly earn their way through college.

Marriage. Before World War II marriage between or among college undergraduates was exceedingly uncommon and was usually forbidden by college regulations. After the war, and the "GI bill," which provided free college education for veterans (somewhat older than the present or previous generations of college students), the percentage of married students on campus rose sharply. Today marriage of college students is generally permitted, and the records show that their academic achievements are as high as, if not higher than, those of their single colleagues. Marriage, therefore, is not an absolute reason for leaving college. More frequently it is the arrival of a family that makes it necessary for the feminine partner in the marriage to interrupt her collegiate career.

Disinterest. College is not for everyone. There are some students who are swept into college only to discover that student life and academic pursuits are not for them. Many of them have creative talents in music, art, dance, design, and other fields; and they will actually succeed better outside of college in specialized schools. Occasionally the student and the college are mismatched. The college has no offerings in the student's particular and possibly offbeat line of interest. Transfer to another institution may solve the problem of *apparent* disinterest.

Incompetence. There are a few students admitted to college who genuinely cannot make the grade, or grades, necessary to meet present-day American collegiate standards. In many cases they should not have been in college in the first place, because their aptitudes (as shown often in psychological tests) lie in other directions. They may, for instance, be mechanically skilled or clerically gifted. Some of these students have struggled painfully to enter college. Under personal, family, or social pressures in their high school days, they have driven themselves tremendously to get into some collegiate institution.

The discovery that they cannot keep up with college academic standards, higher and more competitive than those in high school, may be a bitter experience. On the other hand, for a certain number of students who have been pushing themselves unhappily and unsuccessfully to make the collegiate grade, failure to do so and a subsequent formal dismissal from college comes as a great relief. There is an immediate ego-hurt in all these situations; but the long-range results are more gratifying than damaging.

In considering this problem of academic failure by reason of genuine academic incompetence or ineptitude, it should be recognized that not more than 30 to 40% (some say 10 to 15%) of all high school graduates are real "college material." Some children are forced into college against their own inner inclination and will.

Disease or Accident. Except for automobile accidents, disease and accident are relatively rare problems of college students.

Emotional Disturbances. This is the largest single cause of college dropouts. It is present to some degree in practically all cases. It has innumerable manifestations, which can be—incompletely and inadequately—described in such phrases as emotional immaturity, inability to get along well with fellow students ("peers") or families, inability to sit still (constantly flitting about), lack of appropriate motivation, uncertainty as to role in society (although lack of role is sometimes considered a condition of existence in current American adolescent culture), obstinacy, overdependency, incipient mental illness, and overreaction to family conflict. At least two-thirds of all college dropouts are marked by *poor study habits,* usually dating back a long time.

The underlying emotional disturbances in students who drop out of college are frequently triggered by the experiences, challenges, and situational stresses of college life. It should be recognized, however, that emotional disturbances often subside when the immediate stress causing them has been removed. It has also been demonstrated in college health services, daily, and in more formal psychological investigations,[1] that students with emotional disturbances and handicaps can be helped to control and escape them. In more technical language, the emotional disturbances that lead to college dropouts are "amenable to psychotherapeutic exploration and intervention" (if there is a staff providing psychotherapy available).

Family Conflicts. It is strongly suggested by formal investigation[2] of one specific, but representative, group of college dropouts that the real source of the event more frequently lay in the home environment from which the student had come than in the campus situation to which he was subjected. Indeed, in dropping out of college the student was expressing more resentment and rebellion against his parents than against the college (a substitute parent, as we sense in the phrase *alma mater*). In a certain way the dropout student was repeating his parents' experience; for the family histories showed that nearly 60% of the fathers of such students had themselves suffered from interrupted educations or career setbacks, and a high percentage of mothers too had not completed their educational plans. Perhaps because of their own disappointments these parents tended to be overambitious for their children, thus engendering or heightening an overt or unconscious resistance.

A favorable finding of the investigation here reported was that a very high percentage of the college dropouts whose emotional disturbances reflected deep-seated family conflict could be assisted and restored to school by adequate psychotherapy—sometimes prolonged, sometimes relatively brief in time.

Stress

If one were forced to sum up all the reasons for college dropouts in a single phrase, it might

well be: *inability to handle stress.* Understanding the concept of stress will help give you much deeper insight into the reactions of the human organism, mind, and body, both in health and disease. We shall deal with the more technical aspects of stress and stressors in a later chapter (pages 149–152), but here it is already worthwhile to discuss stress in the terms and situations in which the college student most commonly meets it.

A college career and environment undoubtedly place stresses of a great many kinds on students. However, except for those who cannot cope with the stress physically or intellectually or emotionally and must therefore leave college, the satisfactions outrun the stresses and frustrations. Possibly the most stressful factor that the student faces is the continuing, repetitive series of tests and examinations he must take. And yet these same tests *relieve* stress for a great many students. They are encouraged, buoyed up, and even satisfied by taking the tests. The time sequence of events in college life is especially important and often colors personal feelings. It is quite important for the student to recognize that he may see his whole world quite differently on the day after a final examination than he did the day before.

There are literally hundreds of formal and informal factors of college or university life which produce or relieve stress on individual students. With the exception of the tests, examinations, and *difficult courses,* practically all tend to relieve stress more than to create it. Among the activities which appear to produce relatively great satisfaction (relief) and relatively little stress for those who desire to undertake them are: dating, other social activities, church attendance, receiving reports or grades and academic standing, receiving medical treatment (if needed), attending spectator sports, taking part in athletics, engaging in physical education activities.[3]

No one in or out of college can expect to live without stress. Everyone must learn to live with it, exhibited in manifold ways. Simply defined,

[1] Edgar Levenson and Martin Kohn, "A Demonstration Clinic for College Dropouts," William Alanson White Institute of Psychiatry, Psychoanalysis, and Psychology, *Journal of the American College Health Association,* **12**:4, 382–391 (April 1964).
[2] *Ibid.*

[3] John J. Wright, "Environmental Stress Evaluation in a Student Community," *Journal of the American College Health Association,* **12**:3, 325–336 (February 1964).

stress means extra or extraordinary pressures and your reactions to them. Sometimes you voluntarily choose these pressures, as when you enter college. At other times they are forced on you by, for example, a stormy day in the classroom, a rough day at home, possibly an injury or illness. Not all stress is bad. Some of it has a healthy "conditioning" effect on the person and his body. The important thing is the ability to take the stress, to adapt to it, and thereby to gain new and additional strength.

Any assault on the body, physical or emotional, can engender stress. This will often be expressed as an *alarm reaction* in which various endocrine glands, notably the pituitary and the adrenals, will be set off to perform unusual functions. Strong emotions too can cause bodily changes and racing hormones, because emotions in general are meant to make us act. Under stress, breathing speeds up, muscles tighten up, blood vessels contract, and pleasurable or fearful emotions may be stirred up. Healthy relaxation may follow a short burst of stress and excitement.

It is unfortunate, however, when a period of emotional stress envelopes you in such a way that it is difficult or almost impossible to relax. Such undue emotional stress—intense, bottled-up anger, fear, frustration, and worry—can threaten health. Almost half the people who seek medical help have apparently been made worse by prolonged emotional stress. Frequently it keeps them from sleeping.

You are well advised, therefore, to appreciate your capacities, to know and accept your physical and emotional limitations, to keep a rein on your emotional tensions, and to tone yourself down if you feel that you are getting too keyed up. You may have to find situations and people with whom you can blow off steam.

There are no infallible ways of handling tension and stress, but recognition of the condition is the first step toward alleviating it. Your first move may have to be to learn to accept what you cannot change. In this acceptance you gain a new strength to change things that can be changed. You may also find, as already noted, that physical exercise—walking, tennis, or some other sport—will minimize your emotional tensions. In some stressful situations you may discover that plunging into work and keeping busy takes off the bitter edge.

The basic idea is to keep a balance between activity and relaxation. You may find that you must *schedule* time for recreation. If you can get away from the things that are bothering you, even by such simple devices as going to a movie, reading a book, or talking to a friend, you should not hesitate to make this break with your tensions. You can always come back to your job and your responsibilities.

Do not neglect your physical condition, even going to the extent of having a medical check-up, because good health and physical fitness help give you the zest for living that makes it easier to handle stress and tension. Perhaps the chief thing is not to knuckle under to the stress; to convince yourself that one way or another, and in due time, you will master it.

Chief Causes of Illness and Death at College Ages

College years are among the "healthiest" periods of life. These are normally years of high physical vigor, continuing physical growth, and rapid physical reaction time—in fact, the most rapid at any age of life. The diseases that do occur are more likely to be temporary and acute rather than chronic and disabling. Recovery is usually prompt. The greatest single risk to life is accident. It is astonishing to note that in the 15 to 25 age bracket, which includes high school and college students, three of the first five causes of death are essentially psychogenic in origin: accidents, suicide, and murder. It is the mind rather than the body which requires treatment, preventive and curative, in these cases. (The other two principal causes of death in this 15 to 25 youth-age bracket are heart disease and cancer.)

These cause-of-death statistics also hint at the observed fact that emotional disorders, or psychiatric complaints, are among the principal medical problems of college students. It is estimated that perhaps 10 to 15% of all college students sometimes seek psychiatric help, although higher figures have been recorded at some colleges.[4] It has been observed that there is a higher incidence of psychiatric complaints among college students than among their age-mates who go to work in more or less routine and stable working environments immediately after high school. Many college physicians are of the opinion that there is a greater likelihood of *emergence* of psychiatric problems among college students because of the recurrent challenges of their broad and constantly changing collegiate environment. In other words, the emotional problems, if any, come out sooner. This has its favorable aspect in that these patients receive relatively early treatment, which enjoys greater possibility of success in a shorter period of time.

The emotional disorders, or psychiatric problems, are approximately third or fourth in order of frequency of medical complaints of college students. First come respiratory (lung) ailments, chiefly the cold; second, skin eruptions; thereafter, the emotional problems; then gastrointestinal disorders and a wide variety of miscellaneous conditions. College students are not particularly exempt from any diseases or disorders (a great many of which are described in the short reference catalog of Common Human Ailments in Appendix A), but they suffer from them with relative infrequency.

Medical science has identified enormous numbers of general and specific hazards to human health: for instance, microbes and their means of transmission; such degenerative or chronic illnesses as heart disease and cancer, and their habits of progression; psychiatric disorders and their recurrences. The well-informed individual who promptly seeks medical care greatly reduces his risks of disease, disability, and infirmity. Much information about escaping these health hazards, as well as improving your health status, is woven through this book.

[4]W. G. Smith, N. Hansell, and J. T. English, "Psychiatric Disorder in a College Population," *Archives of General Psychiatry,* **9:**351–361 (October 1963).

Life Expectancy Today

The life expectancy of the present-day college student, heir to the medical progress of centuries, is phenomenal—half a century or better. It was not like this in previous generations and centuries, as the historical graph reveals. You can look forward to fifty or more years of life ahead. And perhaps you had better plan for it in terms of health as well as vocation. The way to become a "dear old lady or gentleman" is to start early —say at about seventeen. While looking at the United States' 1960's life expectancy table, it is also worth observing how rapidly it advanced in this century. In about 50 years the average life span in the United States lengthened by a generation: from around 47 years in 1900 to around 70 years in 1950 and still higher today. A reasonable number of today's college students can expect to live into their eighties.

Life expectancy tables, such as the one given here, are based on experience. They tell you what your chances and your hopes are, but they deal with averages, not with individuals. Life expectancy tables are based on mortality tables. We shoot the life expectancy up when we pull the death rates down. This is especially true at the early ages. The table here shows a very hopeful picture of life expectancy for the average American of the 1970's. It can be improved if every individual takes those wise precautions in living that will place him above the average risk shown in the figures. Incidentally, the United States does not enjoy the best—that is, the lowest— mortality record in the world. New Zealand, beats us; but her record points to improvement possibilities on this continent.

Normal Physiological Changes with Age. Your health status, and indirectly your life expectancy, depends, has depended, and will continue to depend on the physiological changes in your body that normally take place with increasing age. Actually the physical, physiological, and emotional changes we all undergo, occur most rapidly in the very earliest years of life. As we grow older, the rate of change slows down.

From birth to about 15 years of age, we grow

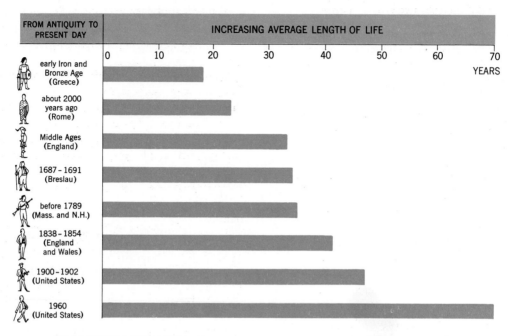

FROM ANTIQUITY TO PRESENT DAY	INCREASING AVERAGE LENGTH OF LIFE						
	0	10	20	30	40	50	60	70 YEARS
early Iron and Bronze Age (Greece)							
about 2000 years ago (Rome)							
Middle Ages (England)							
1687 – 1691 (Breslau)							
before 1789 (Mass. and N.H.)							
1838 – 1854 (England and Wales)							
1900 – 1902 (United States)							
1960 (United States)							

YOU CAN EXPECT TO LIVE LONGER than any of your ancestors, immediate or remote. Average life expectancy in the U.S. increased by nearly a generation (23 years) in the first half of the twentieth century.

rapidly in all dimensions. The peak of human strength and skill, that is, muscular and physiological efficiency, is reached at about age 25. There are exceptions in a few sports; notably swimming, in which teenagers excel.

The ability to withstand physical strain declines after 30, more rapidly in some people than others. As any aging athlete can tell you, the legs are usually the first thing to give out in sports.

Physiological and muscular efficiencies decline slowly from age 25 to somewhere between 45 and 50. They remain at this level for a few years and then tend to pick up again! This pick-up continues for some 10 to 15 years, often up to 70. It corresponds, more dramatically in women than in men, with detectable changes in hormone output. After 70, muscular and physiological efficiency again decline. Perception (the ability to see and hear clearly) which advanced rapidly in the early years of life, also declines in later years, and reaction time increases.

Raising your Health Status

It is the burden of practically all the chapters of this book to tell you how to maintain and improve your health status, and to give you the scientific background for making logical, sensible decisions in health matters. We could partly sum up this plethora of advice as follows:

¶ Eat properly
¶ Exercise sensibly
¶ Get enough sleep and rest
¶ Watch your personal grooming
¶ Cultivate healthy mental attitudes
¶ Learn to play your role as man or woman (father or mother)
¶ Accept some personal responsibility for community health
¶ Utilize medical services promptly and intelligently
¶ Eschew self-medication and quackery
¶ Avoid obvious and known health hazards

YOUR LIFE EXPECTANCY: U.S., 1960's*

At birth you can expect 70.2 years of life remaining

At age 1	71.0
At age 5	67.3
At age 10	62.4
At age 15	57.6
At age 20	52.8
At age 25	48.1
At age 30	43.4
At age 35	38.7
At age 40	34.1
At age 45	29.7
At age 50	25.5
At age 55	21.6
At age 60	17.9
At age 65	14.6
At age 70	11.6
At age 75	8.9
At age 80	6.6
At age 85	4.8

*Estimated abridged life table for the total population: United States, 1961; from U.S. Department of Health, Education and Welfare, Public Health Service, National Vital Statistics Division, *Monthly Vital Statistics Report*, **10:**13, 7 (July 31, 1962).

If your exact age is not given in this table, you can interpolate it by taking a number between the two ages that bracket your own. Thus, at age 38, between 35 and 40, you can figure that you have about 36.5 years ahead of you. White females can add a few years to the numbers given. Negroes must subtract a few years.

This bare summary may serve to mark the road ahead in this book; but it is the information *in detail* in these pages that will sustain your health status. "Eat properly." Yes, of course! But what? When? How much? Why? (See Chapter 10.)

"Exercise sensibly." Obviously! But what kind of exercise? How frequent? How much of it? (See Chapter 7.)

We shall now devote ourselves to a somewhat detailed exposition of the last of the signposts above: how to avoid obvious and well-known health hazards. In other words we shall try to suggest the general and specific courses of action that can save you from the ravages of infectious (communicable), degenerative (chronic), and psychogenic (mental) diseases.

You will find even more specific information in later chapters. What we shall give you here are some valid general principles, widely applicable.

How to Avoid Health Hazards. It is obvious that you can deliberately avoid *direct causes* of disease and accident if and insofar as you know them. You can, for example, deliberately avoid exposure to venereal disease; you can drive your car at a reasonable rate of speed; you can stay away from foods that you know disagree with you; you can keep out of communities (even households!) that are in the throes of an epidemic.

You may cultivate or evolve a mature philosophy of life which can spare you anxieties that are *precipitating factors* in many psychosomatic diseases. You can, by simple planning, avoid the dietary deficiencies (lack of vitamins and minerals, for example) which also precipitate diseases (for instance, scurvy and pellagra). Again, as you understand and take account of the normal reactions of *your* body and mind to various kinds of stress, you can eliminate some of the *predisposing causes* of disease: for instance, the physical and/or emotional fatigue that might predispose to a mental depression; the neglect of a cold which could predispose to pneumonia.

You can escape and *postpone the undesirable outcomes* and effects of many diseases perhaps far more readily than you imagine. For example, a patient under treatment with insulin or tolbutamide (an oral drug) and carefully following his doctor's orders need not die prematurely of diabetes. Even a patient who has suffered a heart attack and thereafter lives under a careful medical regimen that keeps him within the limits of his cardiac reserve may often look forward to a reasonably long (10 to 25 years) and comfortable life. Many people live foolishly for years with nagging diseases that could readily be alleviated, if not cured—skin ailments, hearing difficulties, poor vision—simply because, for some perverse psychological reason, they refuse to seek proper medical attention.

You can *help yourself* toward having adequate

1. *Pain.* Persistent or sharp pain anywhere in the body—head, abdomen, chest, or limbs—particularly if it recurs, is the first of the danger signals. Pain is your friend, for it often drives you to discover and eradicate its cause before it is too late. Pain is a positive indication that something is wrong. Do not play the hero or martyr by enduring or neglecting it. Do not play the fool by masking its effects with some pain-killing remedy.

Special mention needs to be made of *abdominal pain* (or "bellyache" in less elegant language). A number of serious medical emergencies, including appendicitis, are heralded by sharp abdominal pain. With one extremely important exception—cancer—most gastrointestinal disorders manifest themselves by pain in the abdomen. The important thing to remember here is: *Never take a laxative in the pres-ence of abdominal pain.* If it lasts more than an hour, avoid food and drink also (except for a few small sips of water) and consult a physician promptly.

Persistent abdominal pain always demands a medical check-up, but one does not have to run to the doctor with every transient stomach-ache. Physicians call the stomach "the greatest liar in the anatomy" because it reflects and reacts to pain stimuli originating far outside its orbit. Vomiting, for example, may occur as a result of brain injury. Again, motion sickness (air sickness, train sickness, car sickness), which really disturbs the organs of body balance located in the inner ear, may also produce nausea and vomiting.

2. *Fatigue.* "That tired feeling" without immediately obvious cause (such as a late party the night before), that general day-after-day weariness of mind and body, is a second great danger signal. Fatigue wears many disguises. Learn to recognize them. You are probably fatigued if your speech is hesitant and strained . . . if you are ready to snap people's heads off on the slightest provocation . . . if your posture droops and your head and shoulders bow forward . . . if your eyelids are red . . . if dark circles and crow's feet cluster about your eyes . . . if you always get tired in the morning . . . if you are played out by noon . . . if you begin to lose your sense of humor . . . if you find it difficult to concentrate on your work or play . . . if you find yourself failing to "catch on" to things you ordinarily grasp . . . if you feel generally tired, listless, and sluggish, or tense and impatient for a considerable period of time.

3. *Weight Change.* Sudden or extreme change in your body weight, whether gain or loss,

Danger Signals of Disease

always needs an adequate explanation. Sometimes you will first notice a weight change because your clothes no longer fit.

4. *Headache.* There are hundreds of causes for this common symptom. Do not neglect it or mask it with drugs, especially if it recurs.

5. *Fever.* It is practically always a sign of infection. Take your own temperature with a good clinical thermometer if you are in doubt. Anything 1 degree above normal (98.6 degrees Fahrenheit by mouth in adults) suggests prompt medical attention. Learn the easy technique of reading a clinical thermometer.

6. *Bleeding* (hemorrhage) from the skin, nose, or any other body opening.

7. *Indigestion* or malaise, especially if it often occurs. Beware especially of mild but persistent digestive disturbances which you might be tempted to toss off with a dose of "bicarb" or sullen contempt.

8. *Insomnia* (sleeplessness). Don't take sleeping pills. Investigate the cause.

9. *Skin changes.* Every skin rash, unhealed sore, or unexplained change in the color of the skin or complexion—pale face, ruddy face, yellow face (the yellow is a symptom of jaundice)—demands investigation. Warts and moles should be watched to see that they are not enlarging or changing color.

10. *Personality Changes.* If a lion begins acting like a lamb, or vice versa, something's eating someone. Abnormal restlessness, inattentiveness, aggressiveness, or shyness all represent personality changes that bear watching.

11. *Vision Changes.* If you begin to see double, see poorly, see rainbows around lights, or squint, check the cause.

12. *Swelling* —in the abdomen, joints, legs, or any other part of the body. Your shoes may begin to feel tight.

13. *Lumps* or growths—usually painless—on or under the skin in any part of the body, especially if they increase in size.

14. *Breathlessness* —after slight exertion.

15. *Coughing* and hoarseness— if it continues for any period of time.

16. *Sore throat* —which hangs on for more than a day or so.

17. *Loss of Appetite,* or difficulty in swallowing.

18. *Excessive Thirst,* especially when accompanied by excessive or painful urination.

19. *Dizziness,* giddiness, or vertigo. You spin around or the world spins around you.

20. *Bowel-Habit Changes,* notably unaccustomed constipation or diarrhea.

medical and public health facilities available in your community by your own contributions to medical and public health causes before you personally need them. You can support and even take leadership in voluntary health agency drives and service activities, a very educational and heartwarming experience. You can support your local health department and professional societies in your community.

When you or other members of your family are obviously ill, you can promptly seek and accept the best medical advice available in your community. The physician you call or visit will unquestionably be licensed by the state and should at the very least be a member of the local medical society. Conversely, you can stay away from quacks, frauds, and cults who make enormous promises to cure you with their "fake for every ache." Finally, you need not entertain or practice the folly of self-medication, no matter how many self-appointed advisors you accumulate. Remember that he who has himself for a physician has a fool for a patient.

With the help and advice of your doctor you will take advantage of the *immunizations* and occasionally other preventive treatments that are available against some specific diseases. Artificial immunizations ("shots") are now available routinely for infants, on demand for older children and adults—against smallpox, diphtheria, tetanus (lockjaw), paralytic polio, whooping cough, measles, and mumps; also, for either adults or children where the risk warrants it, against cholera, plague, typhus, typhoid, paratyphoid, yellow fever, influenza, "German measles" (rubella), and rabies (for anyone bitten by an animal known or strongly suspected to have rabies).

As a general precaution against disease, and as the measure that you will probably take most commonly for the rest of your life to preserve your health status, you can learn and be alert to the *twenty common danger signals of disease*—and see a doctor whenever one flashes across your consciousness.

Common Problems of College Students. It has already been noted in this chapter that enormous

numbers of students drop out of college for health and psychological reasons; that college students present more psychiatric complaints than their agemates at work; that the three principal causes of death in the college age bracket are of psychogenic origin; that emotional disorders are among the most common medical problems in the college population; and that college students normally endure a considerable amount of psychological stress. College students, therefore, probably have more than their proportionate share of psychosomatic illnesses as well as psychiatric complaints. Cultivation of those practices and factors in everyday living which reduce the risk of primarily physical illnesses will tend to cut the incidence of psychosomatic ailments and will generally improve health status.

There is another path to this important goal and it deserves attention. A college student may be afflicted with anxiety, reflected in a psychosomatic illness, because he is not aware, has not accurately recognized, or has not suitably resolved one or more of the problems that are well known to plague many college students. Here are some of the common and normal problems that you may have to face:

Family Adjustment. Many college students have yet to escape parental domination. A feeling of rebellion and aggression against all authority is a normal part of this drive toward independence.

Social Adjustments. College students naturally want to make new friends, join new groups. But remember that overanxiety to be accepted often defeats its own end.

Sexual Adjustment. Much worry over sexual matters on a college campus is, strangely, owing to unrecognized or unadmitted ignorance in this area. Conflicts between past, family, religious teachings and attitudes, and present collegiate mores and practices often arise. They must be resolved *personally,* but in a broad frame of reference.

Intellectual Adjustment. The comfortable intellectual adjustment achieved in high school may be rudely shaken by the demands of the college classroom, sterner competition, and higher standards. A more serious approach to studying, reading, and thinking may be in order.

Career Uncertainty. This is a foolish worry; for relatively few college undergraduates have *finally* settled on a vocation or career. Fewer than 2 in 5 graduates actually enter the careers they were sure they had "chosen" when they first came to college.

Fatigue. "Free" for the first time to "do what they want," driven by ambition, parents' expectations, desire to be popular, fear of failure, other fears and desires, some students drive themselves unmercifully into a state of fatigue. The remedy: slow down; strike a balance of work, play, and rest.

Personal Appearance. Some students worry about their personal appearance. Too often they have set rigid, unrealistic ideals for themselves; they neglect the simple details of good grooming; they do not appreciate or cultivate their unique, given assets of looks and personality.

Immaturity. Some young men and women at college feel out of place, inferior, and immature. Experience and maturity, it should be recognized, are the very gifts you go to college to find and develop. It may be helpful to think through, work out, and even write down a new, more mature philosophy of life for yourself.

By recognizing and attacking, where they exist, any one or more of these common problems of college undergraduates, the individual student takes positive steps toward improving his health status. In so doing he gains added strength to solve more problems and make strides toward his larger life goals. Good health is a strong bulwark.

From Personal to Community Health

We have begun this book for a course in health education primarily with a discussion of problems and needs that affect the health status of about 2 million college freshmen and 4.5 million upperclassmen in the United States. Although we have spoken of the concept of community health, we have talked principally about you, the college student. This text will move from YOU to

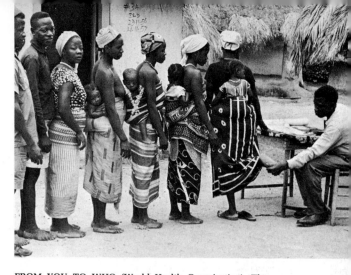

FROM YOU TO WHO (World Health Organization). Three billion people in the world are finally looking forward to solving centuries of health problems. In a Nigerian village the World Health Organization worker is examining the population for yaws. It is estimated that 25 million people are suffering from this disease, and its elimination is a target in WHO campaigns. (Photograph courtesy WHO)

WHO—the World Health Organization—and will pay increasing attention to the gradually larger units in which good health attitudes and practices must be operative: the family, the city, the state, the nation, the globe.

WHO is officially concerned with the health problems of billions—the *3 billion* people who now inhabit the face of the globe and who are multiplying at such a rate that it looks as if the world population may be doubled within a century. We are living in the midst of a population explosion; and this is one of the major health problems, having social and political overtones, with which we shall increasingly concern ourselves. Satisfactory means of dampening the worldwide population explosion have yet to be successfully applied. We shall discuss it more fully in a later chapter.

Suffice it to say that the twentieth-century's population explosion is the outcome of its genius in health matters, the application of which has sliced death rates and shot up life expectancies in every country on earth. We should be well aware of another result of this phenomenon, namely that a radical change in attitudes toward health and disease has already taken place in the twentieth century.

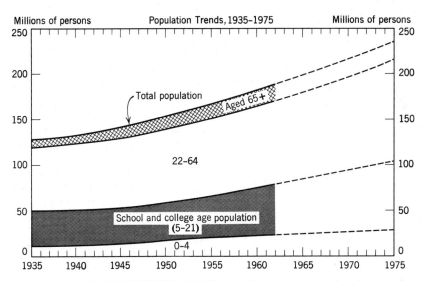

Millions of persons — Population Trends, 1935–1975 — Millions of persons

Total population

Aged 65+

22–64

School and college age population (5–21)

0–4

THE POPULATION OF THE UNITED STATES is trending upward, as is that of many other countries. A total of 230 million people in the United States is forecast for 1975. Relatively speaking, the school and college age population (ages 5–21) is expected to expand most rapidly.

Historians of the future may well regard as the most important single fact about the first half of the twentieth century that men and nations then advanced from a sense of helplessness about disease to an attitude of hopefulness that their ancient scourges and pestilences could in fact be controlled and therewith the average productive span of human life astonishingly lengthened. This has been achieved in large measure through a concentration of medical and scientific research, whose findings made it possible to control adverse factors in man's physical and biological environment, and thus attain a high measure of control over communicable disease in man and animals.

This change in mankind's attitude toward disease, with attendant hopes for improving the *quality* of lengthened spans of human life, is a great new factor in the total historical development of our time. Significant social and political events are already flowing from this fact. A glimpse of this historical significance, but hardly its full impact, was caught at the turn of the century by Harvard's president, A. Lawrence Lowell, who said:

It is hardly an exaggeration to summarize the history of four hundred years by saying that the leading idea of a conquering nation in relation to the conquered was, in 1600, to change their religion; in 1700, to change their trade; in 1800, to change their laws; and, in 1900, to change their drainage. May we not then say that on the prow of the conquering ship in these four centuries first stood the priest, then the merchant, then the lawyer, and finally the physician?

It requires great exercise of imagination on the part of college students today to realize the feelings of hopelessness, dejection, and terror that sometimes gripped the hearts of earlier generations caught in the gales of an epidemic.

In our own time, there may conceivably be widespread epidemics of new strains of communicable disease which medical science has not completely banished. Yet it must be said that young people today are at least free of the dreadful sense of pestilence that weighed down the spirits and colored the life outlook of earlier generations. This change in attitude is a clear gain in the direction of healthier living. We no longer live under the shadow of communicable disease as our ancestors did. The disease risks in the United States have shifted from acute and infectious to chronic and degenerative illnesses; from diseases of childhood to diseases of middle and later life.

SUMMARY

We began with the World Health Organization's definition of health; namely, "Health is a state of complete physical, mental, and social well-being, and not merely the absence of disease or infirmity." We noted the colleges' responsibility toward the health of their students and faculty. We discussed *stress* as the largest single factor leading to college dropouts. We noted psychogenic factors as the principal causes of death in the college age group: suicide, accidents, and homicide. We presented a table of life expectancy in the United States. It showed that the 20-year-old college student could expect to live another 52.8 years.

We introduced the subjects of raising one's health status and avoiding health hazards. We presented the 20 common danger signals of disease and pointed out that when they occur, you should check with a physician in short order. We listed the common problems of college students and discussed what might be done about them. Finally we noted the relationship of personal and community health—the steps from YOU to WHO.

SUMMARY REVIEW QUESTIONS

1. How would you describe or define "health?" What relationships do you see between personal and community health?
2. For the protection and improvement of their health, what does a college owe its students and faculty?
3. Why do so many students drop out of college? What steps do you think might be taken to change this situation?
4. What kinds of stress does a college career place upon students? How might these stresses be ameliorated?
5. What are the principal causes of (1) illness and (2) death at college ages? In spite of these risks, what is the life expectancy of the average junior or senior college student?
6. Outline briefly what you must do to maintain and improve your health status. How, in general, can you avoid obvious and known health hazards?
7. What are the 20 common danger signals of disease?
8. What are the most frequently encountered problems of college students? How, if at all, do these problems affect their health?
9. What significant changes in attitudes toward health and disease have occurred in the twentieth century? Why?
10. Are the following statements sense or nonsense? Why? *Health and disease are complete opposites. . . . All work and no play makes Jack a brighter boy. . . . The best way to conquer stress is to surrender to it. . . . The same factors which make for happier everyday living also make for longevity. . . . Every young woman must choose between college and marriage.*
11. What do the following terms mean to you: alarm reaction, vertigo, immaturity, psychogenic, population explosion, soma, degenerative disease, stress, respiratory, physiological?

Recommended for Further Reading: *Mental Health in College and University* by Dana L. Farnsworth, M.D. *The American College* by Nevitt Sanford. *A History of Public Health* by George Rosen, M.D. *Letters to His Son* by Lord Chesterfield. For more complete references, see Appendix E.

PART ONE MENTAL HEALTH

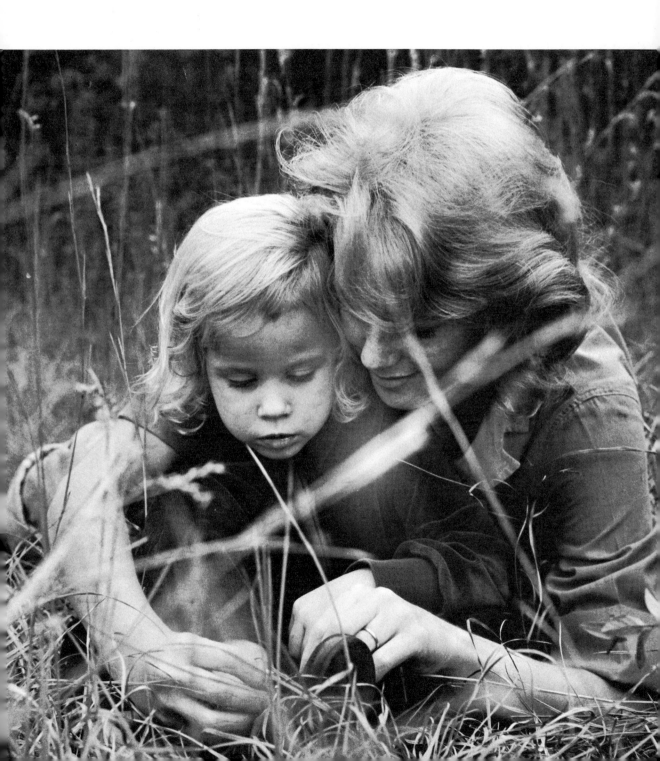

2

MENTAL HEALTH: MIND AND BODY

MANY DEFINITIONS OF "MENTAL HEALTH" have been attempted. A simple and sensible concept is that proposed by Freud: a person is mentally healthy to the extent that he can *love* and *work*. Conversely, he is mentally ill to the degree that he *cannot* love or work. This concept leaves a wide range for normal behavior. It also suggests that, just as perfect happiness comes to no one, even so no one is ever in perfect mental health all the time. Imperfection is the distinctive badge of the human race, and we are wise when we acknowledge this about ourselves.

The mentally healthy person has learned to live with the frustrations of human existence, but they do not disenchant him from continuing the struggle. He accepts the fact that human beings will make mistakes so long as they keep trying. He keeps his tolerance for frustration, disappointment, and grief at a high level. He also realizes that the ancient Socratic doctrine, "Know thyself," is at the heart of mental health but that it is a hard doctrine to apply.

If one really knows himself, he knows his own weaknesses, shortcomings, and failures. Yet the humility to accept these shortcomings is rare. Dr. Karl Menninger has put it this way: "That curious emotional defense which impels some people to believe themselves exempt from all failure, from all weakness, from the taboo of 'abnormality,' is perhaps the greatest enemy of healthy-mindedness."

We must not think of mental health as a sheer abstraction. It has a locale in the body and mind of each individual. But problems arise if we attempt to assign exact bodily locations to the multitudinous functions of the mind and emotions. The best we can say is that these functions occur in or are mediated by the human nervous systems, sometimes assisted by the endocrine system. We shall seek later in this chapter to provide a brief description of the human nervous systems and, beyond that, to offer some explanation of the physiology of thought and feeling.

Mental health is a 24-hour-a-day possession. It is present during sleep as well as waking. Indeed, one of the positive indications of lack of mental health is constantly disturbed sleep—sleeplessness or insomnia. In the mentally healthy man or woman there is a regular cycle of sleep and wakefulness. Throughout all of this the unconscious mind remains in operation. Since sleep and rest are critical factors in mental health, we shall also deal with these subjects later in this chapter.

Toward Conscious Control of Unconscious Forces

Human beings have the power to think and reason and to govern their actions, within limits, by the higher faculties of the mind. 'Schools' of philosophy have exalted man's reason implying that mankind could attain Utopia through the exercise of reason. But it has always been sensed, and twentieth-century research in psychiatry and psychology has clearly demonstrated, that human conduct is never completely reasonable. Motives for conduct are always a mixture of conscious thought and unconscious or preconscious impulses in undiscoverable proportions.

The unconscious motives in behavior are often described as emotional reactions.

The value of conscious thought and reasonable effort in directing our behavior, in opening new horizons, and in illuminating new goals for us should never be discounted or negated. But we must also recognize that deep in the psyche unconscious, emotional forces are constantly at work to modify, influence, and sometimes overwhelm our intellectual powers.

To know this in general, and to pinpoint it as far as possible for our own particular psyche, is to take a great step forward in achieving conscious control of our unconscious drives. The control will never be complete, but it will usually be adequate to get along in the world and sustain reasonable achievement. Serious failure of the conscious mind to control the unconscious forces by which it is besieged and bombarded can result in such life tragedies as mental illness, "purposive accidents," suicide, chronic alcoholism, narcotic addiction, antisocial and even criminal behavior.

The Unconscious Mind. To understand why people think, feel, speak, and act the way they do we must grasp the concept of the unconscious mind. To anticipate a fuller description in the following chapter, we shall give a very brief résumé at this point.

The unconscious mind is the repository of thoughts and feelings of which we are unaware. It files and remembers (but does not necessarily release to conscious memory) *all* our past experience. Indeed, it releases comparatively little, largely because we *want* to forget or repress unpleasant memories. We can assign a *theoretical* structure to the unconscious mind which helps to comprehend its operation.

The unconscious mind is assumed to consist of three parts: *id, ego,* and *superego.* The id may be said to represent the primitive drives and instincts of the human being. The ego represents the conscious self, which makes contact with reality and tries to keep the demands of the id in tune and touch with the real world. The superego is, crudely, the conscience, which also seeks to direct the ego.

The ego has a tough job. It must seek to satisfy the demands of the id, the superego, and external reality at the same time. To protect itself, the ego must adopt defenses; it must find compromise solutions which at least temporarily stabilize conflict in the unconscious mind and permit the individual to carry on. These compromises are often called mental mechanisms. The ego represents that part of the psyche which looks, acts, and builds toward individual satisfactions and socially commendable achievements in human life.

Interaction of Mind and Body

Physical health and mental health are certainly intertwined. For purposes of discussion we may separate mind (psyche) and body (soma), but in the everyday business of living they are indivisible. What we think and feel, consciously or unconsciously, is reflected in the cells of our bodies. Consider, for example, the shiver of fear and the blush of shame. Conversely, damage, deprivation, or disorder of the body affects the mind. Take, for instance, the delirium produced by high fever. Furthermore, our feelings and conduct can be drastically altered by drugs—for example, alcohol, narcotics, tranquilizers, and cerebral stimulants. These are fairly extreme examples. A more subtle interaction goes on all the time under the mediation, regulation, and control of the two important integrative systems of the body—the nervous system and the endocrine system.

The simple principles for maintaining a reasonably good state of physical health—adequate diet, sufficient rest and exercise, attention to warning signals of disease—apply also the quest for mental health. One cannot pursue mental health as if it were a butterfly to be caught in a net. Indeed constant concern over health is itself unhealthy. One attains and maintains mental health by indirection. The positive steps are outward. A person in a good state of mental health is identified by the fact that he enjoys good personal and social relationships with other people. He is not brooding about himself, nor introspectively exploring the state of his unconscious mind. He is living out, within the framework of the culture around him, something that may be called a satisfying and mature philosophy of life.

An excellent summary and overview of the problems of and opportunities for mental health was presented at the International Conference on Health and Health Education held in Philadelphia in July 1962 by Dr. Cyrille Koupernik, of the Children's Clinic of the Neuropsychiatric Faculty of Medicine in Paris. The essence of Dr. Koupernik's observations (originally in French and with some emendations and additions [in brackets] by this writer and translator) is as follows:

The whole idea of "mental hygiene" [or mental health as we prefer to call it in the United States] is relatively recent. It is more difficult to formulate both the methods and limitations of this area of preventive medicine than those of more traditional fields. Smallpox, tuberculosis, and poliomyelitis are ills which afflict mankind without regard to any of cultural, social, or ethical conceptions. But even on questions of diet, as a result of differences in climate around the globe, it is impossible to arrive at a unanimity of opinion. To expect any unanimity on the specific goals of mental health is doubly difficult. [The difficulty in setting standards or criteria to determine who is and who is not mentally healthy is highlighted in an 8-year study, published in 1962 under the title *Mental Health in the Metropolis* in which it is averred that only one out of every 5 adults aged 20–59 living in a particular section of midtown Manhattan can be considered as "essentially well" in terms of mental health.]

Nevertheless there is general agreement on these three points:

1. [Good] mental health permits the healthy development of the individual [his spirit and even soul, if you will; and respects individual differences between people and peoples].

2. At the same time a [good program of mental health] favors the integration of the individual in the group within which he is destined to live.

Since every individual will eventually leave the family group into which he is born, a third valid goal of mental health might well be to teach him gradually how to live in the world outside his immediate family, and to prepare him for the "world of tomorrow" in which he must inevitably live.

3. Finally, it must be recognized that our traditional concepts [in this relatively new discipline of mental hygiene] are applicable principally to Western societies and culture, which have certain [built-in] traditions which it is imprudent to expect to change [overnight]. Optimism about rapidly altering the current concepts of Western civilization are [to put it mildly] unjustified.

The goal of modern mental health has apparently been a [negative one]: not to return to the dogmatic and authoritarian concepts of the Victorian era. But we should not move toward the reverse excess and affirm that truth resides only in the concept of *laissez-faire*.

From the [psychoanalytically oriented teachings of the past half century—the teachings of Freud—viewed as a method of research rather than a method of therapy, and greatly revised since their original pronouncements]—we can accept certain principles as well established. These include:

¶ Most important, the demonstrated need of the infant and child for love and affection. It cannot be repeated too often that the child needs to love and be loved as its natural right, and that no other institution can replace the family for this indispensable end—certain political theories (Spartan and *kibbutzim*, for example) notwithstanding.

¶ Equal recognition of the fact that there are [normal] periods and points of discomfort and inquietude in the evolution of the infant toward maturity. We must accept the facts that infants usually begin to refuse proffered food at about the age of six months (this, however, appears to be a problem principally in the "well-developed" nations of the world); that they develop sleeping difficulties (possibly because their physiologically geared sleeping habits are not in phase with the socially dictated sleeping habits of the older members of their families); that a "negativism" and crisis of opposition to authority usually develops during the second or third year of life; that a [set of feelings] is often crystallized in a refusal to abide by social proprieties; that jealousy of an older child toward a younger brother or sister (an interloper in the family system) is almost inevitable; that children at about the age of three years become notably interested in their bodies, including their sex organs, and in the sexual life of adults.

It is not necessary, however, for parents to give preschool children exhaustive explanations of adult sex relations and the mysteries of procreation—for the intelligence of children at this age cannot comprehend the genuine and mature significance of this subject. However, the young child should not be so shielded from all knowledge of human anatomy and reproduction that he becomes an object of derision to his schoolmates (from whom he is all too likely to obtain distorted versions of sexual matters which may have unforeseen consequences on his later development toward a full heterosexual maturity in love relationships).

Writers, teachers, and parents must avoid creating a sense of anxiety about [sex matters] among their readers, students, and children. They must be equally blameless of inculcating others with a sense of guilt or forcing them into unnatural attitudes about these matters.

In dealing with the problems that agitate adolescents we should not forget that the educative process is a [two-way street], and that unless we listen attentively to their problems and complaints we are more likely to aggravate than to diminish the conflicts between older and younger generations.

Teamwork for Mental Health Is Vital. The concept of teamwork among professional disciplines and cooperation between peoples is vital to any scheme of mental health. The field of mental health and human relations is far from being the exclusive property of the physician or even of "technicians" trained in the methods of psychotherapy—orthodox Freudian, psychobiologic, or somewhere in between. It may even be argued that the physician, trained in objective observations of facts, is less well trained than members of some other professions,[1] notably the social caseworker and the clinical psychologist, in dealing with problems of general psychotherapy and human relations.

Professionals in the field of mental health must thoroughly appreciate what an illness means to its victim. The sick man feels sick, and his feelings must be respected. He must not be looked upon as a field of battle upon which one team (or school) of psychiatric creed will win a "victory" over rival schools.

The revolution in psychiatry and psychiatric treatment which began with Freud is not to be wiped out; but the Freudians (especially since the advent of a new psychopharmacology in the 1950's) can no longer assume the role of the only legitimate priests and prophets in the further development of the mental health of individuals, communities, and nations. The help of all professional groups, psychologists, physicians, social workers, teachers, nurses, parents, and others, and of the people themselves, is necessary if the high goals of mental health are ever to be achieved. With such cooperation mental hygiene is not a vain hope but rather a major weapon in the armament with which mankind can fight successfully against the mounting menace of its mental ills.

Some Principles of Mental Health

There is no "magic formula" for personal happiness or mental health. The positive tenets of mental health can be expressed in the same words as the age-old ethical teachings of all great religions. The Golden Rule—"Do unto others as you would have them do unto you"—is one of the greatest recipes for mental health, unless, of course, this great moral axiom is itself neuroti-

[1] A sign in the window of a busy bar in Washington, D.C., once read: "Quick service inside. Four 'psychiatrists' in constant attendance."

cally abused. The difficulty is not to put the principles of mental health into words but rather to put them into practice. This every individual must do for himself.

We offer the following simple principles for improving mental health and decreasing the burden of what Freud called "everyday unhappiness":

Have faith in something beyond yourself.
Show appreciation to and of other people.
Face your responsibilities.
Live one day at a time—in "daytight compartments."
Set your life in order.
Lead your own life.
Don't take your troubles and your negative feelings out on other people.
Strike a balance of work, play, love, and worship in the daily cycle of your activities.

Emotions

It would be naive to think that any human being can consistently and invariably follow the simple principles of mental health just set forth or any other valid statement of similar "good advice." Emotions, positive and negative, are constantly breaking in upon our conscious striving for a happy, well-adjusted life. A favorable balance can be struck; but we cannot deny the emotional stresses always operating in our unconscious minds.

"Emotion" is a difficult concept to pin down. In the most popular concept "to be in love" is an "emotion," to cry easily or to fly off the handle on the slightest provocation is to be "emotional." In more sophisticated connotations we use such phrases as "emotional reactions," "emotional stability," and "emotional maturity."

All this implies that emotions must be kept under control. This is true enough, but we must also recognize that the powerful, primitive, inner forces that we call emotions animate *all* human behavior—for better or worse. Emotions are feelings. We become consciously aware of them when they are heightened to a certain degree, but they are constantly resident in the unconscious mind. The operation of the emotions offers testimony to the unity of body and mind in the human being.

This was observed by William James, the father of modern psychology, who formulated one of the early theories of emotion in the 1880's and who wrote:

If we fancy some strong emotion, and then try to abstract from our consciousness of it all the feelings of the characteristic bodily symptoms, we find we have nothing left behind. . . . What kind of emotion would fear be left if the feelings neither of quickened heartbeats nor of shallow breathing, neither of trembling lips nor of weakened limbs, neither of goose flesh nor of visceral stirrings, were present, it is quite impossible to think. . . . Every passion in turn tells the same story. A purely disembodied human emotion is a nonentity.

James's theory of emotions has been largely superseded, but his descriptions are still valid. Emotions do not live in thin air; they must have some bodily expression. Certain modern physiologists describe emotions as "visceral actions."

Another important investigator of human emotions was the great Harvard physiologist Walter B. Cannon. He observed that fear, rage, pain, and hunger are emotional reactions that human beings share with lower animals. He explained these reactions in part as a result of the mediation of the endocrine system, particularly the release of adrenalin under conditions of stress, excitement, or danger. He saw these bodily reactions as "purposeful reflexes" designed and developed to assist survival in critical emergencies. He accounted for the similarity in the expression of strong emotions on the part of man and animal on the grounds that there is "an ancient and primitive part of the brain which is the common possession of all vertebrates." Some of Cannon's conclusions have been challenged, but of the central thesis there is no doubt: emotions stimulate the mobilization of body forces for action. When action cannot be taken, harmful effects may result. Emotions may be "converted" into physical illness.

Emotions in general and emotional stress in particular obviously have innumerable effects upon human physiology. Efforts of scientists to study hormonal and other physiologic changes that occur under such types of emotional stress as depression and anger have been hampered by the difficulties of inducing these emotions in realistic experimental settings. Recent studies, however, have made use of hypnosis to study the effect of emotions without situational complications that might distort the findings. Under these conditions of study, some made by U. S. Public Health Service investigators, it has become possible to observe some of the more subtle effects of emotions upon human physiology. It has been demonstrated now, for example, that various types of emotional stress, such as depression, fear, and anger, are associated with an increase in free fatty acids in the blood stream. This finding bears importantly on further investigations both in the field of nutrition (Chapter 10) and heart disease (Chapter 16).

In the brief consideration of the nature of emotions, of which we shall say much more in the next chapter, we have presented them as a kind of "bridge" between purely psychic and essentially physiological reactions of the human being. We turn now to a description of the human nervous system. It is the great integrative system. Through it, assisted by the endocrine system, emotional reactions are transmitted and made manifest.

The Nervous System

Conscious and unconscious thoughts and feelings certainly must have an abode in the human body, but it is not yet possible to specify their "local habitations" with any great accuracy. In the largest sense we feel and "think" with our entire bodies. The "language of behavior" is spoken by every cell in the body. Through the performance of different functions by myriads of separate cells, the total action of the body and the pattern of human conduct become possible. But this is effective and meaningful action only when the activity of the cells, and the organs they comprise, is coordinated and integrated through the nervous and endocrine systems.

The nervous system is the essential communication system within the body, and it also makes possible communication between human beings. We cannot here explore all the marvelous complexities of the human nervous system, of which the brain is the signal part. But we must emphasize the continuing importance of a well-functioning nervous system to the characteristic behavior of the human being. There remain many unsolved mysteries in this area. We do not know, for example, how a nerve cell (or a group of them) transmutes sensation into action. Since the nervous system carries sensation, information, and orders from one part of the body to another, there is some justification for comparing it with a series of interconnected telephone systems—so long as we remember that this description is an oversimplification of its complex functions.

For convenience of understanding and description, it is conventional to divide the single integrated nervous system into three major parts: *peripheral, autonomic, and central.*

The peripheral nervous system includes nerve trunks and end-plates, like the retina of the eye, with which the body perceives and makes contact with the outside world. These end-organs, or end-plates, may be likened to the receivers and mouthpieces of myriads of telephone instruments. The end-plates that pick up sensations are called *receptors;* those that deliver orders are called *effectors.* Sensations are transmitted through *sensory nerves;* orders come back by way of *motor nerves.*

End-organs are specific for their particular sensations or reactions. Thus the eye reacts to light, the ear to sound, the nose and tongue to chemicals in solution (providing the senses of taste and smell). Human beings have far more than the traditional five senses. There are distributed on the body, for example, end-organs for hot and cold, for pressure, for pain; and there are combinations of impacts on end-organs that give a sense of vibration, balance, hunger, thirst, and other feelings.

The autonomic (or vegetative) nervous system is composed of a series of nerve relays or switchboards (ganglia) that run up and down the outside of the spinal column and their interconnecting nerves. This system operates chiefly to help reg-

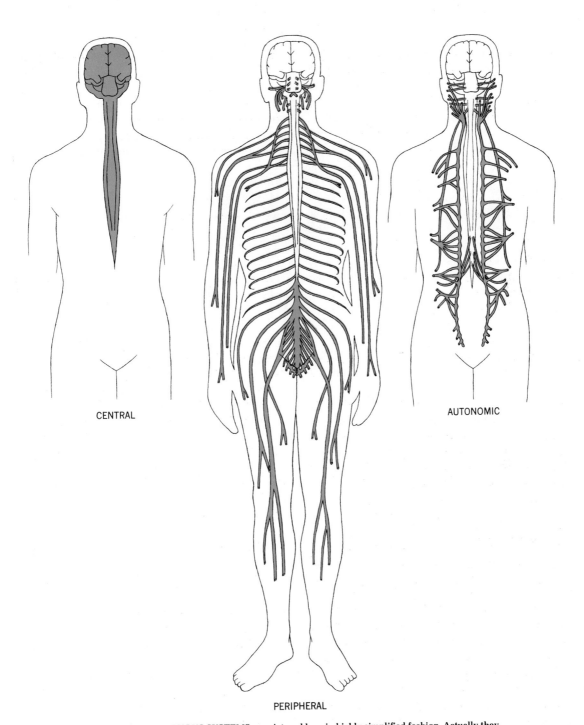

CENTRAL

AUTONOMIC

PERIPHERAL

THE HUMAN NERVOUS SYSTEMS are pictured here in highly simplified fashion. Actually they are all interconnected and integrated with each other. The central nervous system includes the brain and spinal cord. The peripheral nervous system reaches out to the end organs, such as the retina of the eye and nerve endings on the surface of the skin. As shown in the simplified picture above, the nerve trunks originating from the central nervous system have been cut off before branching out and reaching the end organs to which they go. Many fine, complex branches are not shown. The autonomic nervous system, which parallels but lies outside the spinal cord, includes both sympathetic and parasympathetic nerves and their junctions (ganglia). This system "automatically" controls many body functions, such as breathing and digestion.

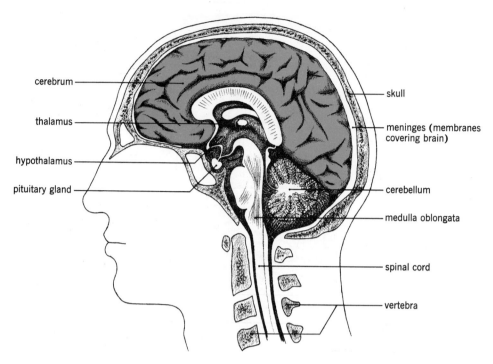

cerebrum

thalamus

hypothalamus

pituitary gland

skull

meninges (membranes covering brain)

cerebellum

medulla oblongata

spinal cord

vertebra

THE HUMAN BRAIN. A midsection of the human brain and the upper part of the spinal cord.

ulate man's basic physiologic functions, such as digestion and respiration, which go on without any conscious thought or effort. There are two parts to the autonomic nervous system; they act as antagonists of one another.

The central nervous system can be considered both the central and executive office of the body's communication system. It includes the spinal cord, the brain-stem, and the brain itself. It is the brain that interprets the meaning of the sensations picked up by the end-organs of the peripheral nervous system. The cerebrum, divided into two cerebral hemispheres, is the largest part of the brain and the seat of man's highest intellectual and rational functions. In it are localized many important brain functions, for example a speech center.

Damage to the Nervous System. The nervous system can be damaged by infection (e.g., syphilis), tumors (e.g., brain tumor), violence (e.g., skull fracture), poison (e.g., lead poisoning, acute alcoholism), and nutritional failure (e.g.,

beriberi). There are also many nervous disorders of obscure or uncertain origin. Indeed it has been calculated that there are more than 300 different disease conditions (clinical entities) which can produce disability in the nervous system, and it is further estimated that there are more than 10 million people in the United States affected with neurological disabilities. Among the common neurological disabilities are epilepsy, cerebral palsy, multiple sclerosis, muscular dystrophy, Parkinson's disease ("shaking palsy"), stroke (which is damage as a result of broken or clogged blood vessels in the brain), poliomyelitis, mental deficiency or retardation, blindness, and deafness.

The Nerve Cell

The nerve cell is the fundamental unit of the nervous systems. Technically it is known as a *neuron.* It has been estimated that the cortex of the brain alone contains more than nine billion neurons. A diagram of a typical neuron looks

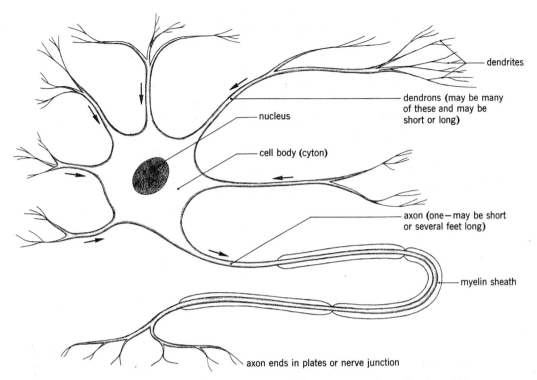

NERVE CELL. A typical nerve cell (neuron). Arrows show the direction of nerve impulses within the nerve cell to and from the cell body (cyton).

somewhat like an octopus. Like all other body cells, the neuron has a central portion called its cell body (cyton) and containing its nucleus.

Extending out from this central portion are two or more (usually more) fibers, filaments, or fingers of nerve tissue. One of these fibers, which carries nerve impulses away from the central cell body, is called its *axon*. The other fibers are called *dendrons;* at their far ends, where they branch off like twigs, the dendrons become *dendrites*. Axons and dendrons can be of any length; some of them are several feet long. A nerve cell has only one axon but may have many dendrons.

As they run the length and breadth of the body, axons and dendrons from the same or different nerve cells often run parallel with each other. Like a number of telephone wires running underground together, they form a cable enclosed in a flexible tube. The separate nerve fibers are protected and "insulated" from each other by a covering called a *myelin sheath*. The whole cable of nerve fibers makes up what we ordinarily describe as a nerve. The nerves follow recognized pathways to all parts of the body.

When you cut a nerve, you are actually cutting a great many nerve fibers. When a nerve fiber is injured or destroyed, it will regenerate in time —slowly—but when a nerve cell is destroyed, it is gone forever. Nerve cells can be distinguished from nerve fibers by color. The cells are gray; the fibers are white. The "gray matter" of the brain is a tight collection of neurons. The difference in color is due to the myelin sheaths.

A collection or concentration of nerve cells in one spot is called a *ganglion*. The plural for these "ganged-up" nerve cells is *ganglia*. Many small ganglia are found in and near the spinal cord, but the brain is the biggest ganglion of them all.

Stimulus Brings Response. We come now to the more difficult, but more fascinating, question of understanding how the human nervous systems normally work.

Let us return to the simple concept of sensory and motor nerves and nerve cells. Sensory or afferent nerves carry messages *to* the central nervous system. Motor or efferent nerves carry messages *away* from it. Now it is important to draw the distinction that sensory messages may be perceived either by the *conscious, preconscious,* or *unconscious* mind and that motor acts may be either *voluntary* or *involuntary*. If the sensation is not registered in the conscious mind and the reaction is involuntary, we have a so-called "simple reflex" response.

Such reflexes, or "nervous reactions," are not limited to man. Elementary forms of life also have them. Prick an ameba with a pin, and it will react by withdrawing from the pinhead. The fundamental principle is: *stimulus always brings response.* The difficulties, at the human level, lie in evaluating the stimuli and ascertaining the exact pathways of the response.

Associative or Intermediate Neurons—Heart of the Mystery. The central mystery about the human nervous systems rests primarily in what is still unknown about the nature and action of *associative,* or *intermediate, neurons.* These "in-between" nerve cells, which are neither motor nor sensory nerve cells, are found in all ganglia up to and including the gray matter of the cerebral cortex. Some of them are bunched together in fairly well-defined tracts, but the most painstaking dissection of the nervous systems has not been able to trace their innumerable interconnections. It seems unlikely that anyone will succeed in doing this in the forseeable future.

Associative neurons connect with each other and with the sensory and motor nerve cells that activate them. By analogy, we can compare them with the switchboards and relays of telephone systems. But in the final analysis they are no more mechanical than the human telephone operator who must pick and choose which wire she will plug into which socket on the switchboard. Or, granting a completely mechanized telephone system, the associative neurons are no more me-

chanical than the human brain which decides what telephone number is to be called.

The associative neurons encompass the human ability to select and interpret sensations conveyed by sensory nerves and to give orders for action conveyed by motor nerves. They determine whether and when a stimulus will appear in the conscious mind. They direct both voluntary and involuntary acts. Beyond that they are the ultimate physical residence of the human mind, will, and soul.

Nerve Impulse—Reflex Arc—Synapse. A great deal of useful information about the operation of the human nervous systems has been obtained by studying them as electrical systems and measuring their reactions with apparatus that records their electrical effect. We can say, therefore, that a *nerve impulse* acts like an electrical wave beginning in some part of the nervous system and communicated to other parts.

The basic mechanism of nerve action is the *reflex arc.* In terms of the simple reflex act, a stimulus to a sensory end plate brings a response on the corresponding motor end plate. This is how it happens.

The stimulus sets off a nerve impulse. The impulse is carried along one or more of the dendrons of the sensory nerve cell to its cell body and then out along the axon. Then it jumps to the dendrons of an associative neuron. This event is called a synapse. In terms of visible electrical phenomena, you might compare it to a spark jumping a spark gap.

In the associative neuron, or group of them, the sensation elicits a response, and, *mysteriously,* is transformed into a type of electrical reaction which can send an appropriate signal for action.

The transformed nerve impulse now jumps again from the associative neurons to the motor nerve that goes out to the spot where the original sensory stimulus arose. This second jump is also a synapse, or it can be considered part of the first one. The end-plate of the motor nerve along which the impulse travels finally gives the muscle or gland an order to carry out the designated reaction.

Kinds of Reflexes. All kinds of nervous activity in the human body, even up to the composition of sonnets and sonatas, involve some reflex actions, require some synapses among the associative neurons. More strictly speaking, however, a reflex is considered to be an *unconscious* reaction to stimuli. Most human movements and activities, such as breathing, digesting, and balancing the body, occur at this unconscious level. It is most probable, however, that every one of these activities is in some way registered and stored up in the "memory" of the associative neurons and can under some circumstances be recalled to the attention of the unconscious or conscious mind.

Reflexes have been classified in several ways. We have the so-called *simple reflex,* whose action was described above. It occurs, for example, when the knee tendon is tapped, the leg jerks. It also occurs when the sole of the foot is scratched; the big toe turns up. Most reflexes, however, are more complex, involving groups of nerves and muscles or glands, such as withdrawing the whole arm when a finger is pricked. These are called *coordinated reflexes* or reaction responses. These coordinated reflexes can continue to occur, sometimes rhythmically, one after the other. Then we have a *chain reflex,* like breathing or walking.

The newborn infant has a number of "automatic" reflexes with which he comes into the world, for example, grasping and sucking. Nobody taught the baby how to perform these acts essential to his survival. Such reflexes are called *inherited reflexes,* or inborn "mass reactions." As the baby grows, he learns and is taught to do a great many other things, "by habit" as we say. Such actions, which may be as complicated as playing a piano, are called *acquired* or *conditioned reflexes.* Conditioned reflexes are acquired by practice and become habits, as long as they are reinforced.

Conditioned Reflexes. The first clear descriptions of the conditioned reflex were given by the Russian physiologist Ivan Pavlov, who arrived at the concept during the course of experiments on the actions of the digestive glands. He characterized a reflex as "a necessary reaction following upon a strictly defined stimulus under strictly defined conditions."

Pavlov's basic experiments were done with dogs. The dog was shown food; his mouth watered. (The amount of saliva was actually measured.) At the same time a bell was rung. This "strictly defined stimulus" was repeated with the same dog several times. Then, under the same "strictly defined conditions," no food was shown to the dog but the bell was rung. The dog's mouth watered at the sound of the bell alone. This was the response which Pavlov described as the conditioned reflex.

The conditioned reflex is actually a very complicated process and depends upon transference of signals up to and around the cerebral parts of the brain. The associative neurons are definitely involved.

Just as the reflex arc is the physiologic unit of the nervous system, so the conditioned reflex is the unit of acquired behavior—or character. It is the cornerstone of our concept of personality reactions.

On the Nature of Stimuli. Reflex actions happen literally "quick as a flash" or "in the twinkling of an eye." That is pretty fast, but it is important to realize that it is not instantaneous. It takes a certain amount of time—just tiny fractions of a second—for a nerve impulse to travel around the reflex arc. When compared with the rate of travel of other electrical phenomena, for example radio waves, nerve impulses appear to travel rather slowly. Their actual speed is 200 to 300 feet a second, depending upon temperature and other factors. The corollary, of course, is that it takes time to react and to think.

In addition to the time factor involved in human thought and action, the strength of the stimuli provoking them must also be considered. An explosion in the same room, for example, can practically shatter the receptor end-plates of the human ear; but a whisper in the next room will not even be heard. To set nerve impulses in motion a stimulus must be strong enough to be noticed or picked up by the end-plate; it must last long enough to be felt; it must build up to a recordable intensity quickly enough to be registered.

We tend to think of stimuli as external forces and events. But, as anyone who has ever been awakened by a nightmare knows, the stimuli that set off gross reaction responses may be internal —hidden residents of the unconscious mind. These stimuli function below the level of awareness; they are, as we say, repressed. The stage is set for trouble when emotional conflicts, lingering in the unconscious mind, arouse deep-seated drives and desires that cannot be consciously accepted or fulfilled. The individual is then stimulated to action that he cannot or dare not take.

The damaging or noxious stimuli of internal origin are resident in the unconscious mind and, by inference, stored in the associative neurons in the body. Forgotten memories of past experience are the grist of these stimuli. They are often evoked, without rising to conscious perception, by symbols of past fears, dangers, and angers.

These stress stimuli are detected and picked up by various parts of the central nervous system— the cerebral cortex above and the spinal ganglia below. Their signals converge on the hypothalamus, the so-called "master autonomic switchboard" in the midbrain. It issues orders to the viscera and the endocrine glands, over a complicated series of relays and switchbacks.

Crucially, this process continues as long as the stimuli are present, or, to put it the other way, as long as the unconscious emotional conflicts are unresolved. The physiological responses in the body may also continue in one form or another so long as the internal stimuli remain.

On the Nature of Responses. The nature of bodily responses to internal, psychic stimuli has already been suggested. These responses are "protective reaction patterns" developed for action in the face of danger or emergency. But, continually evoked by symbolic threats resident in the unconscious mind, the physiologic changes may be perpetuated into chronic states or even chronic illnesses. At first these may be only functional disturbances, such as occasional palpitations of the heart, but after prolonged strain irreversible structural damage to organs and tissues may occur.

It is also possible for an illness apparently organic in its inception to provide a means of discharge for a psychic conflict. The illness may then be perpetuated long beyond its normally expected duration.

There is apparently an optimal amount of stimulus to which organisms, including the human, can respond. An overwhelming stimulus like an electric shock may produce a catastrophic and fatal response. But there are subtle gradations of the kind and amount of response. The optimal stimulus brings just enough response to meet the emergency. This may be called a normal "alarm reaction." The response mechanism, however, tends to overshoot the immediate need and to overreact. If the stimulus keeps up, the response mechanism becomes exhausted, and so does the organism. If the stimulus is unrelenting and the response mechanism gets no chance to recuperate, a state of shock and eventually death of the organism (or atrophy of a part) occur. This can be illustrated on many levels, as Hans Selye has done. (See page 151.)

Deprivation, whether nutritional or emotional, may be regarded as a noxious stimulus or stress. Spitz has brilliantly shown, with motion-picture evidence, that infants in an orphanage deprived of "mother love" for a period of months run a graded, downhill course and often literally die of this lack of love.

Creative Thinking

The interrelationships between the unconscious mind, the central nervous system, and the bodily expression of emotions are not all negative or concerned with the production of illness. On the contrary, there is reason to believe that these interrelationships make possible the highest forms of creative thinking.

Creative thinking may express itself in the composition of music, literature, and painting; in scientific investigation and the formulation of brilliant hypotheses.

We are indebted to the great French philosopher and mathematician, Jules Henri Poincaré, for a most lucid report of how the unconscious mind, or, as he terms it, the "subliminal self," works in achieving mathematical creation. Having established the basic points that the unconscious mind goes to work on mathematical problems only after the conscious mind has labored over them, and, further, that the unconscious mind is not a purely automatic mechanism, Poincaré goes on to say:

The combinations [put together in the unconscious mind must] be exceedingly numerous, useless, and cumbersome. The true work of the inventor [or the artist in any field] consists in choosing among these combinations so as to eliminate the useless ones. . . .

What is the cause that, among the thousands of products of our subconscious activity, some are called to pass the threshold [of consciousness] while others remain below. Is it simple chance which confers this privilege? Evidently not! Among all the stimuli of our senses, for example, only the most intense fix our attention, unless it has been drawn to them by other causes. More generally the privileged subconscious phenomena, those susceptible of becoming conscious, are those which directly or indirectly affect most profoundly our *emotional sensibility.*

Here is the link between thought and feeling, mind and brain, psyche and soma. Psyche projects, feeling selects. The selected thoughts are the conscious thoughts which we can convey to other people in word and act. The ideas which blossom are often the symbols of repressed and condensed memories.

Sleep

Man spends approximately a third of his life in sleep. Yet for an activity so common and universal, we still know surprisingly little about its fundamental mechanisms. The most scientific explanations of the function of sleep hardly surpass Shakespeare's seventeenth-century description:

Sleep that knits up the ravell'd sleave of care,
The death of each day's life, sore labour's bath,
Balm of hurt minds, great nature's second course,
Chief nourisher in life's feast.

During sleep the sleeper becomes unconscious, unaware, and more or less unresponsive to the environment about him. However, this is a relative matter. Some sense and some parts of the body remain more alert and more in function than others. For example, a sleeper may sleep through a loud noise but awake at the lightest touch. Again, while the lungs and heart may work more slowly during sleep, the sweat glands and some parts of the brain and nervous system may become more active. This increased, even though temporary, activity of the nervous system is the explanation of dreams, sleepwalking (somnambulism), and talking in one's sleep. Exactly why these events occur to a specific person on a given night cannot be explained, but the fact of their occurrence demonstrates that sleep and waking are both part of the same cycle of living. It is questionable whether the unconscious mind ever completely rests. Anxiety, certainly, is one of the great enemies of sleep.

Most of the measurable physiological functions of the body are diminished during sleep. The body temperature falls, indicating a general decline in metabolism and a decrease in the tone of muscles. Muscular relaxation is one of the key components of sleep. During sleep also the heart beats more slowly, blood pressure and pulse rate fall, breathing is slower, and secretion from nearly all glands diminishes.

But sleep is more than a time of rest and relaxation. It is also a time of recuperation and repair, of growth and regrowth. During the normal course of living, cells of the body wear out and must be replaced. This regeneration takes place more rapidly during sleep. It has been shown, for example, that the cells of the skin divide and make new cells about twice as fast during sleep.

The amount of sleep a person needs is therefore influenced by his rate of growth. Rapidly growing infants need more sleep than children; children more than adults. Again in old age, when the reparative processes of the body are less active, an increase in sleep may be required. Furthermore during the period of recovery from a debilitating illness or operation (convalescence)

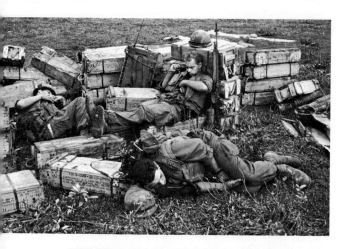

HOW TIRED CAN YOU GET? Three marines fall asleep atop ammunition boxes during pause at Gio Linh, just south of the demilitarized zone in Vietnam. They had been under repeated mortar and artillery attack. (Wide World Photos)

and in some stages of pregnancy, added increments of sleep or rest may be essential.

REM

Experiments undertaken in the 1950's and 1960's have added a great deal to our concepts of the sleeping state. The use of the electro-encephelograph (EEG), which records "brain waves," was one of the best new tools for studying sleep. The new concept pointed out the fact that every sleeper's night is punctuated by regular periods of body change and dreaming accompanied by rapid-eye-movement (REM).

About two dozen sleep laboratories in the United States are now observing the REM characteristics and other bodily changes during sleep. In spite of their research efforts, the exact nature of the sleep phenomenon both in men and animals still eludes analysis.

We have only begun to learn what people mean when they say they slept "well" or "poorly." The differences can be partly determined by brain-wave patterns, heart rates, and temperature changes noted during sleep. The poor sleepers do not seem to follow the 24-hour rhythm of sleep and wakefulness. (This rhythm is sometimes called the "circadian" rhythm, from the Latin phrase *circa dies*, translated to mean "about one day.") The poor sleepers show an unusually small amount of REM sleep. By EEG monitoring of sleeping persons, who are fitted with tiny electrodes on their bodies (including the eyes), it has been possible to detect four stages of sleep. Stage IV is the sleep of the weary, the time when recuperative powers are at their best and sleep at its deepest. This stage comes normally within the first few hours of sleeping.

The treatment for sleep problems, both sleeplessness (insomnia) and oversleeping (narcolepsy), has been made more complicated by these recent discoveries about sleep. Alcohol, barbiturates, and tranquilizers do not enhance sleep: they change the usual pattern of nighttime sleep by reducing the amount of the needful REM sleep. Stimulants, such as the amphetamines, have the same effect.

How Much Sleep? Research and common experience both indicate that sleep requirements are individual, governed by factors of age, general state of health, current activities, emotional outlook and previous sleeping habits.

Most adults sleep 6 to 8 hours out of 24. But some need more; a few less. Occasionally a person "drugs" himself with too much sleep and fails to get his full measure of living. The people who claim to get along on very little sleep at night usually do some of their sleeping during the day. They take short naps and they have usually mastered the art of relaxation.

The test of whether or not you are getting enough sleep is a simple, practical, and individual one. You are getting enough if you wake up in the morning refreshed and ready for the new day. The first half hour after arising can be discounted in applying this test, because it takes varying lengths of time for metabolism to rise to a level of full wakefulness.

Occasional loss of sleep will not have harmful effects. Under conditions of military necessity men have often gone 48 to 72 hours without sleep and recovered with only 12 hours of rest and sleep. Even test subjects, who have been kept awake as long as 200 hours, have not suffered significant physiological changes, although they do exhibit some temporary psychological deficits; they become restless, irritable, and unable to add numbers accurately in their heads.

Sleeping Soundly. There is no best position for sleeping. Any position in which you are comfortable will serve. It is the common practice in Western society to sleep in a bed. But there are some primitive people who sleep in a squatting position. The Japanese sleep on the ground or floor without mattresses. Sailors manage to get a good night's rest in hammocks. And, as every college student knows, almost anyone can learn to sleep sitting up.

It must be recognized that some hours of sleep are deeper or "sounder" than others. These 2 to 4 hours of deep sleep, whether they come before or after midnight, are the important ones in the body's recuperative process. The different levels of sleep can be detected in "brain wave" patterns. The factors that make for sound sleep are many and often highly individual. Darkness, quiet, agreeable room temperature, and an accustomed, comfortable bed favor a good night's sleep. So do regular sleeping habits—that is, going to bed about the same time almost every night—and a balanced pattern of living that is free from repeated, abnormal tensions. A good day is the best prelude to a good night's sleep.

Insomnia. Insomnia (sleeplessness) is a common complaint. Many people who make this complaint are getting more sleep than they think; they remember the hours they were tossing about and forget the time they were asleep.

Everyone has occasional sleepless nights, usually after a particularly worrisome day. But persistent insomnia deserves a medical check-up and not frantic self-medication.

Excessive fatigue is sometimes a cause of insomnia; a person may be just too tired to sleep. On the other hand mild exercise, like a short walk before going to bed, may induce sleep.

Eating habits may be a factor in insomnia. One person may be kept awake because he has had too heavy an evening meal, another because he is really hungry. Coffee, tea, and other cerebral stimulants taken late in the day have different effects on different people. Some will not be bothered by them; others will be kept awake. Personal experience is the only test.

You may not be sleeping because your room is too hot or too cold, too noisy or too light. A change to a more comfortable bed and mattress may also help. If the failure to sleep has deep psychological origins, improvement in the physical factors of the sleeping quarters will not help much.

Relaxation of mind and muscles is the key to falling asleep. That is why many of the time-honored technics of getting to sleep often work. These include: leisurely retiring, reading or listening to music before retiring, taking a warm (not hot) bath, counting sheep (or anything else), breathing deeply and rhythmically, consciously attempting to relax the muscles.

The greatest single cause of sleeplessness is simply the fear that one is not getting enough sleep. Sleep needs differ. When you go to bed, feel confident that you will get enough rest, whether you sleep or not.

Sleeping Pills. Sleeping pills are sedative and hypnotic drugs, usually but not always barbiturates. (More information on barbiturates will be found in Chapter 6.) Addiction to barbiturates is possible and overdoses can be fatal, particularly when the pills are ingested simultaneously with alcohol. Bromides and antihistamines (drugs sometimes prescribed for hay fever) also have sleep-producing effects.

The self-prescribed use of sleeping pills—especially the barbiturates—can be dangerous. The sale of barbiturates and some other kinds of sleeping pills without a physician's prescription is forbidden in all states. Those pills that can be bought without prescription contain ineffective drugs or such small quantities that they can't work, except by suggestion.

SUMMARY

We have introduced the important topic of mental health, dependent both on the human mind and body. We have outlined some simple principles of mental health ("Have faith in something beyond yourself," etc.) and discussed the nature of human emotions, which include bodily reactions. We have given a description of the human nervous systems; peripheral, autonomic, and central. We have elucidated the nature and function of the nerve cell (neuron), the fundamental unit of the nervous systems. These, we have pointed out, can be studied as electrical systems in which stimulus always brings response. Stimuli may be external or internal, resident in the unconscious mind. Responses are of many kinds, beginning with the simple reflex arc and advancing through conditioned reflexes to creative thinking. We have also discussed the phenomenon of sleep, **for it** reflects conditions of mental health. We come to the simple conclusion that mind and **body** are tightly intertwined in helping an individual to reach a goal of good mental health.

SUMMARY REVIEW QUESTIONS

1. What does the term mental health mean to you? How do you think it is achieved? What are valid goals of mental health? What are the principal obstacles in the way of reaching these goals?
2. Cast up your own list of "principles of mental health." How does it compare with the advice along this line you have gleaned from other sources? Why do you think you have given somewhat different emphasis to your "advice to yourself"?
3. How close is the relationship between mind and body in the human being? What specific examples can you give to indicate that this is either a very close or a distant and somewhat casual relationship?
4. What is an emotion? How do human emotions originate and how are they usually expressed?
5. What are the major divisions of the human nervous system, and what is the principal function of each division? Are they truly separate?
6. What is a reflex? How many examples can you give? To what kinds of stimuli does the human organism respond?
7. What, in your own experience, have been the greatest obstacles to restful sleep? How have you overcome them, or how would you expect to overcome them?
8. How, practically speaking, can you tell whether you are getting enough sleep? Are you getting enough sleep? If not, what do you propose to do about it?
9. Are the following statements sense or nonsense? Why? *What is mind? No matter. What is matter? Never mind. . . . The language of behavior is spoken by every cell in the body. . . . A person can be too tired to sleep. . . . Some people have no emotions at all. . . . Man is born, suffers, dies. . . . And they lived happily ever after.*
10. What do the following terms mean to you: insomnia, synapse, conditioned reflex, creative thinking, cerebrum, neuron, peripheral nervous system, psyche, soma, Parkinson's disease, REM?

Recommended for Further Reading: *The Human Mind* by Karl Menninger, M.D. *Managing Your Mind* by S. H. Kraines and E. S. Thetford. *The Revolution in Psychiatry: the New Understanding of Man* by E. Becker. *Psychology: The Briefer Course* by William James. *Understanding Human Nature* by Alfred Adler. For more complete references, see Appendix E.

3

THE UNCONSCIOUS MIND—ANXIETY

PERSONALITY HAS BEEN DESCRIBED AS "THE sum total of our ways of behaving, especially toward other people." Our behavior is controlled not only by apparently conscious thought and decision but also by our emotions, which have roots in the past. We are always influenced more or less by our unconscious mind, which is the dwelling place of our emotions and the matrix of our personality structure.

Personality Development

"As the twig is bent, so the tree inclines." "The child is father to the man." In these old proverbs also is summed up a great deal of the best present-day knowledge of normal personality development. This development begins at birth; the behavior patterns of later life are established in the cradle, the nursery, and the elementary school room.

Despite individual differences, personality development follows a fairly consistent and universal pattern. It normally proceeds step by step, stage by stage toward the elusive, relative, and rarely attained goal of "emotional maturity." Physical growth and biological readiness precede the emotional development. Each intermediate stage in personality development must be worked through before a person can go on to the next stage. No one can leap from infancy to adulthood. Arrested and distorted development, however, is all too common. The relationship of the individual with his own family, from earliest infancy onward, is a crucial factor in personality development (see "Function of the Family" Chapter 11).

The Stages of Love. The newborn infant is helpless, dependent on his mother or her substitute for survival, yet he is born with the will to live and love. This innate will to survive, to grow up and enjoy life is the basic font of vital human energy; it has been given the name of *libido.* As personality development progresses, a large part of the libido evolves into more directed and controlled feelings, which we call love. Fully developed, the libido represents all those inner strivings which tend to preserve and extend life—to "heal, cultivate, protect, and inspire" the human personality. But in the infant this love force appears in a crude, undifferentiated, untutored form.

The infant begins by loving himself. This is called *narcissistic love,* after the Greek legend of Narcissus, the handsome lad who fell in love with his own image in a pool. The infant "loves" and finds pleasurable gratification in different parts of his own body in a regularly observed succession. His first libidinal attachment is to his mouth (he puts everything into it), then to his anus, then to his genital organs.

As he becomes increasingly aware of the difference between himself and other people, the infant gradually shifts his love to objects outside himself. The first libidinal shift is to his mother, then to other members of the household. The young child identifies himself closely with his parents, idealizes them, and seeks to imitate them. This is *imitative love.*

There comes a time, usually between the ages of four and seven, when the imitative child wants jealously and intensely to "possess" the parent of the opposite sex. Little boys naïvely say,

"When Daddy is at the office, I'll be Daddy"; and little girls earnestly assert, "When I grow up, I'm going to marry father." This stage of development, which certainly occurs in Western culture with its ideal of romantic monogamous marriage, is called *oedipal love,* after the Greek legend of King Oedipus, who was fated to kill his father and marry his mother.

In later childhood, as the boy and girl become aware that their oedipal longings are impossible of fulfillment, emotional attachments shift outside the home and become centered in "loyalty" to a gang or a "crush" on a friend. The new libidinal attachment is usually to a person of the same sex. This is sometimes designated as *homosexual love.* In late childhood, a period of sexual latency, this is a perfectly natural emotional attachment—not to be confused with adult homosexuality.

In puberty, love attachments return to the opposite sex. But this usually begins as a kind of *idealistic love* for some distant, unattainable personality—as unattainable in reality as was father or mother, but secretly and subtly cast in the parent images. The idealistic yearnings of hosts of teenagers for the same popular and symbolic figure of the sport or entertainment world is a repeatedly observed phenomenon.

The next and final stage in the development of the capacity to love is *heterosexual love,* love for a person of the opposite sex. This is the fulfillment of the normal course of love development. But it does not wipe out all previous love attachments; some self-love, for example, always remains. Nor does it exclude the simultaneous presence in the psyche of anger and fear.

Anger and Fear—"Negative Emotions." Anger, fear, hate, jealousy, and revenge are in a sense protective reaction patterns, slumbering reflexes evoked by threats or suspicions of danger. They mobilize psychic energy and physical resources for that end. But when too frequently or constantly evoked, particularly by imagined danger, and when unchecked in their operation, they can have a destructive effect on personality.

Anger, or aggression, in its many guises is the normal but primitive response to frustration. It is basically the desire to remove by attacking, killing, or destroying anything that threatens the survival of the individual in body or spirit. All too often anger is destructively turned against oneself.

When you are thwarted or frustrated by yourself, others, or circumstances, you cannot help *feeling* angry. But there is a vast difference between *feeling* angry, *appearing* angry, and *acting* angry. You can learn to do something constructive with your mobilized energy. You should neither swallow it (repress it) nor turn it against yourself. For anger repressed will return in some other emotional disguise.

The seeds of anger, like love, are sown in infancy. Frustrations evoking and nourishing anger begin at birth, when the human being is "continually encountering the painful experience that the world is no longer shaped so exactly to his subjective demands as was the maternal womb."

Infants are born with certain instinctual reactions which are sometimes called "fears." However, the face and substance of fear changes as experience enlarges. For example, people get progressively more afraid of snakes as they grow older. One of the most pervasive human fears is that of loss of parental love, or, more abstractly, fear of rejection or social disapproval.

Fear is the emotion associated with flight from danger which threatens survival. Fear and cowardice are not the same thing; one can *feel* afraid and still *act* bravely, which is what most "heroes" do.

Personality patterns, it should now be plain, reflect the constant interplay of positive and negative emotions. In wholesome personality development the "loving" emotions are encouraged to blossom and modify the effects of the negative emotions. Technically speaking, we seek to "eroticize our aggressions." We turn now to consider the unconscious mind, where these things occur.

The Unconscious Mind

The unconscious mind is a paradox. We become aware of it only when and to the extent that it releases memories, thoughts, and feelings to consciousness. It holds and withholds many secrets. We assume the existence of an unconscious mind because it offers the most rational and scientific way of explaining human behavior. This hypothesis has superseded the animistic explanation that a child is "bad" or his father an alcoholic because the Devil is in him.

There are those who cling to "free will" and reason as the fundamental determinants of human conduct. On this score it can be said that we must act as if our wills were free and as reasonably as our unconscious minds will allow us. But there can be little doubt today that individual reason and will are persistently limited by unconscious forces. We are fundamentally driven by our emotional reactions. We can do only what the structure of our personality permits.

For these and other reasons we must now examine the structure of the unconscious mind. It is the major area of psychic processes and hence the central subject matter of mental health and mental hygiene. To use several figures of speech, the conscious mind is only the facade of the unconscious; it is the part of the iceberg that floats above the water; it is just the skin of the apple. The picture of the unconscious mind that we shall present is of necessity generalized and oversimplified. But it is not merely hypothetical; it corresponds with and explains how human beings actually behave.

The structuring of the unconscious mind here set forth is based on psychoanalytic theory, initiated and expounded principally by the Viennese physician Sigmund Freud. It has acknowedged limitations, but it is far from being outmoded.

The most serious criticism of the psychoanalytic formulation of human conduct is probably that it does not give full enough weight to the physiological factors involved. Freud, who began as a neurologist, anticipated this criticism and worked out his theory precisely because there was not enough information at that time on the physiology or pathology (disorder) of the human nervous system to explain the huge backlog of unhappy people and mental illness that confronted him.

The success of recent drug therapy (e.g., tranquilizers and cerebral stimulants) in treating mild and severe mental illness suggests that physiological modifications of the nervous system can favorably modify the events presumed to occur in the unconscious mind. But the new ability to alter and improve the physiological factors in mental illness does not entirely wipe out the psychic factors.

Those who doubt the existence and importance of the unconscious mind must find a better explanation for such questions as: How can a fact be remembered one minute and forgotten the next? Where do dreams come from? Why do so many people feel uncomfortably anxious and guilty about trivial and unimportant events of their past and present experience? Why do patterns of reaction established in childhood persist throughout adult life?

Although other terminology for the structure of the unconscious mind can be and has been used, the well-accepted (Freudian) construct divides it into three interacting parts: the *id,* the *ego,* and the *superego.*

The Id. A newborn baby, helpless though he is, nevertheless has instincts and aptitudes (like the sucking reflex) for survival. This passion for existence, this inherent vital emotional energy we have pointed out can be described as his libido. In a more impersonal term it can also be characterized as the id. All that we can guess concerning the existence of the id we gain from observations of the conduct of the libido. (We have already traced the normal course of libido attachments to "love objects" from early infancy through adulthood.) In the structure of the unconscious mind, therefore, the id can be construed as the uncontrolled source of the inborn tendencies, the instincts, the unconscious striving of the human organism to live and enjoy life.

The id, however, has characteristics which are not in accord with the best in human conduct. Like a child who "wants what he wants when he wants it," the id constantly seeks its own pleasure and gratification. It acts as if pleasure were the only thing in the world that counts. It operates on the pleasure principle exclusively.

This is the way infants and children behave, and it takes education, maturation, and social pressure before they give up the pleasure principle as the chief guide to conduct. Even in adults, of course, the pleasure-seeking drive persists—but it is under greater control.

The id does not distinguish between good and evil. It is illogical; it holds contradictory wishes and impulses at the same time. In a word, the *id is unrealistic*. The human organism which responded solely to its whims, its sexual and aggressive tendencies, would probably not long survive.

The Ego. The ego represents the conscious self. Through it the id is kept in touch with reality —with the external world about it. Through the perceptual apparatus of the human organism, the ego sees, hears, tastes, smells, and feels what is going on about it. The ego acts in terms of the reality principle, which is an important characteristic of adult behavior. The ego gradually develops and gains strength in the course of the individual's growing up and becoming educated in the ways of the world.

But the ego is frequently under pressure to satisfy the id. This it cannot always do, any more than a parent can completely satisfy all the demands of a child. The relationship of the id to the ego has been aptly described as that of the horse to the rider. The rider directs the horse with more or less success. Sometimes, however, the horse is balky. He runs away; he may even throw the rider. In other words, the pleasure principle often defies and sometimes dethrones the reality principle.

The ego is almost the whole of the *conscious* mind and it is the seat of the higher faculties of the mind. However, a large part of the ego is submerged in the unconscious mind. A traffic of sensations, thoughts, and memories back and forth between the conscious and the unconscious passes over the highways and nerve pathways of the ego. Not all thoughts and feelings pass with equal freedom. The ego places barriers— defenses—against unwelcome impulses entering consciousness. We shall have much more to say

about these ego defenses, or mental mechanisms, later on in this chapter.

The important characteristics of the ego, learned in maturation, are that it is in constant touch with external reality; that it can learn by experience; that it can interpose thought between wish and act; that it unifies, modifies, and integrates thoughts and feelings; and that it can be reasonable.

The Superego. Crudely speaking, the superego is the conscience, the small voice within us that warns against temptation and wrongdoing. But the voice we hear is only the conscious part of the superego. A larger part of it is buried in the unconscious, where it frequently bullies the ego and makes itself felt in vague but distressing feelings of guilt and shame. The superego embraces not only our conscious moral standards but also our "ego ideal"—the picture of ourselves as we would secretly like to be and appear to the world.

While the reality principle restricts the ego to what is possible, the superego tells it what is permissible, or what is socially acceptable. The superego is an essential check on asocial or antisocial conduct.

A peculiarity of the superego is that it is often behind the times. Its sternest admonitions frequently remain those that were formed in early childhood principally between the ages of three and six. At this time the child is strongly identified with his parents (or their substitutes). Their least prohibitions and commands, their values and their attitudes, are etched deeply on the young and weak ego of the child, and these feelings become the essence of his superego.

The unfortunate catch in this is that the parents, impelled by their own superegos, too often urge the child to be better than he can be ("a *perfect* little lady or gentleman") and better than they, the parents, are or were themselves.

Conflict in the Unconscious Mind. This can be understood as battles between the ego and the id, the superego and the id, the ego and the superego, and struggles within the id. The focus of these conflicts is on the ego. It must mediate between the id and superego; it must obey the dictates of the superego; it must control the whimsical demands of the id; it must satisfy the needs of external reality; it must guide the entire personality through the shoals and competitions of the real world. Some egos are stronger than others, but no ego can always meet all the demands upon it. It must sometimes adopt compromises, subtle means of self-protection variously called "ego defenses," mental mechanisms, and mental dynamisms.

When the ego is under stress from the id or being "punished" by the superego, the individual whose ego is being hurt suffers from anxiety—a vague but often powerful feeling for which he has no obvious or immediate explanation. He cannot put his finger on the source of the anxiety because it is concealed and disguised in the unconscious mind. The anxiety may express itself in feelings of tension, guilt, inferiority or even physical symptoms (e.g., a headache). There are always some physical reactions to the stress of anxiety. In one sense anxiety may be considered an admission on the part of the ego that it is temporarily unable to cope with its taxing job.

Later in this chapter we shall deal with constructive ways of handling anxiety. At this point we shall set forth some of the mental mechanisms by which the ego seeks to defend itself against otherwise intolerable anxieties generated by conflicts in the unconscious mind.

The Mental Mechanisms

Mental mechanisms (mental dynamisms, ego defenses) operate solely in the unconscious mind. At the time we are using them, or *overusing* them, we are not aware of the fact. In retrospect we can sometimes recognize how our egos were defending themselves, and we are usually acutely aware of the mental mechanisms grossly employed by other people.

It is possible to identify some types of behavior originating in the use of mental mechanisms; childish behavior in an adult, for example, indicates the use of a mental mechanism called re-

gression. Different people habitually use different mechanisms; most people use several. When one compromise fails, the uneasy ego grasps desperately for another.

We must not blame ourselves or other people for using mental mechanisms; they are sometimes necessary to a particular individual to enable him to deal with his real-life situations. We may, however, fairly question the persistent overworking of one or another mental mechanism. This betrays serious unresolved conflicts in the unconscious mind, or, in other terms, an unsettled personality or a troubled person.

Repression. The most important mental mechanism is called *repression;* it is an emotional block that keeps us from remembering something even if we want to. In brief, the ego buries unpleasant memories and associations and frightening feelings. It also inhibits pleasant feelings, which arouse the threat of the id going out of control and prompting socially unacceptable behavior of a sexual or aggressive nature. Repressed material represents emotional reactions that we want to hide even from ourselves. But this repressed, buried, warded-off, hidden material does not disappear. It seeks expression one way or another. Since it is barred from directly entering the consciousness, it usually appears in a disguised and distorted form.

Among the ways in which repressed memories and experiences may assert themselves are dreams, amnesia, purposeful forgetting, slips of the tongue, and the formation of neurotic anxiety symptoms. In dreams we find disguised images of the circumstances that have been repressed into the unconscious. Dreams usually represent wish fulfillments—but of wishes we would not dare harbor in the conscious mind. Very often they are wishes to harm those we love—parents, spouse, children, brothers, and sisters.

Amnesia means loss of memory—forgetting or repressing whole spans of time. Unpleasant war experiences are sometimes thus blanked out. Again, we do not like to look forward to events that threaten pain, difficulty, or embarrassment. So we purposefully forget a medical appointment; we stand up a date we didn't want in the first place. Of great significance is the universal experience called *infantile amnesia*. Almost everyone "forgets" the feelings of frustration, fear, and other experiences that occurred during infancy and early childhood.

Identification. Identification is the process by which the ego gains strength through attachment to another person, group (notably the family), or institution. The infant, as noted, identifies himself first with his mother, then with other members of his immediate family. The young child feels and behaves as though he were the parents themselves. He *uncritically* imitates their ways; he *unconsciously* adopts their traits, habits, ideas, prejudices, and values. When he is angry at them, he may hit himself!

Identification in later life represents the need for belonging to some group or "herd" and being accepted by that group. Even outcasts huddle together for mutual reassurance. Identification is on the whole one of the most satisfactory adjustment mechanisms. However, *overidentification* with one's family, school, or other group may sharply limit one's personal development, inhibit outgoing feelings toward other people, and indicate unresolved inner feelings of a childlike dependency on others.

Idealization. Identification of the young child with his parents gradually turns into idealization of them. The child's own ego ideals, the inner picture of himself as he feels he would like to be, are permanently established in his superego by this process of idealization.

Idealization, as a mental mechanism, is a device the ego adopts to escape the recriminations of the superego. When it substitutes other ideals for the original parent ideals, it always includes at the core of the new ideals some fraction of the original pattern. "Idealistic love," as we have noted, is shaped in the inner image of one's parents.

Like identification, idealization is usually uncritical. This often leads to overestimation of the people toward whom it is directed. We see idealization blissfully at work in young lovers, who refuse to see the least blemish in their beloveds.

Idealization is also employed at the very highest cultural levels—in religious worship and love of God, commonly idealized as Father, all-powerful and all-loving. We attribute to God all that is best in man.

Regression. Regression means reverting to immature and often childish behavior in the presence of current difficulties and frustrations. In terms of overt behavior it is one of the easiest of the mental mechanisms to observe and identify in other people. We all know the boy who won't play if he can't be captain of the team; the girl who sulks or goes into a temper tantrum if she misses a much-desired date; the tennis player who smashes his racket when he loses a match; the "perpetual undergraduate" college alumnus, yelling himself hoarse at a football game; the child who throws himself on the floor and screams at the top of his lungs when he is denied candy.

Regression is a retreat from the complexities of the present to the fancied security of the past. The ego feels more comfortable—for the moment—in seeking an old solution for a present problem.

Projection. We frequently seek to excuse our own failings by blaming them on someone or something else. The student who is failing a college course may sincerely but erroneously believe that the instructor is down on him. The poor workman blames his tools. Auto accidents are always "the other fellow's fault." When the ego rejects responsibility for failure and projects the blame elsewhere, it is employing the mental mechanism of projection.

But the process of projection may be much broader than merely excusing failure. We may, for example, project our own feelings on other people or the world at large. When we feel "blue," we may see the whole world as black. We often attribute our own most undesirable traits to other people. If we are "bad," they are worse. We are most prone to project on others those feelings which trouble us most. Thus, if we feel secretly hostile toward somebody else, we may imagine that he is equally hostile toward us—which may or may not be the case. Seeing others in a distorted image of ourselves may make us unduly critical, sarcastic, cynical, and pessimistic.

Substitution. Substitution and displacement are mental mechanisms akin to projection. We sometimes substitute one love object for another—as does the childless woman who lavishes maternal affection upon a dog or cat. We may also displace our feelings, sometimes because we are afraid to express them toward the person who aroused them. Thus a man may be angry at his boss but displace his anger upon his wife—for some trivial reason. A girl who is angry at her parents may take it out in a quarrel with her boy friend.

Rationalization. Rationalization is perhaps the most widely and frequently used of the unconscious ego defenses. It reflects a built-in bias, of which we are unaware, in favor of ourselves, our feelings, our own opinions, ideas, and prejudices.

Rationalization is the practice of finding and giving plausible and apparently "reasonable" explanations for thought and conduct that stem from quite different motivations than those we openly express. Rationalization is unconscious self-deception. It usually comes as a great shock to find that others do not see us or our points of view as we see them ourselves. We often rationalize our conduct to cover up our less worthy motives—often our jealousies—toward other people. Thus a teacher or mother chastises children "for their own good"—unaware that she is enjoying her own sense of power.

Rationalization is not valid reasoning. To a certain extent rationalization is inevitable. Since all our strongest personal beliefs—and prejudices—are rooted in emotions, it is not surprising that we defend them by rationalization rather than by critical, logical thought.

Some of the most penetrating observations on rationalization were written more than a generation ago by the late James Harvey Robinson in his brilliant book, *The Mind in the Making*, thus:

We are incredibly heedless in the formation of our beliefs, but find ourselves filled with an illicit passion for them when anyone proposes to rob us of their companionship. It is obviously not the ideas them-selves that are dear to us, but our self-esteem, which is threatened.

We are by nature stubbornly pledged to defend our own from attack, whether it be our person, our family, our property, or our opinion. A United States Senator once remarked to a friend of mine that God Almighty could not make him change his mind on our Latin-America policy. We may surrender, but rarely confess ourselves vanquished. In the intellectual world at least peace is without victory.

Few of us take the pains to study the origin of our cherished convictions; indeed, we have a natural repugnance to so doing. We like to continue to believe what we have been accustomed to accept as true, and the resentment aroused when doubt is cast upon any of our assumptions leads us to seek every manner of excuse for clinging to them. The result is that most of our so-called reasoning consists in finding arguments for going on believing as we already do. . . .

The "real" reasons for our beliefs are concealed from ourselves as well as from others. As we grow up we simply adopt the ideas presented to us in regard to such matters as religion, family relations, property, business, our country, and the state. We unconsciously absorb them from our environment. They are persistently whispered in our ear by the group in which we happen to live. . . .

The little word *my* is the most important one in all human affairs, and properly to reckon with it is the beginning of wisdom. It has the same force whether it is *my* dinner, *my* dog, and *my* house, or *my* faith, *my* country, and *my* God. We not only resent the imputation that our watch is wrong, or our car is shabby, but that our conception of the canals of Mars, of the pronunciation of "Epictetus," of the medicinal value of salicine, or the date of Sargon I, are subject to revision.

Fantasy and Daydreaming. Unconscious fantasy, often translated into fancy daydreaming, is one of the most subtly dangerous mental mechanisms because although up to a certain point it is useful and constructive, beyond that difficult-to-determine point it can be destructive of the personality. Everyone engages in fantasy and daydreaming; the world properly respects the faculty of constructive imagination, as illuminated by artists in every media.

Fantasy becomes dangerous, however, when we no longer distinguish between what is fantasy and what is reality. In the unconscious mind fantasy is the property of the id, which indulges in wishful thinking just as much as it can without restraint from the ego. It is not strange, therefore, that fantasy plays such a large role in childhood. The child acts out his wishes and fantasies in play, but he is deadly serious about his world of make-believe. The id is overwhelming the ego.

Normal fantasizing has been carried too far when it has become a facile substitute for work and effort needed to bring a vision to reality, when wishful thinking about success supersedes all struggle to attain it.

Conversion. The conversion of conflicts in the unconscious mind into physical symptoms of illness is one of the most commonly employed of all mental mechanisms. Physicians estimate that at least half the patients they see are suffering from complaints in which psychic or emotional factors are the prime if not the sole complaint.

The student who always gets a headache when faced with an examination is displaying a conversion symptom. So, too, is the soldier who suffers from hysterical blindness when he sees his buddy blown up a few feet away from him. Conversion reactions are in fact more common in wartime than peacetime, and they are the explanation of such conditions as hysterical paralysis, convulsions, loss of voice and deafness, "shellshock," "soldier's heart," and "battle fatigue."

Illness becomes a way out of an intolerable situation. Physical pain is substituted for inner anxiety. The patient is unaware of the source of his pain. It is just as real to him as if it had a definite basis in a recognizable bodily defect. For example, a patient with a severe backache of purely psychogenic origin feels just as bad as if X-ray evidence actually showed a fracture in his spine.

Conversion symptoms are often difficult to relieve for the added reason that they offer some secondary gains or benefits to the patient. He gets sympathy because he is "sick"; he may be relieved from the pressure of ordinary duties and responsibilities; he may even collect unearned money because of his "affliction." For example, some people who have been involved in accidents do not recover from their symptoms until they receive a substantial cash settlement from an insurance company.

The "chronic invalid," the hypochondriac always worried about his health, and the neurotic who "enjoys" poor health offer further examples of conversion reactions. There is no accounting for their long lists of vague aches, pains, and other complaints except on a psychological basis. Fatigue is one of the commonest complaints.

Nevertheless actual impairment of bodily functions may result from prolonged unconscious conflicts. Practically any organ or system of the body can be affected by "psychophysiological disorders." Many emotional reactions, for example, are visibly expressed in skin troubles. Other diseases which may be initiated or aggravated by unconscious anxiety include bronchial asthma, peptic ulcer, chronic colitis, and heart disease (especially disease of the coronary arteries). Bodily illnesses wholly or partly of psychic origin are often described as "psychosomatic"— from "psyche" for mind and "soma" for body.

Some Other Mental Mechanisms in Operation. From the descriptions and examples of mental mechanisms already given it should be obvious that hidden struggles and conflicts within the unconscious mind create not only psychosomatic illness but also the wide diversity of personalities whom we meet in real life and in fiction. Without going into the complete details of the psychic processes involved in each, we shall give brief descriptions of generally recognizable "stock characters" whose peculiar behavior patterns are controlled by overworking ego defenses and mental mechanisms.

The Extrovert. He turns to the outside world, to fierce rounds of activity, to careless and unreflective action in order to smother his inner conflicts. "The life of the party" is usually running away from himself.

The Introvert. He substitutes thought for action. He shrinks from his social environment. He finds decision painfully difficult. He looks too long before he leaps.

The Perfectionist. He sets his goals so high that neither he himself nor others can reasonably criticize him for failing to achieve them.

The Specialist. He chooses so odd or unique a line of endeavor that there is little competition in it; thus he escapes the normal competitive struggle.

The "Know-It-All." He covers up his inner sense of inadequacy by an attitude of superiority. He appears too cocksure, dogmatic, and positive about his knowledge and opinions. He knows all the answers, he thinks; but he holds only minor jobs.

Mrs. Grundy. She viciously gossips about and criticizes others to compensate for her own feelings of inferiority. She secretely fears that, given the chance, she would behave worse than those she criticizes.

The Alibi Artist. He cannot face overt criticism. He fears that others will discover and confirm the low opinion he has about himself.

The Isolationist. His unconscious mind has fashioned logic-tight compartments so that some parts of his inconsistent, paradoxical, multiple personality are completely isolated from others. This is the Dr. Jekyll and Mr. Hyde character. A more recent portrayal of the multiple personality is to be found in the well-known psychiatric study entitled *Three Faces of Eve.*

The Symbolist. He performs symbolic acts as a bribe to his superego in order to blot out or undo even more painful thoughts lurking in his unconscious mind. A classic example is Lady Macbeth repeatedly washing her hands in the vain hope of washing away her deeper feelings of guilt about having instigated murder.

The Fetishist. He displaces his strong feelings for a person onto a thing. Afraid to express openly a love for a particular woman, he holds some physical symbol of her—a handkerchief, a lock of her hair—in even higher esteem.

Pollyanna. She persistently looks at the world through rose-colored glasses. She childishly denies that life includes struggle and difficulty. Eventually she is tripped up and overwhelmed by it.

Sublimation. Sublimation means directing, channelizing, and converting basic emotional drives, crude instinctual impulses, into *socially acceptable and useful activities.* It is the true taming of the id by the ego under direction of the superego. Sublimations are the most constructive compromises and the happiest solutions to the inevitable frustrations that life sets before us. Though difficult to achieve, they bring social reward and approval which reinforces and strengthens the ego.

Sublimations take many forms. Some serve for a time; others for a lifetime. The lives of dedicated men and women—scientists, artists, missionaries—illuminate how satisfying and creative sublimation can be.

Most commonly the making of a home and the rearing of a family give the opportunity for the sublimation of feelings to a most socially useful end.

Sublimation is not entirely an unconscious process. Conscious effort enters into it. One deliberately chooses realistic goals and activities which he can, step by step, and in spite of frustrations and difficulties, hope to reach.

Doing the Best You Can. It is important for college students to realize that all roads to mental health do not lead through sublimation and the exercise of initiative and creativity to its highest degree (and often with frustrations beyond the tolerance of the individual concerned). There is another type of mental health, found among many college students, which may be described by the simple phrase of "doing the best you can." Psychiatrists Roy G. Grinker, Sr. and Jr., and John Timberlake, affiliated with the Institute for Psychosomatic and Psychiatric Research and Training of the Michael Reese Hospital and Medical Center, Chicago, have offered an elaborate description of this particular type of "mentally healthy" college student (in the June, 1962 issue of the *Archives of General Psychiatry*).

These doctors offer the following description of a group of 65 goal-oriented and mentally healthy young men attending a small college. (The college is deliberately not identified by the investigators, nor do they assume that the type of mental health that these young men enjoyed is to be considered the prototype for all college students. Indeed for many highly intelligent, artistically or scientifically oriented college men and women the kind of "mental health" they discovered and described in their particular study would be deadly.)

On the surface, the investigators point out, this group of 65 young men were free from psychotic, neurotic, or disabling personality traits.

The students, averaging 18 years of age, came from every area of the United States and Canada, from farms and cities. All were working toward degrees in health and physical education, group work, or community recreation, and had strong convictions and motivations about their career choice.

Through interviews, questionnaires and a behavior rating scale, Dr. Grinker found the following conditions characteristic of this group:

¶ Sound health from birth.
¶ Average intelligence.
¶ Relatively low socioeconomic family circumstances.
¶ Affectionate relationship with both parents.
¶ Parental agreement and cooperation in child-raising.
¶ Definite and known limitations on behavior.
¶ Punishment reasonable and consistent.
¶ Sound early religious training.
¶ Held a job early in life.
¶ Externally oriented rather than introspective, with low degree of creativity.
¶ Ideals of contentment, sociability, doing good, and making friends.
¶ Success sought in achieving limited goal rather than ambition to rise higher socially, earn more, or live better than parents.
¶ Strong identification with father and father figures.

Any one, or all, of these factors may be important in the development of this type of personality. Average intelligence with a capacity for honest and accurate self-appraisal is an antidote to useless and disappointing goal-seeking.

In contrast to the plight of students at many modern universities where an infinite number of goals are possible, this group had a single goal, finishing school and starting their chosen work.

Furthermore, most of the students studied had become associated with this type of work in childhood and felt that the college and the future career for which they were preparing was the "right place" for them.

While this type of adjustment is associated with "stability and a special type of happiness," it is also associated with narrowness and limitations of interest, ambition, creativity, and excitement.

These young men cannot be understood apart from the culture in which they were reared. Parental emphasis on early work, sound religious training, and the ideals associated with doing good as well as parental firmness and interest constitute aspects of an ethic acceptable without rebellion because of the sincere manifestations of love and consistency toward the child.

The subjects became more interested in avoiding failure than attaining great success and "doing the best you can" became the essence of their way of life.

Theories of Personality Development

Although Sigmund Freud has left the deepest impress on the fields of psychiatry and psychology, there are many others whose work has fashioned the current concepts in these disciplines. Among them are Alfred Adler, Carl Jung, Karen Horney, Erich Fromm, Harry Stack Sullivan, Henry A. Murray ("personology"), Kurt Lewin (application of "field theory" to all branches of psychology), Gordon Allport ("psychology of the individual"), Kurt Goldstein ("organismic psychology"—the organism always behaves as a unified whole), Abraham Maslow ("holistic-dynamic theory"—an optimistic approach to psychology), William H. Sheldon ("constitutional psychology"—mind and body are "one"; the relationship between body build and behavior), Hans J. Eysenck ("factor analysis," application of mathematics of psychology), Reymond Cattell (measuring personality traits), Ivan Pavlov (stimulus-response theory), John B.

Watson (behaviorism), Edward Thorndike (importance of reward and punishment in the learning process), John Dollard and Neal Miller (reinforcement theory of learning), Carl Rogers ("self-theory" and nondirective counseling), and Gardner Murphy ("biosocial theory"—man is a biological organism in reciprocal relationship with his social and material environment).

To return now to the personality development concepts of Jung, Adler, and the other "social psychologists," Fromm, Horney, and Sullivan.

Although Freud and Jung had been colleagues, in 1914 they broke completely. Jung could not accept Freud's theories of sex. He went on to develop his own "analytical psychology." Jung sees the individual personality as the product and container of its ancestral history, going back into the dim and unknown origins of man as a separate species. Hence he conceives a "collective unconscious," which is a storehouse of latent memory traces inherited from man's ancestral past. From this are derived so-called "archetypes," defined as a "universal thought form" (idea that contains a large element of emotion).

Anthropology and sociology began to emerge as separate disciplines during the latter part of the nineteenth century. These new social sciences held that man is chiefly a product of the society in which he lives. This doctrine seeped into the realms of psychoanalysis and psychology. Among those who used this concept of "social psychology" to modify the traditional outlook of classical psychoanalysis were Adler, Horney, Fromm, and especially Sullivan. Adler established a system called "individual psychology" which conceives of every individual as a unique constellation of motives, traits, interests, and values. Adler fashioned a humanistic, optimistic theory of personality, which was at odds with Freud's more materialistic conceptions.

Fromm's basic viewpoint is that man feels lonely and isolated because he has become separated from nature and from other men. As man has gained more freedom, he has also felt more alone. Fromm stigmatizes a whole society as "sick" (e.g., Nazi Germany) when it fails to satisfy the basic needs of man.

Horney sees her ideas as falling within the framework of Freudian psychology, but she attempts to eliminate some fallacies in his theory. For example, she feels that the Oedipus complex is not a sexual-aggressive conflict between the child and his parents but an anxiety growing out of basic disturbances (e.g., rejection) in the child's relationship with his parents. She feels that anything that disturbs the security of a child in relation to his parents produces "basic anxiety." This manifests itself in later years as "neurotic needs"; for example, irrational demands for affection and approval, for power, perfection, and invincibility.

Sullivan is the creator of the viewpoint known as "the interpersonal theory of psychiatry." He regards personality as "the relatively enduring pattern of recurrent interpersonal situations which characterize a human life." As Sullivan points out, the individual does not and cannot exist apart from his relations with other people. From birth the infant is part of an interpersonal situation. Even a hermit takes with him the memories of former personal relationships, and these continue to influence his thinking and acting. Sullivan views the properly conducted psychiatric interview, the face-to-face situation that takes place between the patient and the therapist, as a crucial point in helping troubled people.

Relief of Anxiety. The legitimate question remains: How otherwise than by sublimation can we reduce or minimize the burdens of anxiety inevitably generated by conflicts in the unconscious mind?

The first step is to understand that anxiety wears many disguises which we have tried to strip away by describing the behavior patterns that result from overworking of the mental mechanisms. The perfectionist, the hypochondriac, the man who continually projects his own failings on others, the woman who always rationalizes her mistakes, and all the rest are motivated by an inner anxiety. This emotion may parade as fatigue, overactivity, homesickness, physical illness, a sense of inferiority, depression, and in scores of other guises. By recognizing that anxiety is the basic motivation for personal conduct which displeases himself and attracts unfavorable reactions from others the individual is in a better position to seek and get help with his problem.

How else do you get rid of anxiety? Essentially by talking it out! University of California Medical School psychiatrists J. Ruesch and A. R. Prestwood[1] made a special study of the problem of relieving anxiety and came to this well-accepted conclusion:

The successful management of anxiety generated in daily life seems possible only through a process of sharing and communication.

The process of communication is essential for healthy functioning. Thus are people able to combine their efforts, to complement and increase their ability to cope with their surroundings. The ability to communicate and hence to share anxiety seems to constitute the process responsible for feelings of personal security on the part of the individual. Alleviation of anxiety comes through personal contacts. This process is basic to all interpersonal relationships from babyhood to old age.

An Age of Anxiety? Anxiety is one of the most common symptoms that a practicing physician encounters in his patients. The range of this anxiety is wide, reflected in patients suffering from simple tension to those with severe mental illness. But is ours really more of an age of anxiety than previous generations? At a symposium on "Anxiety and a Decade of Tranquilizer Therapy" held in New York in April, 1964, Dr. James G. Miller, of the University of Michigan, and Dr. Raymond B. Cattell, of the University of Illinois, expressed grave doubts as to whether this was really an age of anxiety beyond that of earlier eras.

Miller acknowledged the stresses of modern life: the hydrogen bomb, the population and information explosions, the increasing pressures of urban life. On the other hand, he pointed out, fear of sudden death and malignant illness is diminishing because medical research has provided powerful weapons against them.

"Civilization has curbed some of the lawless terrors and removed some of the rudeness of life in previous centuries," Miller continued. "Education has reduced superstition and fears arising from ignorance. A pervading sense of potentially malign supernatural powers has receded. There may even be less anxiety now than in the more brutal past," Miller concluded.

Dr. Cattell reported on the results of psychological studies of anxiety. Of ten nations that he had studied, the lowest levels of anxiety were found in the United States and Great Britain, while the highest levels were found in such underdeveloped nations as India. "It would seem that anxiety is higher where standards of living are lower, and where a country has cultural and political crevasses separating its peoples," Dr. Cattell observed. "But with America and Britain lowest on these lists," he continued, "the view that we live in an unusually anxious culture and age is scarcely supported." Interestingly, Dr. Cattell found the highest levels of anxiety in the United States among newspaper editors and writers; the lowest, for professionals, among university administrators.

There are many definitions of anxiety. Dr. Miller, for example, views it as a "signal-like pain." It reports whether a person has adequate processes of adjustment to cope with actual or threatened stress. Abnormal signs of anxiety, he felt, could cause useless distress; but mild anxiety can sometimes be associated with better performance. Dr. Cattell took a sterner view. He described all anxiety as "a lack of confidence, a sense of guilt and worthlessness, an unwillingness to venture, a dependency, a readiness to become fatigued, irritable, and discouraged, an uncertainty about oneself and a suspicion of others, and a general tenseness." He felt that this kind and degree of anxiety does not motivate but rather disorganizes the psyche.

Speaking from a woman's point of view at the symposium, author Marya Mannes called the "destructive anxieties" of this age the "pressures of society and the mass media to make [women] conform to the classic and traditional image in men's eyes and to be not only the perfect wife, mother, and homemaker, but also the ever-

[1] J. Ruesch, and A. R. Prestwood, *A.M.A. Archives of Neurology and Psychiatry* (November 1949).

young, ever-slim, ever-alluring object of their desire." Miss Mannes also designated the "anxieties engendered by the quest for success [as] relentless, degrading, and corroding. They infect husband and wife and the nature of their love. . . . Whatever is attained is never enough," Miss Mannes continued. "These are the social anxieties which afflict our age," she said.

Dr. Ashley Montague, Princeton anthropologist, described anxiety as "the unspecific fusion of fear and insecurity with uncertainty and helplessness in the face of danger—a generalized fear." He further elucidated, "Fear is usually a response to a specific danger; anxiety is the response to a diffuse, generalized fear. As such, anxiety, like stress, appears to be a concomitant of the very process of living."

There are disagreements on the origins as well as the nature of anxiety. There is (1) a psychoanalytic viewpoint, with many variations; (2) a conditioned reflex theory; and (3) an organic view. In the psychoanalytic view anxiety represents conflict in the unconscious mind, particularly a conflict between instinctual desires and a fear of what will happen if they are carried out. The anxious individual feels trapped between two opposing forces. According to the conditioned reflex theory (originally Ivan Pavlov's), anxiety is a conditioned response or learned habit that follows anticipation of danger. Neurotic symptoms are considered learned patterns of behavior that reduce the anxiety, which Pavlovians feel to be the central and most important motivational force in human behavior. In the organic or biological concept of anxiety, its basis is physical and it is caused by dysfunction of certain structures of the brain.

It should be pointed out that there is such a thing as a "normal anxiety," which is in proportion to the danger that elicits it. When anxiety occurs repeatedly and out of proportion to the threats involved—possibly as a result of unconscious conflicts—a condition of abnormal anxiety is present.

It would be a major, indeed impossible, task to wipe out all the anxieties that afflict the human race. There are available, however, individual treatments for people who are deeply troubled and disabled by their own anxieties. Part of the relief for anxiety comes from "talking it out" either in everyday communication or in professional psychotherapeutic interviews.

In addition to that crucial means of relieving anxiety there are now chemotherapeutic agents —drugs—which aid in the task. This is basically the class of drugs known as tranquilizers, introduced into medical practice in the mid-1950's. According to one definition (by Chauncey D. Leake), tranquilizers are chemical compounds that are specifically useful for the relief of anxiety and are differentiated from other central nervous system depressant drugs by that quality. All of them have somewhat different pharmacological action but their net therapeutic effect on mood and behavior is to reduce anxiety. However, one cannot depend on tranquilizers alone, or any other drug, to dispel his anxieties.

Chronic (Pathological) Fatigue

Closely akin to anxiety, and perhaps another form of it, is the condition often described as chronic, or pathological, fatigue. Chronic fatigue may also be called "emotional fatigue." It is different from the physiological fatigue that follows after strenuous work or exercise.

Chronic, or pathological, fatigue is a symptom that something is wrong with the person who suffers from it. Many people are chronically fatigued without realizing it. This fatigue may be expressed in changed moods, attitudes, and behavior, for example, exceptional irritability, loss of a sense of humor, or even loss of weight, poor appetite, and restless sleep. A constant state of muscular tension—considerably beyond normal muscle tone—commonly accompanies chronic fatigue. This abnormal tension, or hypertonus, arises because the muscles are being constantly stimulated by unconscious motivations to make first this move and then that. However, the stimulus to complete the move is inhibited and countermanded before the muscles can fully obey. These alternating commands keep the muscles constantly on stretch. Fatigue products

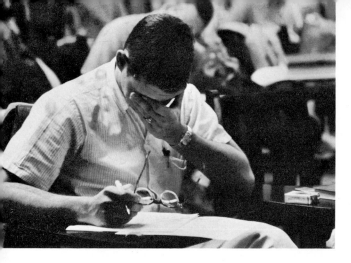

FATIGUE may be simple physiological fatigue resulting from extreme muscular exertion or lack of sleep; or it may be chronic pathological fatigue produced by deeper emotional factors, such as anxiety. (Photograph by Zimbel-MONKMEYER)

are never completely enough dispelled, so the feeling of fatigue persists.

External pressures and environmental circumstances are factors in bringing on chronic fatigue. This has been studied particularly in the field of industrial hygiene. Workers become fatigued and less productive when they must work under conditions of poor light and glare, poor ventilation, too much noise and heat, uncomfortable seating, and exposure to dusts and fumes.

Other factors that induce fatigue are excessive hours of work, lack of properly spaced rest pauses, awkward working positions, "speed-up" of work beyond capacity to perform, and the monotony of simple, repeated operations. Workers are less productive also when they are afraid of and hostile toward their jobs and bosses.

Some of the facts discovered in the study of industrial hygiene can be profitably applied by the wise student in eliminating fatigue factors from his own life. He can arrange to do his studying under the best possible conditions of physical comfort and efficiency. Equally important is a rhythm of work balanced with relaxation. A rest pause of five minutes during each study hour is advisable. There should be some regularity in the student's schedule of study, play, eating, and sleeping. Too much extracurricular pressure should be avoided. Procrastination, delay, and overcrowding of hours bring on fatigue and re-

duce efficiency. Careless students work the hardest.

While fatigue is a symptom of disease, it must also be recognized that fatigue may predispose to disease—for example, the common cold. Sufficient time for recovery from fatigue must be allowed, especially after infectious diseases. Convalescence should not be unduly shortened. For simple fatigue, rest is the sovereign remedy. But in cases of chronic fatigue professional help may be needed, and great effort may have to be exerted to root out its causes.

Why to Stay away from Stimulants. The *wrong way* to fight fatigue is by indulgence in chemical stimulants. The reason? Too often, when taken in sufficient dosage to have any genuine effect, they create a "rebound reaction" and, after a short while, you end up feeling more fatigued than before you took the drug.

Probably the best known and most widely used stimulant drug is *caffeine,* which is the active ingredient in coffee, tea, chocolate drinks, some cola drinks and many nonprescription "stay awake" drugs.

There are, of course, many other drugs known to stimulate the central nervous system, including amphetamines (such as benzadrine) and whole new series of psychic stimulants that were developed in the 1960's. When prescribed by a physician upon proper indications, these are valuable medications.

Many college students, however, have the mistaken idea that they can take these so-called "pep pills" indiscriminately and without harm. "Pep pills" are often used by students to cram for exams or to drive all night to get home or back to college after an exciting weekend. This is a dangerous practice, because all potent stimulant drugs may have side effects (in addition to rebound reactions) and untoward reactions that were not anticipated by the indiscriminate self-medicator. There are better ways than chemicals to deal with fatigue; notably by better organization of one's time, by recreation, relaxation, good sleeping habits, and the control of factors and problems which induce needless psychic stress and muscular tension.

SUMMARY

This chapter has covered the sequence of normal personality development, from infancy onward. It has presented the concept and the construct of the unconscious mind, divided conventionally into id, ego, and superego. It has discussed the conflicts in the unconscious mind and described a number of the "ego-defenses," also called mental dynamisms, by which the ego protects itself; for example, repression, regression, rationalization, etc. The important subject of anxiety has been introduced in this chapter and several ways of relieving it were discussed—notably through sharing and communication and by means of tranquilizers. The topic of chronic, or pathological, fatigue akin to anxiety has also been presented. In conclusion, the unconscious mind is a powerful force in determining human personality and behavior.

SUMMARY REVIEW QUESTIONS

1. What is the relationship of personality to emotions? To the unconscious mind? How do we judge personality?
2. What is the proper sequential order in which the following types of love appear in the course of normal personality development: idealistic, narcissistic, oedipal, homosexual, heterosexual, imitative? At approximately what age does each appear?
3. What are the two chief "negative emotions"? What is their purpose? How should they be consciously managed?
4. What do you understand by the term *unconscious mind?* What is its relationship to the conscious mind?
5. What do you understand by the id? The ego? The superego? What are the leading or peculiar characteristics of each?
6. How do conflicts in the unconscious mind produce anxiety? What can be done to relieve such anxiety?
7. What is a mental mechanism (or dynamism)? Can you name six and explain briefly what each one means?
8. How do you explain in terms of overworked mental mechanisms (or otherwise) the behavior of "stock characters" described in the following terms: the hypochondriac, the alibi artist, the homebody, the absent-minded professor, the perfectionist, the spit-fire, the sarcastic critic, the extrovert, Lady Macbeth, Pollyanna?
9. Do you believe that we live in an "age of anxiety"? Justify your answer, whether positive or negative.
10. What is chronic, or pathological, fatigue? How does it differ from normal, or physiological, fatigue? In what way, if any, is it related to anxiety?
11. Are the following statements sense or nonsense? Why? *Anyone who is afraid is a coward. . . . It is easy to get angry at those you love. . . . The child is father to the man. . . . Fatigue never hurt anyone. . . . The man who knows where he is going is on the road to mental health. . . . Always do the best you can with what you have where you are.*
12. What do the following terms mean to you: libido, infantile amnesia, repression, fantasy, frustration, emotional maturity, neurotic anxiety, ego defense, fetishist, tranquilizer, stimulant?

Recommended for Further Reading: *Discovering Ourselves* by Edward A. Strecker, M. D. and Kenneth E. Appel, M. D. *Love or Perish* by Smiley Blanton, M. D. *The Undiscovered Self* by C. G. Jung. *Anxiety: A Condition of Modern Man* by Henri Steiner and Jean Gebser. *Psychopathology of Everyday Life* by Sigmund Freud, M.D. For more complete references, see Appendix E.

4

MENTAL ILLNESS

Macbeth: How does your patient, doctor?
Doctor: Not so sick, my lord,
   As she is troubled with thick-coming fancies,
   That keep her from her rest.
Macbeth: Cure her of that.
   Canst thou not minister to a mind diseased,
   Pluck from the memory a rooted sorrow,
   Raze out the written troubles of the brain
   And with some sweet oblivious antidote
   Cleanse the stuffed bosom of that perilous stuff
   Which weighs upon the heart?
Doctor: Therein the patient
   Must minister to himself.

Shakespeare: Macbeth

THE LESS A PERSON KNOWS ABOUT MENTAL illness, the more likely he is to consider it a "disgrace." This attitude reflects a fear of the unknown, a defeatist prejudice against false stereotypes, and a true ignorance of the nature of mental illness. Without denying the seriousness of *some* forms of the disease, we can nevertheless begin by recognizing these hopeful facts:

Mental illness today is largely curable. A diagnosis of mental illness is not a clap of doom. "No branch of medical science except obstetrics is blessed by so many recoveries as psychiatry," affirms Karl Menninger. And he speaks from the well-documented records of psychiatrists and hospitals. Furthermore, most attacks of mental illness, properly treated, are of short duration—a few weeks or months.

The introduction of new drugs in the 1950's and 1960's gave fresh impetus and offers still wider hope for cure or relief of mental illness. These drugs, sometimes classified as "ataraxics,"

tranquilizers, or cerebral stimulants, have reversed the long-time trend of increasing populations in mental hospitals. The decline began in 1956.

The management of mild as well as severe mental illness has been improved by the new drugs. This is important when one recalls that at least half the patients who consult physicians are suffering from emotional disorders, which produce psychosomatic illness or psychogenic complaints.

Effective as it is, the treatment of mental disorders with drugs, by psychotherapy, and in many other ways remains largely empiric; they work but no one knows exactly how or why. On the other hand a better understanding of the causes of mental illness has presented new opportunities for its *prevention*.

The key to the fuller understanding of mental illness is to be found in the workings of the unconscious mind and its mental mechanisms.

These offer rational explanations for the queer behavior, the strange feelings, and the otherwise apparently meaningless conduct of the mentally ill, the neurotically disturbed, and even the criminally inclined. This knowledge can be misapplied, but it is a heartening fact that year after year more people are becoming concerned with the prevention of mental illness. Among them are parents, laymen, physicians, deans, social workers, teachers, nurses, psychologists, recreation leaders, and clergymen.

Research in mental illness is being increasingly well-supported, although the financial support is still far from adequate.

In short, there has been steady progress in the treatment and prevention of mental illness since the turn of the twentieth century.

What Really Is Mental Illness

Mental illness can be described as the *exaggeration* of personal feelings, and consequent behavior, to the point where it strikes other people as queer, odd, abnormal, annoying, or dangerous. The distinction between mental health and mental illness is a very practical one: a person is mentally ill to the extent that he cannot love or work. Obviously, then, there are all degrees of mental illness, ranging from the very mild to the exceptionally severe.

Two other practical criteria (but not very accurate ones) for evaluating the severity of mental illness can also be set down: (1) Does the victim feel bad enough to seek professional or outside help for his distress? (2) Does the physician, usually a psychiatrist, who diagnoses his condition believe that he will benefit by hospital treatment or requires hospitalization because he is a risk to himself or a danger to other people?

We have, then, three general classes of mentally ill people. The first, and by far the largest, comprises the millions of odd, emotionally disturbed, continually unhappy people who stumble through miserable lives without getting or accepting real help for their illness. Many of them are actually sicker than those who see physicians or go to the hospital.

The second class of mentally ill are those who have at least identified their need, often desperate, for help and have sought it. Most neurotics fall in this category.

The third group of mentally ill includes those who require or will benefit by hospitalization. A very high proportion of this group are definitely, if temporarily, psychotic. This is the class of patients who are generally thought of as "the mentally ill," but they make up only a small fraction of the total.

The mentally ill are not so evidently different from mentally healthy, or "normal," people. Indeed, they are often the same people at different times. When a person finds he cannot eat, sleep, concentrate, or get along with other people for days on end, he is on the road to or in the throes of mental illness and needs help. Mental illness is emotional rather than mental (or intellectual) in origin and content.

There are, of course, some cases where definite physical damage to the brain can be clearly demonstrated; for example, cases of third stage syphilis, causing general paresis; and advanced cases of chronic alcoholism, in which brain damage appears as "DT's", delirium tremens. There is today a vast amount of brain research seeking to link physiological changes in the brain with various mental illnesses.

It is possible, however, to regard mental illness as an extreme protective device adopted by the ego to shield itself from deeper hurts by unconscious conflicts and bludgeonings. To be sure, the cloak of illness is a very poor form of social adaptation and no shield at all against societal disapproval. But for the individual caught in the trap of his own internal emotional strife, mental illness seems for a time at least the best way out of his unconsciously engendered difficulties.

We say "for a time" because the unconscious threats and situational stresses to which mental illness is the response may in time subside, with a disappearance of the symptoms of illness, or the patient may be gradually educated to a better solution than illness to his deep-seated fears. But when he becomes ill, he is saving himself from the inner threat of unthinkable annihilation or deprivation; the illness is an escape. The mental processes here described are complex and difficult to untangle in individual cases, but they are not mystic and completely unfathomable. Mental illness does not strike without warning. It is the culmination of unsuccessful reactions to life problems and long-time failure to adjust to real-life situations.

A precipitating factor in the illness can usually be identified. Often it is the deprivation of a source of emotional support—a beloved spouse, parent, or child. Psychiatrists also identify an "old-sergeant syndrome." This apparently tough-minded army personality breaks down emotionally when all the individuals upon whom he has previously depended are one by one removed by combat or transfer. The ability to rise above grief and snap back from deprivation is one of the hallmarks of the truly mature person.

As against the precipitating factors in mental illness, there are a host of predisposing factors. The most important of these can be summed up as current physical condition and all previous emotional experiences, especially the emotional conditioning in infancy and childhood.

Causes of Mental Illness

Mental illness is a reaction to external and internal stress. In much the same way fever is a reaction to the presence of infecting microorganisms in the body. The stress goes beyond the breaking point of the individual's particular personality structure. Even the most stable personalities have a breaking point—as war experiences often reveal.

When we seek the causes of mental disease, therefore, we must look first to the underlying personality structure of the individual in whom the disease appears. Of course, the search does not stop here. Whatever else may be said about the causes of mental illness, this much is clear: multiple factors are involved. It is misleading to attribute them to a single cause or to one traumatic event of childhood.

It is sometimes easier to put a finger on the immediate, precipitating causes of mental breakdowns, but even here great caution in the interpretation is necessary. Situational stresses or external events may precipitate the difficulty. In some instances constant exposure to a "psychogenic," "emotionally contagious" individual, like a tyrant boss or parent constantly getting on other people's nerves, may either crystallize or predispose to mental illness.

In tracing the causation of mental illness, physical factors, reflecting the intimate relationships of mind and body, must always be considered. In a certain percentage of the cases actual damage to or destruction of nerve cells in the brain can be located. But in a far larger percentage, and to some extent in all cases, purely psychological mechanisms and stresses are at work.

A distinction is made between "organic" and "functional" mental illnesses. In the "organic" class some definite and presumably primary damage to the nerve tissue of the brain can be demonstrated. In the "functional" cases, no such injury can be found.

Among the causes of direct damage to the brain can be listed infections, meningitis, syphilis, head injuries (trauma), drugs used to excess, poisons, tumors, and hardening of the arteries of the brain (causing "little strokes," which are part of the aging process). Late syphilitic infection is responsible for general paresis. Alcoholic psychoses, which include delirium tremens, are typical of brain damage and malfunction induced by drugs or poisons.

Types and Classifications of Mental Illness

Basically mental illness is classified by the severity of its symptoms, by the degree to which they incapacitate the patient for normal living. We speak of two major categories of mental illness: *psychoses,* which are the severe types of mental illness that often require a period of hospitalization, and *neuroses,* the less extreme forms of personality derangement. The difference between psychoses and neuroses is one of degree.

The words "psychoneurosis" and "neurosis" are used interchangeably.

Psychiatry makes more extensive and exact diagnoses and uses more elaborate descriptions of mental illness. The American Psychiatric Association has a classification of about 60 categories of mental illness, but there is a strong trend toward avoiding categorical diagnosis of mental illness. As Karl Menninger has pointed out, patients recover from their mental illnesses but not from their diagnoses. It is preferable, therefore, to speak of "schizophrenic reactions" rather than schizophrenia. Since the diagnosis of mental illness is a job for the psychiatrist, not the college student, we shall limit the further description of mental illnesses to the few broadest types.

Schizophrenia, sometimes called dementia praecox, is the most common of the serious mental illnesses and the one for which hospitalization is most often required. Literally the term means "split personality." Emotional disorganization is the hallmark of this condition. The victims may be unaccountably sad or happy; they do not respond appropriately to real-life situations; they are withdrawn and usually apathetic; they are ready to daydream their lives away; they often suffer from fantastic delusions and hallucinations. (Delusions are false fixed ideas; hallucinations are imaginary voices or visions.)

Some schizophrenics act and talk silly and childishly, without orientation to time and place; others fall into a stupor or a state of muscular rigidity; still others go into a frenzy of excitement or overactivity. They withdraw from reality, and attempt to live in worlds of their own.

Schizophrenics do not lose their mental capacities, as measured by I.Q. tests, but their intelligence is divorced from other phases of their personality. Schizophrenia usually develops gradually and is generally apparent before the age of 40.

Recent research in the cause and treatment of schizophrenia offers great promise of a "breakthrough" in the management of this illness. For example, an unusual serum factor has been found in the blood of many schizophrenics, which suggests the possibility of an antiserum or other drug to combat the illness. Progress is also being made in acquiring basic information about childhood schizophrenia and ways of treating it—partially through family interviewing and counseling. When the disease appears in young children (under six), it is important to distinguish between childhood schizophrenia and mental retardation. The schizophrenia may be curable.

Paranoia describes a state of mental illness characterized by persistent delusions of grandeur or persecution. It is related to schizophrenia but far less common. Many paranoiacs are "rational" on all subjects except one or two on which they have some irrational fixed idea. There are many paranoid personalities among people who are not hospitalized for mental illness.

Manic-depressive psychoses involve extreme swings in mood, far beyond the essentially normal feelings of elation or depression. (Everyone has some mood swings.) The hypermanic may talk incessantly, pursue a flight of ideas, and sometimes require restraint for his protection. In acute depression the patient may feel so guilty, project so much anger upon himself that he does not want to continue living. He may absolutely refuse to eat and may plan or attempt suicide. The manic stage can be likened to reactions beyond those more commonly observed as extroversion. Manic-depressive reactions often, but not *necessarily,* move in a cycle. For weeks, months or years the person is depressed; then, for no apparent reason he feels unduly elated—and vice versa. The intellectual and emotional faculties are not impaired.

Related to the depressive phase of the cycle is the condition known as *involutional melancholia,* which usually occurs in women at the menopause.

Senile dementia describes the childishness of old age, the deterioration of mental and emotional facilities that *sometimes* accompanies the aging process. Often, however, there is some actual damage to the blood-vessels of the brain. This condition rarely occurs before 60.

Hysteria describes the neurotic reaction characterized by lack of control over acts and emotions and by conversion of inner anxiety into physical symptoms (e.g., hysterical paralysis). *"Shell shock"* was a term used in World War I, as was the term *"combat fatigue"* in World War II, to describe an essentially hysterical psychosomatic reaction to military situations involving danger. The soldier's ego seeks to be removed from and escape the zone of danger without disgrace. "If you're sick, you can't fight," runs the winning argument in the unconscious mind.

"Nervous breakdown" is a popular phrase used to describe almost any kind of mental illness, mild or severe, which incapacitates an individual. The milder breakdowns are often described as *neurasthenia, psychasthenia, anxiety state,* or *mild hysteria.*

Psychopathic personality is a term used to denote individuals who have no particular mental disease but who cannot adjust themselves morally, socially, or legally to their environment. A high proportion of criminals, vagrants, and delinquents fall into this category.

Particularly to be deplored is the label "psycho" on any individual who has ever suffered a mental illness.

Gross Misconceptions about Mental Illness

In the popular mind there remain a number of gross misconceptions about mental illness. Many people still cling to distorted stereotypes of mental illness—"the raving maniac" in the padded cell, the "village idiot," the "daft girl" who thinks she is Queen of the May, the man who believes he is Napoleon. A visit to any well-run mental hospital, and even to its back wards, would quickly dispel this illusion. To correct these and some other misconceptions, we may assert:

Insanity and mental illness, though related, are *not* the same thing. Insanity is a legal rather than medical term and implies that the person is incapable of determining between right and wrong and further that his actions are so unreliable that he is a danger to himself and others. Both circumstances are sometimes the case, but most mentally ill people are *not* insane.

The mentally ill person does *not* "lose his mind," except in rare instances. *Temporary* distortions of some mental faculties, such as memory and power of concentration, frequently occur. Real or permanent deterioration of the intellect is exceptional.

Mental illness is *not* caused by masturbation, is *not* punishment for sin, is *not* directly inherited. There has been much speculation on the subject, but there is no convincing scientific evidence that mental illness is passed along from parent to child in the germ plasm. The appearance of several cases in the same family may represent social and cultural (rather than physical) heredity, since all the members of the family have been exposed to the same anxiety-provoking personalities and environment.

Mental illness is *not* mental retardation, or *feeble-mindedness.* The mentally defective person never develops average intelligence, whereas many people who suffer from mental illness are far above normal in intelligence.

People who consult psychiatrists, psychologists, or other counselors are *not* crazy. A visit to a psychiatrist is *not* an admission of a fatal weakness. There is no more "disgrace" in consulting a psychiatrist than in seeing any other medical specialist.

Treatment of Mental Illness

Lee R. Steiner, who has studied for many years the question of where people take their troubles, points out that they take them not only to psychiatrists and physicians but also to clinical psychologists, psychoanalysts, social workers, ministers, rabbis, priests, marriage counselors, vocational counselors, guidance counselors, bartenders, beauticians, fortune tellers, astrologers, and a miscellaneous assortment of self-appointed experts and charlatans. Steiner's most trenchant observation is that the outcome of treatment appears to depend more upon the *rapport,* or personal relationship, established between the patient and his "healer" (therapist) than on any other factor.

The psychiatrist, is the best-qualified person to treat the whole range of mental illness—and certainly the psychoses. All psychiatrists are doctors of medicine who have taken postgraduate training in their specialty. Most are certified as medical specialists by the American Board of Psychiatry and Neurology. There are, however, only about 17,000 psychiatrists in the whole United States.

The modern psychiatrist has many means of treating both mild and severe mental illness. The oldest is hydrotherapy (water treatment, of which bathing in warm springs and the "ducking stool" are ancient examples). The latest are the new drugs, the ataraxics, introduced in the 1950's. The most disputed is psychoanalysis, which took root in the 1900's.

The type of treatment selected, or attempted, depends on specific diagnosis, length and severity of the illness, and the personality structure of the particular patient.

Central to all types of treatment is *psychotherapy,* which essentially means purposeful conversation between the patient and his therapist. This includes directive and non-directive counseling, reassurance, group therapy, hypnosis, confession, orthodox Freudian psychoanalysis, and theoretical or practical ("shortcut") modifications of it.

Most of the short-range methods of psychotherapy are called *suppressive;* they attempt to drive conflicts so deep into the unconscious mind that they are no longer troublesome. Many so-called "miracles" and faith cures are suppressive psychotherapy. They are usually most effective in cases of conversion hysteria. For example, in hysterical paralysis, a lame patient may visit a famous shrine or get a great shock, throw away his crutches, and walk again.

In expressive psychotherapy the patient is encouraged to talk about thimself, his problems, his thoughts, feelings, dreams, and inner conflicts to the extent that he is or becomes aware of them. The goal here is re-education of the patient, particularly to help him find a changed perspective toward himself and other people.

Psychoanalysis. *Psychoanalysis* is the prototype of all forms of expressive psychotherapy, but it is only one of many kinds of psychotherapy. Pioneered in theory and practice by Freud, it established the vital importance of the unconscious mind and its anxiety conflicts. It remains the basis of all psychodynamic psychology despite modifications by Adler, Jung, Rank, Horney, Sullivan, and many others. But its value as a method of treatment is being called increasingly into criticism. This criticism is especially directed against high-priced, scantily available, "orthodox" Freudian analysis.

Dr. Hans Eysenck, professor of psychology at the University of London, has charged: "Psychiatrists and psychologists will have to acknowledge the fact that current psychotherapeutic procedures have not lived up to the hopes which greeted their emergence 50 years ago. It would . . . appear advisable . . . to discard the psychoanalytic model." This advice goes farther than the present consensus of professional opinion about the value of analytic (or psychodynamic) theory and treatment. Some 200,000 patients in the United States are still treated every year by psychoanalysis (including orthodox analysis), and a great many are certainly helped if not "cured" according to strict scientific criteria. Many times that number of people are enjoying the outcomes of more indirect practice of psychotherapy. Freud is not dead, but he is no longer undisputed monarch of the realms of mental healing. [Sigmund Freud, the man, the Viennese father of psychoanalysis, died in 1937].

Other Types of Psychotherapy. In *directive counseling,* which attacks primarily the patient's conscious worries about his immediate real-life situations, the counselor does most of the talking. He often tells the patient directly what he thinks the patient ought to do. In *non-directive counseling,* at the same conscious level, the patient is left much more to his own devices to determine what steps he must take to shed his apparent difficulties.

In *group therapy,* under a skilled discussion leader, patients are encouraged to talk about themselves and share experiences in such a way that they get better insight into their problems and recognize, at the very least, that they are not alone in facing and striving to meet particular human troubles.

Hypnosis has some limited uses in treating neuroses—but only in the hands of a well-qualified practitioner. Hypnotism can be dangerous when practiced by parlor amateurs or unscrupulous quacks. Approximately three out of four people can be hypnotized to some extent, but only one in five deeply. Women succumb to it more readily than men.

Drug Therapy. Sedative drugs, like bromides and barbiturates, and stimulating drugs, like amphetamine (Benzedrine), have long been effectively used in treating mental illness. The new 1950 ataraxic drugs, tranquilizers, and brain stimulants, have given even more remarkable results. The first of these was reserpine, derived from *Rauwolfia serpentina.* This is the snakeroot plant, which has a long and romantic history in the herbal medicine of India. (Rauwolfia derivatives are also used in treating heart disease.)

The next important tranquilizing drug, discovered in France, was chlorpromazine. A young French doctor, conducting wounded soldiers back by plane from Indo-China, is credited with first observing its significant tranquilizing effect. Both these drugs proved of unexpected value in treating schizophrenia, particularly in quieting and relaxing agitated patients.

Scores of tranquilizers are now on the market and research continues for newer and better ones, free of side reactions. Probably the best-known tranquilizer is the American discovery named "Miltown" (meprobomate).

Such drugs should be taken only under medical supervision. They have been popularly called "don't-give-a-damn pills" and they have raised the seriously interesting question: How tranquil can you get? Cerebral stimulants are drugs which elevate mood, which "cheer up" depressed patients—the effect opposite to that of tranquilizers.

Some Other Psychiatric Treatments. Electroshock treatments, introduced about 1940, have also proved of great value in treating mental illness, particularly depressed and melancholic patients. A mild electrical current is passed between the frontal lobes of the brain. Shock treatment is quite safe; millions of such treatments have been given with very few accidents or untoward reactions. A shock effect can also be produced by injections of insulin and metrazol. The use of the new drugs has cut the need for shock treatment at least by half.

Hospitalization itself, in a properly run psychiatric hospital, is still another important form of treatment for mental illness. The essence of hospital treatment—in addition to the custody which prevents the patient from harming himself or others—is to relieve the patient temporarily of the stress of external reality and give a weakened ego a better chance to get control again of the unconscious mind.

Physical Fitness and Behavior Therapy. A high degree of physical fitness (see Chapter 7), and a liberal engagement in recreational exercise can be recommended as an outlet for tensions of modern living. This prescription is especially applicable to young adults. Dr. Donald J. Erickson of the Mayo Clinic, speaking at the 1962 American Medical Association Convention, pointed out that while "stress disorders are increasing," exercise allays anxiety and is helpful in promoting relaxation. The conveniences of our culture—elevators and automobiles, for example—he said, are "depriving us of exercise that is necessary to maintain physical fitness. As a consequence the great functional reserves of the human organism that have been provided by nature may be diminished—since the body systems readily adapt to changes in functional demand."

"Behavior therapy," or conditioning therapy, based essentially on the principle of the "conditioned reflex" originally popularized by the Russian scientist, Ivan Pavlov, in the early 1900's, obtained renewed attention from research scientists and practicing physicians in the 1960's. Coupled with the new drug therapies, behavioral therapy is making strong claims for renewed clinical attention. At a 1962 conference on conditioning therapies versus psychoanalysis, Dr. A. Hussain of the Yankton State Hospital, Yankton, South Dakota, reported a cure rate of 95% in a series of 105 behaviorally and drug-treated patients suffering chiefly from anxiety neuroses. The series also included patients whose diagnoses were recorded as obsessive compulsive neuroses, hysteria, impotence, homosexuality, and phobic (excessive fear) reactions.

The Extent of Mental Illness

Within the context of a broad definition of mental illness, the number of victims runs into the millions. The National Association for Mental Health estimates that at least one in every ten people—20,000,000 people in all—has some form of mental or emotional illness that needs psychiatric treatment. In at least half of all the millions of medical and surgical cases seen by physicians, there is a component of mental illness.

About 760,000 mentally ill patients are in or under the care of mental hospitals on any one day of the year, more than all other diseases combined. About 500,000 new patients are admitted each year. There are approximately 500 mental hospitals in the United States, of which half are state hospitals. Most of these are large, with 2000 to 12,000 beds, and are overcrowded and understaffed. About 500 community general hospitals have separate units for treating psychiatric patients and another 500 admit psychiatric patients to their regular medical facilities.

With good care at least 70% of the patients admitted to mental hospitals or services can leave partly or totally recovered. About 75% of those admitted for the first time leave the hospital within the first year.

Approximately $2 billion a year is directly spent in the United States for the care and treatment of the mentally ill in the hospitals. Business authorities conservatively estimate that the indirect cost of emotional illness to business runs to many billions of dollars a year.

Availability of psychiatrists is an index of community service for the mentally ill. The number of psychiatrists in the United States is on the increase. Since 1956 the ratio of members of the American Psychiatric Association to the

number of people in the United States has increased by about 30%.

The location of psychiatrists in the United States remains concentrated. Over half of them are in five states—California, Illinois, Massachusetts, New York, and Pennsylvania. In two-thirds of the counties in the country, there are no psychiatrists.

The introduction of new drug and other modern psychiatric treatments has encouraged the development of community-based psychiatric services for prevention, diagnosis, treatment, and rehabilitation. These clinics now take patients of all ages and many treat patients with psychoses. In 1962, they served nearly 750,000 patients. Professional manhours in staffing these clinics is also increasing.

On the basis of past record it may be anticipated that the indices showing improvements in mental health care will continue to rise.

Community Mental Health Centers. Another forward step in providing improved care for the mentally ill in the United States is the development of comprehensive community mental health centers, which enable the mentally ill to be treated at home. Federal grants-in-aid to finance up to two-thirds the cost of construction of these new local mental health treatment centers were authorized in 1963. The development of these community centers is expected to be not only more effective but also less expensive in providing public hospital care for mental illness. Treatment will usually begin earlier, when it is more intensive and effective; will avoid separation from family and commitment to a state hospital; and will offer the support of community resources following treatment.

Community mental health centers, as now visioned, embrace a new concept and a new challenge: comprehensive treatment provided in the community for all who need it. Services provided by the centers will include round-the-clock emergency services, short-term hospitalization, outpatient services, partial hospitalization in day or night treatment programs, aftercare, consultation, and education services for community agencies. Dr. Robert H. Felix, when Director of the U.S. Public Health Service National Institute of Mental Health, said: "Not since the creation of the National Institute of Mental Health in 1949 has such specific impetus been provided by the Federal government for the opening of a new era in dealing with problems of mental illness."

Prevention of Mental Illness

How Can Mental Illness be Prevented? Mental health must be considered not only a personal problem but also a family, community, and public health problem. As an individual, you can make conscious efforts toward leading a well-balanced life, including work, play, love, and worship, and toward understanding yourself.

As a parent, you can help prevent mental illness in your children by bringing them up with a balance of loving care and consistent discipline that sets limits for action. Some roots of mental illness are set in childhood; emotional patterns are crystallized before intelligence takes over. Hence mental health becomes a family affair.

As a citizen you can support the mental-health movement, lend a voice toward adequately staffed and supported mental hospitals, mental health clinics, and child guidance centers. You can speak up for an intelligent, well-informed attitude toward mental illness and break down prejudices against the mentally ill. If a relative, friend, employee, or fellow worker seems to be "losing his grip," you can urge professional psychiatric attention. Since recreation is a defense against mental illness, you can also support recreational facilities.

What's Needed to Improve America's Mental Health. A specific program of "Action for Mental Health" was proposed in 1962 as a result of a thus-titled report which was issued in March, 1961 by a Joint Commission on Mental Illness and Health. This was the culmination of a five-year study in which 36 national organizations, including the American Medical Association and the American Psychiatric Association, took part. Key points in the "action program" for improvement of mental health and prevention of mental

illness (or at least its disabling effects) may be briefly summarized as follows:

¶ *More Medical Leadership.* Individual physicians must join more vigorously in national efforts to promote mental health and must take leadership in keeping their own patients, these patients' families, and the community at large more accurately informed about mental health and illness. The public's lack of understanding and frequent misinformation about psychiatric illnesses are basic causes for the rejection of the mentally ill and the failure of many programs intended to aid them. Physicians in general practice and in specialties other than neurology and psychiatry can do much to change this unfortunate climate of opinion.

¶ *More Mental Health Personnel* (for example, psychiatric social workers, trained psychiatric nurses and aides, clinical psychologists, volunteer workers in mental hospitals). There is an acute shortage of adequately trained personnel in the mental health field, and recruitment of both professional workers and volunteers is sorely needed.

¶ *More Research in Mental Health and Mental Illness.* The 1960's formula of allotting a mere 2.5% of mental health budgets for research and training was vastly inadequate. Research in this area must be fostered and expanded in universities, hospitals, medical schools, and other agencies.

¶ *More Mental Health Services at Local (Community) Levels.* There is a demonstrable shortage of such facilities despite growing awareness of the need for local psychiatric clinics, child guidance centers, and the like. Psychiatric information also should be available to the public on a 24-hour-a-day basis, since emergencies (such as drunken combat and attempted suicides) arise in this field at odd hours of the day and night. The most hopeful development is the increase in psychiatric wards at general hospitals (which usually have emergency and ambulance service available).

The groups for which added mental health facilities are especially needed include (1) *children,* who should be reached through school health services and guidance departments as well as clinics and day centers; (2) the *"juvenile delinquent,"* actual or potential, for whose benefit psychiatric clinics and services should be more frequently associated with both juvenile and criminal courts; (3) *the mentally retarded*—an estimated 5 million in the United States, whose existence constitutes a medical, educational, and social problem of vast dimensions; and (4) *the aged,* who are often left in or shunted off to custodial care in mental hospitals because there is no other place for them among community institutions.

¶ *More Funds to Support the Needed Mental Health Services.* Multiple-source financing, with funds coming not only from public but also from private sources (such as philanthropy and fees), appears to be indicated.

¶ *Greater Awareness of the Effect of the Rapid Changes* of the social and political structure of the world upon individual and group mental health.

Suicide. Mental illnesses are not in themselves fatal, like pneumonia and heart disease. There is, however, one fatal termination of mental illness that occurs more commonly than generally supposed: suicide. Every so often a college campus is shocked by this event, and the question arises, "Why did he do it?"

The "obvious reasons" are never the basic reasons. As Karl Menninger, one of the great students of the subject, points out: individuals always in a measure create the unconscious environment in which they exist. Long before the final act, the suicide is helping to create the very trap of circumstances from which, by suicide, he takes flight. He has reached a delicate point of psychic maladjustment where he at one and the same time (1) wishes to kill (anger), (2) wishes to be killed (expiation for guilt feelings), and (3) wishes to die (find peace without struggle). Fortunately for potential suicides, this delicate imbalance cannot be long maintained. If the suicidally inclined individual can be helped through his darkest moments or months, the fatal mood is not too likely to recur.

Rare, indeed, is the individual who has *never* entertained the thought of suicide. There are times in every life when, as Mark Twain put it, we would like to die—temporarily. But these wisps of a passing thought are not to be confused with the dangerous drive toward self-destruction that may occur in the deeply depressed, unconsciously troubled individual.

Suicide, however, can be prevented. If you are genuinely and persistently troubled by suicidal thoughts, be quick to seek help from psychiatric sources. If a friend discusses such thoughts with you, be sympathetic and tolerant of his problems—and guide him firmly to a psychiatrist, physician, or other responsible source of help. The potential suicide should not be left alone, even for a minute.

The magnitude of the suicide problem in the United States is not generally appreciated. Suicide is three times as common as murder.

Deaths from Psychogenic Causes. It may come as a surprise that three out of the five principal causes of death in the college-age bracket are essentially psychogenic in origin, namely, accidents, suicide, and homicide. The unconscious trap which accounts for suicide itself is also responsible for "purposive accidents," which often end fatally (Chapter 18).

Accidents don't just happen; they are caused; and the cause of a high proportion of these "accidentally on purpose" events is to be found in the unconscious mind. The "accident-prone" individual unconsciously wants to hurt or kill himself. Failing, or even partially succeeding, he feels inwardly impelled to try again.

Automobile accidents frequently occur under circumstances that give rise to the suspicion that the accident was an attempted, or successful, suicide. One can only guess at the actual numbers, but the high toll of motor-vehicle accidents and fatalities in the late teens and twenties suggests that it is not inconsiderable. Maladjusted young men now make a larger share than ever before of the "accident-prone" group. They often use cars as misdirected instruments of power.

We must therefore list unconsciously motivated "purposive accidents" along with psychoses, neuroses, alcohol and drug addiction, gambling, promiscuity, self-mutilation, delinquent and antisocial behavior, suicide itself, and other forms of "partial suicide" as exhibitions of mental illness.

Mental Retardation

Mental retardation, mental deficiency, or (as it was once called) feeblemindedness, is quite different from mental illness. The problem of mental retardation presents a major challenge to our society—to find causes, seek prevention, and provide the best possible assurance for lives of maximum usefulness. The late President John F. Kennedy, appointed a panel of physicians, scientists, educators, lawyers, psychologists, social scientists, and others to review programs and needs, to ascertain gaps, and to prescribe a program for action.

The panel's report[1] showed mental retardation to be a major national health, social, and economic problem, affecting some 5.4 million children and adults and involving some 15 to 20 million family members in the United States. The panel estimated that the cost of care for America's mentally retarded was about $550 million a year, not counting a loss of several billion dollars of economic output to the nation annually.

Mental retardation has been defined as a condition, characterized by faulty development of intelligence, which impairs an individual's ability to learn and to adapt to the demands of society. The failure of intelligence to develop normally may be owing to diseases or conditions that damage the brain, occuring before or at the time of birth, or in infancy and childhood. The retardation may also be owing to factors determined by heredity that affect the development of the brain.

Some infants are born with "inborn errors of metabolism," giving rise to a variety of heredi-

[1]Luther W. Stringham, "Mental Retardation" and Leonard W. Mayo (Chairman), "Report of the President's Panel on Mental Retardation," in *New Directions in Health, Education, and Welfare—Background Papers on Current and Emerging Issues*—1963, The Tenth Anniversary of the U. S. Department of Health, Education, and Welfare (Anthony J. Celebrezze, Secretary), Office of Program Analysis.

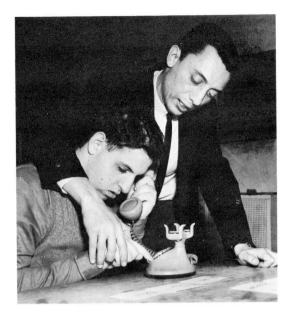

THE PROBLEM of mental retardation is now being attacked with vigor in the United States, in terms of rehabilitation of those afflicted. The retarded boy shown is being taught how to dial his home phone number. (Photograph by Bayer-MONK-MEYER)

tary metabolic diseases. Among them are diabetes, phenylketonuria (abbreviated to PKU), and galactosemia. PKU is caused by the lack of a single enzyme necessary to convert phenylalanine (an amino acid) to tyrosine. The consequence is irreversible damage to the newborn brain, leading to mental retardation. Once a diagnosis of PKU is made, by relatively simple tests initiated soon after birth, the condition can be treated with a diet free of phenylalaine. If begun early enough, diet therapy—that is, a diet free of phenylalanine, can prevent progression of the disease and its effects on the central nervous system. PKU testing is now mandatory in several states.

Galactosemia is another inherited metabolic disease. It is characterized by abnormally high levels of galactose in the blood. It is usually discovered when the infant is 2 to 3 weeks old and cannot tolerate milk. This condition also may result in mental retardation as well as blindness, hardening of the liver, and death. The treatment again is by diet, that is, by providing a diet free of galactose. The affected children can slowly be returned to normal diets.

The magnitude of the problem of mental retardation in the United States may be roughly cast on the basis of standard intelligence tests. It has been generally noted that anyone with an I.Q. below about 70 has significant difficulties in adapting adequately to his environment. About 3% of the population score below this level.

Therefore it can be estimated that of 4.2 million children born each year, 126,000 are, or will be classed as, mentally retarded. Of these it is estimated that 4200 (0.1% of births) will be retarded so profoundly that they will not even be able to take care of their own physical needs. Another 12,600 (0.3% of births) will suffer "moderate" retardation; that is, they will remain below the 7-year intellectual level. The remaining 110,000 (2.6% of births) are those with mild retardation and represent those who can, with special training and assistance, acquire limited job skills and achieve almost complete independence in community living.

If these percentage figures were applied to the population as a whole, it would indicate that there are 5.4 million mentally retarded people in the United States—60,000 to 90,000 profoundly retarded; 90,000 to 110,000 severely retarded; 300,000 to 350,000 "moderately" retarded; and some 5 to 5½ million mildly retarded children, adolescents, and adults who are able to adjust in a limited way to the demands of society, and possibly to play a positive role as workers.

The number of mentally retarded patients who are getting care in residential institutions is minimal—about 200,000 or roughly 4% of the total. It has been estimated that it would cost $1 billion a year to construct adequate facilities and institutions, and to provide special care in the family home for mentally retarded patients. Other services required by the mentally retarded and their families include: (1) diagnostic and clinical services, half of which were established in the last five years; (2) special education for the mentally retarded, a task for which 75,000 specialized teachers are needed; (3) preparation of professional personnel in many areas; (4) vocational rehabilitation (though 25% of those coming out of special classes cannot be placed); (5) parent counseling; (6) social services; and (7) research.

It would be wonderful to put a finger on the chief causes of mental retardation and thus to get some promise of stopping the condition. Unfortunately this is not the case. From 75% to 85% of the retarded show no demonstrable gross abnormality of the brain, and their condition must be regarded as caused by incompletely understood psychological, environmental, or genetic factors. Only in 15% to 25% of the diagnosed cases of mental retardation can a specific disease entity be held responsible (for example, infections of the mother, brain injury during delivery—particularly in premature infants—abnormal grouping of chromosomes). Because of increased survival rates of retarded infants, we are now beginning to see that 75% of the retarded under 6 years of age have some associated physical disability.

It must also be conceded that the improved and more extensive prenatal, obstetrical, and pediatric care in the United States in the last 20 years has brought about the survival of a great many infants who were premature, had congenital handicaps or malformations, and suffered from mental retardation—a frequent concomitant of such handicaps. This fact operates to increase the number of retarded at all age levels. According to one government estimate, unless there are major advances in methods of prevention, there will be as many as one million more mentally retarded persons in the United States in the 1970's. Other problems for the mentally retarded are also foreseen; for example, as machines replace unskilled labor, which is what educable retarded children could be trained to do, opportunities for employment will diminish.

SUMMARY

This chapter has been devoted to two major subjects, mental illness and mental retardation, which are related but essentially different and separate problems. We have described mental illness as the abnormal *exaggeration* of personal feelings, and we have discussed the types, causes, extent, and improved treatment of mental illness. With psychotherapy, new drug therapy, hospitalization and other treatments, the outlook for the cure of those mentally ill patients who can obtain adequate treatment is indeed good. The outlook for the "cure" of mental retardation is at present less favorable, primarily because much less is known about the causes of mental retardation. Nevertheless the problem is now being attacked with vigor in the United States. In the next chapters we shall discuss two serious social problems which are essentially psychiatric in origin and management: alcoholism and drug use.

SUMMARY REVIEW QUESTIONS

1. In what ways, if any, has your attitude toward mental illness and mental retardation been changed by the information you have received in this book (and this course)? What misconceptions that you previously held about mental illness have been corrected?
2. What is the key concept to the understanding of mental illness? How would you now describe or define mental illness?
3. What are the causes of mental illness, so far as they are presently known? What is the distinction between "organic" and "functional" mental illness?
4. What are the principal diagnostic classifications of mental illness and what is the distinguishing mark of each?
5. What methods of treatment are now available for cases of mental illness, ranging from mild to severe?
6. What evidence can you cite to indicate that there has been a genuine improvement in the care of the mentally ill in the United States in the decade of the 1960's? What facts and figures, if any, can you cite to the contrary?
7. What is the present extent of mental illness in the United States? (Cite some specific figures.)
8. What can still be done in the United States to prevent mental illness? What steps can an individual take to avoid serious mental illness or a "nervous breakdown"?
9. What makes people attempt or commit suicide? How can suicide, or the inclination thereto, be prevented?
10. What is mental retardation? How large a problem is it now in the United States? What can be done about it?
11. Are the following statements sense or nonsense? Why? *Anyone who consults a psychiatrist is crazy. . . . Mental illness is incurable. . . . Every mentally ill person requires hospitalization. . . . Mental illness is essentially an exaggeration of normal feelings. . . . Better obstetric and pediatric care is now saving the lives of too many feebleminded infants and children.*
12. What do the following terms mean to you: schizophrenia, paranoia, manic-depressive psychosis, nervous breakdown, ataraxic, group therapy, psychoanalysis, suppressive psychotherapy, I.Q., PKU?

Worth Looking Into: *Man Against Himself* by Karl Menninger, M.D. *Every Other Bed* by Mike Gorman. *Suicide: A Sociological and Statistical Study* by Louis Dublin. *Basic Theory of Psychoanalysis* by Robert Waelder. *Principles of Dynamic Psychiatry* by Jules Masserman, M.D. For more complete references, see Appendix E.

5

ALCOHOL AND ALCOHOLISM

ABOUT SEVEN-EIGHTHS OF AMERICAN COLlege men and three-fourths of American college women have taken a drink of an alcoholic beverage some time in their lives. However, not more than one boy in five or one girl in ten drinks oftener than once a week. Conversation about liquor among college students far outruns their actual consumption of alcoholic beverages. It would have to. The sale of alcoholic beverages to young people is almost everywhere illegal—and most college students are still minors under these laws. (Legal definitions of a "minor"—a definition often linked with the age at which a young man or woman may marry without parental consent—vary from state to state: under 21 in many states, under 18 in others, for example.) This fact in itself may help to explain why boastful attitudes about the amount of liquor they can "hold" persist among many college boys. Their bragging, incidentally, frequently harks back to a one-time experience.

The right to drink alcoholic beverages is considered an adult privilege; and many younger college boys are fighting to prove that they are already fully grown adults. For this reason alcoholic bravado is often unconsciously equated in the minds of the braggarts with their sexual prowess. When they brag to their dates about how much liquor they can drink, they really mean to say, "See what a man I am!"

Why College Students Drink

Unquestionably a certain number of college students drink liquor on some social occasions.

There are indeed in Western civilization certain socially acceptable occasions (and even rituals) for the use of alcoholic beverages. They are, for example, an integral part of certain religious rites and ceremonies. Very few drink heavily; they would not last long on any campus. Some students continue social drinking for the rest of their lives. Others, after a juvenile fling, subside into abstinence. Some drift into chronic alcoholism, and a few end on Skid Row. There is also a group of college graduates who abstain from liquor during youth but begin drinking in later years.

Drinking is less fashionable and not so "smart" today as it was some years ago on American college campuses—particularly during the prohibition era (1918 to 1933), when college students were directly aping their law-breaking elders.

The attitudes and practices of the administration and alumni of any particular college are very likely to determine student attitudes toward the social acceptability of drinking. If the faculty club has a bar on campus and the alumni club a bar off campus, if cocktails are served at official college functions and faculty parties, if alumni turn up half-drunk at athletic events, it will be rather difficult to convince students that drinking is either socially unacceptable or morally wrong.

As long as beer is seductively advertised on television and "hard liquor" in magazines of intellectual stature, it will be difficult to re-establish the picture of Old John Barleycorn, with a noose in his hand, hauling young men and women down the road to perdition. One swallow doesn't make a drunkard. It is only fair to point out that *attitudes* toward alcohol differ not only in different colleges but also in different sections of the United States. There is general and official agreement, however, that college students should not drink.

Why do college students sometimes drink? Some drink to prove they are "men." Others regard their ability to consume large amounts of liquor as a bid for attention, or a point of superiority to assuage inferiority feelings. Still others drink out of a feeling of rebellion against parents or college authorities.

Curiosity is another impetus toward drinking in college. A few young people feel that they cannot afford to miss the "experience" of getting drunk, unpleasant and risky as it and its aftereffects may be. Social pressure is another impulse to college drinking. Many students drink simply because they think it's "the thing to do." Their friends or their fraternity brothers or sorority sisters urge them on. A few college women undoubtedly consent to drinking because they are afraid they will be unpopular or considered "poor sports" if they do not. All such superficial reasons for drinking may, however, lead to a subtle or unconscious desire to utilize alcohol as a means of removing inhibitions related to unconventional behavior.

No amount of exhortation will keep an adult college student from drinking if he is bent on doing it. On the other hand a sober examination of the pros and cons of the facts about alcohol and alcoholism will permit any individual intelligent enough to be in college to make up his or her mind about drinking.

The Risk of Alcoholism. Some authorities, as might be expected, are more vehement than others about the risks of alcoholism. Dr. Marvin A. Block, a Buffalo, New York, physician, for example, and others, have estimated that one out of every 15 teenagers is likely to become an alcoholic. Dr. Block feels that home influences are the decisive factor in whether or not the risk becomes an eventual reality. He calls "kiddy cocktails"—soft drinks served to children in cocktail glasses—"a dangerous procedure." He sees very little alcoholism, however, among individuals who came from homes where drinking was

done regularly with meals. Children from such homes, he finds, look upon drinking as part of their home life and rarely go on to excessive indulgence in alcohol in later life—unless their own parents have set them an unfortunate example of excessive and unruly drinking. Dr. Block concludes:

We should teach our young people that not to drink does not affect them socially, that alcohol is not a necessity of life, that some people may drink if they wish, but that to others it will bring harm. If we could teach people that the real sophisticate never drinks excessively, and that to do so means social ostracism, we'd find less and less alcoholism.

Varying Tolerances to Alcohol

It must also be recognized, however, that varying tolerances to alcohol occur among different individuals. An explanation as to why two people of the same weight who drink the same amount of alcohol may react differently to it was given in the May 19, 1962 issue of the *Journal of the American Medical Association* as follows:

An experienced drinker has learned how to counteract some of the adverse effects of alcohol, whereas a novice, faced with the same situation, would be less capable of compensating for the alcohol-imposed handicap.

This is the answer of the AMA Sub-Committee on Alcohol, given in answer to a question submitted to the *Journal*.

Habitual drinkers absorb their alcohol more slowly and oxidize it more rapidly than do persons who rarely take a drink.

Also, the presence of food in the upper gastrointestinal tract tends to retard the rate of alcohol absorption and thus ameliorates the effect of a given dose.

However, the group said, there is little difference among individuals in ability of brain tissue to resist the effect of a given tissue concentration of alcohol.

All persons show some impairment in driving ability at a blood alcohol concentration of 0.10 per cent, and in some this ability is impaired at a level as low as 0.02 per cent. Regardless of tolerance, the fatal concentration is 0.6 per cent to 0.8 per cent.

BLOOD-ALCOHOL CHART*

Showing estimated *per cent* of alcohol in the blood by number of drinks in relation to body weight

Body Weight	Drinks											
	1	2	3	4	5	6	7	8	9	10	11	12
100 lbs.	.038	.075	.113	.150	.188	.225	.263	.300	.338	.375	.413	.450
120 lbs.	.031	.063	.094	.125	.156	.188	.219	.250	.281	.313	.344	.375
140 lbs.	.027	.054	.080	.107	.134	.161	.188	.214	.241	.268	.295	.321
160 lbs.	.023	.047	.070	.094	.117	.141	.164	.188	.211	.234	.258	.281
180 lbs.	.021	.042	.063	.083	.104	.125	.146	.167	.188	.208	.229	.250
200 lbs.	.019	.038	.056	.075	.094	.113	.131	.150	.169	.188	.206	.225
220 lbs.	.017	.034	.051	.068	.085	.102	.119	.136	.153	.170	.188	.205
240 lbs.	.016	.031	.047	.063	.078	.094	.109	.125	.141	.156	.172	.188

The chart defines a blood alcohol percentage of .050 or less as usually innocuous.

OVER .050 but LESS than .150 results in some impairment of JUDGMENT and VISION.

A concentration of .150 or MORE results in increasingly dangerous INTOXICATION.

However, since the passage of time REDUCES blood alcohol concentration, the actual concentration of alcohol in the blood at any given time may be determined by subtracting .015 per cent from the percentage shown on the chart for every hour that elapses since the first drink.

*This has been reproduced from the New Jersey Department of Law and Public Safety pamphlet "Blood-Alco Chart."

(Blood alcohol per cent means the per cent of the chemical substance, alcohol, to the estimated total volume of blood, about 7 quarts, circulating in the entire body. Thus it may be observed that a very small percentage of alcohol in the bloodstream—indeed as little as $\frac{2}{100}$ of 1%— can have significant effects.)

To set the stage for a more exact understanding, let us briefly consider what alcohol and alcoholism really signify, and how many people we are talking about when we speak of drinkers and alcoholics.

Alcohol is essentially a *depressant drug* which affords a prompt, but temporary, escape from the stresses of external reality or inner turmoil. We speak, of course, only of *ethyl alcohol,* the active ingredient in all alcoholic beverages. Alcoholism, therefore, may be described as poisoning with an overdose of alcohol. Drunkenness is the temporary result.

Chronic alcoholism is the outcome of prolonged and repeated use of alcohol to compensate for deep-seated personality problems. It falls within the category of mental illness, although there is also a biochemical approach to the disease. Some scientific investigators have suggested that alcoholism is a form of allergy; others, that it is a metabolic disease. It is probably fair to say that the causes of alsoholism are multiple and in large measure still undefined.

Well over 90% of 80 million adult drinkers in the United States use alcoholic beverages temperately. They can "take it or leave it alone." Their home, business life, and health are not adversely affected. They are *social drinkers.*

But somewhat over 6.5 million people have gone beyond social drinking and have become what may be loosely termed "alcoholics." About 85% of these alcoholics may be classified as *heavy drinkers.* These excessive drinkers (both men and women) frequently harm themselves physically, psychologically, and socially.

Beyond this group are some 600,000 to 800,000 *chronic alcoholics* (also called *problem drinkers* or *compulsive drinkers*) who no longer have any control over their desire or need for alcohol. They are the true "slaves to drink."

The Pattern of an Alcoholic. The gradual steps by which an individual becomes a chronic alcoholic can usually be recognized. Here, progressively, are some of the warning signs of an insidious drift toward chronic alcoholism:

¶ When you are out drinking with friends, you are always the one who has to have that "last" or "extra" drink.

¶ Your hangovers get worse and worse. You find you are suffering from temporary blackouts. You are plagued with feelings of remorse, anxiety, or guilt.

¶ You discover that drinking means more to you than to other people and you start looking for that alcoholic kick more often than you used to. You begin sneaking drinks at odd times.

¶ You find yourself turning more and more to alcohol. One drink is never enough. You don't want to stop drinking until you are drunk.

¶ You won't admit what's happening to you. You find all kinds of excuses and rationalizations for your drinking. You assert that you can handle your liquor. (The people with whom you associate, however, may not accept your excuses; and you will gradually find yourself excluded from their company.)

¶ You make a great discovery—a cure for hangover; namely, one, two, or more drinks in the morning.

¶ You become a solitary drinker. Alcohol alone is company and pleasure enough for you. But you may feel quite dejected between your sprees. You may begin to brood over yourself. You may feel very self-conscious and afraid of being with other people. At other times you may feel very antagonistic toward and critical of others—often those nearest and dearest to you.

¶ Getting drunk, going on benders, becomes the main goal of your life—even though the results are severe hangovers, terrifying fears, social ostracism, tremors (shakes), and even worse, delirium tremens (DT's). At this point you have become a truly chronic alcoholic. You desperately need the help you should have sought earlier. . . . But you can still be helped, if you make up your mind.

The Effects of Alcohol

The effects of all alcoholic beverages depend upon the amount of alcohol, ounce for ounce, that they contain. Hard liquors—whiskey, brandy, gin, vodka, and rum—have the highest concentration of alcohol by volume; "100 proof" means the beverage contains 50% alcohol. Light wines run from about 7 to 12% alcoholic content, and beer much less.

A bottle of beer and a shot-glass of whiskey are roughly equivalent in their alcoholic content.

Beer often tends to be fattening. In caloric value and vitamin content a glass of beer is about half as nutritious as a glass of milk. Inasmuch as it is rapidly metabolized in the body, alcohol does have some little food value.

The concentration of alcohol in the blood stream determines its effect. Behavior of the "average" drinker can be correlated with percentages of alcohol in his blood stream approximately as follows:

Blood Alcohol 0.01%. The drinker feels his head clear; he breathes more freely through his nose; there is a mild tingling of the mucous membranes of the mouth and throat.

This primary physiological kick is one of the reasons why alcohol is so commonly regarded as a stimulant. It does stimulate the sensory organs in the mouth and digestive tract. For a few minutes this leads to more rapid circulation of the blood and with it a clearing away of some fatigue products of the body. Hence the drinker "feels better," momentarily. The depressant effect begins when the alcohol in the blood stream reaches the brain.

Blood Alcohol 0.02%. The drinker enjoys a pleasant feeling and is willing to talk freely. He has a sense of warmth and physical well-being. This is the appeal of alcohol to the social drinker. Still there may already be a touch of dizziness, a slight throbbing, and sense of fullness in the head.

Blood Alcohol 0.03%. The drinker has a feeling of mild euphoria. "All's right with the world." He doesn't worry. He has in effect lost the capacity to worry because the depressant effect of the alcohol has already impaired his judgment and memory.

Blood Alcohol 0.04%. The imbiber displays lots of energy. He talks freely—and loudly. But his hands begin to tremble and his movements are a bit clumsy. Beyond this point he is legally intoxicated as shown by "drunkometer" tests.

Blood Alcohol 0.05%. Now the drinker is "sitting on the top of the world." His inhibitions are almost all removed. He says he can "lick anybody in the world"—but he has difficulty in lighting a match.

Blood Alcohol 0.07%. Now the worm has begun to turn. A feeling of remoteness steals over the drinker. His pulse is strong and his breathing heavy. His energy is abated.

Blood Alcohol 0.1%. Now the drinker staggers perceptibly. He talks to himself. He feels drowsy.

Blood Alcohol 0.2%. The drunkard now needs help to walk. He is easily angered. He feels nauseated. His bladder control is poor.

Blood Alcohol 0.3%. The victim is now in a stupor. He does not understand what is said to him. He may sleep and vomit by turns.

Blood Alcohol 0.4%. The patient is now completely unconscious—"out cold." The depressive effect of alcohol has wrought a deep anesthesia.

Individual Differences in Effect. Despite the similarity of effects in terms of blood concentration of alcohol, it should be pointed out that individuals differ greatly in the amount of alcoholic beverages they need to yield a similar degree of intoxication. Heavier people can stand larger doses of alcohol than smaller people. Some may be drunk on one-quarter of the amount of alcohol that it takes for others. A teetotaler will respond to a far smaller dose of alcohol than a chronic alcoholic. As with many other drugs, a certain amount of tolerance to alcohol is developed—which means that the intake doses must be increased.

The circumstances under which alcohol is taken may also modify its effects. It is, for example, more intoxicating on an empty stomach than when taken with a meal. Alcohol is one of the few substances that is directly absorbed into the blood stream from the stomach. Furthermore, it passes more rapidly from the stomach into the intestines when there is no food present to delay this passage. From the intestines also alcohol is rapidly absorbed and carried to the brain.

Some Psychological Effects of Alcohol. Under the influence of alcohol, even in "safe" concentrations, mental processes are altered. Fantasy increases; alertness diminishes. Many carefully devised psychological tests have proved this point—for example:

Thirty to 60 minutes after drinking 1 to 3 ounces of alcohol, reaction time is significantly increased. It takes an experienced auto driver half again as long as normal ($3/10$ instead of $2/10$ second) to get his foot on the brake. A professional typist makes 40 to 50% more errors in her typing. A bricklayer lays only 90% as many bricks as he could while completely sober. Ability to add simple numbers decreases 10%. Capacity to do problems involving mathematical reasoning falls 10 to 20%. Ability to match words with opposite meanings decreases by one-third to one-half.

Throughout all these tests, the subject is usually under the impression that he is doing better than he would when cold sober. He is fooled because his judgment as well as his reaction time is impaired. In an experiment with 20 automobile drivers, all thought they were driving more slowly than usual when the fact was that they were driving faster. Long-experienced British bus drivers, with two shots of whiskey under their belts, were willing to try to squeeze their buses through a gap 14 inches narrower than the bus!

Physiological Effects of Alcohol. In the past, gruesome physiological effects were pointed out as the effects of alcohol. Cirrhosis of the liver, with the showing of a "hobnailed liver" in a bottle, was a prize demonstration. Every ailment to which the alcoholic—or even the moderate user of alcohol—was subject was attributed to this one cause.

Today it is the consensus of medical opinion that the *temperate*, moderate and occasional use of alcoholic beverages has little, if any, residual effect on the health of the user. Statistical records show that moderate users of alcohol live as long as total abstainers. This would indicate that temperate use of alcohol does not result in bodily harm. On the other hand the immediate after-effects of alcoholic indulgence—hangover, headache, and nausea—and the more frequent risk of accident or contraction of venereal disease while under the influence of alcohol must be accounted as bodily risks due to alcohol.

The continued excessive use of alcohol brings physical and mental deterioration and often untimely death. Excessive drinkers shorten their lives; their resistance to disease, notably pneumonia, is decreased; their nervous and digestive systems are impaired; they are subject to alcoholic psychoses, such as delirium tremens (DT's).

Alcoholics often skip meals and generally neglect their diet. Bloated with liquids, they blunt their normal hunger pangs. Since they eat so poorly, chronic alcoholics often suffer from nutritional deficiencies, especially lack of vitamin B, which exaggerates their nervous difficulties.

Alcohol—Medicine and Drug. Alcohol is sometimes prescribed as a medicine by physicians. Its judicious use is generally confined to elderly patients suffering from chronic disease. It eases their pain and discomfort and gives them a welcome sense of temporary well-being. In small doses it is a spur to appetite.

Alcohol also has the pharmacological effect of a vasodilator; it causes the blood vessels to expand. This is why a feeling of warmth follows alcohol ingestion, and why alcohol is not forbidden—in moderation—to patients suffering from some forms of heart disease or high blood pressure. The therapeutic uses of alcohol are, however, very limited. It is *not* good for snakebite.

Alcoholism as a Mental Illness

In recent history alcoholism was regarded as a sin, or a weakness in the moral fiber. Indignant citizens insisted that the alcoholic could stop drinking if he wanted to. Many drunkards were hopefully lured into "signing the pledge" by earnest temperance workers who had no real idea of the underlying reasons for alcoholism.

Today we know enough about alcoholism to describe it properly as a mental illness, or at least as the primary symptom of an illness.

Here is the testimony of an ex-alcoholic on the nature of the sickness: "I remember—I can never forget—the years in which I suffered from acute chronic alcoholism. They were the most painful years of my life. I suffered constantly, not just one kind of pain, but all kinds of pain. I suffered

physically, mentally, emotionally, financially, and socially—in every department of my life." The writer of these lines is Mrs. Marty Mann, now executive director of the National Council on Alcoholism.

What Makes An Alcoholic? What makes an alcoholic? Why do some people cross the line from social drinking to problem drinking? Since research in alcoholism is still comparatively young, there are no final answers, but psychiatric studies have given some powerful hints.

First, there is the possibility that many chronic alcoholics have physical constitutions which are especially sensitive to alcohol—just as other people are peculiarly allergic (sensitive) to different foods (e.g., strawberries) and drugs (e.g., penicillin).

Second, the psychological reasons for compulsive drinking undoubtedly differ to some extent in each individual case. The personality and the history of each chronic alcoholic supplies the clues to his particular reasons for excessive drinking. Yet there are some permissible generalizations.

Alcoholics are preponderantly males. However, in comparatively recent years there has been uncovered a considerable number of female alcoholics, who use alcohol primarily as a bulwark against loneliness. Women find it easier than men to conceal addiction to alcohol. Three-fourths of known alcoholics are between the ages of 35 and 55. They come from all walks of life, and they exhibit all degrees of intelligence. Many are outwardly jolly and sociable creatures. Others may be just the opposite: dour and sour. They seem to want and need to be popular with their fellow men. Here is the fallacy. Underlying this need, which is a wish to be loved, the alcoholic has a deep, vague, sometimes unknown (to him) feeling of insecurity. It is this dreaded feeling which he tries to drown and deny with alcohol.

The alcoholic suffers from a deep-seated neurosis, whose origin far antedates the excessive drinking. Regardless of the actual circumstances of his life, the alcoholic lives with unconscious, painful, neurotic conflicts. He wants to run away from himself. Alcohol seems to temporarily float him away from his problems and give him respite from his emotional conflict.

The origins of the neurotic conflicts of the alcoholic probably go back to childhood. They often embrace feelings of long-repressed anger against parents who betrayed, rejected, or frustrated him as a child. Alcohol temporarily releases this dreadful inner feeling of guilt, frustration, and insecurity, so the alcoholic resorts to it more and more. His drinking may also represent a secret revenge against his parents.

The alcoholic is not consciously aware that he is responding to a clash of forces in his unconscious mind. Indeed he can rarely be persuaded to recognize that he has inner conflicts. Yet his unspeakable secret terror and his inner burden make the alcoholic in greater need of release than the ordinary person. *The difference is quantitative, not qualitative.* Alcohol does ease emotional tensions; the alcoholic stands in greater and more constant need of such relief. Obviously all neurotics do not become alcoholics. They find other outlets (for example, obesity or gambling) or happier solutions for their inner torment.

Treatment of Chronic Alcoholism. The treatment of chronic alcoholism in the past was generally disappointing. The patient was sobered up, remorsefully "went on the wagon" for varying lengths of time, then plunged into another stuporous alcoholic spree. This cycle was repeated many times. Recent approaches to treatment are much more hopeful. Any alcoholic who really wants to free himself from the affliction of compulsive drinking can probably succeed in this attempt.

The basic approach to the treatment of alcoholism now concerns itself, first, with raising the alcoholic's ability to tolerate the tensions that drive him to drink, and second, with reducing or eliminating his stress situations. The alcoholic often desperately needs psychotherapy to understand himself—but he is not always ready for it. Meanwhile, he usually requires supportive therapy. Here the new tranquilizing drugs, chlorpromazine and meprobomate, for example, are often of great help.

Complete medical care (medical rehabilitation) is also usually necessary, for the alcoholic is likely to be suffering from conditions which place additional stresses on his psychological and metabolic weaknesses. Malnutrition—particularly lack of vitamins—chronic indigestion, fatigue, chest and abdominal pains, and neuritis are common symptoms that require attention. Massive vitamin therapy, particularly with the vitamin B group, is sometimes effectively prescribed.

The aversion treatment, combined with psychotherapy, is sometimes helpful. In one such method the patient takes a drug (like antabuse) which makes him exceedingly sensitive to alcohol. He becomes ill and vomits whenever he takes a drink. This reaction enforces sobriety for many months while the patient is in the process of acquiring an improved attitude toward his inner problems.

In the final analysis, however, the alcoholic requires a high degree of social rehabilitation. He is particularly responsive to his social environment. Here, Alcoholics Anonymous (AA), an organization of recovered alcoholics started in the United States in 1935, has done great service in saving chronic alcoholics. They estimate that 50 to 75% of those who join their ranks and make a real effort to free themselves from compulsive drinking succeed in doing so. The alcoholic can never take another drink if he wants to stay "cured."

Alcoholism as a Social Problem

Even a single episode of intoxication can plunge an individual into folly of far-reaching consequence. However, it is the heavy drinkers and chronic alcoholics who create the social problems associated with alcohol. Crime, accident, and divorce rates are significantly higher among alcoholics than among the rest of the population. Many homes and families are wrecked by the neurotic illness exhibited as alcoholism. The social consequences on wives (sometimes husbands) and children is tragic and enormous.

The cost of alcoholism in the United States, in terms of care and treatment of alcoholics in hospitals and jails, crime, accidents, lost wages, support of dependents and so forth is estimated at well over $1 billion a year. This may perhaps be charged against the $3 to $4 billion a year collected in federal, state, and local taxes on the sale of alcoholic beverages. Actually between 4 and 5% of the national income, a sales figure now over $10 billion annually, is consumed in the purchase of alcoholic drinks.

Alcohol is a traffic hazard of the first magnitude. One of every five fatal auto accidents involves either a drunken driver or a drunken pedestrian. Legal interpretations obscure many of the official statistics on drunken driving, but its frequency is far too great for comfort. The drunken driver is often under the impression that the *other fellow* is on the wrong side of the road.

A past president of the American Automobile Association declared: "A person who has been drinking is fifty-five times more likely to have an accident involving personal injury."

There can be but one safe motto: *If you drink, don't drive. If you drive, don't drink.* You are also well within your moral rights to refuse to ride with a driver who has been drinking.

Prevention and Control of Alcoholism

The prevention and control of alcoholism is still a world-wide problem. It is an ancient and repetitive problem too. The Greeks of antiquity used wine as a weapon of conquest over barbarian tribes in the Mediterranean just as the

IF YOU DRINK**			Effects	Alcohol concentration in the blood	Before you drive WAIT***
Cocktails OR	Highballs OR	Beer			
WITHIN FIFTEEN MINUTES			If even one cocktail is taken on an empty stomach, absorption may be so rapid that alcohol piles up in the blood stream for a brief period and produces an exaggerated effect for a short time.	.03%	½ hour
WITHIN ONE HALF HOUR			Warmth—mental relaxation—decrease of fine skills—less concern with minor irritations and restraints.	.06%	1 hour
WITHIN ONE HOUR			Buoyancy—exaggerated emotion and behavior: talkative, noisy or morose. Perceptible loss of fine coordination.	.09%	2 hours
WITHIN TWO HOURS			Clumsiness—unsteadiness—tunnel vision.	.12%	3 hours
WITHIN THREE HOURS			Intoxication: Obvious and unmistakable impairment of bodily functions and mental faculties. Even after considerable alcohol has been eliminated, acute hangover symptoms remain.	.15%	5 hours

*Based on a person of average size—150 lbs. The effects will increase or decrease with corresponding weight differences.

**The body reacts quicker to alcohol taken when the stomach is empty.   ***After finishing the last drink.

Driver WAIT Meter* (Time Allowance Chart)

white man, some 23 centuries later, employed "firewater" to the destruction of American Indian tribes. The Greek philosopher Plato noted that "drunkenness is an important subject and it takes no mean legislator to understand it."

One fact, however, appears to be established by centuries of experience with alcohol: you cannot legislate it out of existence. In 1918, for example, the United States was politically manipulated into passing a national law (actually a constitutional amendment) intended to eliminate any use and all possible abuse of alcohol by legally prohibiting the manufacture, transportation, and sale of all alcoholic beverages. This "noble experiment" was a dismal failure. Bootleggers, moonshiners, racketeers, and their respectable customers nullified the law within a few years. In 1933 the national prohibition laws were formally repealed. The practical control of alcoholism in the United States is still left mainly to police departments. Arrests for drunkenness make up a large proportion of the total arrests in any metropolitan area.

Since chronic alcoholism is an illness, one of the first steps in the prevention and control of this illness is to keep the patients out of jails and put them in hospitals adequately equipped and staffed for this purpose. Such complete programs are rare, although over 3000 general hospitals will now admit patients for the treatment of acute alcoholism. Out-patient clinical facilities must also be made available. All this requires considerable outlay of money and continuing public support. It is, however, a less expensive way of dealing with the problem than jailing drunks.

The full and practical cooperation of the medical profession in managing the problems of alcoholism must also be obtained. This has been difficult to get because alcoholics have always been unsatisfactory and refractory patients for the doctor in private practice. With better methods of treatment, however, the professional attitude is gradually changing. Finally, programs of research and education in the field of alcoholism must be relentlessly pursued to bring the vast problem more clearly into focus.

The individual as citizen can do much to help meet the expensive and often heart-breaking problem of alcoholism. In the last analysis, however, his own temperate use of or abstinence from alcoholic beverages will provide the basis for effective community control. The individual who has a strong personality, inner spiritual resources, and a sensible working philosophy of life rarely needs alcohol to escape rather than face up to the normal stresses of everyday living.

SUMMARY REVIEW QUESTIONS

1. Why do college students sometimes drink alcoholic beverages? Do you consider any or all of these reasons valid?

2. How do you distinguish between social drinkers, heavy drinkers, and compulsive drinkers? Approximately how many people in the United States fall into each of these categories?

3. To what extent do you regard alcoholism as a moral weakness? A sin? An illness? A crime? On what outside opinion or authority do you base your own judgment?

4. What are the immediate effects of drinking alcoholic beverages? What determines these effects and what factors serve to modify these effects? What are the long-range effects of (a) temperate, moderate use of alcoholic beverages and (b) excessive use of alcohol?

5. What are the steps by which an individual gradually descends the scale from social drinking to chronic alcoholism? What are the clues or warning signs by which the stages of this descent can be recognized?

6. Since chronic alcoholism is a sickness, what kind of sickness is it? What makes an alcoholic? How can chronic alcoholics be treated? Can they be "cured?"

7. In what respects is alcohol a social problem? How can this problem be met? Do you believe that chronic alcoholism can be prevented or controlled? If so, how? If not, why not?
8. Are the following statements sense or nonsense? Why? *Anything is worth trying once. . . . Alcohol is a stimulant. . . . Tolerance for alcohol is the same for everybody. . . . If you drink don't drive; if you drive don't drink. . . . "I wonder often what the vintners buy/One-half so precious as the stuff they sell."*–from the *Rubaiyat of Omar Khayyam.*
9. What do the following terms mean to you: ethyl alcohol, 100 proof, blood alcohol, AA, cirrhosis of the liver, "noble experiment," aversion treatment, social drinker, DT's tolerance (to alcohol)?

Worth Looking Into: *Marty Mann's New Primer on Alcoholism* by Marty Mann. *The Neutral Spirit: a Portrait of Alcohol* by Berton Roueché. *Alcohol and Alcoholism,* produced by the Public Information Branch of the National Institute of Mental Health. *The Lost Weekend* by Charles Jackson. For more complete references, see Appendix E.

Sociological Factors as Causes of Alcoholism

Although intensive research has so far failed to identify a simple chemical, physiological or emotional cause of alcoholism, studies in a different area are now yielding new findings regarded by many scientists as particularly illuminating and potentially practical. Largely in the field of sociology, but also involving physiology, psychology, nutrition, cultural anthropology and epidemiology, these new studies have been aimed at determining why alcoholism is widespread in some national and cultural groups but rare in others.

Those with the highest reported rates of alcoholism are classed as high-incidence groups. They include particularly the northern French, the Americans—especially the Irish-Americans (but not the Irish in Ireland)—the Swedes, the Swiss, the Poles and the northern Russians.

By contrast, the relatively low-incidence groups include the Italians, some Chinese groups, Orthodox Jews, Greeks, Portuguese, Spaniards and the southern French.

Differences among some of these cultural groups are reflected in the composition of groups of alcoholics studied in the United States. In one group analyzed in New York City, where available figures indicate that roughly 10 percent of the total population is Irish, 15 percent is Italian, and 25 percent is Jewish, 40 percent of the alcoholics were Irish, 1 percent Italian and none Jewish. In an extensive California study, in an area with large proportions of Irish, Italian and Jewish inhabitants, 21 percent of the alcoholics were Irish, 2 percent Italian and 0.6 percent Jewish.

It does not seem likely that genetics can adequately explain these variations. Various investigators have reported that alcoholism is decreasing among Irish-Americans and Swedish-Americans but rising among second- and third-generation Italian-Americans. Some workers claim that the rate may be rising among Italians in Italy, especially in Rome and other major cities, apparently paralleling the rise in personal income. A slight but distinct rise has been noted among Jews, particularly as they tend to change from Orthodox to Reform attitudes.

Similar studies have shown that the low rates of alcoholism exhibited by some groups cannot all be attributed to abstinence. Most Mormons and Moslems, for example, do not drink because of religious beliefs, and their alcoholism rates are low. But other groups—especially the Italians, Greeks, Chinese and Jews—contain very high percentages of drinkers, and many of them use alcohol abundantly. For example, the per capita alcohol consumption in Italy is rated second only to that in France, but the rate of alcoholism among Italians is relatively low.

In a study published by the American Medical Association in its manual on alcoholism, Dr. Selden D. Bacon of Rutgers University compares two American groups as follows:

For the Orthodox Jews

"The social functions of drinking are strikingly clear. Drinking is to draw the family together, to cement the bonds of larger group membership, to activate the relationship between man and deity. This is understood by the participants. The rules and procedures of drinking are about as ritualized as those of a university football game or a church service. Violations of the rules, or violations of propriety while drinking, are quickly and severely penalized.

SOURCE. From *Alcohol and Alcoholism,* U.S. Department of Health, Education, and Welfare, Public Health Service Publication No. 1640.

"The custom is learned from infancy; it is instilled at the time that basic moral attitudes are learned and is taught by prestigeful members of the group (parents, rabbis, elders). The custom is closely entwined with family and religious constellations. No great emotional feeling about drinking as such is particularly noticeable; there have never been experiences with prohibition; there are no abstinence movements; there is no Dionysiac cult or worship in drinking. Members of this group sneer at other groups that exhibit drunkenness . . . All members of this society drink, they do so hundreds of times every year, they use beer, wine and distilled spirits . . . Alcoholism is practically unknown."

For the Anglo-Saxon Protestant Group

"The social functions of drinking are rather vaguely and somewhat defensively described; they concern drawing people—both family members and also complete strangers—together, often for purposes of 'fun,' often to allow relaxation from (rather than, as in the preceding case, closer adherence to) moral norms. The rules and procedures are on occasion rather specific, but also show enormous variability so that a given individual may follow one set of rules with his family, another with business or professional associates, and a third on holiday occasions, and show even different patterns when away from the home town. Sanctions for violations are extremely irregular, ranging from accepting laughter to violent physical attack . . . The custom is generally learned between the ages of 15 and 20. Sometimes the learning stems not from parents, ministers, physicians, elders, and teachers, but from other adolescents. There is great emotional feeling about the problem on the mass level as well as by individuals. Activating the custom, especially by the young, is often attended with feelings of guilt, hostility, and exhibitionism, and may occur as a secretive practice insofar as parents or employers or elders are concerned . . . Perhaps three-quarters of the males over 15 years of age and perhaps over one-half of the females over 15 years of age use alcoholic beverages, there being not too much use of wine, relatively greater use of beer by men, and use of distilled spirits . . . Alcoholism is not rare in this group. Perhaps 3 to 7 of every 100 users of alcohol are alcoholics."

Dr. Albert Ullman of Tufts University has suggested that the rate of alcoholism is low in those groups in which the drinking customs, values and sanctions are well-established, known to and agreed upon by all, and consistent with the rest of the culture. By contrast, the rate tends to be high in groups with marked ambivalence toward alcohol—with no agreed-upon ground rules. When such conflict exists, with resultant pressures, guilt feelings and uncertainties, the alcoholism rate may be very high. This has been noted among the relatively few Mormons who drink, among moderate drinkers who feel forced to over-indulgence to prove their "manliness," and especially among children of parents with conflicting attitudes—such as a father who sees drinking as a virtue and a mother who feels drinking is a sin.

The full significance of such ambivalent feelings as a cause of alcoholism is yet to be determined. It may be at least hypothesized, however, that they play a significant role.

6

DRUG USE AND ABUSE

STUDENT DRUG USE IS INDEED A COMMENTARY on American society, but it is above all an indirect criticism of our society's inability to offer the young exciting, honorable, and effective ways of using their intelligence and idealism to reform our society.

Thus does Kenneth Keniston, of the Department of Psychiatry of the Yale Medical School, conclude a report on "Heads and Seekers: Drugs on Campus, Counter-Cultures, and American Society."[1] This same article begins:

Students who use drugs are usually treated by the mass media as an alien wart upon the student body of America. . . . Few subjects arouse feelings as intense and irrational as does the topic of student drug use; in few areas is there greater tendency to distort, to perceive facts selectively, and to view with alarm. Few topics are treated with so much heat and so little light.

A distinction may be made between drug users and drug abusers. Practically every American *uses* psychoactive drugs—for this list includes aspirin, sleeping pills, stimulants, tranquilizers, anti-depressants, ethyl alcohol, caffeine (in coffee and tea), and nicotine (in tobacco). Any of *these* drugs is subject to abuse, for taken in excess they become poisons. "The dosage makes the poison," runs an old medical axiom.

What is new in the pattern is the use by college students (and even occasionally high school students) of new or at least newly recognized drugs which change moods and alter consciousness. Student drug use—and abuse—usually involves

[1] K. Keniston, M.D., "Heads and Seekers: Drugs on Campus, Counter-Cultures, and American Society," *The American Scholar*, 97–112 (Winter 1968–1969).

hallucinogenic drugs; they produce hallucinations, that is, sense perceptions not based on objective reality. The victim of hallucinations sees, hears, smells, tastes, or feels things that aren't there.

Most commonly used of the hallucinogens is marihuana. Others are LSD, DMT, psilocybin, mescaline, and peyote. Student use of the hallucinogens is increasing. However, it does not reach anywhere near the exaggerated figures that have been used in some debates. A recent Gallup poll arrived at an estimate that only 5 to 6% of all college students have "ever tried" any of the hallucinogenic drugs. Keniston estimates that fewer than 10% of American college students have ever tried such drugs.

Drug use and abuse seems to be more common at colleges and universities where there is a high "intellectual climate"—such as the Ivy League colleges, some of the Big Ten universities, and a few small, liberal arts colleges. At these colleges, a drug use rate (at least one try at the drugs) ranges between 10% to 50% of the student body. Use of drugs is lowest in the vocationally oriented departments of a university; that is, schools of business administration, engineering, agriculture, and education (of teachers).

Keniston divides "drug users" into three separate classes: (1) *tasters,* who have tried a drug no more than three times and do not intend to continue; (2) *seekers;* and (3) *heads.* The *seekers* makes up the largest contingent of college drug users. Relatively speaking, they have used drugs only a few times, but they plan to continue use in their search for relevance both within and without their college experience. These students can be called seekers because they seek in drug use some way of "intensifying experience, expanding awareness, [and] breaking out of deadness and flatness [of their current pattern of life]."

Heads is shorthand for "pot heads," users of marihuana, and "acid heads," users of LSD and other, less potent, hallucinogens. This is a relatively small group of students who use drugs often, for example, every weekend. To quote Keniston again:

For such young men and women drug use is not just an intermittent assist in the pursuit of meaning, but a part of a more general "turned-on" ideology.

But even among the heads, drug use does not invariably constitute the deeply psychopathological and self-destructive phenomenon it is sometimes said invariably to be. . . . Many students who use marihuana routinely do *not* experience the ominous personal deterioration, the "bad trip," or loss of motivation that is sometimes thought to accompany even casual drug experimentation.

There exists, however, a small but highly publicized group of drug-takers for whom even a single experience with the hallucinogens produces serious ill-effects. Marihuana, rarely, and LSD, more often, can elicit panic states or transient psychotic reactions. The real risk for these students, however, is that they will temporarily drop out of the college scene into some "hippie" subculture. However, many of those who drop out eventually find their way back to the mainstream of society.

In the late 1960's the *New York Times* conducted a nationwide survey on drug usage. The survey revealed that for many students the use of drugs—particularly marihauna—was considered a part of growing up, perhaps "as common as the hip flasks during the Prohibition era." Many students sample drugs simply because they are available. Others want to appear daring or sophisticated. Some do because it is "the social thing to do, like sipping a cocktail." Others say, "It's not addicting, it's cheaper than booze, and the high is better."

The college drug user tends to be rather bright but introspective. He often has deep personal or family problems and appears alienated from the values of his fellow students and his family. However, it should not be assumed that all college drug users fit this pattern.

Some Definitions

By *medical* definition, a narcotic is a drug that will put you to sleep or into a stupor and, at the same time, relieve pain. By *legal* definition, narcotics are a defined group of addictive (habit-forming) chemical substances whose indiscriminate use renders the user useless to himself and often dangerous to society.

In the practice of medicine, narcotic drugs, prescribed by a physician who understands both their effects and side-effects, have a legitimate place. Morphine, the pain-killer, is one of the sovereign remedies in the doctor's bag.

The "true" narcotics are drugs derived from opium, that is, opiates and synthetic substitutes for morphine, such as meperidine and methadone. The true opiates are all derived from the poppy plant, *Papaver somniferum*. Opium itself is a crude, gummy resin which can be smoked in a pipe. The most important drug derived from opium is morphine; the most dangerous, heroin; others are codeine and papaverine. Chemists and pharmacologists have tried for decades to formulate a synthetic drug that would have the painkilling effects of morphine without its addicting property. Hundreds of such drugs have been tried; those that relieve pain also produce addiction.

The opium poppy is now grown in such countries as India, Turkey, China, Egypt, and Mexico, where the climate is hot and dry and where land and labor are cheap. The unripe seed pods of the poppy contain a juice from which crude opium is extracted.

Although cocaine is legally defined as a narcotic under United States law, it is actually a stimulant drug. Marihuana is also regarded as a narcotic, though strictly speaking it is not. The distinction between true drug addiction and drug habituation has been defined by the World Health Organization as follows:[2]

Addiction is a state of periodic or chronic intoxication produced by the repeated consumption of a drug and involves tolerance, psychological dependence, usually physical dependence, an overwhelming compulsion to continue using the drug, and detrimental effects on both the individual and society. *Habituation* is a condition, resulting from the repeated consumption of a drug, which involves little or no evidence of tolerance, some psychological dependence, and a desire (but not a compulsion) to continue taking the drug for the feeling of well-being that it engenders. Detrimental effects, if any, are primarily on the individual.

However, since these two terms have been used interchangeably, the World Health Organization had suggested that the term "drug dependence" be used, with the modification of the particular drug added. As an example, "drug dependence of the barbiturate type."

Historical Perspectives

The use and abuse of drugs that reach the central nervous system and affect behavior have been known since antiquity. The most widely used of such substances is probably ethyl alcohol.

Still other psychoactive drugs—opium, marihuana, and cocaine—were discovered by prehistoric man. These intoxicating substances were often employed as part of a religious ritual. The Chinese knew about marihuana as early as 2700 B.C.; the ancient Egyptians were acquainted with opium as early as 1500 B.C. There is also a reference to the use of opium in Homer's *Odyssey* (9th century B.C.).

The Greek and Roman physicians of antiquity used opium for its ability to induce sleep and relieve pain. In the early Christian era its use spread to many parts of Europe, and it was fur-

[2]From *Drug Abuse: Escape to Nowhere*, Smith Kline & French Laboratories, in cooperation with the American Association for Health, Physical Education, and Recreation, 1969.

ther used medically to suppress cough and relieve diarrhea, usages which still prevail.

The use of opium either as a medicine or as an intoxicating agent gradually spread throughout the world. American physicians in the eighteenth century used it to relieve pain associated with venereal disease, cancer, gallstones, some fevers, and as a remedy for diarrhea, vomiting, and the pains of childbirth.

In spite of its widespread medical use, physicians were slow to realize the fact that opium was an addictive substance. The same opinion was held about two alkaloids of opium discovered early in the nineteenth century—morphine in 1805, codeine in 1832. Physicians who were aware of opium addiction thought they could remedy the condition by prescribing morphine or codeine. All they did was to transfer patients from one addicting drug to another. The addicts preferred the morphine to the opium—it was ten times as strong!

Another factor that promoted the use of opiates was the invention in 1843 of the hypodermic needle and syringe. This instrument was used widely during the American Civil War to administer morphine not only for relief of painful wounds but also for the treatment of dysentery. As a result, many thousands of soldiers returned to civilian life addicted to morphine. Their addiction was intensified by the fact that opium and its derivatives were freely and cheaply sold in pharmacies and even rural stores; as laudanum (1 grain of opium to 15 drops of alcohol) and paregoric (1 grain to 480 drops).

In 1898 still another alkaloid of opium—heroin—was derived synthetically from morphine. This turned out to be the most powerfully addicting drug of all. At first heroin was used as a treatment for morphine addiction; but the error of this was soon discovered. Heroin has no legitimate medical uses.

The medical viewpoint on the hazards of opium and its derivatives gradually crystallized during the nineteenth century. In general, until late in the century, physicians thought of opiate addiction in about the same category as alcohol addiction. In 1889 one physician wrote, "The use of morphine in place of alcohol is but a choice of evils, and by far the lesser." The use of narcotics spread in America by their use in advertised "patent medicines." There was no control at that time over such medicines, since the first Federal Pure Food and Drug Act was not passed until 1906.

Public opinion did not then harshly condemn opiate addiction. Except for smoking opium in Chinese "opium dens," its use—at least orally—was considered an unfortunate habit rather than an affront to public morals. The use of opiates was more prevalent in the upper classes. Distinguished men of literary and political stature were acknowledged "opium eaters." Among them were Edgar Allan Poe, the American author; John Randolph, an American statesman; Samuel Coleridge and Francis Thompson, English poets; and Thomas De Quincy, who wrote "Confessions of an English Opium Eater."

The risks of narcotic addiction came to be more sharply understood in the early part of the twentieth century. In 1909 a federal law was passed prohibiting the importation of opium or its derivatives except for medical purposes. In 1914 the Congress of the United States passed the *Harrison Act* to control narcotic addiction. It did not make addiction per se illegal but put controls on the production, manufacture, and distribution of narcotics. Physicians were permitted to dispense or prescribe narcotic drugs. (Included among the "narcotic" drugs was cocaine, which is actually a stimulant.)

It soon became evident that private physicians could not succeed in treating narcotic addiction on an outpatient basis because the patients were so unreliable. For a brief time (1919–1923) local and state health departments set up clinics to dispense drugs to addicts as a part of treatment. But this effort also proved unacceptable because it was feared that narcotics were being dispensed too freely, and the clinics were closed.

At this point, the drug addict who could not break his habit turned to the underworld "black market" for his drugs, which had previously been a minor source of supply. The money cost for drugs in this market was high. A large number of addicts therefore became involved in criminal activities to support their addiction.

A number of additional federal laws to control the narcotics traffic were subsequently passed, and many states and cities passed laws and ordinances based on the federal models. The federal laws included:

Marihuana Tax Act (1937). This law provided the same controls over marihuana as the Harrison Act did for narcotics. (Again, marihuana is a hallucinogen, not a "narcotic" in the same sense that opiates are; but the extension of terms of Harrison Act to marihuana has suggested that it is.)

Narcotic Control Act (1956). In the face of increased juvenile use of narcotics after World War II, this act provided heavy penalties for the unlawful sale of narcotics and marihuana to minors. For example, an adult who furnishes heroin to a minor may be subject (for a second offense) to imprisonment from ten years to life, an optional fine up to $20,000, or the death penalty if a jury so directs.

Drug Abuse Control Amendments (1965). These enactments extended the Federal Food, Drug and Cosmetic Act to control stimulant, depressive, and hallucinogenic drugs which may be subject to abuse. Barbiturates, amphetamines, LSD, and comparable drugs are included in these categories.

The enforcement of these antidrug laws was formerly vested in the Federal Bureau of Narcotics, operating under the United States Treasury Department; the Food and Drug Administration (FDA); and the Bureau of Customs. In 1968 these enforcement agencies (except for the Bureau of Customs) were merged into the Bureau of Narcotics and Dangerous Drugs in the United States Department of Justice.

Even as wider and stricter enforcement of laws against narcotics and other dangerous drugs were enacted, a somewhat different picture of the addict appeared. He was regarded not only as a criminal, but as a sick, tortured person, desperately in need of help.

A White House Conference on Narcotics and Drug Abuse, in 1962, helped further to establish this new image. One panel of this meeting referred to the addict as "an inadequate personality . . . unable to cope with the stresses of normal life."

The conference also noted the increase in the abuse of stimulant, depressive, tranquilizing, and hallucinogenic drugs on the part of young people in high school and college.

Heroin

Heroin, variously known as "H," "hard stuff," etc., is the most dangerous narcotic in terms of producing addiction. It is an outlawed drug that has no approved medical use. Addicts may at first take this narcotic orally or by sniffing it. Later, however, they usually inject it into their veins ("mainlining") for quicker effect. The injections or "fixes" are made with a hypodermic needle and syringe, but in a pinch a vein and an eye-dropper to insert the drug often serve a desperate addict.

Probably three-quarters of confirmed narcotic addicts use heroin. They may be "hooked" in a few weeks or even days. No one who begins to use drugs would choose to become an addict. In fact, no one really believes it will happen to *him*. Among the fallacious arguments for "just trying" narcotics are: "You'll get a thrill out of it." "You'll feel good." "It peps up your sex appeal." The truth is that opiates do not increase sex desire; in fact, they are likely to diminish it. And the temporary "good feeling" or "high" is purchased at a high price.

The initial, early effects of the opiate drugs (depending on the dose) are to relieve pain and produce a false sense of well-being (euphoria). Addicts have said that heroin "makes my troubles roll off my mind" and "it makes me feel more sure of myself." But the dosages must be continually increased to achieve this "desirable" end. Soon, however, the user becomes physically and psychologically dependent on the drug; the craving is relentless. A this point the addict does

not feel supernormal with the drug. He is miserable and subnormal without it. (Some of his physiological processes cannot function without the drug.) His total preoccupation with getting the next doses of the drug he craves almost always prevents him from either continuing his education or holding a job. His health is likely to be poor, causing his life expectancy to be considerably shorter than that of the nonuser.

One characteristic of addiction to heroin and other opiates or their synthetic substitutes is *withdrawal sickness* (also known as the "abstinence syndrome"). Beginning about 18 hours after the last dose of the narcotic, the withdrawal symptoms occur. These include sweating, shaking, chills, vomiting, diarrhea, and severe stomach pains. These symptoms may remain acute for as long as 36–72 hours. Modern treatments have eased some of the pangs of the withdrawal symptoms, but so-called "cold turkey" withdrawal remains a painful experience.

"Street" supplies of heroin are uncertain as to dosage, since the drug is "cut"—diluted—with milk sugar. Therefore it is possible that in some cases true physiological dependence has not occurred, causing comparatively mild withdrawal symptoms. On the other hand, the uncertain dosage may have a sufficiently high percentage of heroin to cause death.

The addict is almost always in trouble with his family and with the police. At least half the known addicts have police records even before they become addicted. Since an addict may have to spend $75–$100 for a day's supply, he finds that he has no other avenue except crime to raise that amount. Women addicts usually become prostitutes; men become thieves, muggers, and "pushers."

Most addicts begin young. A third of them are under 20, and two-thirds under 30. They are generally found in large cities among socially and economically depressed groups. Of the 60,000 heroin addicts known to the Federal Bureau of Narcotics and Dangerous Drugs, more than half live in New York State, and most of these in New York City. But no age, class, or profession is exempt from the risk.

Chart Listing Drugs, Medical Uses, Symptoms Produced and Their Dependence Potentials*

Name	Slang Name	Chemical or Trade Name	Pharmacologic Classification	Medical Use	How Taken
Heroin	H., Horse, Scat, Junk, Hard Stuff, Harry, Joy Powder	Diacetylmorphine	Depressant	Pain Relief	Injected or Sniffed
Morphine	White Stuff, Miss Emma, M, Dreamer	Morphine sulphate	Depressant	Pain Relief	Swallowed or Injected
Codeine	Schoolboy	Methylmorphine	Depressant	Ease Pain and Coughing	Swallowed
Methadone	Dolly	Dolophine Amidone	Depressant	Pain Relief	Swallowed or Injected
Cocaine	Speed Balls, Gold Dust, Coke, Bernice, Corine, Flake, Star Dust, Snow	Methyl ester of benzoylecgonine	Stimulant	Local Anesthesia	Sniffed, Injected or Swallowed
Marijuana	Pot, Grass, Locoweed, Mary Jane, Hashish, Tea, Gage, Reefers	Cannabis Sativa	Stimulant Depressant, or Hallucinogen	None in U.S.	Smoked, Swallowed or Sniffed
Barbiturates	Barbs, Blue Devils, Candy, Yellow Jackets, Phennies, Peanuts, Blue Heavens	Phenobarbital Nembutal, Seconal, Amytal	Depressant	Sedation, Relieve high blood pressure, epilepsy, hyperthyroidism	Swallowed or Injected
Amphetamines	Bennies, Dexies, Co-Pilots, Wake-Ups, Lid Proppers, Hearts, Pep Pills	Benzedrine, Preludin Dexedrine, Dexoxyn, Methedrine	Stimulant	Relieve mild depression, control appetite and narcolepsy	Swallowed or Injected
LSD	Acid, Sugar, Big D, Cubes, Trips	d-lysergic acid diethylamide	Hallucinogen	Experimental Study of Mental Function, alcoholism	Swallowed
DMT	Businessman's High	Dimethyltriptamine	Hallucinogen	None	Injected
Mescaline	Cactus, Peyote	3, 4, 5-trimethoxy-phenethylamine	Hallucinogen	None	Swallowed
Psilocybin	Mushrooms	3 (2-dimethylamino)-ethylindol-4-ol dihydrogen phosphate	Hallucinogen	None	Swallowed

*Reprinted with permission of the New York Times, January 9, 1968.

Usual Dose	Duration of Effect	Initial Symptoms	Long-Term Symptoms	Physical Dependence Potential	Mental Dependence Potential
Varies	4 hrs.	Euphoria Drowsiness	Addiction, Constipation Loss of Appetite Convulsions in overdose	Yes	Yes
15 Milligrams	6 hrs.	Euphoria Drowsiness	Addiction, impairment of breathing	Yes	Yes
30 Milligrams	4 hrs.	Drowsiness	Addiction	Yes	Yes
10 Milligrams	4–6 hrs.	Less acute than opiates	Addiction	Yes	Yes
Varies	Varies	Excitation Talkativeness Tremors	Depression, Convulsions	No	Yes
1 or 2 Cigarettes	4 hrs.	Relaxation, Euphoria, alteration of perception and judgment	Usually none	No	?
50–100 Milligrams	4 hrs.	Drowsiness, Muscle relaxation	Addiction with severe withdrawal symptoms, possible convulsions	Yes	Yes
2.5–5 Milligrams	4 hrs.	Alertness, Activeness	Delusions Hallucinations	No	Yes
100 Micrograms	10 hrs.	Exhilaration, Excitation Rambling Speech	May intensify existing psychosis, panic reactions	No	?
1 Milligram	4–6 hrs.	Exhilaration Excitation	?	No	?
350 Micrograms	12 hrs.	Exhilaration, Anxiety Gastric distress	?	No	?
25 Milligrams	6–8 hrs.	Nausea, Vomiting, Headaches	?	No	?

Cocaine

Cocaine comes from the leaves of the coca plant, grown in Peru and Bolivia, where the leaves are chewed for their intoxicating effects. Though legally classed as a narcotic, cocaine is actually a stimulant drug. It stimulates the central nervous system and thus temporarily banishes feelings of fatigue. The user becomes excited and talkative. Later he is afflicted with hallucinations and sleeplessness. Addicts to cocaine take it by injection or by sniffing the white power, which is called "snow." (Its takers are referred to as "snow birds.") Occasionally cocaine is mixed with heroin to provide a potent injection called a "speed-ball."

Cocaine is not widely used in the United States. Its original usage as a local anesthetic has been supplanted by synthetic drugs, such as novocaine and procaine.

Cocaine is a highly toxic drug and has been recognized as such even by potential users. Its abuse leads to rapid weight loss, extreme weakness, and mental deterioration.

Barbiturates

Barbiturates are depressant or sedative drugs. Popularly they are known as "sleeping pills," and in drug jargon as "goofballs" or "barbs." They act to relax the central nervous system. Over 2500 barbiturate drugs have been formulated since they were first introduced in Germany in the early twentieth century. However, only about 30 of the known barbiturates are actually in medical use.

Barbiturates have an important place in medical practice. They are widely used to treat high blood pressure, epilepsy, insomnia, and some mental illnesses; to relax patients before and during surgery; and for a host of other conditions. Of all the prescriptions doctors write for psychoactive (mind-affecting) drugs, about one in four is for a barbiturate. There are short-starting, fast-acting barbiturates and also slow-starting, long-acting ones.

In the higher dosages, which the abusers of these drugs habitually take, their effects resemble those of alcoholic intoxication—confusion, slurred speech, staggering; reduced ability to think, concentrate, or work; and finally a deep sleep (coma). Overdoses can be fatal.

Barbiturates are physically and psychologically addicting. Some experts think barbiturate addiction more difficult to cure than narcotic dependency. Convulsions following sudden withdrawal can be fatal.

The combination of barbiturates with alcohol, even in moderate doses, is especially dangerous. The two drugs, working together, synergize each other, and the total result is greater than that of either drug acting alone. Hence barbiturates are a factor in causing auto accidents, and are a leading cause of fatal accidental poisoning in the United States.

Amphetamines

Amphetamines, popularly known as "pep pills" or "bennies", are stimulants to the central nervous system. They are prescribed in proper doses by physicians to combat fatigue and sleepiness and to depress appetite (in people on weight-reduction programs). Self-prescribed and misused, they can be dangerous. Sometimes they are used in connection with depressant drugs, such as barbiturates, to get a chemical "up" followed by a chemical "down." This is a serious misuse of these drugs.

In heavy doses the amphetamines cause jitteriness, irritability, unclear speech, and tension. People on very heavy doses are withdrawn, dull, and disorganized in their thinking. The sudden withdrawal of amphetamines from the heavy abuser can result in deep and possibly suicidal depression.

Amphetamines are misused in various ways. Truck drivers take them to keep awake on long hauls. This dangerous practice may often result in serious traffic accidents. College students sometimes take amphetamines to keep them awake when cramming for exams. There are two dangers in this: (1) the effect of the drug may wear off and they will fall asleep during the examination; or (2) if increased dosages are used, they may cause a degree of intoxication which will make it practically impossible to write an acceptable examination paper.

Amphetamines and similar stimulant drugs do not produce physical dependence the way narcotics do. However, psychological dependence may result. Tolerance for the drug also develops, which means that larger and larger doses are need to obtain the desired effect.

Marihuana

Marihuana is a drug derived from the Indian hemp plant, *Cannabis sativa*. The flowering tops and the leaves of this plant, as well as its somewhat stronger cousin, *Cannabis indica*, are used to make the drug. It has been known and used for several thousand years, all around the world. It is known as "kief" in North Africa, "hashish"[3] in Arabia, "bhang" in India, and "ma jen" in China.

The drug can be taken in various ways—by chewing the leaves, by sniffing it in powder form, by mixing it with honey or candy for eating or drinking, or—as is most common in North America—by smoking it. The dried leaves and tops of the plant are chopped or crushed and fashioned into thin-paper cigarettes. These are called "reefers," "joints," or "sticks." The drug itself is known in the jargon of drug abusers as "pot," "tea," "grass," "weed," or "Mary Warner." The smoke from a marihuana cigarette smells like burnt rope or dried grass and has a characteristic, sweetish odor.

The strength of the drug varies from time to time and place to place, depending how and where it is grown, how it is prepared, and how it is stored. The kind grown in North America—largely in Mexico—is much weaker than the kind harvested in Asia, Africa, and the Near East. Traffic in marihuana is restricted in almost all

[3] The possibly violent result of using this drug may be judged by one of the words derived from it—*assassin*, from "hashish," a stronger form of marihuana. In some Oriental countries young men were deliberately inspired to commit murder by feeding them hashish.

civilized countries but its use continues. Immense quantities are smuggled into the United States across the Mexican border.

Marihuana was introduced into the United States as an intoxicating drug in the 1920's. Its general use was outlawed by the Federal Marihuana Tax Act of 1937 because it was believed to be a narcotic. This was followed by strict laws and enforcement in almost every state. Arrests on marihuana charges in the United States have doubled in the past decade (since about 1960).

Effects of Marihuana. When smoked, marihuana quickly enters the blood stream and proceeds to the brain and nervous system, bringing about changes in the mood and thinking of the user. The effect on emotions and senses varies widely, depending on who the smoker is as well as how much and what kind of marihuana is used. Also involved are the social setting and what results the smoker expects. Marihuana is commonly smoked in a social setting—at a "pot party" or "tea party."

In some respects the early effects of marihuana are like those of alcohol. The first effect is stimulation, during which time inhibitions may be loosened. Soon afterward the smoker drifts into a state of euphoria. His sense of time and distance is often distorted; a minute may seem like an hour. Because it sometimes produces hallucinations, marihuana is classified as a mild hallucinogen. However, it often produces vivid, visual imagery in the user. The drug effect begins about 15 minutes after the marihuana is smoked and may last from two to four hours.

The marihuana user finds it harder to make decisions which require clear thinking—and he is quite responsive to other people's suggestions. He should not be driving an automobile while under the influence of the drug.

The physical effects of marihuana use are less important than the psychological dependence which it induces. The early physical effects may include dizziness, dry mouth, more rapid heart beat, lower body temperature, red eyes, and occasionally hunger, especially for sweets.

Marihuana does not produce the physical dependence that the true narcotics do. Once an optimal amount is taken, the user does not find it necessary to take increased dosages. There are no withdrawal symptoms when the drug is stopped. These facts have led to the opinion that marihuana is "no worse than alcohol." To evaluate this opinion, we must consider the tragic effects that heavy drinking or alcoholism can have on the individual and upon society.

There is a strong consensus of opinion that marihuana produces a difficult-to-cure psychological dependence if it is taken regularly.

In a 1967 study of narcotic addicts from big city areas, it was revealed that four out of five had previously used marihuana. On the other hand, there are immense numbers of marihuana smokers who do not go on to use morphine or heroin. No cause-and-effect link between marihuana and narcotics has been found.

Federal and state laws deal with marihuana as strictly as if it were a narcotic. To *possess,* give, or sell marihuana in the United States is a felony. The federal penalty for a first offense may be 2 to 10 years' imprisonment and a fine of up to $20,000. Young people tempted by marihuana should remember that an arrest or conviction on a marihuana charge can seriously cloud their future educational and employment opportunities.

A new chapter in the marihuana story was opened in 1966 when an Israeli chemist, with United States support, succeeded in synthesizing the active ingredient in marihuana; namely, tetrahydrocannabinol (THC). This new synthetic drug makes it possible for researchers to determine more exactly the effects of marihuana.

LSD and Other Hallucinogens

A hallucinogen, as was already noted, is a drug that causes hallucinations. These are trancelike states of mind in which an individual may see, hear, taste, smell, or appear to touch something that is not really there. In other words, the hallucinogens alter perceptions. For example, a doll might appear as a frightening monster. The drug-taker may also suffer from delusions (false

beliefs), and imagine that someone is out to "get" him (a delusion of persecution). The great appeal in taking hallucinogenic drugs is the alteration of the state of mind in the direction of believing oneself a more sensitive, powerful, and important person than he really is.

LSD, lysergic acid diethylamide, is an hallucinogenic drug and, at present, one of the most potent of them. There are 300,000 doses to the ounce! The hallucinogens are also called psychedelic—or mind-expanding—drugs, but this is usually a false designation. These drugs are as likely to constrict consciousness as to expand it. Among the other known hallucinogenic drugs are: psilocybin, derived from a "sacred mushroom" used for centuries by Mexican Indians to produce visions and hallucinations as part of their religious ceremonies; mescaline, derived from seed-pods, "buttons," of the peyote cactus; morning glory seeds; nutmeg; and Jimson weed.

LSD is a late comer to the field of hallucinogens. It was first discovered in 1938 by Albert Hofman, a chemist working in the Sandoz Research Laboratory in Switzerland. Five years later, in 1943, he accidentally discovered its special property of changing sense perceptions, that is, of producing hallucinations, illusions, and delusions.

A spate of research with LSD followed this discovery. There was some early hope that it might prove useful in treating some kinds of mental illness. Two-and-a-half decades and some 2000 scientific papers later, however, the drug still had no approved place in medical practice. Within that time, though, the use of LSD escaped from the field of careful scientific investigation and was taken up by some presitigious persons. The English author, Aldous Huxley, in a book, *Doors of Perception,* published in 1954, praised LSD's unusual properties.

Among the other early proselytes and proselytizers of LSD were two former members of the Psychology Department at Harvard, Timothy Leary and Richard Alpert. They called LSD a "sacred biochemical," which brought mystic understanding. They claimed that normal consciousness is a dim, dull thing in comparison with the aura of understanding and insight that results from taking LSD or any of the half-dozen other psychedelic drugs. Among these may be mentioned DMT (dimethyltryptamine), derived from the seeds of certain plants found in South America and the West Indies.

Lysergic acid, from which LSD is made (by relatively simple chemical processes), is derived from ergot, a fungus that grows on rye and wheat. LSD may be obtained as a pill, a powder, or a tasteless, colorless, odorless liquid in ampules. It is often taken on a lump of sugar, a cookie, or a cracker.

The negative effects of LSD were not recognized until the early 1960's. In 1965, by an act of Congress, it was declared an illegal, dangerous drug. The manufacture or sale of LSD or similar drugs was made illegal. In some states laws were passed making even the possession of the LSD-type of drugs illegal. Taking these drugs is called "taking a trip." Commonly these trips are pleasurable, but sometimes they are horrible experiences verging on panic. It should be noted that LSD is an *unpredictable* drug or at least that it has unpredictable results on some takers. People who have taken it many times may suddenly find themselves on a disconcerting "bad trip." In some instances, hallucinations have continued, or reappeared, over long periods of time after the drug was taken. In some cases, also, LSD has provoked psychotic reactions.

That LSD is a dangerous drug can be adduced from the testimony of physicians who have treated patients for the results of its effects. Dr. Donald B. Louria, president of the New York State Council on Drug Addiction, has said:

There is no other drug used promiscuously under uncontrolled circumstances that is as dangerous as LSD. It is absolutely unpredictable.

In the 114 cases hospitalized by Bellevue Hospital [New York City] in the past 18 months [1966–1967], the average age was 23 years. Thirteen percent entered the hospital with overwhelming panic. There was uncontrolled violence in 12 percent. Nearly 9 percent had attempted either homicide or suicide, none successfully. Of the 114, one out of seven had to be sent on from Bellevue to long-term mental hospitalization,

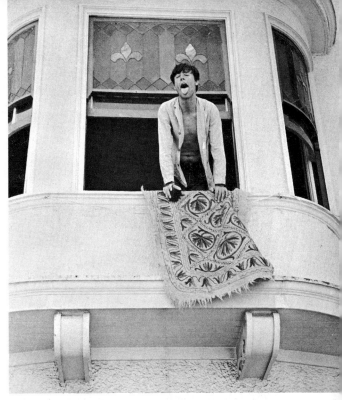

IN HAIGHT-ASHBURY a young hippie on a bad trip cries out in defiance (or for help). (Photograph by Miller-MAGNUM)

and half of these had no history of underlying psychiatric disorder.

A study entitled "[College] Student Use of Hallucinogens" was undertaken by Dr. Herbert D. Kleber in the mid-1960's. He noted that 24 percent of those using the LSD-type drug were judged to have adverse reactions. These included anxiety reactions, persistent hallucinosis, worsening of psychiatric symptoms, and psychic dependence on the drug. On the other hand, he reported that half the students who took the drugs claimed that they "had improved their lives." Many people including musicians, who have taken an eight-to-ten hour trip on LSD, have the impression that they are giving tremendously better performances than usual. The playing of a group of musicians under the influence of LSD was tape-recorded. The musicians felt that they were playing more brilliantly than ever before. When they had recovered from their LSD trance and heard their performances being played back to them, they said, "How could we have played so badly!" In short, LSD fools you.

Whether or not LSD has long-range adverse effects on the brain has not been definitely determined, but that it has some danger is suggested by the effects of the drug on test animals. Short-term dangers may also result from the strange effects of LSD. Some users of the drug think they can fly or walk on water, and are injured or killed when they attempt such feats. Recent scientific evidence has demonstrated the damaging effect of LSD on the chromosomes.

Identifying the Drug Abuser

We shall review here some of the signs and symptoms that may be part of the pattern of identification of students in the habit of using dangerous drugs. Sudden changes in behavior always deserve attention. When this altered behavior becomes the new pattern, drug abuse should be considered as a possible factor.

Among the common behavioral signs that may suggest drug abuse in college (or even high school) students are the following:

Significant changes in class attendance; changes for the worse in work turned in; unusual flare-ups and outbursts of temper; unusual activity or indolence; poor personal appearance, since serious drug abusers generally become indifferent to and neglect their appearance as well as their health habits; furtive behavior because the drug abuser fears discovery; wearing sunglasses at inappropriate times to hide dilated or constricted pupils; constantly wearing long-sleeved apparel to hide needle marks on the arms; begging, borrowing, or stealing money or other items, such as radios and jewelry, which can be converted quickly into cash, in order to pay the expenses of the drug habit; frequenting odd places, such as closets, storage rooms, or parked cars, in order to take drugs; and associating with other known drug abusers.

In addition to these behavioral clues common to abuse of all kinds of drugs, each specific category of abused drugs has some special manifestations associated with it, as follows:

The glue or solvent sniffer generally retains on his breath or clothes the odor of the substance inhaled. Furthermore, his nose runs and his bloodshot eyes water. He lacks muscular control, as if he were intoxicated. He may see double or complain of hallucinations. Finding a handkerchief or paper bag with dried plastic cement is a telltale sign of glue sniffing.

The abuser of depressant drugs, notably barbiturates and some tranquilizers, exhibits most of the symptoms of alcoholic intoxication—except that there is no odor of alcohol on his breath. He may stagger and stumble. He is usually drowsy and sometimes falls into a deep sleep in the classroom. He lacks interest in school activities and may appear disoriented.

The abuser of stimulants, especially amphetamines, is characterized by excess activity. He is often irritable, argumentative, and nervous. He has difficulty in sitting still. Because amphetamines have a drying effect on mucous membranes, those who abuse these drugs have bad breath, a dry mouth, and an itchy nose. They can be observed scratching their noses and licking their lips with their tongues. They are often chain smokers; they talk incessantly about any subject at hand; and they frequently boast about going long hours without food or sleep.

The abuser of narcotics (heroin, morphine, and synthetic substitutes) is rarely seen in the classroom. If he is, he will usually appear lethargic and drowsy or display symptoms of deep intoxication. Sometimes narcotic addiction begins by drinking paregoric or cough medicines containing codeine. The presence of empty bottles of such substances in wastebaskets or on school grounds is a tell-tale sign. Other "beginners" in narcotic abuse may inhale heroin in powder form. This leaves traces of a white powder around the nostrils, which become red and raw.

The "mainliner" most commonly uses the veins on the inner surface of the arm, at the elbow. Here scar tissue ("tracks") appears after numerous injections and identifies the narcotic abuser. (Hence he wears long sleeves.)

The narcotic abuser needs equipment, called "works" or "outfit," to "mainline" his drugs. This equipment consists of a spoon with a bent handle or a bottle cap, a small ball of cotton (called "satch cotton"), a syringe or eye-dropper, and a hypodermic needle. Heroin powder is dissolved in a little water in the bent spoon or bottle cap and heated over a match or lighter. The cotton acts as a filter as the narcotic is drawn up through the needle into the eye-dropper or syringe. The "mainliner" must keep his equipment handy. Hence it is likely to be found on his person, in his desk, or in his locker. Finding such an "outfit" is almost a sure sign of narcotics abuse.

The marihuana smoker is sometimes betrayed by the odor of marihuana ("pot")—something like the odor of burning rope—on his breath or clothing. He may also be identified by the possession of marihuana cigarettes, often called "sticks," "reefers," or "joints." These cigarettes are usually smoked in a group situation; after one or two puffs, the joints are passed on to another member of the group.

The marihuana user is difficult to detect unless he is under the influence of the drug at the time he is being observed. He is unlikely to be recognized in the classroom. In the early stages of the marihuana effect, when the drug acts as a stimulant, the smoker is likely to be animated, talking loudly, and bursting into laughter. In later stages he is sleepy or stuporous.

The abuser of hallucinogenic drugs, such as LSD, is not likely to be detected in a classroom. The taking of such drugs, usually called "taking a trip," also usually occurs in a group situation under special conditions. The users generally sit quietly in a dream or trancelike sleep. One member of the group does not take the drug at the time and looks after those others who may be suffering from a "bad trip." Sometimes a user of hallucinogenic drugs may become terribly frightened and seek to escape from the group. Someone must prevent him from taking dangerous or even fatal actions.

Treatment for Drug Addiction

Although there has been some progress, the treatment of drug addiction (or dependence) re-

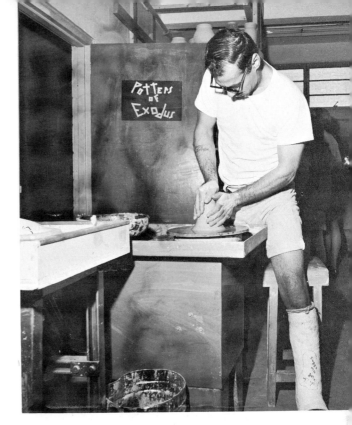

THIS EX-ADDICT is undergoing occupational therapy in the pottery shop at Exodus House, a private, voluntary agency for rehabilitation of addicts who have already been detoxified. (Photograph by Bijur-MONKMEYER)

mains far from satisfactory. Addicts are no longer considered as altogether incurable. The feeling that addiction was largely untreatable arose from the fact that so many patients on opiates went back to drug use after long periods of hospitalization.

The first step in the treatment of the drug abuser is usually detoxification, that is, drug withdrawal. There are several treatment methods, however, in which the patient is carried along for some time on lowered doses of drugs. Sudden withdrawl of addicting drugs is called "cold turkey" and is usually a highly painful process for the addict. Controlled and gradual detoxification is best done in a hospital setting under medical supervision.

The total pattern of treatment, however, goes far beyond detoxification. It includes psychiatric evaluation and treatment, continuing medical supervision, and counseling, especially after the patient returns to the environment from which he has come.

This is the most critical step in the rehabilitation process. The old neighborhood pressure on the former addict to go back to drugs is tremendous. He needs guidance and support during this period. He may be required to remain in contact with a social caseworker or specially trained probation officer, keep psychiatric as well as other medical appointments, and attend group therapy sessions. This kind of supervision may be needed for several years. Unfortunately, it is rarely available. Hence the "hard core" drug abuser may return to drug use even after a long period of "keeping clean," that is, not taking drugs.

Some Special Treatment Programs. Several kinds of special treatment programs have sprung up in different communities. All of them have interesting possibilities, but they must still be characterized as experimental. For example:

The Methadone Program was initiated in New York City by Drs. Vincent Dole and Marie Nyswander, associated with the Rockefeller Foundation. It provides for carrying along on methadone—a long-acting, synthetic narcotic—former heroin addicts with a history of relapse. The drug is reputed to satisfy narcotic hunger without producing euphoria, the drug-induced feeling of superb well-being.

The British System permitted physicians to carry narcotic addicts along on usually small, main-tenance doses of narcotics after all other treatment methods had failed. The treatment was revised in 1968 and patients are now referred to treatment centers.

Synanon consists of a number of residences in the United States where ex-addicts manage the program and admit other addicts to take part in their drug-free project. Once admitted, the ex-addict is expected to work hard toward his own rehabilitation.

Daytop Lodge is another residential facility designed to help ex-addicts take the big step toward transition into community life. Located on Staten Island, in New York, it is directed by Synanon "graduates."

Narcotics Anonymous, modeled after Alcoholics Anonymous, has chapters in many large cities. Spiritually oriented, it relies for its effectiveness on mutual inspiration, discussion, and the therapeutic value of confession.

The California System provides for sending addicts to a rehabilitation center and thereafter to "half-way houses", where outpatients may stay for up to three months. The unique feature of this plan is that all outpatients must submit to periodic tests with Nalline, a synthetic antinarcotic. This drug brings about withdrawal symptoms if the person taking it is using narcotics.

In general, it may be said that methods of treatment which bring favorable community and peer pressure to bear on ex-addicts are more successful than those in which they must go the route alone.

SUMMARY

We have noted the presence of narcotics and other potentially dangerous drugs on the American scene, particularly on the college campus and in the urban ghetto. Figures for once-tried, casual, or regular use of drugs by college students are difficult to obtain.

We have tried to set the problem of drug abuse in historical perspective, reaching back to antiquity. We have detailed the actions taken and the laws passed in the United States to control traffic—especially underworld traffic—in narcotics and other dangerous drugs.

The narcotics include opium and drugs derived from it: notably *morphine,* medically of great use as a pain-killer, and *heroin,* an outlawed drug on which many young addicts are often "hooked." Among other potentially dangerous drugs discussed here are:

Cocaine, a stimulant drug from South America.

Barbiturates, sleeping pills especially dangerous in overdoses or when combined with alcohol.

Amphetamines, "pep pills."

Marihuana, commonly known as "pot," next to alcohol the most widely abused drug on the American scene.

LSD and other hallucinogens, whose risks have become apparent only recently—in the 1960's.

We have also reviewed some of the signs and symptoms by which drug users, especially students, can be identified. Finally, we have discussed present-day treatments for drug addiction and some of the systems employed for keeping "cured" addicts from drifting back to drug abuse.

SUMMARY REVIEW QUESTIONS

1. What are the differences between medical and legal definitions of narcotics? What was the public attitude toward narcotics in the United States during the nineteenth century? What changes have taken place in the twentieth century?

2. What are "dangerous drugs" other than true narcotics, as discussed in this chapter? Name four such drugs and describe their origin.

3. How does *narcotic* addiction usually occur? What kind of life does the drug addict live? What is the relationship between drug addiction and crime?

4. What are the effects, physical and psychological, of marihuana? From what and from where does marihuana originate? Is it to be regarded as a true narcotic? What is its relationship to other forms of drug dependence?

5. What are hallucinogenic drugs? Name four and state their origin. What arguments in favor of their use are put forth by the proponents of these drugs? What are the dangers of these drugs, as noted by physicians?

6. Are the following statements sense or nonsense? Why? *Anything is worth trying once . . . . You don't know what living is until you've tried reefers. . . . Barbiturates are not dangerous; doctors prescribe them. . . . Once you're hooked on narcotics, you're hooked for life. . . . Smoking marihuana is no worse than heavy drinking of alcoholic beverages. . . . Overdoses of sleeping pills are frequently fatal. . . . There can be no harm in "taking a trip" with LSD once in a while.*

7. What do the following terms mean to you? psychedelic, heroin, "snow," barbiturate, amphetamine, psychic dependence, "cold turkey," "mainlining," "bad trip," "pot party," hallucinogen?

Worth Looking Into: *Drug Abuse: Escape to Nowhere* published by Smith, Kline & French Laboratories. *Confessions of an English Opium Eater* by Thomas de Quincy. *Drugs on the College Campus* by Helen H. Nowlis. *The Drug Scene* by Donald B. Louria. For more complete references, see Appendix E.

Factors Leading to Drug Abuse

George D. Demos, Ph.D. and Mary P. Frazer, R.N.

During the past several years there has been a great deal of interest regarding the use and abuse of drugs among young people throughout the United States. This interest has led to realistic concerns about the effects various drugs are having not only on college–age youth but on high school and junior high students as well. Perhaps the following incident will help to describe the problem which those concerned with student health are facing today.

A sweet-faced girl of twenty-two came into the student health center, very frightened and anxiously asking for help. She told us that, since taking LSD with a group of friends approximately two months ago, she had been having nightmares. At times she felt detached from her body. Frequently while talking to people, or even just looking about, the faces would appear to melt and run together as if they were made of warm wax. These experiences were horrifying to her and she said, "I don't know why anybody would try LSD."

What is the appeal? Why are young people resorting to such potentially dangerous behavior? What are the motivations? Who are the people who are searching for these experiences and, more importantly, what can be done about helping them in ways that are not potentially destructive? These are difficult questions to answer and we have very inadequate research to substantiate what, at this time, appear only as hypotheses. At any rate, the following are some tentative answers to this most perplexing of problems— the use and abuse of drugs:

1. We are living in a drug-oriented society. It is a rare home that does not have a medicine cabinet packed with every conceivable kind of drug. Through widespread advertising we have literally been brainwashed into believing that whenever we have the slightest problem, it is absolutely essential that we take something for it.

2. We are living in an age of anxiety. The rate at which life is moving creates anxiety in as-similating the new with the old, particularly in the area of values. This leads to confusion, uncertainty and frustration in individuals relative to the disparities that exist around them and leads to impatience with regard to what life should be like. In addition, and perhaps more important, a clash of cultural mores and values occurs.

3. The pressures on young people toward achievement is widespread. One can easily note the pressures to succeed beginning as early as nursery school and continuing through graduate school. The pressures toward the development of professional career aspirations have many concomitant effects which can lead to a pattern of drug abuse among young people.

4. We are living in an age in which individuals in our society are flooded with stimuli, both inwardly and outwardly. As a result, our young people are bombarded with stimulation that they increasingly find overwhelming. The knowledge explosion that has occurred in recent decades is also of such magnitude that it gives a What's the use? Why try? impression to

SOURCE. George Demos, Ph.D., is Dean of Students at California State College, Long Beach, Calif. Mary Frazer, R.N., is a member of the staff of the Student Health Center at California State College.

She originally presented this paper at the Fifth International Congress for School and University Health in Prague, Czechoslovakia in July 1967. This article is reprinted with permission from the *Journal of the American College Health Association* (April 1968).

some people. With this fantastic pace, young people cannot seem to find themselves. In the search, many panaceas are brought forth which attempt to simplify the complexities of the world. They frequently take the form of *drugs*.

5. Organized religion does not play so important a role in the lives of our young people as it once did. To many of the drug users, organized religion represents the establishment—that body of individuals dedicated to perpetuating the status quo and serving as an aversive reinforcer for those who do not conform and who transgress the traditional or stereotyped. Other forms of religious experiences have had greater appeal, primarily those of an introspective character with emphasis on contemplation and isolation [e.g., Zen Buddhism].

6. Youth appears extremely critical of adults, and the disparity between the feelings of young people and adults is particularly noteworthy. Never before have the young people been so diverse in their points of view and in their attitudes and feelings in comparison with their elders.

7. Adults find themselves playing roles, being phony, and not genuine. Young people are painfully aware of these shortcomings, and strive in every way possible not to emulate the adult culture. Drugs provide a quick way for this kind of breakthrough.

8. The spirit of rebellion is very apparent in working with adolescents and young adults.

Rebelliousness as a factor in achieving identity is one of the developmental tasks of youth. It is necessary to work through one's feelings of hostility and rebelliousness toward society. Much of this rebelliousness is projected to authority figures which, in some cases, represent Dad or Mom; in other cases, it may represent the authoritarian or dictatorial aspects of our society.

The use of LSD is, to a considerable degree, centered around the young. Rarely does one find individuals over 30 years of age utilizing this drug.

9. A new morality has been developing among our younger generation, which accepts, essentially, the premise that anything goes, just as long as it doesn't hurt any one. What I do to my own body or to someone else's if he is willing and accepting, is not a matter for anyone else to be concerned about, providing the consequences are not deleterious to others. This, then, becomes a rationalization for young people to experiment with drugs.

10. One of the most powerful movements of our time is the search for authenticity. What young people seem to value most is the truth. When they cannot obtain it, they lose confidence in those elders who seek arbitrarily to perpetuate fiction or error. Eventually this leads to rejection. Many young people feel that modern society, to which they refer as the establishment, is rampant with games, myths, empty slogans, hypocrisy and misdirection. Drugs repre-

sent a way of pacifying the disappointment while searching for their authentic and true selves.

Unfortunately, there are no simple answers to the perplexing problems facing man; if only a pill existed that would answer all of our problems—but this thinking is fantasy—wishful thinking that is far from reality. We solve our problems by facing them head-on, squarely and realistically confronting one another with the real world, and not through a prism that distorts reality in the "eye of the beholder."

Perhaps this is the lesson that young people must eventually find out for themselves; it is desirable to search for the truth, and there is no better way than reality confrontation and hard work. The wishful thinking or magic formula surrounding the pill may temporarily cause one to focus less on the real world. The problems however, do not go away but, in most cases, reappear in more complex forms. The key words of the psychedelic cult: "turn on, tune in, and drop out," represent irresponsible and defeatist attitudes—a fatalism that is pure and simple escapism. A more vigorous, dynamic and viable approach would be to *turn on* one's potential to cope with the problems facing us in a dynamic society, *tune in* to what others are saying and become more sensitive to the world around us, and *drop in* to the real world and take a more active role in ameliorating its shortcomings.

The Campus Drug Problem

Anthony F. Philip, Ph.D.

Illicit drug use by college students, whether as "casual" experimentation or as habitual use, is being viewed increasingly by educational, governmental and medical authorities as a problem approaching public health proportions. Whereas in the past, illicit drug use by students may have been confined largely to amphetamines ("pep pills") and barbiturates ("goof balls") around final examination time, more recently there has been emerging, along with the popularization of psychedelic ("mind-expanding") experiences, a proliferation in the use of psychoactive drugs, especially marihuana and LSD. Although reliable statistics on the extent of such contact with drugs by students are meager, estimates by some college administrators (a group presumably loath to overstate the case for their own campuses) have put the figure as high as 40 per cent. Other equally authoritative campus sources report figures as low as 1 per cent. The range and variability of these estimates seem to reflect a "numbers game" in which the "imprudent and unwary" guess at the high or low incidence of drug use where, in fact, the degree of incidence is uncertain.[1] This "numbers game," incidentally, seems to involve behavior on the part of the participants not unlike what one sees on projective tests of personality, such as the Rorschach. That is, the "guess-timates" of the severity of the problem, as well as college officials' general attitudes and attempts at solution, can be easily influenced, indeed distorted, by their personal strategies for coping with an ambiguous, emotionally-loaded situation.

All this is not to suggest that any and every student who has had contact with drugs necessarily warrants counseling or psychotherapy. Indeed, students argue, like it or not, that casual use of marijuana in the context of social camaraderie is not unlike their grandparents' flouting *their* elders' prohibitions against visits to a speakeasy in the 1920's. In this sense, at least part of the drug problem seems like "old wine in new bottles." While this use of marihuana may constitute a social and legal problem, ordinarily it would not seem to be a psychiatric one. Too many psychologically well put-together, emotionally sound young people report casual use of marihuana in social settings—analogous to their parents' social drinking—to consider all of them as manifesting significant psychopathology. At the same time, however, it should be emphasized that *habitual* dependency on marihuana or other hallucinogens, or so-called "casual" use of LSD are quite another matter.

This raises the question of what one means by drug "use," for to speak merely of drug use is to beg the question. There are varying degrees of drug involvement, and one can distinguish a continuum along which they exist. This ranges from relatively benign, casual experimentation, through habitual use, to the more malignant extreme of drug supplying or pushing.

As with most typologies, however, there is the difficulty of squaring clinical observation with the discrete types. Or, put differently, one may be hard pressed to fit real people into these perhaps overdrawn descriptive pigeonholes. Consider

SOURCE. Anthony F. Philip, Ph.D., is director of Columbia College Counseling Service, Columbia University, New York, N.Y. This article is reprinted with permission from the *Journal of the American College Health Association*, **16**: 2 (December 1967).

[1]S. Pearlman, Drug Experiences and Attitudes Among Seniors in a Liberal Arts College, *NASPA* 4: 121, 1967.

the casual experimenter, for instance. Does one include here only those whose dealings with drugs are on an I-can-take-it-or-leave-it basis? Or what of those whose contacts with drugs primarily are a function of occasional whim and a search for "kicks"? Does one also include those who, although fascinated by the drug mystique, "turn on only with pot" and at that, paralleling the "social drinker," only at social gatherings? Or again, consider the academically well functioning, intellectually precious, gifted student who smokes routinely but sporadically, say several times a month over a period of years. Although all of these cases may involve a certain continuity and longevity regarding their involvement, such drug use does not seem so habitual or maladaptive, as that of the "pothead" or "acid head," to use the users' language. To be sure, the chronic casual experimenter shades into the category of the habitual user. Yet I would argue that habitual use also should be defined in terms of the degree of a student's commitment to the drug mystique. Thus the student who has taken LSD only a few times is more dangerously involved with drugs than are those marihuana smokers just cited as examples of casual experimenters. *Put another way, there is no such thing as "casual" experimentation with LSD.* This is so, not only because of the almost "nuclear" power of LSD (just over two pounds of LSD contain ten million doses, each of which is capable of triggering a psychotic

reaction) but also because the subjective intensity and unpredictability of the LSD experience preclude its being taken lightly.

To return to my unsatisfactory typology, I should like now to present a thumbnail sketch of the habitual student user, in his own jargon, the "pothead" or "acid head." Although there certainly are differences among individuals within this group, in general the common characteristics of habitual users seem to include the following aspects: their renunciation of ordinary values and societal institutions is an expression of what Deane has called the "anarchistic attitude," or the "new student nihilism," an increasingly fashionable one among certain groups of young people, epitomized by the Hippies.[2] More often than not they put on a show of nonconformity in personal hygiene as well as in their attire, mannerisms and attitudes toward what they regard as "the system." They see "the system" as hopelessly mired down in its own anachronistic traditions and, along with this, see themselves as utterly impotent to do anything that will change it. In terms of psychopathology, typically there is intolerable, chronic, low-grade depression including (1) a subjective sense on their part that somehow they have been cheated by life in general and by their parents in particular in a very fundamental way and (2) a smoldering, tense, brooding sort of resentfulness, and a sense that again, somehow, they have not been taken

seriously as individuals who matter. Along with all this, they seem to have more than their share of the average expectable adolescent narcissism, indeed their "pot parties" have the quality of a sort of collective narcissism; they congregate in groups to smoke pot but as soon as they "turn on" and become "high" each is alone, quite absorbed with himself. Finally, they seem preoccupied with issues of personal identity, autonomy and freedom of expression. Indeed most of them seem to see "turning on" or taking an "acid trip" as avenues of self-discovery and as ways of liberating themselves. In most cases I have seen, however, the student appears to be driven by motivations beyond his conscious awareness and control. The subjective sense of "freedom" in these cases invariably has been illusory; the student is being driven rather than really being in the driver's seat himself.

Along with all this, the habitual user seems to need to talk repeatedly about and around drugs. It is almost as if such individuals are trying, by their repetitive talk, to come to terms with the experience. This is not unlike what one sees clinically in patients who have experienced traumatic events such as an automobile accident, major surgery, a death in the family, and the like. Such patients, in their compulsion to relive the experience vicariously by repeatedly talking about it, also are attempting, through this repetition—compulsion to master the traumatic experience by

[2]H. A. Deane, On the New Student Nihilism, *The Graduate Faculties Newsletter* (New York: Columbia University Press, June 1967), p. 2.

repeatedly having another go at coping with it. All this is not to say that the drug experience is necessarily traumatic. Indeed, Bowers and Freedman point out that the psychedelic experience "is clearly a multipotential state with many factors influencing the final outcome, which can range from excruciating anxiety and paranoid delusion to an experience of intense self-knowledge."[3] I would add, based on my own clinical experience with student drug users, particularly marihuana users, that for the majority, perhaps, the drug experience is intensely pleasurable at times bordering on the ecstatic. Dynamically, this drug-induced euphoria often serves to deny or otherwise negate the user's underlying depression. In such cases, drug use becomes a chronic, compulsive defense against intolerable depression.

But what then of the repetition-compulsion as a way of accounting for the habitual user's repetitive drug talk and fascination with the drug mystique? One way of answering this is to recognize that, although traumatic and ecstatic experiences superficially look like polar opposites, on closer look they have an essential feature in common: namely, that both are intensely emotional experiences. In line with this, Silber has suggested that, in this sense, the ecstatic experience itself can be "traumatic."[4] This is to say that from an ego psychological point of view, both the traumatic and ecstatic experiences have in common the fact that in either case there is a relatively sudden, massive increase in psychic excitation. Moreover, this surge of stimulation severely taxes—indeed with the more potent hallucinogens goes beyond—the ordinary capacity of the ego to modulate, control, or otherwise assimilate the experience. Given this ego-state and the implied necessity to cope with the excessive stimulation, the drug user's consequent repetitive talk about and around drugs does seem in the service of the repetition-compulsion.

I should like to make one more general point regarding the habitual user's fascination with the drug mystique, namely, that it involves a narrowing and focusing of his reality experience that is perhaps more profound in effect than the widely touted "expansion of consciousness." This retreat from reality, incidentally, as well as the conspicuous narcissism it nurtures, is promoted explicitly by Timothy Leary and other spokesmen for the psychedelic cult in their injunction to "turn on" (with drugs), "tune in" (to another kind of reality), and "drop out" (of an increasingly ugly, and unsatisfactory adult world).[5] The habitual user's reality as it filters into him through his subculture indeed does seem different. This is not merely the "tuning in to another kind of reality" experience that occurs during the altered state of consciousness immediately following drug ingestion. Instead, it has to do more generally with the everyday life of the habitual user, that is, with the bulk of time when he is *not* under the direct pharmacological influence of drugs. For even during these "drug-free" periods, habitual users seem to be narrowly preoccupied with the drug mystique, to speak in a parochial jargon, to see the ordinary world as a nightmarish place and, in short, to be in a world of their own, emotionally apart and insulated from the ordinary problems of men. Mamlet also takes note of this when he holds that habitual drug use, rather than being a "consciousness *expanding*" experience, perhaps more importantly, seems instead to be a "consciousness *limiting*" one.[6] That is, the scope of the habitual user's reality experience is constricted in that other more ordinary and conventional reality encounters, such as commitment to work, school, heterosexual as well as more general social relationships either are grossly avoided or otherwise severely

[3] M. B. Bowers, Jr. and D. X. Freedman, 'Psychedelic' Experiences in Acute Psychoses, *Arch. Gen. Psychiat.*, 15: 244, 1966.

[4] E. Silber, Chevy Chase, Maryland, personal communication, November 1966.

[5] J. Siegel, "The New Sound: Tune In, Turn On, and Take Over," *The Village Voice*, Nov. 7, 1966, p. 3.

[6] L. N. Mamlet, 'Consciousness Limiting' Side Effects of 'Consciousness Expanding Drugs', *Presented at the Annual Meeting, American Orthopsychiatric Association*, Washington, D.C., 1967.

limited. Put another way, the habitual user's life space is so filled by the drug mystique that little room is left for anything else.

To turn now to the question of why they use drugs, students offer a tantalizing variety of answers. Whether these answers really explain why they use drugs is another question. Many of the students' answers serve only to raise more questions.

Before listing some of the answers students do give, it should be noted that reasons for using drugs seem to vary depending on (1) whether the student involved is a casual experimenter or an habitual user; (2) whether the drug involved is an hallucinogen or an amphetamine or barbiturate and (3) the adequacy of the student's personal and social adjustment.

Without attempting to categorize them in terms of these three factors, reasons students have given for using drugs include:

(a) to make a show of independence from parents or the "bourgeois, middle-class" establishment generally;

(b) to show their contempt and disdain for the older generation and to shock adults in general and their parents in particular; [As an interesting sidelight, sexual promiscuity, for some students, has become such a commonplace that it no longer has shock-value.]

(c) curiosity ("just to see what it's all about") and influence of friends;

(d) and for using marihuana:

(1) it is a "cool" thing to do and shows that one is a "swinger"; for "kicks"

(2) its illegality shows that one is not afraid to challenge "authority" and to take "risks"

(3) compared to liquor, marihuana is less harmful, is a "cheap date," gives a cleaner "high," is easier to "come down" from, and has no hangover

(e) and for using LSD and other hallucinogens (to some extent including marihuana as well) their reasons include:

(1) self-help, that is, a sort of "magic pill" do-it-yourself psychotherapy. Such students assume, almost always erroneously, that self-exploration leads to self-discovery, particularly regarding repressed childhood traumatic experiences. They further assume that uncovering such experiences will solve virtually all of their problems.

(2) self-exploration of a "creative" sort, that is, use of drugs to increase one's understanding and appreciation of the arts.

(3) seeing an "acid trip" as an adventure in brinkmanship, that is, as a counterphobic, whistling-in-the-dark sort of confrontation of repressed material in one's unconscious.

(4) A cultist sort of religious belief in its magical powers.

(5) a belief that sexual sensation is enhanced by these drugs.

I wish to suggest that the reasons students give for using drugs seem related to issues of ego identity, values and autonomy and more generally to the complex tasks of late adolescence as a whole. Consider, for instance, such reasons as self-exploration, self-discovery, and self-help; or consider the search for adventurous or creative experiences. Are these not ill-conceived manifestations of a quest for identity and a sense of personal meaning? And is not drug habituation itself an attempt at resolution of the identity crisis by flirting with, if not in part choosing a negative identity, that is, an identity perversely based on elements that had been presented to the youngster as most undesirable?[7] And is not the "Hippie" movement iself a collective attempt to institutionalize negative identity elements on a grand scale?

Such students tend to regard even the most toned down, patently nonmoralistic medical statements on the dangers of drug abuse as just one more example of older generation propaganda aimed at brainwashing them. Others may take a less explicitly negativistic position but nonetheless dismiss such educational approaches, for example, as the misguided efforts of misinformed "squares who really don't know what the drug scene is all about."

Aside from the small number of potential habitual users, however, there is the vast majority of students who either have not yet tried drugs, or whose involvement with drugs is as yet

[7] E. H. Erikson, The Problem of Identity. *Psychol. Issues*, 1: 131, 1959.

only casual. Such students know relatively little about drugs beyond what they have learned via campus rumor mills or the public news media. With some notable exceptions, these sources of information either exaggerate the hazards of drugs or, on the other hand, extol their magical powers. The student who is exposed to these claims and counter-claims ordinarily has little in the way of responsible, balanced, authoritative information on which to base a decision as to whether or not he will use drugs. And, for better or worse, it *is* the student's decision.

In line with this, I would argue that the college administration has a responsibility, indeed an obligation, to inform students of the potential hazards of drugs and of *administration policies* about illicit drug use. This is based on the assumption that availability of facts enhances responsible choice and possible mastery of a situation otherwise fraught with misinformation or unknowns.

PART TWO PERSONAL HEALTH

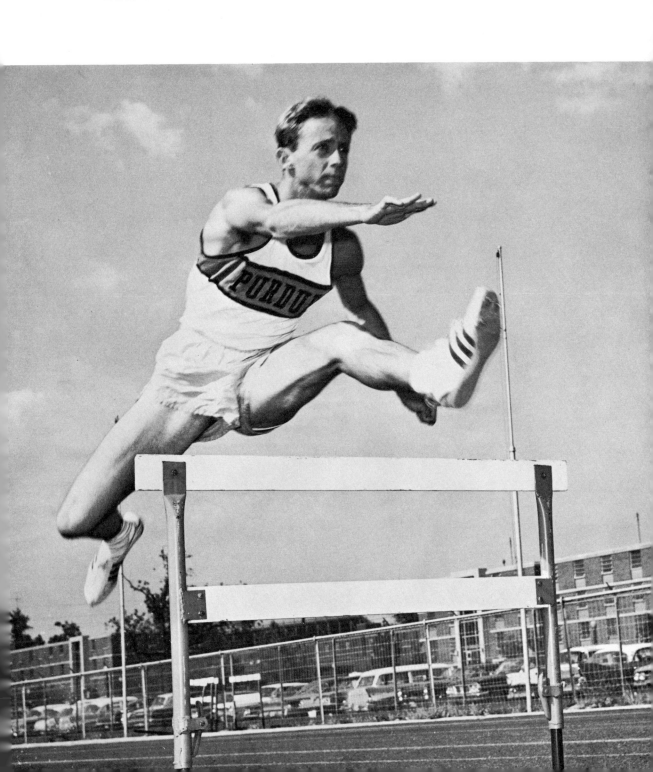

OVERLEAF
Physical fitness, a significant aspect of total well-being, has exercise as one of its essential elements. (Purdue University Photographic Services)

7

PHYSICAL FITNESS—
PERSONAL FITNESS

GOVERNMENTAL CONCERN WITH THE PHYSICAL fitness of its youth has often, but not always, been stimulated by military considerations. Rejection rates of young men deemed medically unfit for military service have aroused considerable alarm about the "flabbiness" of American youth.

In response to this widespread attitude, President John F. Kennedy, in 1961, appointed a President's Council on Youth Fitness and issued a Presidential Message on this subject. (See page 105.)

He further defined physical fitness as ". . . a broad quality involving medical and dental supervision and care, immunization and other protection against disease, proper nutrition, adequate rest, relaxation, good health practices, sanitation, and other aspects of healthful living. *Exercise* is an essential element to achieving physical fitness."

In this chapter we shall pay particular attention to exercise as a means of achieving those desirable physical qualities of strength, stamina, and endurance.

It should be noted that there is a more limited standard of physical fitness than the one quoted at the beginning of this chapter. In this narrower concept physical fitness is equated with ability to meet standardized physical fitness tests, and emphasis is placed upon neuromuscular development through strictly defined periods of "vigorous activity" and rigorously outlined sets of exercises.

There is no achieving physical fitness or personal fitness simply by talking about it. The muscles of the body, supported by its other organs, must be put to work or into play in order to attain measurable increases in physical fitness. (Maximum oxygen intake per unit of body weight provides one such objective measurement.) It has been adequately demonstrated that 8 to 12 weeks of rigorous physical conditioning for the "normal" but relatively inactive individual will significantly augment his physical fitness, as measured by the oxygen intake and other tests. Very few college students are prepared to sacrifice 2 or 3 months of their life solely to achieving a measurably high degree of physical fitness. Other more gradual and educationally coordinated methods are in order.

Physical Education is Part of a Great Tradition

One of the opportunities of college life is to learn how to improve and maintain physical fitness for a lifetime. The primary responsibility for this teaching is usually charged to the department of physical education, although other departments may share in the task.

It is significant to realize that physical education in its broad sense is part of the great tradition of education and learning. It has an ancient classical and a chivalric background too. Greek sculpture evoked the ideal of the strong, graceful body; Olympic games their interest in physical

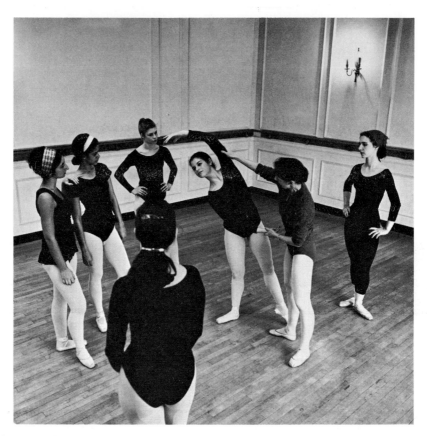

THE AMOUNT AND KIND OF EXERCISE you take will be determined by your own motivations. Dancing is a fine example of recreational exercise. (Photograph by Rogers-MONKMEYER)

fitness. Training for knighthood in the Middle Ages included that phase of physical education which we would today call physical training. The battle of Waterloo, said the victorious Duke of Wellington, was won on the playing fields of Eton. The rise of modern Germany, following the Napoleonic wars, was linked with the development of the gymnastic *Turnverein* (turners or tumblers) movement. The memoirs of World War II's Field Marshal Montgomery are full of analogies from the world of sports.

The tradition of the dance, which is part of physical education combined with esthetics, goes back farther and earlier than any of the rest. Dance is among the most ancient of art forms. Understanding the meaning of dance forms helps us to perceive the cultures in which they originate.

Physical education, is an integral part of human learning. Its primary though not its only goal is to help students attain and maintain that degree of physical fitness which leads to academic and later-life accomplishments. Today the subject area of physical education draws upon the same scientific disciplines that are the basis of the art of medicine and other academic subjects catalogued as biology, psychology, nutrition. Physical education in college has important practical aspects, such as the supervision of athletics and the provision of sports programs for many (or most) students. In conducting these and other programs in which "learning by doing" is the basic methodology, physical education provides for the mental health, social and recreational needs of students. It should be understood therefore that physical education does not preach or

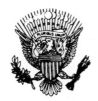

A PRESIDENTIAL MESSAGE
On the Physical Fitness of Youth

The strength of our democracy is no greater than the collective well-being of our people. The vigor of our country is no stronger than the vitality and will of all our countrymen. The level of physical, mental, moral and spiritual fitness of every American citizen must be our constant concern.

The need for increased attention to the physical fitness of our youth is clearly established. Although today's young people are fundamentally healthier than the youth of any previous generation, the majority have not developed strong, agile bodies. The softening process of our civilization continues to carry on its persistent erosion.

It is of great importance, then, that we take immediate steps to ensure that every American child be given the opportunity to make and keep himself physically fit— fit to learn, fit to understand, to grow in grace and stature, to fully live.

In answering this challenge, we look to our schools and colleges as the decisive force in a renewed national effort to strengthen the physical fitness of youth. Many of our schools have long been making strenuous efforts to assist our young people attain and maintain health and physical fitness. But we must do more. We must expand and improve our health services, health education and physical education. We must increase our facilities and the time devoted to physical activity. We must invigorate our curricula and give high priority to a crusade for excellence in health and fitness.

To members of school boards, school administrators, teachers and pupils themselves, I am directing this urgent call to strengthen all programs which contribute to the physical fitness of our youth. I strongly urge each school to adopt the three specific recommendations of my Council on Youth Fitness:

1. Identify the physically underdeveloped pupil and work with him to improve his physical capacity.

2. Provide a minimum of fifteen minutes of vigorous activity every day for all pupils.

3. Use valid fitness tests to determine pupils' physical abilities and evaluate their progress.

The adoption of these recommendations by our schools will ensure the beginning of a sound basic program of physical developmental activity.

In our total fitness efforts the schools, of course, will not stand alone. I urge that in all communities there be more coordination between the schools and the community, parents, educators and civic-minded citizens in carrying forward a resourceful, vigorous program for physical fitness—a program that will stir the imagination of our youth, calling on their toughest abilities, enlisting their greatest enthusiasm—a program which will enable them to build the energy and strength that is their American heritage.

John F. Kennedy (1961)

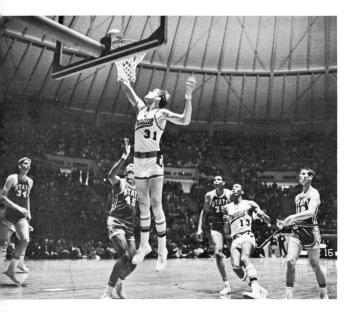

IN COLLEGIATE SPORTS the motions of the body frequently reach their summit of strength and endurance. (Purdue University Photographic Service)

make at least the following "passing" scores on the three tests:

Men	Women
3 pullups	8 modified pullups
14 situps	10 situps
4 "squat thrusts"	3 "squat thrusts"
in 10 seconds	in 10 seconds

Advantages and Values of Physical Fitness

Underlying most current discussions on the advantages and values of physical fitness is the assumption that the conditions of American civilization have generally reduced the need for physical activity almost to a vanishing point. Machines do most of the work that used to be done by human muscle power. To mail a letter, one jumps into an automobile and drives around the block. The basic argument here is that better programs are necessary for assuring the adequate amount of physical activity that used to be part of everyday living. (A busy housewife or a farmer still gets plenty of daily physical activity!) For many people, and some college students, however, "regular exercise, adapted to one's physical potentialities, represents a return to the wisdom of the ages" (Jean Mayer).

The best reason for developing the strength, stamina, and endurance that mark a high degree of physical fitness is the personal satisfaction one gets in doing it. The immediate reward is a sense of physical and mental well-being. As C. B. ("Bud") Wilkinson has put it: "We now recognize [physical fitness] as a quality which contributes to our social and intellectual effectiveness. We are awakening to the realization that man's physical function is subtly related to his mental, moral, and spiritual processes. What affects one affects the other."

Another, less appreciated outcome of programs of physical fitness, physical education, and *dance* is that it develops one's *kinesthetic* intelligence. (*Kine* means movement; *esthetic,* beautiful. The word as a whole may be taken to mean "pleasure in movement.") In the conclusion of a brilliant essay, based on studies of "stylized" (that is,

teach exercise for its own sake; it simply uses this as one of many modalities for helping students to develop their total personalities. This is in the best academic tradition.

Are You Physically "Underdeveloped"? You may not care whether you are physically "developed" or "underdeveloped." Or you may possibly be afraid that you are *not* up to standard in physical fitness and development when in fact you are above it. The President's Council on Youth Fitness has developed three standard screening tests for "physical fitness." If you take these tests you can quickly and easily classify yourself as up to, above, or below par in physical fitness, defined as physical strength, flexibility, and agility.

The three screening tests are (1) *pullups,* testing arm and shoulder strength (there is a modified pullup for women), (2) *situps,* testing flexibility and abdominal strength, and (3) *"squat thrusts,"* probing your agility. The tests are fully pictured and described on pages 108 and 109.

If you are at the "freshman stage" of personal and physical development (age 17), you should volitional) human movements and inquiring into the nature of movement as a significant form of human experience, Drs. Eleanor Metheny and Lois Ellfeldt declare:

Kinesthetic intelligence is one of the significant forms of human intelligence and kinesymbolic knowledge makes a unique contribution to man's comprehension of reality by adding to the store of meanings that are the basis of the significance man finds in his life as a human being. . . . In this context physical education—as we prefer to call it, "movement education"—can be identified as one of the forms of liberal education, comparable with music and the other nonverbal arts as a source of one of the kinds of meaning that enrich man's comprehension of reality as he knows it.

This point may perhaps be emphasized by an anecdote about the great Russian physiologist, Ivan Pavlov. When asked why he spent so much time working in his garden, he answered: "To give joy to my muscles."

Participation in athletics, sports, and games requires at least a minimum degree of physical fitness or physical readiness; yet more desirable qualities are developed *through* participation. Dr. Leonard A. Larson, of the University of Wisconsin, has stated:

The team is a miniature society, containing all the elements of democratic human relations, ranging from respect for the individual personality to group self-government.

Physical education and athletics draw upon and contribute to the philosophies of American culture and contribute to some of the important goals of education: the development of confidence through achievement, understanding of human relations, knowledge and care of the body, and preparation for effective use of increased leisure time. Opportunities in these areas should be offered to all individuals from their early years, when they may begin the foundations for sports participation throughout their lifetime.

Another potent set of arguments for physical fitness and physical activity is that they may decrease a tendency toward the onset of certain diseases and thus increase human longevity. In particular, it is argued that long-term exercise

may have a protective effect on the cardiovascular (heart and blood vessels) system and possibly reduce the level of cholesterol in the blood serum. Two distinguished physicians, Dr. Hans Kraus and Dr. Wilhelm Raab, have written a useful book on the role of physical *in*activity as a causative factor in the origin of a variety of diseases. The book is titled: *Hypokinetic Disease.* The term "hypokinetic," coined by Dr. Kraus, is from Greek roots and means "caused by insufficient movement or motion." An American heart specialist, Dr. Joseph B. Wolffe, of Philadelphia, confirms their point, with which many physicians would agree, thus:

After more than three decades of experience as a cardiologist, I am convinced, from empirical as well as clinical observation, that there is a direct correlation between the sedentary, pushbutton character of our culture and the constantly rising incidence of coronary artery disease and other forms of cardiovascular disturbance. . . .

We, of both the medical and non-medical disciplines . . . are duty-bound to imbue the present and growing generation with knowledge for fitness—for *total* fitness, physical, moral, intellectual and emotional. . . . Too many sectors of our leadership reveal a tragic myopia on the subject of fitness. . . . Even among some educators there is a compulsion, in our mechanized, materially oriented era, to place all emphasis on the physical sciences, on mathematical and technological training, at the expense of the healthy development of the nervous, cardiovascular, and other systems of the body so vital for successful coping with one's environment.

Exercise: How Much? What Kind?

A great variety of graded programs and corresponding tests for physical fitness, in its narrower sense, have been developed and applied. For example, a complex series of rating scales for physical capacity (fitness) are included in the *5BX (Five Basic Exercises) Plan for Physical Fitness,* a program originated and promulgated by the Royal Canadian Air Force. The *5BX Plan* and its companion program for women, *XBX,* a ten exercise plan, became internationally popular in the early 1960's. The use of *5BX* and *XBX* pro-

Three Screening Tests for Physical Fitness (arm and shoulder strength, flexibility and abdominal strength, and agility)

IA: Pullups—Men

Equipment.—A bar of sufficient height, comfortable to grip.

Starting position.—Grasp the bar with palms facing forward; hang with arms and legs fully extended. Feet must be free of floor.

Action:

1. Pull body up with the arms until the chin is placed over the bar.
2. Lower body until the elbows are fully extended.
3. Repeat the exercise as many times as you can.

Rules:

1. The pull must not be a snap movement.
2. Knees must not be raised.
3. Kicking the legs is not permitted.
4. The body must not swing.
5. One complete pullup is counted each time you place your chin over the bar.

To pass: 3 pullups.

IB: Modified Pullups—Women

Equipment.—Any bar adjustable in height and comfortable to grip. A piece of pipe, placed between two stepladders and held securely, may be used.

Starting position.—adjust height of bar to chest level. Grasp bar with palms facing out. Extend the legs under the bar, keeping the body and knees straight. The heels are on the foor. Fully extend the arms so they form an angle of 90 degrees with the body line. Brace your heels if necessary to prevent slipping.

Action:

1. Pull body up with the arms until the *chest* touches the bar.
2. Lower body until elbows are fully extended.
3. Repeat the exercise as many times as you can.

Rules:

1. The body must be kept straight.
2. The chest *must* touch the bar and the arms must then be *fully extended.*
3. No resting is permitted.
4. One pullup is counted each time the chest touches the bar.

To pass: 8 modified pullups.

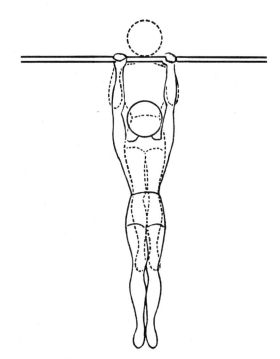

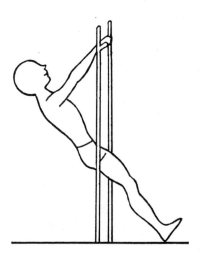

II: Situps (Men and Women)

Starting Position.—Lie down on your back with your legs extended, feet about one foot apart. Your hands, with fingers interlaced, should be grasped behind your neck. Keep your heels on the floor. This can be accomplished by having a partner hold your feet down (as shown in the illustration), or by placing a heavy sofa cushion or gym mat on your feet, or by putting your feet under the edge of a low sofa.

Action:

1. Sit up and turn the trunk to the left. Touch the right elbow to the left knee.
2. Return to starting position.
3. Sit up and turn the trunk to the right. Touch the left elbow to the right knee.
4. Return to the starting position.
5. Repeat as many times as possible.
6. One complete situp is counted each time you return to the starting position.

To pass: Men—14 situps.
        Women—10 situps.

III: Squat Thrust (Men and Women)

(You will need either a partner or an automatic timer to time yourself in this exercise.)

Equipment.—A stopwatch, or a watch with a sweep-second hand.

Starting Position.—Stand at attention.

Action:

1. Bend knees and place hands on the floor in front of the feet. Arms may be between, outside or in front of the bent knees.
2. Thrust the legs back far enough so that the body is perfectly straight from shoulders to feet (the pushup position).
3. Return to squat position.
4. Return to erect position.

Scoring.—Your partner gives the starting signal, "Ready!—Go!" On "Go" you begin. Your partner counts each squat thrust. At the end of 10 seconds, he says, "Stop".

Rule: You must return to the erect position of attention at the completion of each squat thrust.

To pass: Men—4 squat thrusts in 10 seconds
        Women—3 squat thrusts in 10 seconds

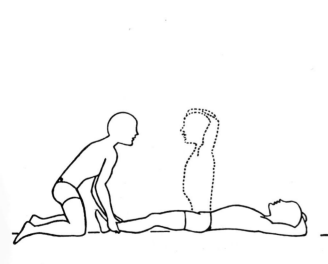

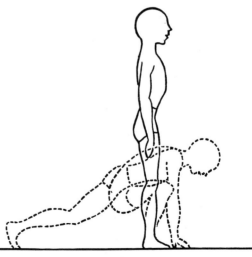

grams, as outlined in slim printed manuals, was claimed to have eliminated "desk-bound flabbiness" in many parts of the world.

The *5BX* plan presents a graded series of relatively simple calisthenic exercises which are to be self-administered in only 11 minutes a day and can be done without equipment other than the determination to keep up with them. Since all exercise is (by definition) physical effort, and since the human animal often resists such effort, the eventual value of *5BX*, like Walter Camp's "Daily Dozen" of the 1920's, cannot be judged.

Over half of the *5BX* time is devoted to "running in place" (stationary run) with various intermittent kicks and leaps. Also included are various bending and stretching exercises, starting from the erect position and from several floor positions.

It takes a great deal of motivation and willpower to keep up a solitary program of calisthenic exercises. It has also been demonstrated that the presence of spectators or, even more so, participation in a group or class steps up performance of muscular tasks.

How much and what kind of exercise to take each day is a question that has confronted you, and that you have answered, from the time you were learning to walk. When you were a toddler, exercise was the main business of your life. You considered it play. You have been making decisions about exercise, whether work or play, all through your education. Some exercise was probably forced on you—in the form of household chores and compulsory "gym" classes. But basically you have been deciding for yourself how much physical activity and what kind of exercise you were willing to seek or accept. We may divide this exercise into three categories: (1) the inescapable exercise of *daily living;* (2) exercise accepted by reason of *occupation;* and (3) exercise chosen for *recreation.* As a college student you are still making these daily decisions about exercise, and you will continue to do so for the rest of your life. By studying the facts about exercise, physical fitness, and physical education, you will be able to make more rational choices.

Perhaps the only bit of general advice that can be given is this: take *enough* exercise, with pleasure, to feel that your body is toned up to a pitch of well-being. But do not take so much that physical fatigue constantly overburdens your capacity for the enjoyment of life. A moderate amount of exercise daily is far better than sporadic bursts of physical activity.

The amount and kind of exercise you take will be determined by your own motivations, or necessities. You can exercise (1) for fun, (2) to keep in shape, (3) to do your job, (4) to gain strength, (5) to improve your figure or physique, or (6) to reduce. You should know that exercise *alone* will not take off weight, although it may be employed (especially as "spot" exercises) to change body contours. Nor will exercise *alone* maintain health, although it is a step in the right direction.

Regular exercise in moderation keeps the body flexible and supple. The abdomen, for example, can be kept reasonably flat and smooth by bending and stretching. Exercise also keeps up "muscle tone" (see page 120). A further advantage of regular exercise is that it stimulates the general physiology of the body, especially the functions of the circulatory system, the respiratory system, and the excretory system (all of which we shall consider in the next chapter.)

Vigorous exercise can be considered useful up to about the ages of 35 to 40. Increasing age should be no bar to *some* regular physical activity. Older people should be encouraged to take exercises within the range of their physical capacities.

We have by no means reached a complete pushbutton stage of civilization, but the ever-increasing introduction of labor-saving devices, linked with a growth of specialization of occupation among the white collar classes, is producing a more sedentary civilization. There is a limit to the amount of sitting a person should do for his own good. On the other hand there is evidence, adduced by Raymond Pearl and others, that lifetime occupations which demand continuous output of physical energy tend to shorten life.

The "student life" can be an extremely sedentary occupation, and students must often be urged to make special efforts to tone up their muscles and bodies generally by taking some agreeable exercise. Curiously, the students who protest most about compulsory physical education are usually the ones who need it most.

Respect the Fatigue Point. For a different group of college students and adults the problem of exercise resolves itself into the problem of not overdoing it. A rule of thumb for this group is: exercise to the point of mild fatigue, but not beyond it.

The amount of fatigue produced is probably the best measure of the amount of exercise that ought to be taken. On this score a statement prepared by the American Association for Health, Physical Education, and Recreation offers sound guidance.[1]

"The ability to recuperate after exercise is a good guide at any age. Recuperation should be reasonably prompt. If (1) breathing and heart rate are still greatly accelerated at the end of ten minutes after exercise, and if (2) there is marked weakness or fatigue persisting after a two-hour rest period, (3) restlessness with broken sleep after retiring for the night, or (4) a sense of definite fatigue the day following, the exercise has been too severe or too prolonged for that person in his present stage of physical training and strength."

Choice of Exercise for Recreation. The best choice of exercise is that which gives the most satisfaction. Many factors must be considered to determine suitability of physical activity, but one should certainly like the sports he chooses. There is little to be gained in teaching a girl who wants to go swimming how to swing a pair of Indian clubs instead.

Exercise should be fun! Exercise is part of the normal desire for play that inhabits the human psyche. In young children play and exercise are nearly synonymous.

Several important studies have shown that sports and games are definitely better than calisthenics and apparatus work in conditioning men for physical fitness. Wilbur's study of college freshmen, for example, indicated that games were better than formal gymnastics in building strength in the arms and shoulder girdle, in establishing body coordination, agility, and control, and in reaching a higher degree of general physical fitness.[2]

Recreation has been defined as "activity for pleasure." It achieves relaxation of mind and muscle. The range of recreational exercises is far broader than most people think. Here are some of the possibilities: walking, swimming, dancing, skating, rowing, canoeing, fencing, bicycling, horseback riding, tennis, squash, handball, softball, volleyball, badminton, skiing, sailing, hunting, pingpong, archery, bowling, fishing, gardening, croquet, shuffleboard, horseshoe pitching, hiking, jogging, climbing, and golf. How many of these recreations have you tried? All of these can be coeducational if desired.

Walking is the most flexible and natural of all forms of exercise. Dancing also is a beneficial form of exercise, especially folk-dancing and "modern dance." Social dancing has its place too. It is believed that the rhythms of dance can afford release of emotional and psychosexual tensions rather than unduly heightening them.

There is an advantage in learning sports and obtaining reasonable proficiency at games that you can play for fun for many years after college.

A contrast between work and play activity is also advisable. People whose occupations are generally sedentary and indoors should choose games and sports that take them out of doors and offer opportunity for the exercise of trunk, leg, and arm muscles. Conversely, the man who stands on his feet all day should select recreations that require a minimum of leg work.

Two New Exercise Hobbies. The late 1960's saw the introduction of two new exercise hobbies: jogging and aerobics.

Jogging has three meanings: (1) a steady or an easy-paced run alternating with breath-catching periods of walking; (2) a kind of running, generally a slow regular trot that has been described

[1] Committee report, *The Role of Exercise in Physical Fitness,* American Association for Health, Physical Education, and Recreation (Washington, D.C., 1943).

[2] E. A. Wilbur, "A Comparative Study of Physical Fitness Indices as Measured by Two Programs of Physical Education; the Sports Method and the Apparatus Method," *Research Quarterly* (October 1943).

as the next step up from walking; (3) an entire program of physical fitness, as set forth in a book by William J. Bowerman, track coach at the University of Oregon, W. E. Harris, M. D., a heart specialist, and others. They have provided a detailed instructional guide to jogging, which is one effective kind of physical fitness program. Among the advantages of jogging as a pleasant form of exercise are that it is free, easy, relaxing fun; it can be done alone or in groups; and it is especially good for the heart and lungs.

Schedules are at the heart of the jogging program. It moves from the short and simple to the gradually more difficult. Train, don't strain, say the originators of the system. Here, by way of example, is the schedule for the first week's program for men and women in less than average physical condition:

Week I

Pace 1 equals 110 yards at 55 to 60 seconds, or 25 to 30 seconds, for 55 yards.

Monday, Wednesday, and Friday
(Total distance ½ mile)

			Pace
(1) Jog 55 yards	Walk 55 yards	4 times	1
(2) Jog 110 yards	Walk 110 yards		1
(3) Jog 55 yards	Walk 55 yards	2 times	1

Tuesday, Thursday, Saturday, and Sunday

A 5 to 10 minute walk and some easy stretching exercises.

From this primary program, the distance, speed, and amount of jogging are gradually increased. By the final (twelfth) week of jogging for men or women of better than average physical condition, the following schedule has been reached:

Week XII

Pace 4 = 110 yards at 25 to 30 seconds
Pace 5 = 110 yards at 20 to 25 seconds

Monday
(Total distance 4 to 5 miles)

			Pace
Jog 110 yards	Walk 110 yards	2 times	4 or 5
Jog 880 yards	Walk 110 yards	2 times	4 or 5
Jog 330, 220, 110 yards	Walk as needed	4 times	4 or 5
Jog 110 yards	Walk 110 yards	3 times	4 or 5

Jogging is not a competitive sport. It is a simple method of training for improved physical condition. You should, therefore, avoid overtraining and strenuous *daily* jogging. Work hard one day and rest the next.

Aerobics. Aerobics is the second of the recent plans put forward for increasing physical fitness. It has been described in some detail by the man who developed it, Major Kenneth H. Cooper, M.D., of the U.S. Air Force Medical Corps.

The key to the concept, he states, is oxygen. Aerobics means literally "with *oxygen.*" It is the antonym of the word "anaerobic" which means "without oxygen." (Certain bacteria can live only in an anaerobic environment.)

The human body can store food, but it cannot store oxygen. Cutting off his oxygen supply for a few minutes will cause a man to die.

In some bodies, Major Cooper points out, the means for delivering oxygen is weak and limited in resources. Hence the energy demands of the body surpass the body's capacity to produce it.

Most, if not all, people can produce enough energy to perform daily activities. However, when they are forced into more vigorous exercise, they can't keep up. They become "winded" and fatigued at very low levels of effort. The aerobic pattern of exercises which Major Cooper recommends has the special virtue of building up the cardiovascular and respiratory systems of the body so that they will supply oxygen in whatever amount it is needed.

The aerobic system is a *point* count for different physical activities. You have to make 30 points a week to keep up with the system. You win points by exercising within a definite time limit. The categories of exercise are: running, swimming, cycling, walking, running in place, and engaging in fast games of handball, squash, or basketball. Cooper provides standards against which you may gauge your own condition. What is the distance, he asks, that you can cover in 12 minutes running or running and walking?

If you cover:	you are in fitness category:
Less than 1.0 miles	I Very poor
1.0 to 1.24 miles	II Poor
1.25 to 1.49 miles	III Fair
1.50 to 1.74 miles	IV Good
1.75 or more miles	V Excellent

Answers to Some Practical Questions about Exercise. *What good are reducing exercises?* They help to distribute body fat, cutting down hip measurements, for example, but they are of little value for losing weight. You would have to walk or scrub floors for about half an hour to work off as many calories as you get in a slice of bread. You would have to chop wood hard for about an hour to get rid of the caloric energy in a malted milk (around 500 calories).

Dare a woman exercise during her menstrual period? Yes, but not too strenuously. Both violent exercise and extreme fatigue should be avoided.

What about exercise after illness or accident? Follow your doctor's orders and advice. Present practice is to avoid abuse of bed rest and get patients, including surgical, obstetrical, and even heart patients, back on their feet as soon as possible. However, some infections (notably virus infections, such as hepatitis) leave their victims in a weakened condition for a long time and prohibit anything but minimal physical activity even though the patient thinks he "feels fine." The acute or convalescent stages of most diseases interdict vigorous exercise.

What about exercise and meals? Among the effects of exercise are changes in the distribution of the blood and depression of gastric secretion. These effects are related to the excitement of competition as well as to sheer physical activity. Heavy exercise immediately after meals, therefore, appears to interfere with digestion.

Therapeutic Exercise The range of exercise is wide and certainly not just recreational or solely for physical development or for training in sports and dance. The experts in rehabilitation, physical therapy, and corrective physical education have developed large batteries of specialized exercises and apparatus to retrain, strengthen, and restore to normal (or nearly normal) and useful function muscles ravaged by a disease, such as poliomyelitis, or by an accident.

Therapeutic exercise as an adjunct to other methods of medical treatment has been developed to a point where once hopeless, bedridden invalids are again able to walk, work, and live almost normally. This field of rehabilitation as a "third phase of medicine" was pioneered and enhanced in veterans' hospitals during World War II, especially by Dr. Howard Rusk. "Dynamic therapeutics," including therapeutic exercise, often achieves heartening results with shattered human bodies. Corrective and therapeutic exercise is administered under close supervision for definite, graded, medical purposes; and it serves high ends. It is not, however, the type of exercise a healthy young adult would normally undertake for pleasure.

Isometric Versus Isotonic Exercise. No current discussion of exercise would be complete without some exposition of isometric exercise and comparison of it with isotonic exercise. Isometric exercise, under that name, gained popularity in the 1950's and 1960's. In some respects it is a rationalization and amplification of certain body-building techniques introduced almost two generations ago to help create the image of the heavily muscled male physique. Isometric exercise has also been commercialized and undignified to the extent of advertising it as "instant exercise," promoted with such promises as "Imagine a 6-second exercise that helps keep you fit better than 24 pushups!"

The essence of isometric exercise is the practice of muscular *contractions* to the utmost of one's ability—maximum, all-out bursts of effort for a brief period of time, usually 6 to 15 seconds. You push, pull, press, or lift against an object that does not move. This object might be as simple as a door-frame;[3] it could also be an isometric

[3] "Isometric Exercises To Build Your Strength "in *Your Guide to Physical Fitness,* 16 pp., n.d. Distributed jointly by the American Football Coaches Association and the Tea Council of the United States (16 E. 56th St., New York 22, N.Y.).

A SIMPLE SERIES OF ISOMETRIC EXERCISES, ILLUSTRATED

The simple series of isometric (static) exercises pictured here was developed by the American Football Coaches Association. It is primarily for developing added strength, when used in conjunction with isotonic (dynamic) exercises, calisthenics, weight-lifting (graded resistance exercises), and regular football drills.

Each of the 10 isometric exercises shown here is performed for only 6 seconds, once a day, later twice a day. The crux of the system is that each push, pull, press, or lift against the immovable object must be done with *maximum, all-out effort*. The equipment needed is simple—a convenient doorway, a towel, possibly a box or stool—and the time required is short.

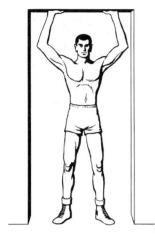

Exercise 1
PRESS IN DOORWAY: Stand in the doorway (on a box or stool if necessary). Bend your arms. Lock your knees and hips. Push with all your might, maximum effort, against the top of the doorway.

Exercise 2
LEG PRESS: Stand in doorway (on box or stool if necessary). Keep arms straight, legs bent. Legs press upward with maximum force against the top of the doorway.

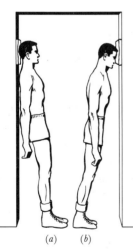

Exercise 3
NECK DEVELOPER: Place a folded towel between the back of your head and the door jamb, while you lean slightly backwards (*a*). Press the back of your head against the door jamb. Next put the folded towel between your forehead and the door jamb and press forward (*b*).

Exercise 4
NECK DEVELOPER (2): Put the unfolded towel around the back of your head and grasp the loose ends with both hands. At the same time push back with your head and pull forward with your arms.

(*a*) (*b*)

Exercise 5
ARM DEVELOPER: Rest one elbow against the door jamb. Then press against it as hard as you can with the opposite arm. Reverse arms. The purpose of this exercise is to develop the pushing muscles of the arm and shoulder.

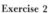

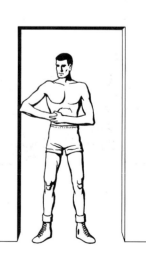

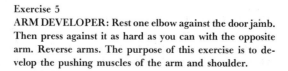

Exercise 6

SIDE PRESS: Place one hand on each side of the door frame. Push outward with both arms.

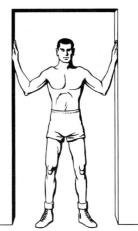

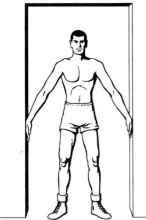

Exercise 7

LATERAL RAISE: Place the backs of your hands against the door frame, one on each side. Push outward with both hands. Purpose here is to develop shoulder muscles.

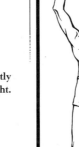

Exercise 8

PULL DOWN: Grasp the top of the door frame as tightly as you can with both hands. Keep arms and legs straight. Pull down as hard as you can.

Exercise 9

LEG PRESS: Sit in the door frame, back straight against one side, feet (complete heels and soles) tight against the other side, so that you are in a semi-sitting position. (See illustration). Press your back against one side of the door frame at the same time that you press your legs away from the other side.

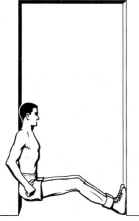

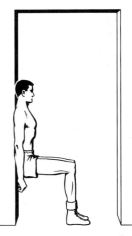

Exercise 10

STATIC WALL SIT: Place your back flat against the wall (door frame). Let your arms hang loosely at your sides. Bend your knees to assume sitting position. (See illustration). Press backwards.

rack,[4] a spring dynamometer for elbow flexion exercise,[5] a back dynamometer for spine extensor exercise,[6] bar bell or other weights too heavy to lift, or a fellow-student on your back.

Because of the lack of or little movement connected with them, isometric exercises are also called "static" exercises. In this they are in contrast to the better-known types of calisthenics, described as "dynamic," "ballistic," or "isotonic" exercises, all of which involve considerable free body movement. A simple example of the difference between isometric and isotonic exercise can be put this way:

Suppose your car is stuck in the mud. To release it, you get out and push against the back frame or bumper of the car as hard as you can, using (contracting) primarily your back and leg muscles. So long as the car does not move, thus requiring repeated contractions of a few sets of muscles, you are doing an isometric exercise. However, as soon as you manage to push hard enough to start the car moving out of the mud, you have crossed over from an isometric to an isotonic exercise. You are also moving many more muscles.

The principal and unquestioned outcome of isometric exercise is to increase the *strength* of the muscles exercised; it does so by an increase in tension; but exactly why the increments of strength increase as a result of tension has not been settled. Neuromuscular performance is not augmented along with the increase in strength, and may even be diminished.[7] Isometric training

did not improve performance in either the high jump[8] or the broad jump,[9] under controlled experiments. It has been concluded that there is a certain limited specificity to improvements in muscular proficiency achieved by isometric training. One investigator reports: "For example, if elbow flexion strength is tested with the elbow at the waist and also with the elbow overhead, then an [isometric] training program instituted with the elbow exercised at the waist, the result afterward will be an increased strength of the performance with the elbow at the waist, but no increase with the elbow overhead."[10] For training of athletes and for general physical conditioning isometric exercises are used along with isotonic exercises, skill trials, and other methods (sometimes graded resistance).

If they work, the isometric exercises increase the muscular strength factor in relatively little time. They do not always work, however, because the person doing them cannot always be sure that he is exerting maximum effort in his contractions. This subjective factor may be why some investigators have found an insignificant increase or no increase in muscular strength attributable to isometric contractions.

However, it is also possible that sufficient time to permit adequate test of the exercises has not been allowed. A person's rate of strength improvement, in isotonic as well as isometric exercises, depends primarily on the extent to which he *overloads* his muscles. It may be that in many reported studies of isometric exercises the overload principle has not been adequately applied. The work done per unit of time is the critical variable in extending muscular strength and also muscular endurance. Isotonic exercises are superior to isometric in developing muscular endurance; for the isometric exercises constrict blood and oxygen supplies.

There was a great burst of popularity for iso-

[4] F. A. Lindeburg, D. K. Edwards, and W. D. Heath, "Effect of Isometric Exercise on Standing Broad Jump Ability," *Research Quarterly,* 34: 4, 478–483 (December 1963).

[5] G. T. Adamson, "Effects of Isometric and Isotonic Exercise on Elbow Flexor and Spine Extensor Muscle Groups," p. 172 in *Health and Fitness in the Modern World,* a collection of papers presented at the Institute of Normal Human Anatomy in Rome, Italy. Chicago: The Athletic Institute (in cooperation with the American College of Sports Medicine), 1961.

[6] *Ibid.*

[7] W. Harrison Clarke, "Development of Volitional Muscle Strength as Related to Fitness," p. 200 in *Exercise and Fitness,* a collection of papers presented at the colloquium on exercise and fitness sponsored by the University of Illinois and the Athletic Institute, December 1959. Chicago: The Athletic Institute, 1960.

[8] Richard A. Berger, "Effects of Dynamic and Static Training on Vertical Jumping Ability," *Research Quarterly,* 34: 4, 419–424 (December 1963).

[9] Lindeburg, Edwards, and Heath, *loc. cit.*

[10] Laurence E. Morehouse, "Physiological Basis of Strength Development," in *Health and Fitness in the Modern World, op. cit.,* p. 193.

metric exercises in 1953, when two German investigators, Th. Hettinger and E. A. Mueller, announced that a single 6-second a day contraction against two-thirds strength resistance would increase muscle strength by 5% a week, by 50% in ten weeks![11] Later studies have not verified this percentage gain, and a more realistic figure is said to be nearer 2% per week.

The apparent simplicity and quick results of isometric exercises, as reported by the early investigators, have attracted considerable research attention. Some negative results have occurred; for example, decrease in muscular strength, muscular pain and damage. Pierson and Rasch reported the injurious consequences of maximal (twice a day) isometric arm exercises, undertaken experimentally by 15 upperclass medical students, 11 of whom soon developed sore arms.[12] On the other hand some investigators, notably Flint, consider isometric exercises safer than conventional "ballistic" (body-movement) exercises, especially for children.[13] With controlled static (isometric) movements, she believes, there is less risk of going beyond the limits of extensibility of the muscle. Pain would stop the movement before any injury occurred whereas ballistic movement cannot always be stopped the instant pain is felt.

Isometric exercises play an important part in another field of usefulness, namely in *corrective* physical education, physical therapy, and rehabilitation practice.

Collegiate Sports and Athletics

The incessant motions of the human body reach their summit of strength and endurance in competitive athletics and their peak of grace in ballet dancing. There are some interesting borderline events, like bullfighting and figure skating, which are both esthetic and athletic.

The interest in sports and competitive games, especially among young men, is nearly universal. Early American Indians had their lacrosse and other games; soccer teams draw millions of spectators in Europe; and American colleges and universities have their football and other varsity teams. Interest in athletics would persist whether it was formally under the jurisdiction of universities or outside their scope—as in professional sports.

College athletics, however, periodically come under fire as being "overemphasized." While abuses are possible, colleges and college students appear to have far more to gain than to lose by maintaining a high interest in varsity-athletic and intramural-sports programs. Sports for all is a better program than athletics for a few, but both programs could be carried through in most colleges and universities.

There are values in intercollegiate athletics beyond the direct benefits of the comparatively few varsity athletes engaged. They provide a rallying point for "school spirit," which means a sense of belonging to a recognized group. They help bridge the gap between successive generations of college men and women, for alumni are often as much interested in college teams as undergraduates. Something also can be said for college sports, as William James put it, as "moral substitutes for war." When 50,000 or more people of all ages, on a brisk Saturday afternoon, concentrate on the outcome of an intercollegiate football game and feel with one another in victory or defeat, a psychotherapeutic event of some magnitude occurs.

Athletics, sports, and dance undoubtedly increase the physiological capacities of those who engage in them, particularly heart, lung, and muscle power. The trained athlete is capable of supporting the following changes in his circulatory system during vigorous competition: the stroke volume of his heart may be increased threefold; the total output of the heart may be increased tenfold; his heart rate may double; his blood pressure may increase by half; the total volume of his blood (and the red cells in it) may increase by perhaps 10%.

[11] Th. Hettinger and E. A. Mueller, "Muscle Testing and Muscle Training," *Muskelleistung und Muskeltraining, Arbeitsphysiologie,* **15**: 2, 111 (October 1953).

[12] W. R. Pierson and P. J. Rasch, "The Injurious Consequences of Maximal Isometric Arm Exercises," *Journal of the American Physical Therapy Association,* **45**: 582–583 (1963).

[13] M. Marilyn Flint, "Selecting Exercises," *JOHPER,* **35**: 2, 19–23 (February 1964).

All these changes are for the purpose of supplying blood and oxygen to the active muscles. In times of sustained, vigorous output of energy the skeletal muscles may demand 15 or more times as much oxygen as they need at rest.

The respiratory system of the trained athlete is also more capable of meeting the demand of the tissues for more oxygen, that is, of satisfying the "oxygen hunger" that accompanies vigorous exercise.

Muscle Training and Efficiency. In training muscles for quick reaction and for strength, the principle of overload can be applied. Thus, a batter usually swings several bats before he goes to the plate, but he hits with only one. Constant practice is essential for the attainment and maintenance of muscular efficiency at specific tasks. This is as true of small muscles as of large ones. A famous pianist once said, "If I fail to practice one day, I know it. If I skip practice two days, the critics know it. If I don't practice for three days, the public knows it." Grace of body requires regular, though moderate, exercise of the muscles.

The Musculoskeletal System

It is in the muscles of the body, of course, that the results of intelligently planned exercise become most evident. In them are seen and felt the grace and strength that make for an attractive figure, a useful physique, and an agreeable posture. The courage that Hemingway called "grace under pressure," and the skills that make an athlete or performer, take expression through educated muscles. The graceful body is generally an efficient one, because the muscles and their underpinning bones, joints, and sinews are coordinated under a system of positive control from the brain and nervous system.

We have come to an appropriate place to take a closer look at the musculoskeletal system of the human body. The system consists of some 650 muscles, 206 bones, and 250 joints, plus tendons and ligaments which bind them together. You should have a good general idea of this framework and supporting system of the body; but you

certainly do not have to know the names of all the muscles, bones, and joints to use them efficiently.

Bones. Exceedingly diverse in size and shape, the bones of the human body provide the scaffolding upon which the rest of the body is hung. The ligaments of connective tissue, the tendons, and the muscles, all of which help to keep the bones in their proper position, are equally important in determining the size and shape of the body. An unsupported skeleton (its joints wired together to provide skeletons for study) would collapse in a heap under its own weight.

Bones are living tissue. The long bones of the body are hollow and contain marrow, where red blood cells are manufactured. This is true also of some flat bones, namely, breastbone and ribs. From an engineering standpoint, the long bones represent a great triumph of efficiency, for they combine great strength and weightbearing ability with comparative lightness. It has been estimated that human bones are twice as strong as oak wood and can resist a load of 2 tons per cubic inch. The outside of the bone is covered with a closely fitting membrane, called the periosteum, through which nourishment from blood and feeling through nerves are brought to the bone.

The bones are subject to some disease, for example osteomyelitis, but they are far more commonly injured by accident. The knitting, or healing, of a broken bone when its ends are placed in apposition and "set" together remains one of the great mysteries in the operation of the body. How do the bone cells know that they must throw out extra cells to bridge the break, forming a callus, and by what token do they know when to stop?

Joints. The bones of the body are articulated in several kinds of joints, all of which provide for greater or lesser degrees of movement. The joints at the knees, fingers, toes, and wrists are hinge joints, which permit flexion and extension of these parts. The shoulder joints and the hip joints are of the ball-and-socket variety, which provide for a much wider range of motion, in-

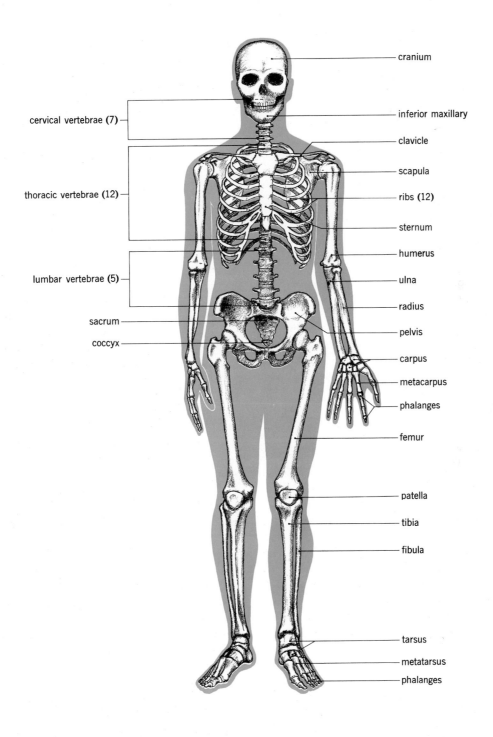

cranium

inferior maxillary

cervical vertebrae (7)

clavicle

scapula

thoracic vertebrae (12)

ribs (12)

sternum

humerus

ulna

lumbar vertebrae (5)

radius

sacrum

pelvis

coccyx

carpus

metacarpus

phalanges

femur

patella

tibia

fibula

tarsus

metatarsus

phalanges

THE HUMAN SKELETON. The bones of the human body, its skeletal framework or system, are shown here in frontal view.

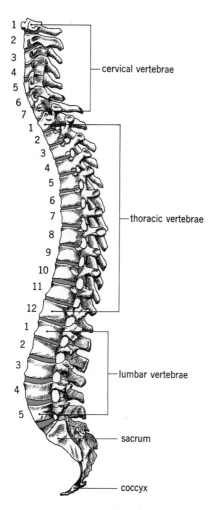

1
2
3
4 — cervical vertebrae
5
6
7
1
2
3
4
5
6
7 — thoracic vertebrae
8
9
10
11
12
1
2
3
4 — lumbar vertebrae
5

— sacrum

— coccyx

SPINAL COLUMN, shown here in extreme backward (dorsal) curvature, includes 24 separate vertebrae.

cluding rotation. The articulations of the ribs allow for only a small range of motion in the chest cavity during respiration.

Between the 24 vertebrae of the spinal column are to be found discs of cartilage (intervertebral discs). These sometimes herniate and press on the nerve trunks with particularly painful results. This situation is sometimes inaccurately called "a slipped disc." Also, low in the back, the joints between the sacrum and the ilium are frequently disturbed, producing a troublesome "sacroiliac pain."

Practically all joints, except the most solid

ones, are subject to dislocations, strains, and sprains. Joints may also become infected, and they may degenerate or calcify, producing "rheumatism" or arthritis of various kinds and degrees.

Muscles. Muscles are the "meat" of the body and make up between 40 and 50% of the body weight. The skeletal muscles give the body form, substance, and grace; they round out its normal shape and characteristic contours. They also give the body its power; their contraction is the motive power which provides for motion of the parts and locomotion of the whole.

Several kinds of muscle tissue can be distinguished. When viewed under a microscope, the tissues of the skeletal muscles, such as the biceps of the upper arm, appear striped, or striated. Similarly observed, the muscle tissue taken from visceral organs, such as the intestine, appears smooth or non-striated. Striated muscles are also called voluntary muscles, and smooth muscles called involuntary muscles.

All muscle tissue has these properties: it can contract; it can be extended; it is elastic, snapping back after being stretched; and it has "tone." To say that a muscle has "tone" means that it is not completely relaxed. It is partially contracted and "on the alert" to contract more. Even in this partial contraction, the muscle is in a sense "at work." It is consuming energy and producing heat necessary to preserve total body heat. Hence the large skeletal muscles can be considered the heating plant of the body. Cold can stimulate muscle tone to the point of involuntary contraction, such as shivering.

Muscle Metabolism. As an engine for the conversion of fuel (chemical energy) into work (motions performed) the muscles of the human body are about 25% efficient. Yet this is more efficient than the best steam engine and about equal to a good gasoline engine.

The skeletal muscles are the principal storage place of glycogen (body sugar) in the body. When the muscle fiber contracts, oxygen and glycogen combine. This combustion, or burning, in the muscles supplies heat to maintain body temperature and the energy needed for muscular action. It also leaves some waste products: carbon di-

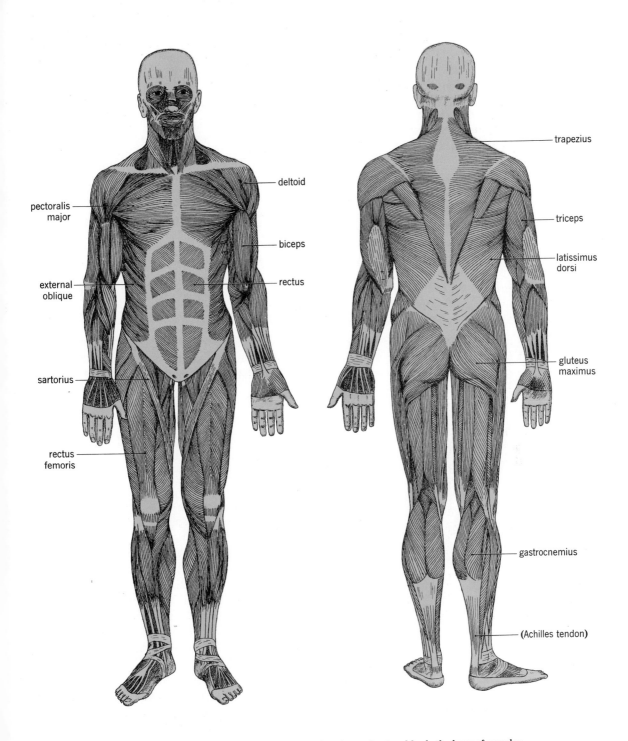

pectoralis
major

deltoid

biceps

external
oblique

rectus

sartorius

rectus
femoris

trapezius

triceps

latissimus
dorsi

gluteus
maximus

gastrocnemius

(Achilles tendon)

MUSCLES OF THE HUMAN BODY. This drawing shows, front and back, the layer of muscles directly under the skin. Only a few of these muscles, the largest and most familiar, have been labeled. There are many other muscles underneath this top layer. It would require a great number of drawings to show all the muscles of the human body.

oxide and lactic acid. The carbon dioxide must be removed by the blood corpuscles. The lactic acid (or salts of the acid, such as sodium lactate) must also be taken away to the liver or otherwise acted upon to be reformed into glycogen.

When the amount of exercise or number of contractions a muscle is forced to perform goes beyond a certain limit, the lactic acid cannot be disposed of as fast as it is formed and some of it spills over into the bloodstream. The accumulation of lactic acid in the bloodstream and in muscle tissue, where it interferes with the chemical reactions required in muscular contraction, is associated with true muscular fatigue. Other waste products of metabolism are also present.

The difference between mild and vigorous exercise may be measured by the concentration of lactates in the bloodstream. If sufficient time elapses between muscular contractions, the fatigue effects are abated, because the waste products are removed. Many other factors enter into the problem of fatigue; but the chemical factor gives us a handhold for understanding the nature of muscular fatigue.

Fatigue

Fatigue arises from many causes and appears in many disguises. The margin between fatigue and disease is often narrow and, indeed, fatigue is a symptom of many diseases.

It is important, however, to distinguish between normal, or physiological, fatigue and pathological fatigue. In pathological fatigue the feelings of lethargy reflect some illness of body or mind. Sheer muscular fatigue, following exercise, is the common form of physiological fatigue which everyone has experienced at one time or another.

Fatigue manifests itself in all organ systems of the body as well as in the mind. In extreme fatigue the alimentary system is almost always involved, and loss of appetite usually occurs. Muscular tenseness is commonly present; the sense of fatigue diminishes as the muscular tensions are reduced.

A simple experiment will illustrate the nature of muscular fatigue. Flex and relax the index finger of your hand as rapidly as possible as many times as you can. After a while, a feeling of discomfort will arise in the finger and then in the forearm. This discomfort will increase to a feeling of pain so intense that you will have to stop the finger exercise.

Some general inferences can be drawn from this simple experiment. In the first place, the more rapidly the exercise is performed, the sooner muscular fatigue ensues. In other words, the more concentrated the output of muscular energy, the more quickly fatigue comes on.

Second, fatigue in one set of muscles affects other sets of muscles; forearm as well as the finger became uncomfortable. This explains, for example, why eye fatigue, excessive use of the ocular muscles, or tired feet can induce lethargy in the whole body.

Third, the feeling of fatigue becomes a sensation of pain, which must always be regarded as a warning that physiological limits have been reached. Hence fatigue is a protective mechanism. The attempt to exercise the finger again before it has recuperated will quickly bring on the warning sign of pain.

Age and general state of health and training have effects on the onset of fatigue. Children both tire and recuperate faster than adults. In older people recovery from fatigue may be quite slow. Hence even mild degrees of fatigue should be respected as signals for stopping muscular exercise.

Physiological fatigue occurs when the demand is put on a muscle to consume more oxygen than is available to it. Waste products of muscular fatigue, such as lactic acid and carbon dioxide, accumulate in the blood stream. The fatigued muscle does not recuperate until the waste products are removed. Practically speaking, this means rest for the fatigued muscles. Anything that stimulates the blood circulation—including mild "toning-down" exercise—will also help get rid of waste products of muscular fatigue.

Posture

The human body is constantly at work against an invisible force—gravity. To maintain an erect and upright posture, many of the muscles of the body must be constantly at work overcoming the normal and forever-insistent force of gravity. This is a fundamental though sometimes neglected fact to be taken into consideration when discussing posture.

Much nonsense has been preached about posture in times past. Let us adopt the modern, dynamic view of posture education. We must begin by noting that posture is an individual matter. Among the many factors that influence it, certainly the skeletal constitution of the individual—his hereditary bone and joint structure and muscular relationships—plays a significant, if not a dominating, role. It is impossible to attempt to set one rigid standard of "normal posture" for all people. It is even more foolish if this standard is taken to be something equivalent to the military position of "standing at attention." Except perhaps for a few minutes at a time, under the watchful eye of a drill sergeant, all men and women are not going to stand alike, walk alike, or sit in just the same position.

What, then, is good posture? Briefly, it is natural posture, expressed in a person's attitude toward handling his body at all times. Posture is not like a cloak, to be put on and taken off as we choose; it comes from within. It is the ability to manage the body efficiently under a great variety of circumstances. We must think not of one posture, but of many.

For each individual there is a comfortable, natural, easy, and therefore probably graceful way of standing, sitting, reclining, and walking. Above all, posture should not be a pose. Human beings were not born to emulate statues in the park or mannequins in store windows.

Psychological Factor in Posture. Since posture reflects attitude toward managing the body, it also at times becomes a reflection of personality, "character," or at the very least, mood. The same is true of gait and carriage, which we might call posture in action. When we see a person furtively slinking down a street, we suspect, perhaps wrongly, that he is up to no good.

Stand Tall. Practically all advice for developing a conventionally good posture, when *standing,* can be summed up in the phrase, "Stand tall." Of course, you should not actually stand on your toes. It should be recognized, however, that the young man or woman of college age has already long passed the "golden age" for materially altering posture. That time came in childhood. Nevertheless a series of so-called posture exercises, under supervision, may effect some changes. Such a program will not be devoted merely, or even directly, to altering the mechanical use of the body. Perhaps four out of five college freshmen do not handle their bodies as efficiently as they could.

Posture and Health. The relationship of posture to health has often been grossly overemphasized. Perhaps the fairest thing to say is that poor posture is sometimes a symptom of poor health rather than a cause of it. What is poor posture? It is a failure or inability to use the body to its best advantage as a mechanical instrument. But we shall have to look far beyond mechanical causes for the reasons.

Fatigue is almost always a part of the poor-posture cycle. Fatigue may be induced by such environmental factors as poor illumination or bad seating. You should "try on" your chairs as you do your clothes. In many cases rest, to overcome the weakening effects of fatigue, rather than exercise will correct the underlying cause of poor posture. Poor eyesight and poor hearing, which require an individual to cock his head to one side to see or hear, may also affect posture. Mental attitude can induce displeasing posture, for example, the "debutante slouch" or the "gangster's swagger."

Good posture is natural posture, or grace and ease of bodily stance and movement within the limits of one's natural frame. It bespeaks self-confidence and reflects good health.

Structure and Care of the Feet

While good posture involves all muscles of the body, it is nevertheless true that a good foundation for standing, walking, or running posture (stance, gait, carriage, and "form") must be supplied by the bones, muscles, ligaments, and tendons of the feet. One of the really controllable factors in improving posture is adequate attention to and proper care of the feet. Tired, aching feet can suffuse the entire body with fatigue and definitely unfavorable effects upon total body posture. This fact is popularly expressed in the exclamation: "My feet are killing me."

Podiatrists (foot specialists) estimate that 70% of the people in the United States born with normal feet will have something wrong with their feet before they reach middle age.

The human foot is ingeniously designed for weight-bearing and for taking up the fatiguing shocks incident to walking, running, and jumping. The two arches of the foot are in effect springs. Each foot has twenty-six bones, bound together by ligaments, cushioned in some places by little sacs of fluid (bursae), and operated by muscles attached to the bones by tendons. The longitudinal arch of the foot runs lengthwise, from the heel to the toes. The metatarsal arch, just back of the toes, runs crosswise.

If the arches sag or break down, the condition known variously as "flat feet" or "fallen arches" occurs. Flat feet, however, are not necessarily either weak or painful. The integrity of the arches can be roughly measured by the footprint. Anyone can see his own footprint by stepping lightly on a flat surface with bare, wet feet. If the arches are normal, the footprint will be wide at the heel and the toes and narrow across the instep. With flat feet, the footprint is the same width all the way along. The height of the instep does not guarantee the strength of the arch. In fact a high arch is often subject to difficulties.

An occupation that demands an excessive

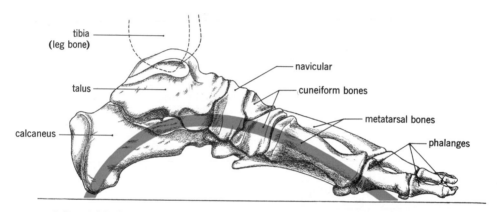

A. Bones of the foot as seen from the inner side of the foot. The superimposed thick line shows the curve of the longitudinal arch of the foot.

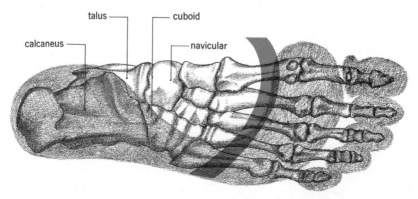

B. Bones of the foot as seen from below. The superimposed thick line shows the curve of the metatarsal arch. The shaded area shows the footprint in relation to the overlying bone structure.

amount of standing, which is often more tiring than walking, may be responsible for weak or fallen arches. A common fault in the use of the feet is "toeing out" instead of toeing slightly inward or preferably straight ahead. When the toes are pointed out, the foot tends to become pronated (rolled in) and its line of weight-bearing is off center. For strong feet, it is better to walk slightly pigeon-toed.

Selection of Shoes. Badly fitted shoes are responsible in large measure for flat feet, corns, bunions, calluses, and ingrown toenails. Shoes should be flexible enough to adapt to the feet, not vice versa. When you buy shoes, make sure they fit. Try on *both* shoes of the pair; the shape and size of your two feet are not exactly alike. Stand and walk in the shoes before you buy

them. The feet spread and become longer when the weight of the body falls upon them. Choice of footwear should be made with consideration of the occasions when the shoes will be worn. It would be pretty silly to wear high heels on a hike or rubber-soled sneakers to a dance.

Energy Costs

Throughout this chapter we have stressed the role of exercise and physical activity in aiding the individual to attain the desirable goals of physical and personal fitness. We have noted that exercise alone is not enough to achieve these ends; we have warned against fatigue; and we have pointed out that no matter how much fun exercise and physical activity may be, they are

THE HUMAN FOOT: Three views of its gross anatomy.

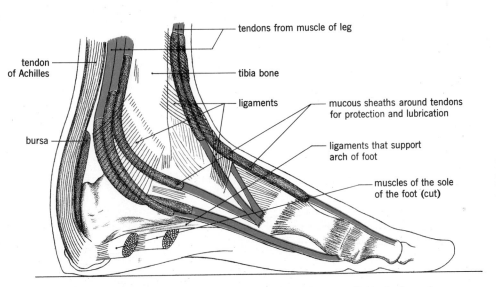

C. Tendons and ligaments in the foot. The tendons extend from muscles in the legs whose contractions bring about the movements of the foot. The ligaments hold the bones in position and thus maintain the arches of the feet.

CALORIE EXPENDITURE (ENERGY COST) FOR DIFFERENT KINDS OF ACTIVITIES

calories per minute	type of activity
	self-care
1.0	
1.2	
1.4	
2.3	
2.5	
3.6	
3.6	2.5 mph
4.2	
4.7	
5.2	

calories per minute	type of activity
	housework
1.5	
1.7	
2.9	
3.3	
3.6	
3.7	
3.9	
4.2	
4.4	
4.5	

always work. There is no quick and easy road to physical fitness, to a good figure, or a strong body. To reach these goals there must always be some output of muscular energy. In one peculiar respect the expenditure of physical energy is like love: the more you expend, the more reserves of it you develop.

The output of physical effort by the human body may also be described and measured as an "energy cost." One interesting way of measuring the energy cost of various forms of human activ-

ity is in terms of *calorie*[14] *expenditures per minute.* A comparison of the energy costs of various types of human activity (self-care, housework, occupation, and recreation) is provided in a chart[15] on these two pages. It may be observed that even

[14] A calorie is a unit of heat. The large calorie, used in exercise and nutritional studies, is the amount of heat necessary to raise 1 kilogram of water 1 degree C.

[15] Chart adapted from special article, "Energy Costs in Prescription of Activity" by Edward E. Gordon, M.D., in *Modern Medicine* (December 15, 1957).

CALORIE EXPENDITURE (ENERGY COST) FOR DIFFERENT KINDS OF ACTIVITIES

calories per minute	type of activity occupation
2.2	
3.2	
4.0	
5.0	100 lbs. / 2.5 mph
6.8	
7.3	
7.7	
8.0	
9.0	27 ft. per min. / 17 lbs.
10.2	

calories per minute	type of activity recreation
2.0	
2.5	
2.8	
4.4	
5.0	
5.0	
5.5	
8.0	trotting
9.9	
10.2	

the person at rest in bed uses up a calorie a minute just to get the "internal work" of his body done (this is also described as basal metabolism, page 199). For each calorie burned he must have an intake of about 200 cubic centimeters of oxygen. (We shall have much more to say about calories in a later chapter on nutrition and diet). A careful study of the calorie expenditure chart will suggest and reveal many things, for instance: . . . housework is hard work . . . feeling hungry after a dance has good reason . . . athletes and lumberjacks need good lungs and stout hearts . . . laborsaving devices (e.g., automation) will always find a welcome market.

Larks and Owls. Energy levels vary within the framework of a day and you have to respect and live with your own. Many years ago the great physician Sir William Osler observed the difference between "student-larks" and "student-owls" in a passage from "The Student Life":

There are two great types, the student-lark, who loves to see the sun rise, who comes to breakfast with a cheerful morning face, never so "fit" as at 6 A.M. We all know the type. What a contrast to the student-owl with his saturnine morning face, thoroughly unhappy, cheated by the wretched breakfast bell of the two best hours of the day for sleep, no appetite and permeated with an unspeakable hostility to his vis-à-vis, whose morning garrulity and good humor are equally offensive. Only gradually, as the day wears on and his temperature rises, does he become endurable to himself and others.

But see him really awake at 10 P.M. While our blithe lark is in hopeless coma over his books, from which it is hard to rouse him sufficiently to get his boots off for bed, our lean owl-friend, Saturn no longer in the ascendant, with bright eyes and cheery face is ready for four hours of anything you wish—deep study or "heart affluence in discursive talk"—and by 2 A.M. he will undertake to unsphere the spirit of Plato. In neither a virtue, in neither a fault, we must recognize these two types of students, differently constituted.

SUMMARY

This chapter has covered a wide variety of topics directed toward a better understanding of the efficient and satisfying use of the human body as a "physical instrument." We have pointed out the role of physical education; reviewed the values of physical fitness both for the individual and the nations; elaborated in detail the subject of exercise, isotonic and isometric; touched on college athletics; described the musculoskeletal system; and presented the subjects of fatigue, posture, and physical "energy costs." One conclusion is simple: We must pay attention to a broad range of subjects to arrive at valid concepts of physical and personal fitness. In the next chapter we shall seek to provide an equally comprehensive picture of the human body in health and disease.

SUMMARY REVIEW QUESTIONS

1. Give at least two definitions of "physical fitness." Describe valid tests, if any, for physical fitness as you have defined it.
2. What are the values and advantages of physical fitness?
3. What is the best criterion for determining when you have had enough exercise? Why is it such a good criterion?
4. Of what great traditions in education is physical education a part?
5. What are two or three of your favorite recreations? How would you rate them (highest first) in terms of their "energy cost?"
6. What are isometric exercises? Give some examples. How do isometric exercises differ from isotonic exercises?
7. What are the arguments for and against intercollegiate athletic competitions? How do athletics, sports and dance increase physiological capacity?
8. What are the essential parts of the human musculoskeletal system? What are the principal functions of each?
9. Discuss fatigue.
10. What is good posture? What is the relationship of posture to health?
11. This is a "trick question." Arrange the following list of occupations in the order in which you think posture would be most important to success—then tell why this is a "trick question": model, dress designer, architect, actor or actress, soldier, teacher, ballet dancer, salesman or saleslady, pianist, circus acrobat, baseball player.

12. What criteria would you employ for the selection of new shoes? In what ways would the use of these criteria reflect your knowledge of the structure and function of the human foot?

13. Do you think "larks," as described by Sir William Osler, should marry "owls?" How do you justify your answer?

14. Are the following statements sense or nonsense? Why? *No exercise is the best exercise. . . . The battle of Waterloo was won on the playing fields at Eton. . . . My feet are killing me. . . . Physical education activities in college should be conducted as far as possible on a coeducational basis. . . . When a muscle has tone, it will sound a musical note if struck.*

15. What do the following terms mean to you: 5BX, hypokinetic, kinesthetic intelligence, aerobics, muscle metabolism, flat feet, calorie, calisthenics, sacroiliac, periosteum?

Worth Looking Into: *Youth Physical Fitness* (Blue Book) by the President's (John F. Kennedy) Council on Youth Fitness. *How To Be Fit* by Robert Kiphuth. *Guide to Physical Fitness* by Justus J. Schifferes. *5BX Plan for Physical Fitness,* from the Royal Canadian Air Force. *The Alabama Student* (and other essays) by Sir William Osler. For more complete references, see Appendix E.

8

THE HUMAN BODY
IN HEALTH AND DISEASE

FOR HEALTHIER LIVING, PERSONAL AND physical fitness, it is not necessary to know human anatomy and physiology in intricate detail. To appreciate the functions and reactions of the human organism in health and disease, it is essential to know in a broad and general way the "working parts" of the human machine (to take one of many possible points of view toward the living human organism), their interrelationships and interactions with each other. *Not* to know this is to be biologically illiterate and to miss the satisfaction of understanding why certain courses of conduct are more sensible than others in raising and maintaining your health status.

You may already have studied basic anatomy and physiology; we shall therefore present a brief recollective summary of these topics—largely in pictures. An accurate summary of gross human anatomy is provided for you in the colored anatomical transparencies following page 144. Other illustrations in this and subsequent chapters will give you an equally graphic picture of different systems, organs, and parts of the human body at work or in action. In spite of all these "breakdowns" of the human organism into specific systems and parts, it must always be remembered that the human body and mind work together as an integrated whole. You will be discovering a host of "things I never knew till now" as you descend the scale from bones and muscles to cells and molecules and study the amazing interactions of body systems under normal conditions and under *stress*. This may often be the fundamental difference between health and disease. Obviously you need not know anywhere near as much about anatomy and physiology as your physician; but you should know enough to make you a good patient.

The Systems of the Body

For purposes of study the classical division of the human body includes the eleven following body systems:

1. *Skeletal.* Made up of some 206 different bones; the framework of the body.
2. *Muscular.* Including several types of muscle tissue; the locomotive system.
3. *Tegumentary.* Including skin, hair and nails; the shielding system. The skin itself is the largest single organ in the body.
4. *Circulatory.* Primarily heart and blood vessels; the fluid distribution or transportation system, widely dispersed.
5. *Respiratory.* Lungs and other organs necessary for breathing; the oxygen acquisition system, quite compact.
6. *Blood-forming.* A system which includes the spleen and scattered areas of bone marrow and lymph node; manufactures blood cells.
7. *Excretory.* Waste disposal system; primarily kidneys, bladder, and lower bowel, but also including lungs and skin (sweat glands).

8. *Digestive.* Food supply and processing system; a 24- to 36-foot channel leading from the mouth to the rectum.

9. *Nervous.* Complex, comprehensive communication and control system; a network packed in the brain and reaching out to all parts of the body.

10. *Endocrine.* A scattered system of ductless glands, whose secretions (hormones) are also part of the control system of the body.

11. *Reproductive.* A relatively small but crucial system.

Many smaller systems and subsystems of the body have been defined and studied; for example, the lymphatic system, a part of the excretory system, including lymph channels, glands and nodes; the biliary system, part of the digestive system, including all the organs that handle the bile secreted by the liver. *Combinations* of major and minor systems can also be studied. These combinations represent complex interrelationships of the parts and systems of the human body. A few of these combination systems are noted below:

Cardiovascular and cardiovascularenal system, including the heart (cardio), blood vessels (vascular), and kidneys (renal), which function together and react on each other in complex ways.

Genitourinary system, including the reproductive (genito) and urinary systems, linked together because of their close anatomical relationships.

Musculoskeletal system, muscles and bones and joints studied together because of their mutual interrelationships in effecting movement and locomotion.

Neuroendocrine system, a linking of the two major control systems.

Reticulo-endothelial system, a linking of the lymphatic network (reticulo) and the endothelial cells of the skin and glands on the premise that this interrelated combination helps provide *immunity* against infection.

Each one of the major systems, subsystems, and combination systems of the human body can be further broken down for study into different parts and specific organs. We speak, for example, of the *upper* respiratory system and the *lower* bowel. We divide the nervous system, grossly, into a central nervous system, an autonomic nervous system and a peripheral nervous system. We name the major organs of the urinary system as kidneys, bladder, ureters, and urethra, but each one of these organs has further anatomical structure and description (as do all other organs).

We know that the different systems are composed of different and specific kinds of *tissues,* regardless of what part of the body they appear in. We know further that tissues, glands, and organs are all composed of *cells.* Cells were first observed with the crude, early optical microscopes of the seventeenth century and so named by the secretary of the Royal Society of London, Robert Hooke. However, it is only with the advent of the electron microscope and other complex instruments of the twentieth-century laboratory that the true and complex structure and nature of cells is gradually being revealed.

Tissues may be considered as groups or configurations of more or less the *same* kinds of specialized and differentiated cells. The many different kinds of cells that make up the tissues of the human body (with corresponding names) have been more or less arbitrarily classified into the four following major categories:

1. *Epithelial* cells or tissues are the cells which (1) cover, protect, and line parts of the body, such as the top inner layer of skin; or (2) are grouped or compacted together to form specific organs or glands, such as the liver or pituitary gland.

2. *Connective* tissue is composed of cells which either themselves, or by means of the substances which they contain or produce, serve to support and sustain the framework (bones) of the body. Among the cells which make up connective tissue are those which produce bone and bone cartilage and, in some classifications, fats cells, blood cells, and certain others.

3. *Muscle tissue* is made of a variety of cells which are the substance of smooth and striated muscles in all parts of the body. (The heart, incidentally, is primarily a muscle, composed of a special kind of muscle tissue.)

4. *Nerve* cells or tissue have their own unique shape and function wherever nerve (or nervous) tissue appears in the body. The nerve cells make up the governing systems of the body in the brain, and the communication system elsewhere. They carry impulses, electrically measurable, from one part of the body to another and correlate these impulses in the brain and spinal cord.

The present structure and functions of the human body are the product of long evolutionary development from the time that life as a natural phenomenon (or an act of God, if you prefer) first began on Earth—itself some 4 billion years old. It is interesting to observe that all the basic materials out of which the human body and all other living matter is composed are present in solutions of *seawater*. It has been suggested that these same substances may have been present in the primeval seawater wherein life on Earth is presumed to have begun.

In our understanding of the human body and its functions, we now descend the scale of size from the objects of study of gross anatomy, visible to the human eye, and tissue structure, evident with the optical microscope, to cellular physiology and to molecular biology, where only the electron microscope and other advanced instrumentation will serve to discover new truths. In addition to decreasing size of the molecules and other particles under study it should also be recognized that there is a rapid *increase in the speed* with which reactions occur at a cellular and molecular level. Many of these molecular reactions occur at speeds faster than a millionth of a second, which is the present limit of time within which events can be accurately recorded or studied.

Based in part on the seawater studies, it is now fairly well established that, *chemically speaking,* the human body and other living organisms are constituted out of about 20 amino acids, 6 pyrimidines, 12 vitamins, 6 monosaccharides (simple sugars), and some 12 to 18 mineral elements. These particular chemical elements and compounds are synthesized into all the substances living cells require; notably proteins, nucleic acids (found in the nucleus of the cell), polysaccharides (complex sugars), and other metabolic substances (metabolites).

Cellular Physiology (Inside the Cell)

Advances in the physical sciences have made possible many of the significant and spectacular developments in the biological sciences. Until the effective use of the electron microscope in the study of the cell became possible, around 1950, the cell looked like nothing more than a practically empty blob of jelly-like protoplasm. Nobody knew what, if anything, was really inside it. True, it was known that every cell had a nucleus, and it had been observed that certain parts of the cell would show up when a particular chemical stain or dye was applied to it. Even before 1925 an Italian histologist, Camillo Golgi, had discovered within cells a delicate network of fibers (since called Golgi bodies or Golgi apparatus) that would stain black with osmic acid and were destroyed by fatty (lipoid) solvents. But he did not know what purpose this "apparatus" served.

Under electron microscope magnifications of about 10,000 times and more, and with laboratory techniques which make it possible to slice individual cells into extremely thin sections, the interior of the cell has become visible. Its structure and function (cellular physiology) are gradually being revealed. The cell is *not* empty. It contains a number of different parts, each with a purpose. The internal organs or parts of the cell, analogous to the much larger organs of the human body, are called organelles (tiny organs). We shall list below the organelles existing within the flexible wall or tegument of every cell and briefly describe the principle function of each organelle, as presently understood:

1. *Cytoplasm.* The fluid part of the cell in which the other parts are suspended.

2. *Nucleus.* The center, "heart" and "brain," of the cell, its governing body, whose molecules give the directions that determine the exact nature of

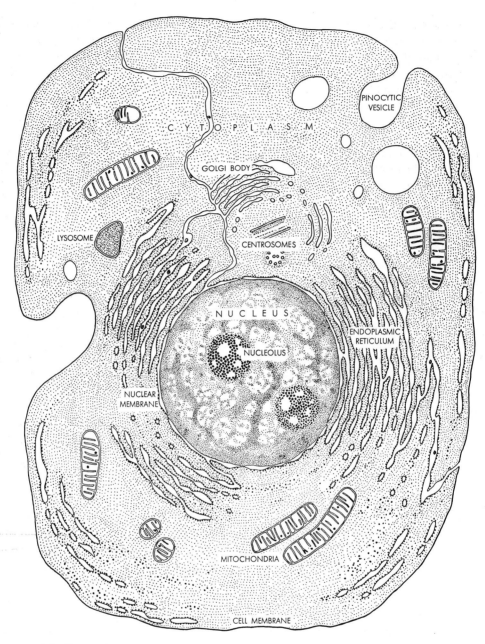

The diagram above, adapted from the *Scientific American,* is a schematic representation of a typical cell. It is based upon the appearance of a cell section magnified about 10,000 times with an electron microscope. The cell's organelles, analogous to a body's organs, are suspended in the cell fluid, called the cytoplasm. Directions that determine the nature of the cell come from the nucleus. Two bodies inside, called nucleoli, are believed to be a major center for the production of molecules that direct the synthesis of proteins. Most protein synthesis takes place in the labyrinthian endoplasmic reticulum, the membranes for which are believed to be made of secretions from the Golgi body. Raw materials to sustain the cell are broken down by digestive enzymes of the sort found in bodies called lysosomes. The materials are then in a form from which energy can be extracted by other enzymes found in the mitochondria and made available to various energy-consuming processes of the cell. Among those is the process of cell division in which structures called centrosomes perform an important function.

each cell. [In dissecting the nucleus into its molecular parts, of which the molecules labeled DNA and RNA are most important (and of which we shall say more later), we descend the size scale radically and move down from the area of cellular physiology to that of genetic or molecular biology.]

3. *Nucleoli.* Two smaller bodies within the nucleus. They are assumed to be the "factories" in which takes place the production and reproduction of the molecules (corresponding to genes) that direct the synthesis of proteins. The proteins, of immense variety, compose the fundamental and truly vital cells and tissues of living organisms.

4. *Endoplasmic reticulum.* A labyrinthine network (reticulum) of organelles suspended inside ("endo") the cytoplasm. The actual synthesis of proteins takes place principally in this network.

5. *Golgi bodies or apparatus.* Apparently the secretions from this apparatus form the membranes which become the endoplasmic reticulum.

6. *Lysosomes.* Bodies ("soma") which break down ("lysis") the raw materials necessary to sustain the cell. They contain digestive enzymes of a sort—catalysts of chemical reactions. Further understanding of the complex nature of enzymes represents one of the great forward steps in biochemistry in recent years.

7. *Mitochondria.* Small, thread-like ("mito") granules or "cartilages" ("chondria"), rod-shaped structures, which, like Golgi bodies, were discovered by differential staining of the cytoplasm of cells. The enzymes or catalysts found in the mitochondria can extract energy from the raw materials broken down by the enzymes of the lysosomes. This energy is made available to the various energy-consuming processes within the cell. A highly important one of these processes is cell division, by means of which cells reproduce themselves. One "mother cell" breaks up into two "daughter cells."

8. *Centrosomes or centrioles.* Tiny organelles, centrally located, which perform an important function in the process of cell division.

The study of the organelles reveals the parts of the cell that are responsible for the functions long known to be common to all cells. Cells have these properties in common: They can move within limits; feed themselves on raw materials, "foodstuffs," that are let in selectively through the cells walls; get rid of waste products; respond to stimuli from an outside environment or from other cells; grow up to their genetically prescribed limits; and reproduce themselves.

Both the area of cellular biology and the more vaguely defined field of *molecular biology* are on the research frontier. A great deal yet remains to be discovered about how cells, composed of molecules, function. There is a gap in knowledge between what the physiologists know about cells and the biochemists about molecules. But here again new tools of research developed in the physical sciences are coming to the aid of biology.

With these new instruments, and new techniques evolving from their use, it is now possible to "operate" on the minute organelles, and in so doing to learn a great deal more about their structure, function, and composition. Possibly the most useful of these new tools introduced from the physical sciences is the *laser* beam. (The word laser is an acronym for the phrase: *Light Amplification by Stimulated Emission of Radiation*.) The tremendously powerful laser beam can be focused down to less than a pinpoint and its stream of energy directed against cell components selectively stained with chemical dyes. The laser beam will instantly destroy the stained particles on which it is focused. Also useful as an "electric knife" in an operative field so small it can only be visualized under an electron microscope are beams of X-rays and ultraviolet light and streams of atomic nuclei. Modern light microscopes, closed-circuit television, and time-lapse cinematography further contribute to this advanced biological and chemical research.

An extremely graphic description has been supplied by John A. Osmundsen (*New York Times,* April 19, 1964, page E-7) of an experiment in cellular physiology conducted and photographed by Dr. Marcel C. Bessis, director of research laboratories of the National Transfusion Center in Paris, France, as follows:

The films showed cells which were exploded, or coagulated instantly, fatally injured with death coming only after agonized contortions, slightly hurt, and apparently completely unaffected by the laser beam.

For example, a tiny white dot of light blinked on and off in a field of white blood cells, showing where the laser beam would strike (when fired). When a cell moved under the dot, the destructive ray was released.

Instantly the cell went through a dance of death, sending out blobs of protoplasm and minutes later stopping in what appeared to be a congealed state.

Then there ensued a grisly scene of other cells seemingly fighting over the remains of the "corpse" (the destroyed cell), devouring its substance in an activity which, in the body, helps maintain health and life.

Molecular Biology— Genes are Molecules

In the semifinal analysis the human body is composed not of cells but of the molecules that make up the cells. In the final analysis it is constructed of the atoms and parts of atoms (e.g., protons and electrons) that shape the molecules. Molecular biology is still a rather vaguely defined field of study, pursued primarily by biochemists who are interested in the chemical synthesis of the crucial DNA and RNA molecules. Molecular biology, therefore, closely parallels the field of *genetic biology;* is related to the study of abnormal cell growth, which is a part of *cancer research;* and draws generously from studies in *virology,* whose research problems deal with particles (?) that are on the borderline of live and inanimate matter. There are many other areas of investigation in molecular biology: for example, the studies in the composition of seawater, noted on page 133; the structure of enzymes, the chemical catalysts that exist inside and outside cells; the relationship of molecular aberrations to specific diseases, such as sickle-cell anemia, a brilliant observation by chemist Linus Pauling.

It is now thoroughly established that genes are molecules. Genes are the specific molecules, in sperm and ova, that *determine* the genetic constitution, the hereditary characteristics, the heredity, of all living matter, including the highly individualized human being. The genes, or genetic molecules, appear in every living cell of the body and determine *its* specific structure and function.

Carrying this *up* the line, as the cells go, so go the tissues, the organs, and the various parts of the body systems that make up the integrated whole human being.

Genes have the remarkable—indeed vital— capacity to reproduce, duplicate, or (in more technical language) replicate themselves, according to an exactly established pattern. The relatively few genetic molecules present in the minute substance of the reproductive cells, sperm and ova, evolve into literally billions of such molecules (genes) present in the cells of the grown human body. The molecular pattern of the later genes in the growing human embryo, fetus, unborn infant, newborn babe, growing child, and adult is established by the very first ones. Here we are entering the field of genetic biology, which, as we have said, closely parallels molecular biology. We shall deal with these closely related areas in more detail under the headings of "Genetics" and "Heredity" in a later chapter (see pages 275–286). Here we shall provide only a brief summary of key points common to both genetic and molecular biology.

It is one of the great triumphs of mid-twentieth-century biology to have discovered the specific molecules which are the genes and which determine the genetic constitution of living matter. These molecules are known to be nucleic acids, found in the nuclei of cells. They are commonly designated DNA, standing for deoxynucleic acid, and RNA, standing for ribonucleic acid. Several forms of each are known to exist. The accepted, though simplified, formula which explains their basic importance to the propagation and continuation of life is this:

$$DNA \rightarrow RNA \rightarrow Protein$$

Proteins, of which there are enormous varieties, are the fundamental substances of which living cells are built; and the kinds and habits of the particular proteins in each cell permit it to perform the essential functions necessary to the enormous congregation of cells which make up the living creature. (There are a few one-celled creatures, such as the ameba.) Proteins are made up of amino acids, about 20 of which are commonly found in nature.

Both DNA and RNA are exceptionally long spiral molecules. A suggested and accepted model of the DNA molecule was provided by the young American biologist, James Watson, and the British biologist, Francis Crick. It is a double helix (looking like a pair of coiled springs interlaced), composed of two chains of nucleotides. A nucleotide (or nucleoprotein) is one of a total of *four* subunits which comprise both DNA and RNA. The nucleotide unit contains an amino acid *base*, the crucial element, to which are attached (in most instances) a sugar molecule and a phosphate group.

The four regular bases of the nucleotides are the chemical substances known as *g*uanine, *t*hymine, *c*ystosine, and *a*denine, commonly abbreviated to G, T, C, and A. Now in linking these nucleotides together to form the nucleic acid chain, DNA, it is obvious that they can be varied in a mathematically infinite order (A, C, G, T; T, G, C, A; AACCGGTT . . . *n*). This would mean DNA "blue-printing" of an *infinite* number of proteins. This is a condition contrary to fact. Furthermore it has already been demonstrated that there is some order in the bonding of nucleotide (or nucleoprotein) bases. It appears that the *sequence* of bases on the nucleic acid chain must form some sort of a *code*. Biologists all over the world are now trying to break the code.

Some progress toward breaking the amino acid code has been made. In 1962 it was discovered that a protein composed entirely of a *single* amino acid, phenylalanine, could be produced in the laboratory under the direction of an artificially synthesized RNA chain made up of a *single* base (poly-U for *u*racil, a fifth base peculiar to RNA). In 1964 it was announced by Dr. H. G. Khorana and his associates at the University of Wisconsin's Institute for Enzyme Research that short biologically active chains of DNA with a predetermined sequence of bases, or code letters, could be put together in the laboratory. The first of these man-made strands of DNA were limited to 15 or 20 bases in length, as compared to natural DNA chains running into thousands and hundreds of thousands of bases in meaningful sequence. As longer chains are developed, the chances of breaking the amino acid code—which is apparently universal among all living organisms—improve. This is one of the fruitful frontiers of research in molecular biology.

Oxygen

There are many chemical elements essential to the life and health of the human body. Some are needed only in minute quantities, such as iodine, essential to the proper functioning of the thyroid gland. Others are requisite in relatively large and regular amounts, like oxygen (O_2).

A human being can live months without food, days without water, but only minutes without air (oxygen). All living creatures require oxygen for survival. It is the combustion (oxidation) of tissue, derived from foodstuffs, that makes life possible. This process provides the energy for all the activities of the human body, both the voluntary ones like studying or dancing and the autonomic or unconscious ones like breathing and digesting food. The significance of this is reflected in the fact that in the tiny embryo growing in the egg or womb the circulatory system is the first one to be formed. Heart, blood vessels, and blood are developed before bones, joints, and muscles. The first of human needs is the need for air—more precisely oxygen—which makes up about one-fifth of the earth's atmosphere. Internal and external respiration are oxygen cycles.

The Circulatory System

The circulatory system may be considered the transportation system of the body. Among its specific functions are the following:

It transfers oxygen and carbon dioxide between the respiratory system (lungs) and the body cells.

It carries nutriments from the digestive system to the body cells.

It removes the waste products of body metabolism (broken-down tissues and some unassimi-

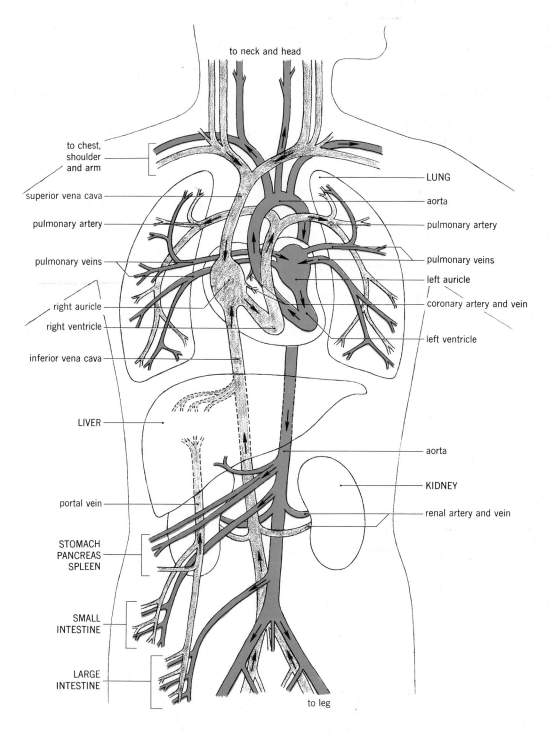

to neck and head

to chest,
shoulder
and arm

superior vena cava

pulmonary artery

pulmonary veins

right auricle

right ventricle

inferior vena cava

LIVER

portal vein

STOMACH
PANCREAS
SPLEEN

SMALL
INTESTINE

LARGE
INTESTINE

LUNG

aorta

pulmonary artery

pulmonary veins

left auricle

coronary artery and vein

left ventricle

aorta

KIDNEY

renal artery and vein

to leg

THE HUMAN CIRCULATION SYSTEM. The essential elements of the human circulatory system are presented here in semidiagrammatic fashion. Arrows show the direction of blood flow to and from the heart.

lated food particles) and conveys them to the organs of excretion.

It transports the "chemical messengers of the body," the endocrine-gland secretions, from the place of their origin to the site of their action and effect.

It helps to regulate body temperature.

It provides help in the form of white blood cells as well as immune bodies for fighting off bacterial invasions and other diseases of the body.

The Blood. Blood itself is obviously the final functioning "tool" of the circulatory system; the rest of the system evolved to get the blood where it is needed. Blood is an extremely complicated substance, and more new things are being learned about it every year. For example, the refinement of blood types, which began with simple O, A, B, and AB, then took on Rh and other factors, goes on apace.

The adult human body contains about 5 to 6 quarts, 4500 to 5500 cubic centimeters, of blood. This amounts to approximately $7\frac{1}{2}$ pounds or 5% of the body weight. Loss of one-third of the blood is usually fatal. Smaller amounts, for example a pint as given at blood donor stations, can be safely spared at proper intervals.

The bloodstream contains many elements. These include *plasma*, the liquid part, which is about 90% water; *red blood cells*, bearers of oxygen; *white blood cells* (leukocytes) of various sizes and shapes; and *blood platelets*.

Deficiency in red blood cells, from a variety of causes, is described as *anemia*. Disorder of white blood cells is called *leukemia*.

White blood cells are scavengers of waste products that come into contact with the blood stream and "devourers" (phagocytes) of many types of invading bacteria in the body.

Normally white blood cells are present at the rate of 6000 to 8000 per cubic millimeter of blood. In the presence of severe infection, however, the white blood count may rise to as high as 40,000 per cubic millimeter. A high count is almost invariably a sign of infection.

Red blood corpuscles (erythrocytes) are the most commonly recognized element of the blood. The typical "red-blooded man"—a normal, healthy adult—has about 5 million red corpuscles per cubic millimeter of blood, which means he has literally billions upon billions in his body. The equally healthy female normally has about 10% fewer red blood cells in an equal volume of blood.

Actually, red blood cells are comparatively fragile; the body destroys and replaces them at the rate of about 1% a day. Red blood cells are formed primarily in the bone marrow and destroyed in part in the spleen. The red blood cells carry oxygen from the lungs to the body tissues. These cells contain hemoglobin, which requires iron for its formation. The oxygen from the lungs is loosely combined with hemoglobin.

The athlete has special need of oxygen in his muscular tissues during competition. The average person, at rest, absorbs and consumes around 200 to 250 cubic centimeters of oxygen per minute. A trained athlete, however, can consume 4000 or more cubic centimeters per minute, all delivered via the blood stream. Athletic training, therefore, aims in part to increase the delivery of oxygen—actually the number of red blood corpuscles—to the muscles as needed. This is accomplished in part by stepping up the pumping action, specifically stroke volume, of the heart.

Blood Vessels. The blood vessels in general may be described as a series of pipe lines or elastic tubes, decreasing in diameter and wall thickness the farther away from the heart they are located. Except for the capillaries, they appear to be constructed in layers like cables, with an inner lining (intima), a muscular sheath, and an outer layer of connective tissue.

The arteries are thicker walled than the veins, because they must support the pumping thrust of the heart. Blood pressure is the pressure exerted by the blood against the walls of the arteries. On the other hand many veins are equipped with valves, whose purpose is to prevent backflow of the blood traveling upward against the force of gravity on its way back to the heart.

The blood vessels do not remain constant in diameter. The arteries, for example, contract to

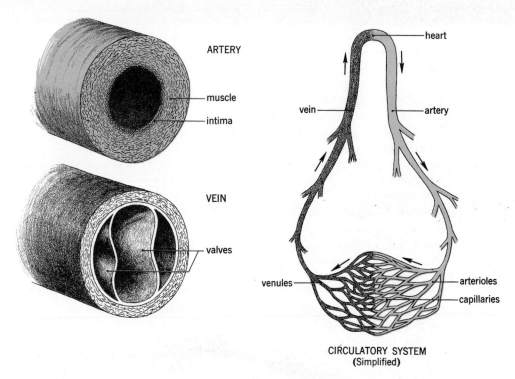

ARTERY
— muscle
— intima

VEIN
— valves

heart
vein —
— artery
venules —
— arterioles
— capillaries

CIRCULATORY SYSTEM
(Simplified)

BLOOD VESSELS. Blood vessels include veins and arteries, venules and arterioles, and capillaries, gradually decreasing in size (diameter) the farther away from the heart they are located. Arteries are thicker-walled than veins, but many veins have valves. At the far end of the circulatory system, shown here in a very simplified diagram, the arterioles and venules join together in minute capillaries so that the blood pumped from the heart eventually returns to the heart. Damage to and deterioration of the blood vessels is now recognized as the chief cause of heart disease and stroke. See Chapter 16.

help speed along the flow of blood. The small veins and arteries, and the capillaries, are especially subject to dilation and contraction under the influence of the autonomic nervous system. Psychic influences, and some drugs, can control the phenomenon of dilation and constriction. Blushing is a typical example of dilation of blood vessels of the face. The evolutionary purpose behind this nervous control of the blood vessels is to assure adequate supplies of blood to those parts of the body that most need them at the time—to the digestive tract after a meal, to the skin for temperature control, to the muscles during exercise. A complete circuit of blood through the entire circulatory system takes less than a minute.

Circulation Systems. Basically, there are two major circulation routes in the body. These systems are described as (1) the pulmonary circulation, which operates between the lungs and the heart, and (2) the systemic circulation, through which blood reaches all other parts of the body. In the systemic arrangement, there are at least three special circulation routes of which we must take note: the coronary circulation, the portal circulation, and the renal circulation.

The main single-trunk artery leaving the heart to begin the course of the systemic circulation is called the *aorta*. It is about an inch in diameter. It arches upward from the heart, then curves in descent. All the arteries branching from the aorta themselves divide and subdivide until they become capillaries and coalesce into the venous return system.

From the capillaries, where the blood has given off its nutrients and oxygen and taken a new load of carbon dioxide and waste products, the venules recombine, just as the arteries subdivided, into larger and larger veins. Eventually they become two large veins, called the superior and inferior vena cava, which enter the right side of the heart.

The heart muscle itself must be supplied with blood—through the coronary arteries. Failure in this system is the common cause of heart attacks. The renal circulation represents a shortcut circuit through the kidneys. There some water and waste products are filtered out. The portal circulation is a blood-return route which runs from the intestines through the liver.

The Heart. Many common idioms of speech testify to the importance of the heart not only in the physiological scheme of the body but also to human endeavor generally: "of stout heart," "good-hearted," "heart and soul," "lost his heart."

Actually, the human heart is a comparatively small organ, about the size of the clenched fist. It is located in the chest, just above the diaphragm, near the midline of the body with its apex (lower point) directed slightly to the left. The heart is a hollow muscle formed of its own special kind of muscle tissue. In function it is a four-chambered, double-acting pump. Like all muscles it is designed to work, and its work is to pump blood incessantly through the various circulatory systems of the body. The left side of the heart (left heart) does most of the work.

Approximately down the middle of the heart is a wall, or septum, which divides into a right and left side. In so-called "blue babies," this septum, which is normally open before birth, has failed to close. Each side of the heart is further subdivided into two chambers each, separated by valves. Thus we have a right auricle and a right ventricle, a left auricle and a left ventricle.

The auricles are in a sense the intake chambers of the heart; the ventricles, the real output or pumping chambers. The pumping action is accomplished by the contraction of the heart muscle (myocardium).

Heart Rhythms. The wave of contractions in the beating heart starts with the auricles and ends with the ventricles. There are timed pauses in this process. The ventricles are at rest while the auricles contract; the auricles rest while the ventricles work; and the entire heart takes a brief rest between beats. It has been estimated that *during sleep* the heart rests for about 28 seconds out of each minute.

The heart is accustomed to keeping its own rhythm and does not need help from the conscious mind. If it occasionally drops or skips a beat, that is no cause for alarm.

Blood Pressure. A person has *two* measurable blood pressures: systolic and diastolic. At the instant that the heart contracts, it is said to be in systole; when at rest, in diastole. Obviously there is more pressure on the arterial vessels at moments of systole. Hence the systolic pressure is always higher than the diastolic. When measured in millimeters of mercury by means of a blood-pressure apparatus, a normal systolic pressure at age twenty is 120; a normal diastolic pressure, 80. Arterial blood pressure usually increases slightly with age and with increase in body weight.

The Respiratory System

The vital function of the respiratory system is to deliver oxygen to the blood. It also eliminates waste products, notably carbon dioxide and water. A mirror becomes clouded when you breathe upon it because there is always some moisture (water) in expired air.

The upper respiratory tract includes the nose, which acts to screen impurities out of inspired air and to warm that air; the mouth; the throat, which is designated as the naso-pharynx and the pharynx proper; and the larynx, or voice box, which houses the vocal cords. Accessory to the nose are the various nasal sinuses, hollow recesses in the facial bones, which also warm the inspired air and may perhaps serve as resonators for the voice.

The tonsillar ring, consisting of lymphatic tissues, lies in the back of the throat. The Eusta-

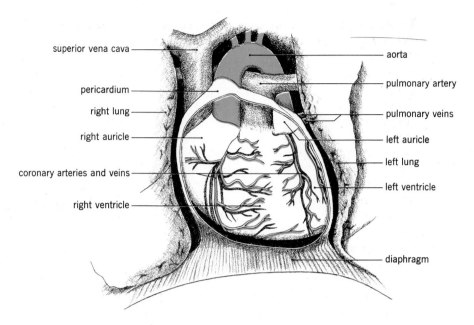

superior vena cava —

pericardium —

right lung —

right auricle —

coronary arteries and veins —

right ventricle —

— aorta

— pulmonary artery

— pulmonary veins

— left auricle

— left lung

— left ventricle

— diaphragm

THE HUMAN HEART I. This drawing presents the exterior appearance of the human heart as it lies in the chest cavity. This is a view from the front, with the pericardial sac opened up.

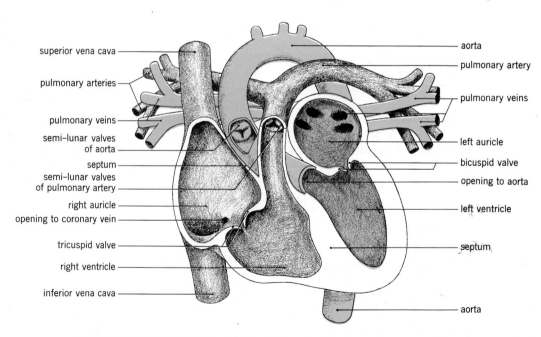

superior vena cava —

pulmonary arteries —

pulmonary veins —

semi-lunar valves of aorta —

septum —

semi-lunar valves of pulmonary artery —

right auricle —

opening to coronary vein —

tricuspid valve —

right ventricle —

inferior vena cava —

— aorta

— pulmonary artery

— pulmonary veins

— left auricle

— bicuspid valve

— opening to aorta

— left ventricle

— septum

— aorta

THE HUMAN HEART II. This drawing shows the interior of the human heart. A semidiagrammatic drawing, it reveals the internal structure of the heart, including its chambers and valves.

chian tubes conduct air from the throat to the middle ear, so that air pressure inside and outside the ears can be equalized.

The lower respiratory system fills the chest or thoracic cavity. It begins with the trachea, or windpipe, a semi-rigid tube, about 4 to 5 inches long, supported by rings of cartilage. (These rings are not quite complete.) At its lower end, the trachea divides into two bronchi: one entering the left lung, the other the right. Inside the lung, the bronchi continue to subdivide into smaller bronchi and bronchioles and finally into tiny, thin-walled air sacs, called alveoli.

Under a high-power microscope, the alveoli look somewhat like a miniature bunch of grapes. There are many millions of these air sacs in each lung. They give the lung its characteristic spongy feeling. The walls of the alveoli are only one cell thick. Each alveolus is in contact with one or more capillary blood vessels coming from the pulmonary circulation.

Respiration. It is at this juncture that the essential work of the lungs is performed. Oxygen from the air diffuses through the alveolar membrane to be caught up in the iron-bearing hemoglobin of the red blood cells waiting and scurrying through the capillaries. At the same time carbon dioxide carried by the venous blood diffuses in the opposite direction back to the alveoli, which might be called "gas exchange stations."

The lungs themselves and the inner walls of the chest are covered with a membranous sac, called the pleura, which secretes a kind of lubricating fluid that prevents friction as the layers glide over one another in the process of breathing. The "floor" of the thorax, which is at the same time the "roof" of the abdominal cavity, is formed by the diaphragm. This is a powerful, dome-shaped muscle which is of great importance to the act of breathing.

Mechanically considered, the lungs act like a pair of bellows, of which certain muscles can be considered the "handles." Quite a number of muscles are involved in the act of breathing.

The total volume of air that the lungs can hold ranges between 3 and 5 quarts, that is, between 3000 and 5000 cubic centimeters at the sea-level pressure of 15 pounds per square inch. This total amount is called the individual's "vital capacity." With each normal breath, however, only about a pint of air (500 cubic centimeters) passes into and out of the lungs. A reserve supply of air, residual air, remains in the lungs, even after expiration.

Both the rate and the depth of breathing are controlled by the respiratory center, located in the medulla oblongata of the brain. The respiratory center is remarkably sensitive to the chemical content of the blood stream, principally to the amount of carbon dioxide in the blood. When the carbon dioxide content of the blood is low, which is usual during sleep because less tissue metabolism goes on, the respiratory center tends to slow up the rate of breathing. Vigorous muscular exercise increases the carbon dioxide content of the blood so that deep and rapid breathing is automatically stimulated.

The Excretory System

The excretory system is the multifaceted waste-disposal system of the body. As cells, tissues, organs, and the body as a whole oxidize or metabolize foodstuffs, water, and oxygen, they accumulate waste products which they must get rid of. This is where the excretory system takes over. The urinary system is primarily concerned with waste-disposal (urine), but parts of at least four other body systems are involved in the excretory process. The lower bowel, or rectum, part of the digestive system, excretes undigested foodstuffs and other things, as feces, through the anus, its lower terminus. The sweat glands of the skin also dispose of waste products and the water in which they are dissolved. The lungs, as noted, eliminate water and carbon dioxide. The lymphatic channels, related to the venous system, transport waste products of cells to points where they can be picked up for external elimination.

The kidneys are the key organs of the urinary system; they also have an intricate physiological relationship with the circulatory system. The two kidneys, right and left, each bean-shaped and

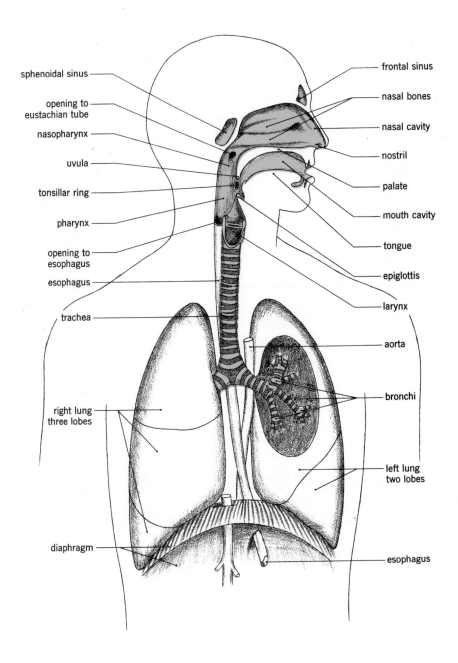

sphenoidal sinus

opening to
eustachian tube

nasopharynx

uvula

tonsillar ring

pharynx

opening to
esophagus

esophagus

trachea

right lung
three lobes

diaphragm

frontal sinus

nasal bones

nasal cavity

nostril

palate

mouth cavity

tongue

epiglottis

larynx

aorta

bronchi

left lung
two lobes

esophagus

THE HUMAN RESPIRATORY SYSTEM. In this illustration the heart and most of the blood vessels have been eliminated. The left lung has been cut away enough to show the branches of the bronchi.

HUMAN BODY
Seeing through the

IN COLORED ANATOMICAL TRANSPARENCIES

The accurate anatomical drawings, reproduced on transparent acetate film by "Trans-Vision®" process on the following pages, give you a unique opportunity to see through the human body. Each of the following anatomical plates (I-VIII) permits you to see a great many different parts of the human body from both their front and back views and in relationship to neighboring anatomical structures. By this unusual method of presentation you get a more accurate and intimate view of the interior of the body than you might otherwise ever obtain (at least outside a dissecting room).

The right-hand plates (II, IV, VI, and VIII) show you the front views, and the left-hand plates (I, III, V, and VII) show you the back views of the same organs. Each plate carries a list of a great many body parts visible on it. The body parts are numbered both on the drawings and in the list for quick identification.

An *alphabetical index* to the pictured and numbered body parts on all eight plates has been provided on the back of plate VIII, at the end of this special insert, for easy reference to the many body parts revealed in detail on the plates.

PLATE I shows the front skin of the body seen from its underside along with networks of veins which course between the skin and muscles. The veins are cut at points where they penetrate to deeper levels to join other veins returning blood to the heart.

PLATE II shows muscles of the face, neck, chest, and abdomen. On the figure's right side, muscles of the chest and abdomen are removed to show the front of the rib cage. Also shown are the thin membranous coverings, called fascia, of the thigh, arm, and forearm muscles.

PLATE III shows (from within) the cranial cavity, parts of the face, the rib cage, and muscles of the chest and abdomen. Note how the diaphragm separates the chest cavity from the abdominal cavity. As you follow the levels of the diaphragm on the succeeding plates, you will notice how much lower is its attachment on the back of the abdominal wall than on the front.

PLATE IV shows the brain and eyeball exposed and deeper muscles of the pharynx. Also shown are the three lobes of the right lung and the two lobes of the left lung. Below the diaphragm are the liver, gallbladder, stomach, and large and small intestines. Note the appendix hanging from the cecum.

PLATE V shows a mid-line (sagittal) section through the head revealing details of the brain, nasopharynx, and larynx. The lungs are cut through in a frontal section to show the space occupied by the heart between the two lungs. Below the diaphragm are back views of the abdominal organs whose front views appear on plate IV.

PLATE VI shows the septum that separates the two hemispheres of the brain, the nasal septum, the heart, and major blood vessels of the trunk and limbs. Now exposed below the diaphragm are the kidneys, pancreas, spleen, and duodenum.

PLATE VII shows the back views of the structures shown on plate VI. Note that the left kidney is located slightly higher than the right kidney and that the ureters empty into the bladder from behind.

PLATE VIII shows the left half of the head seen from a mid-line (sagittal) view, an inside view of the back of the rib cage, the front of the vertebral column and pelvis, and some of the major nerves emerging from the spinal cord. On the figure's left side are shown the deep muscles of the trunk, arm, and thigh. On the figure's right side these deep muscles are removed to show the underlying bones.

Drawings by ERNEST W. BECK, B.S., M.A., in consultation with Harry Monsen, Ph.D., Professor of Anatomy, College of Medicine, University of Illinois.

"Trans-Vision" ®Milprint, Inc. Copyright 1963, John Wiley & Sons, Inc.

PLATE

I

This view shows the skin of
the front of the body seen
from its underside along
with networks of veins
which course between the
skin and muscles. The veins
are cut at points where they
penetrate to deeper levels
to join other veins returning
blood to the heart.

Basilic vein (10)
Cephalic vein (27)
Cubital vein, median (35)
Epigastric vein,
superficial (40)
Saphenous vein, great (120)
Thoracoepigastric vein (139)

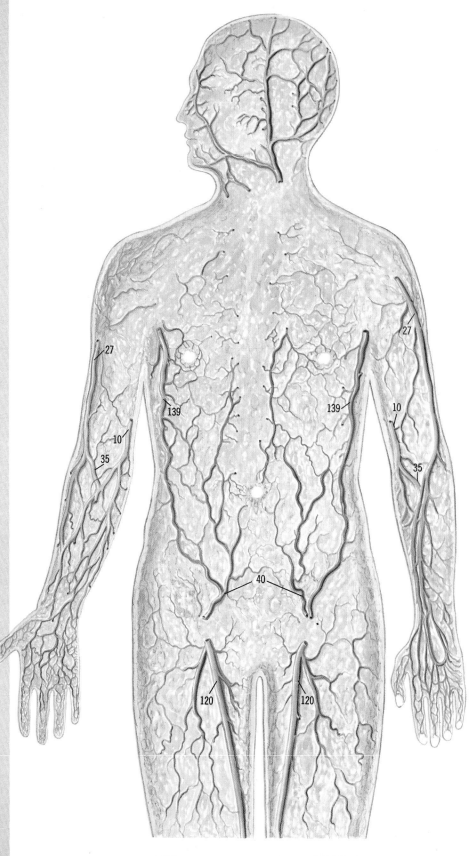

PLATE

II

Abdominal muscles (1)
a. External abdominal oblique
b. Internal abdominal oblique
c. Rectus abdominis
Antebrachial cutaneous nerves (4)
Antebrachial fascia (5)
Brachial cutaneous nerves (15)
Brachial fascia (16)
Buccinator muscle (23)
Clavicle (collarbone) (30)
Deltoid muscle (36)
Fascia of the thigh (45)
Femoral cutaneous nerves (47)
Fossa ovalis (51)
Frontalis muscle (54)
Mandible (78)
Masseter muscle (79)
Orbicularis oculi muscle (92)
Orbicularis oris muscle (93)
Parotid (salivary) gland and duct (98)
Pectoralis major muscle (99)
Rib (114)
Rib cartilage (115)
Serratus anterior muscle (124)
Sternocleidomastoid muscle (129)
Sternum (breastbone) (130)
a. Manubrium
b. Body
c. Xiphoid process
Submandibular (salivary) gland (134)
Temporalis muscle (136)
Trapezius muscle (144)
Umbilicus (navel) (149)
Zygomatic bone (cheekbone) (154)

PLATE

VII

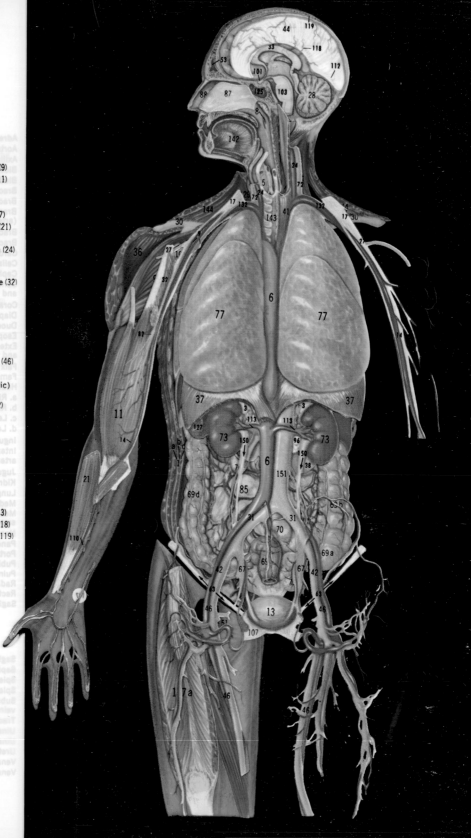

PLATE

VIII

Adductor muscles (2)
Auditory (Eustachian) tube opening into pharynx (8)
Brachial nerve plexus (17)
Brachialis muscle (18)
Brain (22)
Carpal (wrist) bones (25)
Cerebellum (28)
Cerebrum (29)
Corpus callosum (33)
Deltoid muscle (36)
Diaphragm (37)
Femoral nerve (48)
Femur (49)
Forearm muscles (deep flexors of hand) (50)
Frontal bone (52)
Frontal sinus (53)
Gluteus medius muscle (56)
Humerus (60)
Iliacus muscle (61)
Ilium (62)
Intercostal (rib) artery, vein and nerve (64)
Intercostal (rib) muscles, external (65)
Intercostal (rib) muscles, internal (66)
Intervertebral disc (cartilage) (68)
Ischium (71)
Jugular vein, internal (72)
Larynx (75)
Mandible (78)
Maxilla (80)
Medulla oblongata (83)
Metacarpal (hand) bones (86)
Nasal turbinates (88)
Occipital bone (89)
Parietal bone (97)
Pituitary gland (101)
Phalanges (finger) bones (102)
Pons (103)
Psoas major and minor muscles (105)
Quadratus lumborum muscle (109)
Radius (111)
Rib (114)
Sacral nerve plexus (116)
Sacrum (117)

Scapula (122)
Sciatic nerve (123)
Sphenoid sinus (125)
Spinal cord (126)
Subscapularis muscle (135)
Thigh muscles (137)
b. Vastus intermedius
c. Vastus lateralis
d. Vastus medialis
Tongue (142)
Trapezius muscle (144)
Triceps brachii muscle (145)
Ulna (146)
Vertebral column (backbone) (153)

INDEX

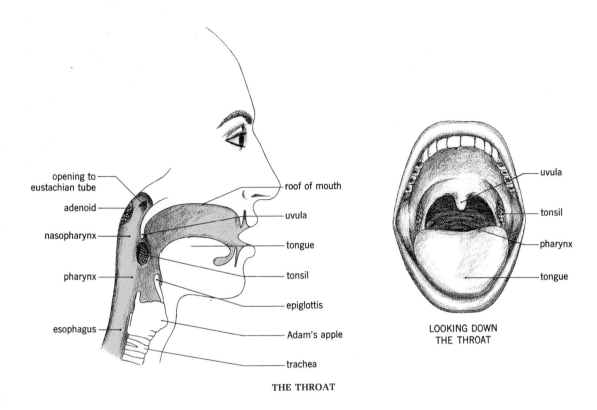

opening to eustachian tube
adenoid
nasopharynx
pharynx
esophagus
roof of mouth
uvula
tongue
tonsil
epiglottis
Adam's apple
trachea

THE THROAT

uvula
tonsil
pharynx
tongue

**LOOKING DOWN
THE THROAT**

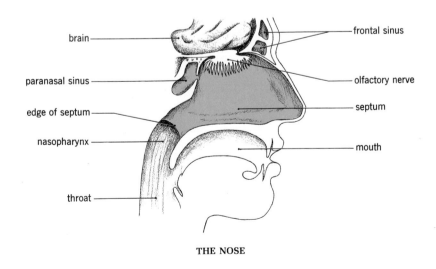

brain
paranasal sinus
edge of septum
nasopharynx
throat
frontal sinus
olfactory nerve
septum
mouth

THE NOSE

about the size of a fist, are located just below the small of the back. They are primarily *filters*—but that is not all. The entire blood supply of the body circulates through them every three minutes or so to be freed of its burden of waste products picked up elsewhere.

Each kidney contains about 2 million little filtering units, clusters of blood vessels called glomeruli. Waste products are there selectively transferred from the circulating blood into tiny funnel-like tubes, called kidney tubules. In addition, large quantities of water and essential body chemicals pass into the tubules. These necessary substances, however, are normally *reabsorbed*, as needed, through the walls of the tubules in order to maintain a normal balance of body fluids and chemicals.

Waste products dissolved in water, that is to say urine, trickle out of the kidneys down two narrow tubes, called ureters, into the bladder. Upon signals from the autonomic nervous system, the urine accumulated in the bladder is externally voided through another tube called the urethra. In the male the urethra is also the terminal channel of the reproductive system, through which sperm is ejaculated. Infection (nephritis) or other damage to the kidneys practically always throws stress on the heart and blood vessels—the other members of the cardio-vascularenal system.

The Endocrine System

The endocrine system, like the nervous system, operates to regulate and integrate the functions of separate cells, organs, and tissues of the body to act as one harmonious whole. This system comprises at least seven endocrine or ductless glands which elaborate an even greater number of biochemical substances. These substances are called *hormones* (after the Greek word meaning to "excite" or "awake"). They are discharged directly into the blood stream for circulation to all parts of the body. They do *not* pass through ducts or channels, like the secretions of the sweat glands, the salivary glands, the mammary glands, and others. Hence the endocrine organs are called ductless glands, or sometimes "glands of internal secretion."

Practically all bodily activities are controlled to some extent by the endocrine glands, and there is a complex interrelationship between them. The hormones themselves have been aptly termed "chemical messengers." This term properly suggests that, like the nervous system, the endocrine system conveys the needs of one part of the body to another. Certainly the hormones act as stimuli to many bodily functions in a very complex pattern. Different hormones have different specific functions and effects, but they appear to interact.

Among the bodily functions which hormones most evidently help control or regulate are growth and development, nutrition of body tissues (metabolism), rhythms of sexual function, muscle tone, and resistance to fatigue. But even beyond that the hormones are concerned with human feelings and emotions and mediate between mind and body. This is especially apparent in the case of the adrenal glands. It has been justly stated that hormones govern "the tides of life."

Reading downward from skull to groin, the seven acknowledged endocrine glands of the human body are: (1) pituitary, (2) thyroid, (3) parathyroids, (4) thymus, (5) adrenals, (6) islet cells of the pancreas, and (7) gonads, appearing as testes in the male and ovaries in the female. Their location is shown in the accompanying illustration. Generally speaking they are small organs, and their importance and effect are out of all proportion to their size.

When the endocrines are in good working order, they enhance the smooth, normal functioning of the body. When the endocrine system fails to work properly, some strange and damaging results occur. The amounts of hormones produced are very small, but too little or too much secretion operates to produce some bizarre effects. For example, extreme endocrine disorders can produce such circus freaks as the giant, the dwarf, the fat lady, the bearded lady, and the "man turning into stone."

The Pituitary Gland. *The pituitary gland,* about

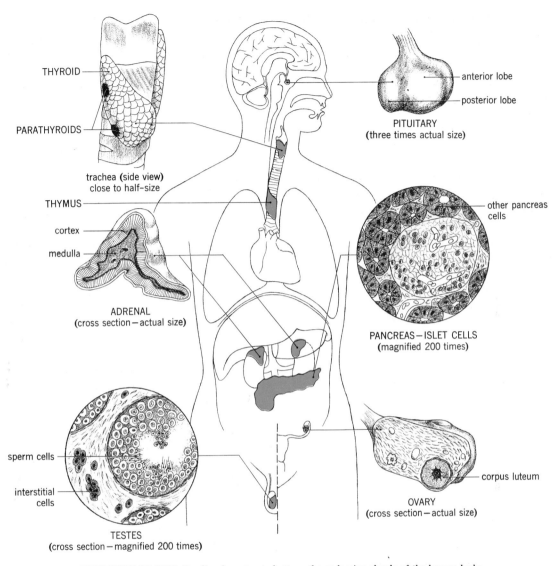

THYROID

PARATHYROIDS

trachea (side view)
close to half-size

THYMUS

cortex

medulla

ADRENAL
(cross section—actual size)

sperm cells

interstitial
cells

TESTES
(cross section—magnified 200 times)

anterior lobe

posterior lobe

PITUITARY
(three times actual size)

other pancreas
cells

PANCREAS—ISLET CELLS
(magnified 200 times)

corpus luteum

OVARY
(cross section—actual size)

ENDOCRINE GLANDS. Reading from top to bottom, the endocrine glands of the human body are pituitary, thyroid, parathyroid, thymus (its endocrine status is questionable), adrenals, pancreas (the islet cells only), and ovaries or testes.

the size of a pea, hangs from a short stalk at the base of the brain. It is sometimes called the "master gland" because it has a legion of functions and appears to exert a controlling and coordinating influence over other glands, which respond to the hormones it secretes. The pituitary is divided into three lobes and secretes at least nine known hormones.

Hormones from the posterior lobe (e.g., pituitrin) act to stimulate smooth-muscle tissue, regulate water balance and help control kidney function. Dysfunction in this lobe can initiate the "thirsty disease," *diabetes insipidus,* in which a patient may drink and void as much as 10 gallons of water a day.

The intermediate lobe of the pituitary gland

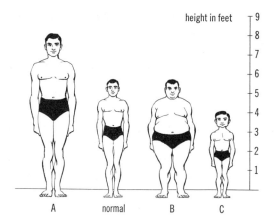

height in feet

9
8
7
6
5
4
3
2
1

A   normal   B   C

ENDOCRINE BODY TYPES. Too much or too little secretion of hormones from the endocrine glands can affect human growth and development in strange ways and distort bodily proportions as contrasted with normal structure. Some of the more extreme variations resulting from endocrine imbalance are illustrated here. A. Giant—too much of certain pituitary hormones in early life. Proportions of the body are normal, however. B. Obesity, pituitary type, due to imbalance of pituitary hormones. Note the disproportion and distribution of fat in the body as compared to thin wrists, hands, ankles, and feet. C. Dwarf (infantilism)—too little growth hormones. However, the proportions of the body are normal.

secretes one known hormone, which possibly helps regulate skin color.

The anterior lobe of the pituitary supplies the hormones that spark normal growth and development and that specifically stimulate other endocrine glands. One of these, for example, influences body size. Too much of it can produce a gigantic stature; too little, a dwarf. Other anterior pituitary hormones have to do with the distribution and storage of body fat; imbalance here can cause the gross obesity of the "fat lady."

The complicated interaction of the pituitary with other glands should be kept in mind. Not only do pituitary hormones stimulate other endocrine glands; their hormones also act upon it. ACTH, for example, is a pituitary hormone. It stimulates the adrenal glands. Furthermore, hormones produced by the ovaries act upon the pituitary gland and vice versa.

Gonads. The testes produce sperm and the ovaries mature ova, but both the male and the female gonads also function as endocrine glands.

Their role in the reproductive process will be discussed in a later chapter (page 287). To summarize briefly: the testes produce the male sex hormone, testosterone, which promotes the development of the secondary sex characteristics of the male. The ovaries elaborate several female sex hormones. These are concerned not only with the development of the secondary sex characteristics of the female but also with the rhythmic regulation of the menstrual cycle and the whole process of readying the female body for reproduction and childbirth.

Adrenals. The adrenals are a pair of glands, each about the size and shape of a Brazil nut, that cap the upper pole of each kidney. These glands have an outer shell (cortex) and an inner core (medulla). The outside and the inside parts elaborate distinctly different hormones with different functions.

The adrenal medulla elaborates the hormone epinephrine, more commonly called by its trade name adrenalin or its nickname, "the emergency hormone." This hormone greatly influences those parts and processes of the body which operate under the control of the autonomic nervous system, with which the adrenal glands have direct connection.

Adrenalin is one of the most important chemical mediators between mind and body. Under the stress of danger or excitement, extra quantities of adrenalin are released into the blood stream. This quickens the heart beat, mobilizes energy-releasing sugar into the blood stream, slows up or stops digestion, sluices blood into the big muscles, dilates the pupils of the eye, and may even cause the hair to stand on end. The purpose of all this is to help the body prepare itself for meeting emergencies—by fight or flight.

Dr. Walter Cannon of Harvard was one of the first to show that the bodily changes which take place under the influence of strong emotions are mediated by adrenalin.

The adrenal cortex produces an entirely different set of hormones, including cortin and cortisone. These adrenal hormones, essential to life, help regulate the metabolism of sodium, potassium, and chlorine. Adrenal hormones can also have some effect on secondary sex characteristics. An overfunctioning adrenal tumor, for example, can masculinize a woman and be responsible for her growing a beard.

Thyroid. The thyroid gland has two parts, weighing about an ounce apiece, that snuggle up against the front of the windpipe and look something like a small butterfly. This gland secretes a very important hormone called *thyroxin*. This hormone is concerned with the activity or metabolism of body cells. It helps control the rate at which cells consume oxygen and utilize foodstuffs. Too much thyroxin (hyperthyroidism) speeds up metabolism; too little (hypothyroidism) slows it down.

Thyroxin is essentially an iodine compound, containing about 65% iodine. Deficiency of iodine in the body or in the diet makes it impossible for the thyroid gland to elaborate thyroxin adequately. Actually very small amounts of iodine are needed, probably not more than 50 to 100 milligrams a year. Iodine is plentiful in seawater and seafood; it is lacking in the soil of many inland areas. To escape the risk of iodine deficiency in the diet one can use *iodized salt.* This is common table salt to which a small amount of potassium iodide is added.

Iodine deficiency is associated with enlargement of the thyroid gland, the condition known as *goiter.* It is also responsible for cretinism. A cretin is a dwarfish, misshapen, flatnosed, often deaf, and usually mentally retarded human creature, born without an adequately functioning thyroid gland. This condition usually results from failure of the child's mother to have a diet adequate in iodine before and during pregnancy. The prevention of cretinism lies in making sure that the mother's prenatal diet is adequate in iodine.

Thyroid extract is a dry, powdered substance derived from the glands of meat animals. Since it speeds up metabolism, it is sometimes used as a weight-reducing remedy. It should never be used, however, except under the direct supervision of a physician.

Overactivity of the thyroid gland (hyperthyroidism, usually accompanied by goiter) causes patients to lose weight, breathe rapidly, have a fast pulse, often become extremely nervous and excitable, and sometimes have bulging eyes. Relief of this condition may require surgery, cutting away part of the thyroid gland, or medical treatment with drugs that tend to slow down its activity.

Other Endocrine Glands and Functions. *The parathyroid glands,* each about the size of a pea, are located at the four corners of the thyroid gland. They secrete parathormone, which helps regulate the body's use of calcium and phosphorus. Too little of this hormone reduces the calcium level in the blood. Too much parathormone, on the other hand, may prompt excessive calcium deposits in other than bone tissue, which is what is happening to the circus freak said to be "turning into stone."

The islet cells of the pancreas are only one part of this much larger internal organ, which also manufactures digestive juices released through ducts. The hormone elaborated by the islet cells is *insulin.* It is essential to the carbohydrate metabolism of the body. Without adequate insulin supply, the body cannot properly utilize starches and sugars. The failure of the islet cells to produce enough insulin is the direct cause of the disease *diabetes mellitus.*

The thymus gland, situated on the windpipe, is classified as an endocrine, but it has no acceptably proved function. Large at birth, it generally withers and shrinks until at puberty it has practically disappeared.

One more observation about the endocrine system as a whole is pertinent. Since it influences so much the course of physical growth and development—as, for example, the advent of sex characteristics—it can also be said to underlie the psychological development of the individual, which waits upon biological readiness.

Stress, Stressors, and Disease

It can be categorically stated that the causes of disease in the human body (and mind) are numerous and multiple. Many causes, intermediate if not final, have long been known. In recent years much emphasis has been placed on stress and stressors as important though not sole causes of disease. In an earlier chapter we discussed obvious stresses and stressors, largely psychological and situational, to which a college student might be subjected (e.g., tests, examinations, difficult courses, family conflicts). Here we shall go more deeply into the subject of stress; but to clarify its role, we shall first have to look at other causes of disease and bodily defenses against them. We shall define "disease" as any departure from a state of health; an imbalance of functions that produces abnormalities or disabilities, temporary or permanent, mild to severe.

The occurence of disease requires conjunction in time and space of three factors:

1. A susceptible host.
2. One or more specific causative (etiologic) agents.
3. An environment both *inside and outside* the host in which the agents of disease can flourish.

The Host. An individual human being may be the host of a disease, but whole communities of men, animals, or insects may also be hosts of disease. Typhus fever is an example of an infectious disease whose host and reservoir is an insect, the louse, most often the body louse. This insect is in man's external environment; and man has learned how to get rid of it (principally with DDT). He has also learned to control many other factors in his external environment—for instance, water supply, room temperature, waste disposal— which make life safer and healthier. Man's internal environment is something else again.

Agents of Disease. Germs—microorganisms—are still the most commonly recognized agents of disease. But there are many others, some not as obvious. Poisons and toxins can obviously produce disease states. So can starvation and semi-starvation; that is, lack of foodstuffs containing chemical elements essential to life and health. Vitamin and mineral deficiency diseases are well known. Scurvy, resulting from lack of vitamin C in the diet, is a classic example. Psychological deprivations also cause disease; it has been shown, for instance, that infants deprived of their

mothers for five or more months, with no adequate substitute, literally sicken and frequently die of emotional deprivation. Finally, stress causes disease. Stresses can be written with either a plus or minus sign. Thus we can say that the body will be damaged by too much cold or too little heat.

Stress, deprivation, and infections (or their toxins) are not completely separate agents of disease. They are usually part of a complete cycle that breaks through the defenses of the body, overcomes its tolerances, and perhaps fatally upsets the constancy of its internal environment. No matter which one of the three phases of the cycle—stress, deprivation, or infection—initiates the disease process, the other two are sure to appear in one guise or another. For example, following the shock and stress of an acute burn, infection and imbalance of body fluids are soon likely to occur, unless corrected by medical treatment.

Internal Environment. Every living organism, every potential host of disease, including man, obviously has an internal environment (within which all the physiological, cellular, and molecular phenomena of the living creature occur). For the individual to be healthy this internal environment must be in good, normal working order. One of the first men to recognize the importance of this internal environment was the famous nineteenth-century physiologist, Claude Bernard, who pointed out that the healthy human being is "a piece of constancy living and moving in a world of variables." When the constancy of the inner environment or milieu is upset, the individual falls ill. Bernard's work emphasized the importance of the endocrine glands and the nervous system in "automatically" regulating the internal environment. In more recent twentieth-century language we might say that the body has a built-in "feedback" or "cybernetic" system to regulate—within limits—its internal environment. Stress and stressors of sufficient magnitude can push it beyond these limits.

Homeostasis. In the 1920's and 1930's Walter Cannon picked up and extended Bernard's concepts. He coined two phrases to sum up his extended findings and concepts; a popular phrase, "the wisdom of the body," and a technical term, "homeostasis." Both these terms describe the tendency of the internal environment of the body to return to normal whenever it is disturbed or assaulted. Some very delicate and complex mechanisms perform and assist with this function. Two examples: blood clots prevent further loss of blood when the surface of the skin is grazed or cut, and broken bones, their ends placed in apposition, immediately begin to knit and heal. And the process begun with the need for healing stops when it is completed! Cannon further pointed out that the internal constancy—the homeostasis—of the human being could not be maintained unless he had access to the elements essential to balancing his internal environment, for example, air, water, essential vitamins, and amino acids. Lacking them, he would fall ill of a "deficiency disease" which may be considered as another form of stress.

Cannon gave the name "stress" to any conditions of the internal or external environment which placed stress on the regulating mechanisms of homeostasis (notably the endocrine system and the autonomic nervous system) and which tended to disturb the steady state of the fluid matrix of the body. Among such stresses Cannon included cold, oxygen deficiency, loss of blood, low blood sugar, infections, and emotional disturbances. It should be noted that homeostatic reactions can be considered *protective* reactions, called into play when the body or mind is placed under stress.

We now recognize that the homeostatic process must not only maintain an inner constancy of the body at any given time but must also meet the changes that occur with normal growth and development of the individual. As Galdston has expressed it: "Dynamic homeostasis can be likened to a man walking a tightrope from one end to the other, balancing himself even while he changes clothes and takes on and discards a variety of other objects."

Thanks to his protective, "built-in" homeostatic mechanisms, man can handle and adapt to a great variety of "normal" stresses. The difficulty arises when an individual is subjected to

stress, physical or emotional, in excess of his *tolerance* for stress. What might be quite beyond the range of one person's tolerance may be well within the range of another's. Stress beyond tolerance creates what has been called the "stress syndrome," an important factor in the causation of many disease conditions, especially the so-called degenerative and chronic diseases. (A "syndrome" is a set of symptoms of disease or bodily disturbance which occur *together;* a symptom complex.)

The Stress Syndrome. Dr. Hans Selye is generally credited with establishing, in the 1950's, a basic concept of the stress syndrome, as it is now understood. He has also called it the "general adaptation syndrome," for reasons which will soon become apparent. The general adaptation syndrome, although resulting from encounter with stress, is nevertheless a set of reactions apart from and beyond those of homeostasis. In making emergency adjustments to stresses and environmental changes, the homeostatic mechanisms provide immediate and *specific* defense reactions; as in the example of blood clotting, cited earlier. In contrast, the general adaptation syndrome evokes *non-specific* reactions in many systems, organs, and parts of the body. These reactions are adaptive; that is, they represent the whole body's attempt to adapt to continuing and even future stress stimuli. However, as Selye himself has pointed out, "The general adaptation syndrome never occurs in its pure form, but is always complicated by superimposed specific actions of the stressors."

The General Adaptation Syndrome. The general adaptation syndrome proceeds in three steps or stages: (1) alarm reaction, (2) resistance, (3) exhaustion.

1. The alarm reaction, which has two phases, "shock" and "countershock," represents the whole body's reaction to *sudden* exposure to stresses and stressors to which it is not adapted.

2. The resistance phase represents the body's continuing attempt to develop defenses to *prolonged* stressful stimuli. Sometimes, however, these continuing defense reactions themselves produce

disease conditions; these are the common "diseases of adaptation." For example, repeated kidney damage (say by chronic infection) evokes a condition of hardening of the kidney tubules and glomeruli (nephrosclerosis) as the body defends itself against this particular stress. Resistance to other types of prolonged stress could have the same effect.

3. Exhaustion is the stage in which the systems of the body can no longer maintain either adaptation or resistance to the stresses to which it has been *overexposed*. In this stage bodyweight decreases; erosions and ulcers may appear in the gastro-intestinal tract; degenerative changes commonly occur in the heart, blood vessels and kidneys.

Selye has provided a long list of alarming stimuli—stressors—that may invoke the general adaptation or stress syndrome. In addition to emotional stimuli, such as fear, rage, worry, anxiety, which are probably the most common, Selye notes the following stimuli:

Trauma, such as fractures, crushing of tissues, surgical interference with vital organs, wounds.

Infections and the toxins produced by bacteria.

Bleeding.

Burns.

Exposure to excessive heat or cold.

Obstetric shock.

Nervous stimuli, such as spinal transection.

Some drugs, such as colchicine.

Deep anesthesia.

Temporary occlusion of blood vessels.

Excess of certain hormones.

Reduction of oxygen tension (lack of oxygen).

Diet factors, such as fasting, overfeeding, vitamin deficiencies.

Overexposure to radiation, such as X-rays, radium, (atomic energy) and even the sun's rays.

The channels through which stresses and stressors operate to produce the general adaptation syndrome are the integrating pathways of the nervous and endocrine systems. In particular it is believed that any important stressor or "noxious agent" directly or indirectly stimulates the anterior pituitary gland to discharge the hormone known as ACTH. This hormone, in turn, stimulates the adrenal gland to release an excess of corticoid hormones that help raise the resistances of the body.

In these last few pages we have delineated the role of stress and stressors in the causation of disease. We have emphasized it because it is a new, well-accepted and *unifying concept* in understanding the reactions of the human body and mind in health and disease. It may be argued that in emphasizing stress as a cause of disease we are simply calling anything that causes disease—infection, vitamin deficiencies—a stressor. In a way that is true; but it is also valuable in arriving at the new and helpful unifying concept of disease. In emphasizing stress we do not mean to negate the numerous other specific causes of disease.

Classification of Disease. In the long history of medicine innumerable classifications of disease have been proposed. At one time, indeed, it was mistakenly believed that the science of nosology, the naming and classification of diseases, was the key to diagnosis and successful treatment of all diseases. Possibly the simplest modern classification is the following threefold but overlapping one:

1. Infectious and communicable diseases—the so-called germ diseases created by the uncontrolled invasion of the body by disease-producing microorganisms. Malaria, pneumonia, syphilis, and measles are examples.

2. Degenerative diseases—in which some part of the body "wears out" or fails to function properly (usually, it may be observed, as the result of prolonged stress). Diseases of the heart, blood vessels, and kidneys; cancer; diabetes; and avitaminoses, like scurvy, fall into this category.

3. Psychosomatic ailments—in which mental or emotional factors (stresses) act to disrupt body functions. Hysterical paralyses, "irritable colon," and probably peptic ulcer provide examples.

SUMMARY

In presenting to you, as we have in this chapter, such fundamental and advanced topics as stress and stressors, molecular biology, cellular physiology, the systems of the human body, and a detailed description of four of the more generalized systems—circulatory, respiratory, excretory, and endocrine—we have sought to give you a picture of the structure and function of the human body in health and disease. This may not be easy to learn, but it is certainly worth knowing if you wish to understand yourself and the causes of your particular reactions to stressors in your own lifetime. In the next chapter we shall give you descriptions of the crucial sense organs of the human body and suggest how to take care of them.

SUMMARY REVIEW QUESTIONS

1. What are the eleven major systems of the human body, as traditionally defined?
2. Name at least six so-called minor systems or subsystems of the human body.
3. What are the four major categories of tissues (or cells) that make up the human body?
4. What properties do cells have in common? In what way do the tiny organelles within the cells resemble the larger organs found in the structure of the human body?
5. What are DNA and RNA? Where are they found in the human body? What is meant by the "amino acid code"?
6. What are the important parts of the human circulatory system? How, in general, does the circulatory system operate? What are its principal functions?
7. What is the structure and function of the human respiratory system? Exactly how does oxygen in the atmosphere get to the large muscles of the body?
8. What organs compose the excretory system of the human body? How do the kidneys perform their function of waste removal?
9. Name the seven endocrine glands of the human body and describe the principal functions of each.
10. Discuss the statement: "The causes of disease are multiple."
11. What is the homeostatic mechanism of the human body as delineated by Walter Cannon? How does it function?
12. What is the stress syndrome, otherwise known as the "general adaptation syndrome," as described by Hans Selye? What happens in each of the three stages of the stress syndrome?
13. What are some of the stressors (name at least six) which may be responsible for disease in the human organism?
14. Are the following statements sense or nonsense? Why? *Stresses can be written with a plus or minus sign. . . . The ryhthms of the heart are controlled by the blood vessels. . . . Every cell has a nucleus. . . . All diseases are fundamentally caused by germs. . . . The first of human needs is oxygen. . . . The physical and biological sciences have grown more and more apart in the past decade.*
15. What do the following terms mean to you: hormone, reticulo-endothelial, molecule, laser, Golgi bodies, molecular biology, cellular physiology, alveoli, genito-urinary, leukocyte?

Worth Looking Into: *The Human Body* by Logan Clendening, M.D. *Atlas of Human Anatomy* by Franz Frohse, Max Brodel, and Leon Schlossberg, *Anatomy of the Human Body* by Andreas Vesalius (Facsimile Editions). *The Wisdom of the Body* by Walter Cannon, M.D. *Beyond the Germ Theory* edited by Iago Galdston, M.D. *The Genetic Code* by Isaac Asimov. *The Physics and Chemistry of Life* by the Editors of the *Scientific American*. *The Double Helix* by James Watson. For more complete references, see Appendix E.

9

SENSE ORGANS:

EYES, EARS, NOSE, MOUTH, SKIN

IT IS THROUGH THE SENSE ORGANS—CHIEFLY eyes, ears, nose, mouth (tongue), and skin— that the brain comes in contact with the reality of the external environment which we inhabit. Without senses—vision, hearing, touch, smell, taste, and others—a human being can hardly be said to exist.

Perception of reality finally takes place in the brain, but the impressions which make this possible come via the nerve pathways of the sensory organs. The brain "dwells in utter darkness" in the cavity of the skull; but it is the brain that sees, hears, feels, and makes interpretations of all the sensory impressions brought to it.

In this chapter we shall place emphasis on the principal sense organs. There are several practical reasons for this. Eyes, ears, and skin, particularly, are complex and specialized organ systems, each of which demands its own specialized kind of care and attention. Furthermore, all the sensory organs (with the exception of the eye) have functions beyond reporting sense impressions to the brain. For a complete understanding of the human organism, these specialized systems deserve to be studied in their own right.

Eyes and ears are two of the greatest assets a human being possesses. Yet many people fail to make the most of them. Eye specialists (ophthalmologists) constantly encounter people with faulty vision who have accepted the blurred, imperfect images of the world they half-see as perfectly normal. "Oh, I see fine," they say until

they surprisingly discover how much better they can see when their visual defects have been properly corrected. Ear specialists (otologists) similarly report that patients have usually lost a full third of their hearing before they take any steps to overcome their partial deafness.

End-Organs of the Peripheral Nervous System

To provide a more exact picture of the operation of sensory organs, we must briefly describe the operation of the peripheral nervous system. As its name implies, it is located at the periphery or outside ends of the nervous systems. It consists primarily of nerve trunks, attaching to the central and autonomic nervous systems, and end-plates, or end-organs. These end-organs pick up specific types of stimuli (light, sound, heat, cold pain, pressure, etc.). They also deliver back messages or orders to the organs to which they are attached. End-plates that pick up sensations are called *receptors;* those that deliver orders are *effectors.* The end-plates are *specific* for their particular sensations. Thus the eye reacts to light, the ear to sound, the nose and tongue to chemicals in solution.

The specificity of the end-plates explains some peculiar reactions. Why do you sometimes "see stars" when you get a punch in the eye? Because the receptors serve only one function. The end-plates on the retina of the eye connect directly with the visual center in the brain. Stimulating the end-plates of the retina with a powerful blow can be translated by the brain only in visual images, that is, the flashes of light we describe as "seeing stars." Similarly a blow on the ear may come as an explosive sound.

Man has far more than the traditional "five senses." There are end-organs for hot and cold sensations, for pressure, for pain, and combinations of impacts on end-organs that give a sense of vibration, a feeling of fullness or tension, a sense of balance, and even the most basic feelings of hunger, thirst, and sexual desire. The end-organs for hot and cold are irregularly distributed on the skin and in the mouth and esophagus; there are many of them on the feet and very few on the chest.

The Eyes

The eye is an extremely complex organ, and we need not enter into all the technical details of its structure and function. *Seeing,* however, depends on the relationship of the eye with that even more complicated structure, the brain. Mechanically speaking, the eye functions as a camera whose images are relayed to the visual centers of the brain.

Protected by eyelids and eyelashes, the eye itself, set in the sockets of the skull, is a globe or sphere filled with fluid. Three coats or membranes enclose the fluid. The fluid in the rear part of the eyeball is called the vitreous fluid; it has a jelly-like consistency. That in the front bulge of the eye is known as the aqueous fluid.

The outer membrane of the eyeball is known as the sclera. A tough, fibrous membrane, it covers the entire eyeball and appears as "the white" of the eyes. However, at the front of the eye, this coat is crystal clear and is called the cornea.

The middle layer of membrane, called the choroid, also encloses the whole eyeball except altogether at the front of the eye, where the pupillary opening is found. The middle layer is pigmented and makes up the iris or colored part of the eye. The iris has tiny radiating and circular muscle fibers which enable it to expand when

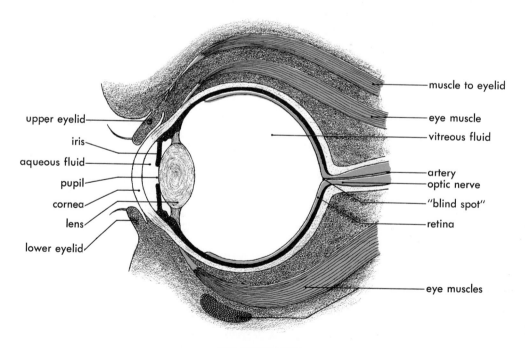

THE HUMAN EYE

light is dim and to contract when light is bright so that light can enter its central opening, the pupil, in the right amount.

The inner layer of the eyeball is the retina; it lines the entire inner (posterior) chamber of the eye except in the region of the iris. This layer is composed of nerve tissue and millions of light-sensitive receptors, known as rods and cones. These are connected with the optic nerve, which attaches to the back of the eyeball. Where the optic nerve connects with the retina, there is a small "blind spot." The optic nerve conveys images to the brain, where they are "interpreted."

One more crucial part of the human camera must be mentioned, namely the crystalline lens of the eye. It is situated immediately behind the iris, which lies between the two chambers of the eye. It is held in place by suspensory ligaments and can be flattened or thickened by the operation of ciliary muscles. The lens is transparent and refracts light. The changes in its shape (degrees of convexity) serve to focus light rays on the retina.

Professional Eye Care. Here are the "danger signals" from the eyes that should prompt you to see a doctor at once: seeing double, seeing blurred outlines around objects that you formerly saw sharply, seeing rainbows or halos around lights, or seeing poorly in the dark.

In some cases your doctor will further recommend that you see an eye specialist. The *opthalmologist,* formerly called oculist, is a physician, licensed to treat all diseases and disorders of the eye and, of course, to use all diagnostic methods. In addition to his regular medical training, the eye specialist has taken postgraduate courses of study in his specialty. His competency is in many instances certified by the American Board of Ophthalmology, founded in 1915, the first of the specialty examining boards in American medicine.

The *optometrist* is also a licensed, professional person who has taken special college and graduate courses in optometry. Optometrists are licensed in all fifty states to examine the eyes for errors of refraction in the lens system, to prescribe

lenses (glasses) to correct these errors, and to prescribe eye exercises and other nonmedical measures in eye care. The optometrist, however, is not a physician. Perhaps three-fourths of all prescriptions for glasses in the United States are written by optometrists.

The *optician* is a technician; he grinds lenses to the prescription of the oculist or optometrist and fits them to the eye in a properly adjusted frame. The adjustment of the glasses to the eye must be accurate, and this requires proper fitting of frames.

Defects in Focus. The eye has a power of accommodation which permits it to focus on objects at varying distances from it. This ability to focus depends on the action of its small ciliary muscles. In near vision, they contract and make the crystalline lens of the eye thicker. For distant vision, the opposite process occurs and the lens becomes flatter. There is a limit, however, to the power of accommodation. When the ciliary muscles are constantly overworked, the effect is eyestrain or eye fatigue, which may be reflected in other parts of the body.

In order for a clear image to be seen, the rays of light proceeding from the visible object must pass through the cornea and crystalline lens and must be focused more or less exactly on the retina. Defects in focusing often occur as a result of weakness or strain on the ciliary muscles, abnormalities in the shape of the cornea and lens, rigidity of the lens and too-great or too-little depth (or length) of the eyeball.

The four common defects in focusing are myopia (nearsightedness), hyperopia (farsightedness), presbyopia ("oldsightedness"), and astigmatism. These conditions account for most cases of poor eyesight. The correction of these defects is made by fitting and wearing the proper kinds of glasses, which compensate for refractive errors of the eye itself.

Nearsightedness (Myopia). In myopia the eyes can focus on nearby objects but distance vision is blurred. The reason for this is almost always that the eyeball is too long in relation to its focusing power. The light refracted by the lens, even with the utmost accommodation, falls in

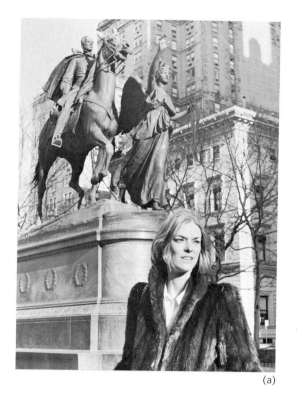

(a)

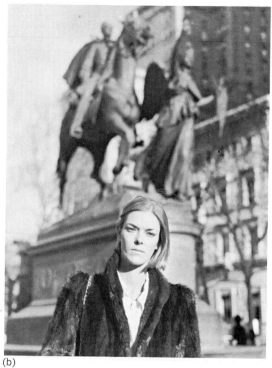

(b)

(c)

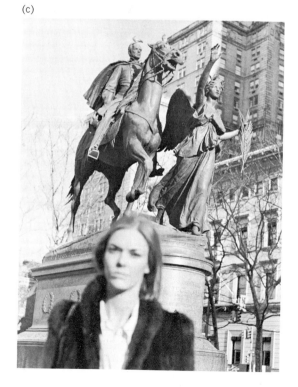

(a) NORMAL VISION. The girl and the statue are both clearly seen. (b) NEARSIGHTEDNESS OR MYOPIA. The girl is clearly seen, but the statue is blurred. The eye focuses the image in front of the retina. (c) FARSIGHTEDNESS OR HYPEROPIA. The statue is clearly seen, but the girl is not. In this case, the eye focuses the image behind the retina. (Photographs by J. P. Goeller) front of the retina. Myopia is corrected by wearing concave (thinner in the middle) lenses in glasses. The light rays coming from a distance are thus spread so that the lens of the eye can focus them on the retina. The cause of myopia is unknown, but it seems in some persons to have an hereditary basis.

In childhood and youth myopia often tends to progress, that is, to get worse. This usually occurs during spurts of rapid growth, especially at puberty. Over a summer a boy may outgrow his glasses, and need new stronger glasses, just as he may swiftly outgrow clothes. Except in cases of truly "progressive myopia," the gradual progression toward shortsightedness stops in the late teens or early twenties. Most nearsighted college students are already as nearsighted as they will ever be.

Close Work. It was formerly advised that nearsighted people should limit the amount of close work, like reading and sewing, that they wanted to do on the theory that close work either aggravated or "caused" nearsightedness. Most eye specialists today have found no acceptable evidence that close work aggravates myopia.

Of course all close work, whether for the nearsighted, farsighted, or so-called normal eye, should be done under proper conditions of illumination and with occasional rest periods. To prevent needless eyestrain, it is a good idea to look away from the book or work every 30 minutes or so and focus on a more distant object.

Farsightedness (Hyperopia). Hyperopia is the type of farsightedness that occurs when the length of the eyeball—the distance from the crystalline lens to the retina—is too short in relation to its focusing power. As a result, the "camera-image" refracted by the lens falls be-

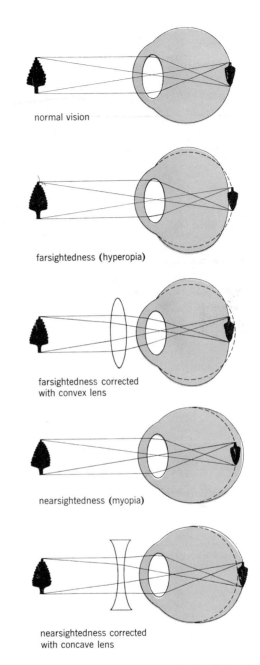

normal vision

farsightedness (hyperopia)

farsightedness corrected
with convex lens

nearsightedness (myopia)

nearsightedness corrected
with concave lens

SIMPLIFIED OPTICS OF VISION. This series of illustrations presents the simplified optics of normal and defective vision, uncorrected and corrected with glasses. In each drawing light rays are shown entering the eye and being bent (refracted) by the crystalline lens of the eye as well as by glass lenses in the two corrected cases. To provide normal vision, the light rays entering the eye are focused by the crystalline lens to fall exactly on the "screen" of the retina. In farsightedness, the point of focus of the light rays falls behind the retina. The rays must therefore be refracted so that their point of focus comes forward. This is done with convex glass lenses. In nearsightedness, the light rays converge in front of the retina. The light rays must therefore be refracted by glasses with concave lenses so that the focal point moves backward to the retina.

hind the retina. In hyperopia, distance vision is usually clear but close vision is likely to be blurred. It is not always blurred, however, because the ciliary muscles can correct the difficulty by persistently contracting. Farsightedness is far more common than nearsightedness.

Eyestrain. The overwork of these muscles at close work, however, results in their fatigue, causing one of the most common forms of eyestrain and being reflected in such symptoms as pain in the eyes, headache, and nervous tension. Since the farsighted person expects to see well, he is likely to overtax his ciliary muscles before he realizes it.

The correction of hyperopia is achieved by wearing glasses with convex lenses, which converge light rays and hence bring the image forward on the retina. By wearing his glasses, at least for close work, the farsighted person can save his ciliary muscles from undue strain. Most babies are farsighted at birth; but the length of the eyeball increases as they grow, and near vision improves.

Oldsightedness (Presbyopia). Presbyopia is a type of farsightedness that almost everyone can look forward to in middle age. It occurs gradually, because the crystalline lens of the eye tends to lose its earlier elasticity as age creeps on. Even though the ciliary muscles do their work, the lens itself fails to thicken adequately to converge light rays from nearby objects on the retina. As in hyperopia, the image falls behind the retina.

The person in his forties or early fifties comes to recognize that he needs "reading glasses" when he has to hold a newspaper or other fine print farther and farther away from his eyes in order to read it. "Reading glasses" for the middle-aged are made with convex lenses. "Bifocal" lenses, which permit easy accommodation to near and far vision in the same pair of glasses, are often a convenience.

"Second Sight." Elderly hyperopes, and presbyopes who required reading glasses, are sometimes in for a pleasant surprise—so-called second sight. They unexpectedly discover late in life that they can read and see better than they have ever been able to do before. Some of them actually throw away their glasses when they get this "second sight."

This condition is the result of a thickening of the lens of the eye so that its refractive index is materially heightened. Actually the thickening of the lens is usually a forerunner of a cataract. Nevertheless the elderly individual may actually enjoy his second sight for many years before definite, and perhaps surgical, treatment of the cataract is necessary.

Astigmatism. Astigmatism to a greater or lesser degree occurs in practically all human eyes because the eyeball is never perfectly round; rather it is a little out of shape. The irregularities occur both on the cornea and on the crystalline lens. In some spots they are uneven and perhaps too flat or too curved in one direction or another. Because of these irregularities, some of the light rays entering the eye may be scattered ahead of the retina, and other rays may be scattered behind the retina.

Astigmatism produces distorted images, fuzzy and out of shape. This common but peculiar error in the refractive powers of the eye is corrected for by eyeglasses ground with "compound lenses." These are made to counteract each specific optical distortion and refractive defect of the eye. The lenses curve the light rays to the proper degree opposite to the abnormal curvature produced by the ocular defect. Some people with astigmatism never know they have it until they get glasses. They have taken it for granted as "normal" vision before it was corrected. Astigmatism can, and usually does, occur together with nearsightedness or, more frequently, farsightedness. Uncorrected, it can lead to severe eyestrain.

Artificial Light. For comfortable use of the eyes in artificial light, the source of light should be steady (no flicker), uniform, nonglaring, and of adequate intensity. Intensity of illumination is measured in terms of foot-candles by photoelectric instruments called light meters. A footcandle is the amount of light projected at a distance 1 foot from the flame of a standard candle.

The critical distance for seeing is the distance between the light source and the observed object.

Where close work such as reading, writing, or sewing is to be done, the light falling on the book or paper or threads should be of an intensity of about 15 to 30 foot-candles, or more.

The major source of light on the printed page or other close work should come from behind. Direct glare of light into the eyes should always be avoided. Lamps should be well shaded, and bulbs should be frosted. It is better to work in a room that is reasonably well lighted throughout than to depend on "pinpoint" lighting on the work itself. In this respect modern, indirect lighting is an advantage. Position while reading —for example, reading in bed—makes little difference provided that the proper conditions of illumination are maintained. The book should be about 14 inches in front of the eyes.

You are the best judge of the amount of light you need to read or do other work. If there is not enough light, you will start to squint and frown and become uncomfortable. If there is too much light and glare, you will begin blinking and turn away from the light source.

Glare requires eye muscles to make constant and extensive readjustments, resulting in eye-strain. "Snow blindness" is an extreme example. Use of tinted glasses, optically correct, can be a help in avoiding undue glare.

Fashion has made sunglasses and dark glasses more popular items of feminine beauty accessories than is physiologically warranted. However, they should be worn for the purpose for which they are primarily manufactured: to protect the eyes from discomforting exposure to the sun's rays. They should not be worn for night driving, that is, to protect the driver from the glare of oncoming head lights. One observer has said of light-tint sunglasses (those that transmit more than 30% of visible light): "[They] are a cosmetic, a decoration—a palliative for neurotics."

Color Blindness—Night Blindness. The retina of the eye is lined with millions of rods and cones. The cones permit us to distinguish shapes and colors in bright light. Millions of shades, hues, and tints of color can be differentiated. In some individuals, however, the cones (and other color-perception apparatus, including the brain connections) fail to distinguish certain colors; most commonly, they fail to sort out reds and greens. This creates the condition of color blindness. So far as is known, color blindness is an hereditary defect and there is no treatment for the condition.

The ability to see in dim light and to distinguish movement depends on the rods in the retina. Since the rods are less plentiful at the dead center than on the sides of the retina, vision at night is usually improved by looking obliquely rather than directly at the objects to be seen.

To see in dim light, the rods must contain a chemical substance known as visual purple. The elaboration of this pigment, which goes on constantly, requires the presence of vitamin A. In the presence of light, the visual purple disappears rapidly and must be re-formed. If it is not, owing to a deficiency of vitamin A or other cause, ability to see at night and in twilight is seriously and in some instances, such as piloting an automobile or an airplane, dangerously curtailed. Night blindness can usually be prevented and alleviated by a diet rich in vitamin A, provided no disease process exists.

Prevention of Blindness. Total blindness in both eyes is a human calamity of top magnitude. But any degree of blindness is a physical handicap that can be economically and emotionally crippling.

The National Society for the Prevention of Blindness, a voluntary health agency founded in 1908, has long attempted to chart a nationwide program for the conservation of vision. Its record of achievement includes the promotion of the practice, now compelled by law, of putting silver nitrate (or equivalent medication) in newborn infants' eyes to avoid blindness from possible gonorrheal infections; the celebration of Fourth of Julys, without eye-damaging fireworks; the sponsoring of "sight-saving" classes in schools and other facilities for partially seeing children; recommendations for school lighting; and a public and industrial educational program in methods of saving sight and preventing blindness. Prevention of eye accidents has an important focus in industry.

It is estimated that there are something over 260,000 "legally" or "industrially" blind persons in the United States and that perhaps half of these cases were readily preventable. The leading causes of blindness are infectious and degenerative diseases and accidents.

Eye Injuries. First aid for eye injuries, even trivial ones, is another important consideration in sight conservation. The eye is easily infected, and scratches on the cornea can become scarred and cloudy, interfering with vision. Foreign bodies—dust, cinders—in the eye must be managed properly.

When you get something in your eye that cannot be immediately dislodged, shut both eyes for a few minutes—and do not rub them. The accumulation of tears will often wash out the particle. This failing, you can try instilling a few drops of clean water in the eye. Washing out the eye with an eye-cup filled with boric acid solution is the next step.

As a last resort, an attempt can be made to remove the particle—if it is visible, and not on the cornea—with the corner of a clean handkerchief or piece of sterile cotton. To find the particle, the lower lid may have to be pulled down or the upper lid everted by taking hold of the lashes and pulling gently upward and outward.

All these procedures should be done with clean hands and in as sterile a manner as possible. If none of these simple measures succeed, a physician should be consulted. Removal of metal or glass particles may require special procedures.

Diseases of the Eye. Just as the eye can affect the entire bodily system, as in general fatigue from eyestrain, so, conversely, systemic infections can play particular havoc with the eye. Syphilis, gonorrhea, and tuberculosis are three top offenders in this role; they have localized ocular effects, but they must be attacked systemically. Some of the childhood diseases, especially measles and scarlet fever, may affect the eyes. Some drugs or poisons taken internally have disastrous effects upon the eyes, especially quinine and methyl (wood) alcohol.

Any part of the eye may be subject to infection. The most serious are those which affect the cornea (keratitis), the iris (iritis), or the retina (retinitis).

Usually less serious but often very annoying infections can afflict the external portions of the ocular system. Most frequently affected is the conjunctiva, the membrane lining the eyelid and covering the front of the eyeball. A mild form of *conjunctivitis* often accompanies a common cold. Very severe infections may be encountered, such as gonorrheal ophthalmia.

Pink eye is a form of conjunctivitis that usually occurs in epidemic fashion. The eyes become bloodshot and inflamed, feel itchy and irritated, often feel as if something was in them, and may be stuck shut at night. Conjunctivitis is generally a communicable and contagious disease.

A *stye* is an infection of the lash roots and associated glands lining the margin of the eyelid. In certain respects it resembles a boil along a hair root. Persistent and repeated styes usually reflect a poor state of general health and are often associated with uncorrected errors of refraction and eyestrain.

The most serious infection of the eyelids is the condition known as *trachoma*, a highly communicable infection. It frequently causes blindness and has been the scourge of many oriental countries. Fortunately the modern sulfa drugs have proved effective in its treatment.

Diseases other than infection can afflict the eyes and cause blindness. Two important disabilities of this type are glaucoma and cataract. Both occur most commonly in middle life or later. Of neither are the basic, underlying causes known.

Glaucoma is a serious disease whose locale is within the eye itself; probably 1 in every 8 or 9 cases of blindness is a result of this disease. In glaucoma the pressure of the fluids within the eyeball unaccountably rises. This intraocular tension makes the eyeball hard, and the pressure, if unrelieved, destroys fibers from the optic nerve to the retina. At first the condition may be painless; sometimes it makes its appearance in red and bloodshot eyes. Other early symptoms are blurred or steamy vision, loss of peripheral vision, and frequent need for changing glasses. Occasionally glaucoma is not discovered until the individual finds that he can hardly see out of one eye. The blinding effects of the disease can often be prevented by prompt and early treatment. Glaucoma can be discovered early by routine testing of the eyes with the instrument known as the tonometer, which records pressure within the eyeball.

Cataract is a clouding of the crystalline lens of the eye or its capsule. Light fails to reach the retina in sufficient quantity to make seeing possible. Cataracts usually develop in one eye before the other and progress gradually. They can usually be relieved—that is, failing sight can be restored—by a delicate operation removing the clouded lens.

Common Questions about the Eyes. *Will looking at television harm the eyes?* No. Commercial television is more likely to produce cultural than ocular blindness. Prolonged viewing of a television screen which flickers and on which images are in poor focus may induce a temporary eyestrain, but this is easily remedied by finding a clearer channel or turning off the set.

Are "drops" in the eyes safe? Yes, when used by a physician for eye examinations. Indiscriminate use of belladonna or similar eyedrops, which make the eyes look big by relaxing the muscles of the iris, is to be deplored.

Can eye exercises make it possible to "see without glasses"? Not if glasses are needed. There is a legitimate place for eye exercises (orthoptics), but not as a substitute for glasses.

What about contact lenses? Contact lenses have been in use since about 1910. They are small lenses that fit directly over the cornea and under the eyelids. They must be very carefully fitted to the exact shape of the cornea, and they have proved most useful in people with marked abnormalities of the cornea. Various improved types are now available, and a suction cup is no longer needed for inserting them and taking them out. Unfortunately, contact lenses usually become uncomfortable after a few hours' wear.

The Ears

Next to the eyes, the ears are the most important sense organs and avenues of communication with the world about us. Like the eyes, they are complicated anatomical structures whose receptor end-organs communicate with the brain. The sensation of sight is carried by light waves, capable of traveling in a vacuum. The sensation of sound is transmitted to the ears through vibrations in the air. You cannot hear in a perfect vacuum.

The value of good hearing can hardly be overestimated. Cover your ears with your hands tightly for two minutes and you will begin to understand what a lonesome world apart the deaf and partially deaf inhabit. It is no wonder that they often become seclusive and suspicious. In human experience danger is usually *heard* before it is seen.

All ears are divided into three parts: an outer, a middle, and an inner ear. The middle ear is a small, irregular chamber, lined with mucous membrane. It is connected with the throat through the narrow, short ($1\frac{1}{2}$ inches long) mucus-lined opening called the auditory or Eustachian tube. The purpose of this tube is to permit equalization of air pressure in the middle ear, so that the pressure on the eardrum will be the same on both sides. Air is forced into the Eustachian tube whenever you swallow, as you do automatically every few moments. You can "open" your Eustachian tubes by yawning. The inner ear is a very small, delicate, and complicated structure set deep in the temporal bone of the skull. It consists of two parts: (1) a series of three semicircular canals, which are essential to the maintenance of equilibrium, and (2) the cochlea, a snail-shaped bony structure about the size of a pea, which carries the end-organ receptors of the hearing process.

Overstimulation of the receptors of the semicircular canals—confusion of them, one might say—can produce dizziness, vertigo, and concomitant nausea and vomiting. This is what happens in motion sickness, when riding in a tossing ship, a bumpy airplane, a fast automo-

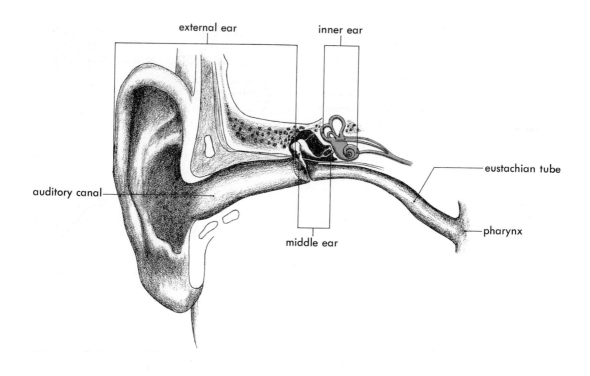

external ear　　　inner ear

eustachian tube

pharynx

auditory canal

middle ear

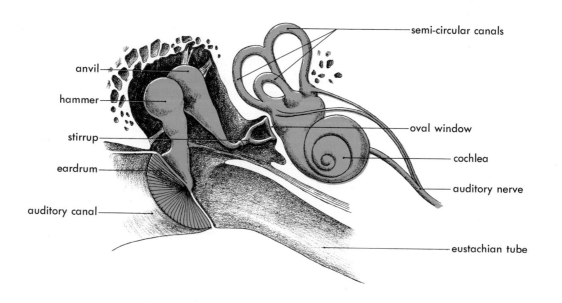

semi-circular canals

anvil

hammer

oval window

stirrup

cochlea

eardrum

auditory nerve

auditory canal

eustachian tube

THE HUMAN EAR is divided into three parts: outer ear, middle ear, and inner ear, as drawn above. The details of the inner ear, including the three little bones of the ear (called hammer, anvil, and stirrup bones) and the semicircular canals, which help maintain our sense of balance, are also shown greatly enlarged in the lower drawing.

bile, or an ordinary merry-go-round. Many *changes* in the direction of motion overstimulate the receptors in the semicircular canals. It is *unaccustomed* motion that produces motion sickness. Seasick individuals recover when they become used to the motions of the boat. With experience in riding, people outgrow carsickness.

The middle ear is the most vulnerable to serious infections. These often travel up the Eustachian tube from the nose and throat. Swimming and diving can encourage such infections.

Two self-inflicted complications must be mentioned: indiscriminate use of nasal drops or sprays and improper blowing of the nose. Infectious material from the running nose or sore throat is often forced up the Eustachian tube by noseblowing. When you blow your nose, especially if you have a cold, blow it *gently*. Do not close both nostrils at the same time.

Wax in the Ear. The accumulation of wax in the external auditory canal on occasion forms a plug which temporarily impedes hearing. This can be a frightening sensation, but it is not a serious condition. The important thing here is not to try to get the wax out by digging into the ear with a hairpin, matchstick, nail file, or paper clip. Such effect may force the plug in tighter, and may even result in scratching or perforating the eardrum and doing other damage. Gently syringing the outer ear with warm water or bland oil will often get rid of the wax.

Causes of Deafness. A few people are born deaf; many more become deaf as a result of accident, infection, or aging. As one grow older, the eardrum tends to become thicker and less flexible in the transmission of sound waves. In some persons, also, irrespective of age, there is an increase in bony tissue so that the stirrup bone becomes firmly fixed in the oval window and is no longer able to function in the transmission of sound. This condition is called otosclerosis. In some such cases, carefully selected, deafness can be alleviated by a surgical operation (fenestration operation) in which a new "window" or opening into the middle ear is cut.

This method works because the bones of the skull can conduct sounds to the cochlea. If

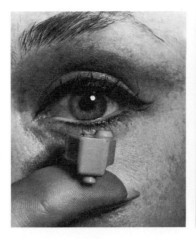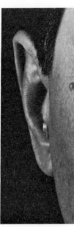

THE "SECRET EAR" is a miniaturized all-in-the-ear hearing instrument, weighing just over a tenth of an ounce with battery. It has neither cords, wire, nor tubes. (Photograph courtesy of Maico Co.)

you do not believe in the effectiveness of this bone conduction of sound, plug your ears—but gently!—and hold a tuning fork to your teeth. Hearing aids that convert sound waves into vibrations work on this principle.

Many theories concerning the development of otosclerosis have been advanced. It is estimated that 10 million people in the United States—women twice as frequently as men—are more or less affected by this condition and the type of middle-ear deafness that it may invoke. According to Dr. Edmund Prince Fowler, of New York, this type of deafness may be of endocrine origin and related to the body's production of the female sex hormone, estrogen.

When the delicate structures of the inner ear or the auditory nerve itself is affected by disease, such as syphilis, meningitis, or scarlet fever, a condition of "nerve-deafness" results and very little can be done about it. Continuing loud or sudden overwhelming noise can damage the auditory apparatus, sometimes irreparably.

Other possible causes of at least partial deafness include localized or systemic infectious diseases, notably measles, mumps, chicken pox, and whooping cough; diseased tonsils and adenoids; uncontrolled or improper swimming;

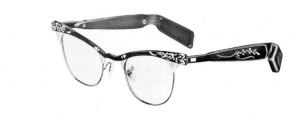

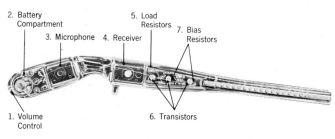

2. Battery
Compartment

5. Load
Resistors

7. Bias
Resistors

3. Microphone   4. Receiver

1. Volume
Control

6. Transistors

GLASSES TO HEAR WITH . . . The most interesting—and extremely effective—new hearing aids for the deaf and partially deaf are "hearing glasses," which can be ornamented in high style and fitted with whatever lenses the wearer needs (clear glass if there are no vision difficulties). The electronic hearing-aid parts are installed in the bows (earpieces) of the glasses. Each bow contains a complete hearing aid, allowing the wearer to hear better in one or both ears. Everything is included—from a miniature microphone that picks up sound to a receiver that delivers it greatly amplified to the ear. (Photograph courtesy of Maico Co.)

and blows on the ears. Frequent colds and neglected "running ears" are also associated with deafness.

Smell and Taste. The special senses of smell and taste, which operate together when it comes to eating food, add to man's pleasures of living, but they are not so important to his existence as they are to most lower animals. Both senses may warn of danger, as in smelling smoke or biting into some foodstuff that just "doesn't taste right."

The sensory end-organs for smell (olfactory chemoreceptors) are located at the top of the inner surface of the nose. These olfactory cells are imbedded in mucous membrane; from them other nerve fibers pass up to the olfactory lobe in the brain, where the smell is "interpreted." The olfactory cells pick up odors from molecules or small particles released by various substances. These particles are present in the air we inhale; and when they come in contact with the olfactory cells, they stimulate the appropriate end-organs.

Human beings can distinguish about 60,000 odors; but these are combinations of a relatively

few specific classes of odors to which the olfactory cells directly respond. According to one classification, these cells respond to only seven odors, described as burnt, acid, putrid, spicy, fragrant, fruity, and resinous.

Taste is the sense by which we perceive the flavor of substances placed in the mouth. The end-organ receptors through which this is accomplished are called *taste buds.* The impulses from these receptors are, of course, conveyed to the brain, where they register as taste sensations. For practical purposes the taste buds may be considered to be located on the *tongue,* though there are a few scattered in the pharynx.

Human beings can actually distinguish only four different tastes: *sweet* and *salt,* in the buds at the tip of the tongue; *sour* (or acid), along the sides of the tongue; and *bitter* at the back of the tongue. The taste buds are reacting to chemicals in solution. The combinations of the four basic taste sensations provide a wide variety of flavors. Whether a food tastes "good" or "bad" to an individual is not based on the intrinsic nature of the foodstuff but rather on his past (learned) experiences with the particular food or flavor.

Stimulation of the taste buds brings about an important unconscious reflex reaction. It induces the secretion of saliva in the mouth and gastric juices in the stomach, thus aiding the process of digestion.

While the nose and tongue, as we have noted, are sense organs, they also serve other functions. The nose and paranasal sinuses are important adjuncts to the respiratory system. The tongue, used for mixing foods in the mouth and for swallowing, assists the digestive system. Both tongue and nose are involved in the process of human speech.

The Skin

Like the nose and tongue, the skin is a sense organ with many other functions. Covering approximately 17 square feet of tangible surface in adults and weighing altogether about five pounds, the skin is the largest single organ of the human body. It is a vital organ. Destruction of a little more than one third of the skin area, as by burning or scalding, is usually fatal.

Clendening speaks lyrically of the skin as "one of the most interesting and mystic of structures." He calls it "that outer rampart which separates us from the rest of the universe, the sack which contains that juice or essence which is me or which is you, a moat defensive against insects, poisons, germs. . . . The very storms of the soul are recorded upon it."

The variety of sensations recorded and reported to the brain by the skin is undoubtedly one of the factors that make it so "interesting." Tactile sensation—touch—is only one of five types of sensation to which the specific end-organs of the skin respond. They can also be stimulated by pain, pressure, heat, cold, and combinations of sensations. Pain is apparently registered by bare nerve endings; but for each of the other sensations there are specific types of end-organs, called corpuscles and discs. Meissner's corpuscles, located mainly in the hairless parts of the skin, are the chief end-organs of the

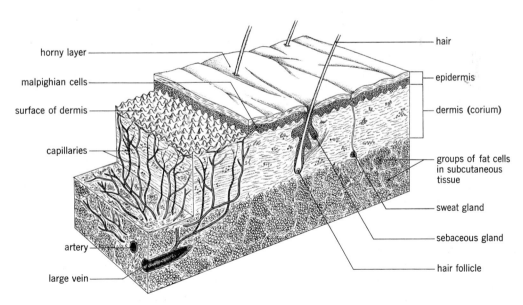

horny layer

malpighian cells

surface of dermis

capillaries

artery

large vein

hair

epidermis

dermis (corium)

groups of fat cells in subcutaneous tissue

sweat gland

sebaceous gland

hair follicle

THE HUMAN SKIN has a more complicated structure than appears on the surface of the body. This neatly blocked-out piece of skin tissue reveals the various layers and underlying structures of the human skin. The blood vessels reaching the skin are numerous; however, they are shown only on the left side of the drawing.

sense of touch. They react individually to touch and collectively to pressure. Another type of tactile sense organ surrounds the individual hairs on the skin. These end-organs are highly responsive to the slightest movements of the hairs, such as those caused by a light touch or a draft of air.

The end-organs for touch are distributed unevenly on the total skin surface of the body. Most sensitive areas are the lips and the tip of the tongue. Fingertips are quite sensitive; back, arms, and legs much less so.

Structure of the Skin. The structure of the skin is far more complex than appears on first glance. Most astonishing, perhaps, is the fact that the outer skin, the visible surface of the body, is composed of dead rather than living tissue. This same fact is true of the fingernails and toenails and the hair. They grow, obviously from the inside out. The cells thus appearing on the outer surface of the body are no longer alive. They have turned into a highly insoluble form of protein, called keratin, which is also found in the horns and hooves of lower animals.

The outer layer of the skin, composed of dry, dead cells, which are more or less flattened out and overlap each other somewhat like shingles on a roof, is sometimes called its "horny layer." These cells are constantly being shed and replaced by new cells, which take their origin in the germinative layer of the skin. This growing layer is made up of what are called Malpighian cells, named after Malpighi, the Italian anatomist, who first identified them.

The pigments which largely, though not altogether, determine the color of the skin are found in the Malpighian layer of cells. The color differences among the races of mankind, and many of the social implications which follow, are thus crucially determined by the amount of skin pigment in the Malpighian cells.

The outer layers of the skin are called the epidermis. Beneath is the dermis or true skin, also called the corium. This is tough, fibrous living tissue with undulating surfaces which penetrate into the epidermis above and into the subcutaneous tissue below. These undulations form series of ridges which are evident on the epidermis, especially on the hands and feet. They create the unique pattern of the individual's fingerprints.

The dermis is well supplied with blood vessels, small capillaries which can greatly expand and contract under nerve impulses and thus help control body temperature. Blushing is the phenomenon that occurs when the blood vessels expand. In the true skin layer are also to be found lymph vessels, nerve endings, sweat glands, sebaceous glands, and hair follicles.

The sensory nerve endings in the skin are capable of reporting a variety of sensations to the brain—as we have already pointed out.

The hair follicles are tiny tubes which harbor the hair roots, one hair to a follicle. As long as the follicle is not atrophied (worn out), injured, or diseased, the hair continues to grow.

The sebaceous glands usually lie close to the hair follicles. Their function is to secrete an oily substance, called sebum, which helps to keep the hair lustrous and the skin soft. An excessive secretion of sebum will produce such appearances as the shiny nose and may be responsible for acne. The glands of the outer ear canal, which secrete ear wax, are similar to the sebaceous glands.

Perspiration. There are from 2 to 3 million sweat glands in the human body. They are most plentiful in the armpits, on the hands and feet, and on the forehead. These tiny coils extract water and some other substances such as salt and urea from the blood flowing through the capillary vessels in the true skin. The extracted water, that is, sweat or perspiration, is then released to the surface of the skin through the minute tubules or openings which we call body pores.

The quantity of perspiration released daily varies greatly and depends on many factors. The sweat glands are never entirely idle. The body, even though it does not feel wet, is constantly releasing some water through the skin. This so-called insensible perspiration may amount to a quart a day.

Loss of body heat through perspiration, both visible and invisible, involves not the blood vessels but the sweat glands. The perspiration that exudes from the pores is removed from the surface of the skin by evaporation. A stream of warm, dry air speeds evaporation. That is why the warm breeze from an electric fan on a hot day still produces the sensation of cooling.

Underneath the true skin is a layer of subcutaneous tissue, which is usually largely infiltrated with fatty tissue. This layer gives the body its more delicate curves and contours. It serves as a cushion between the tegumentary covering of the body and the underlying muscles and permits the free rippling of the skin during muscular activity.

The Functions of the Skin. The skin serves many vital functions for the body. It is, first of all, a protective covering, a barrier against the invasion of pathogenic bacteria. Second, it is the important regulator of body temperature and is provided with the mechanisms with which to perform this task. Third, it is an organ of sensation that provides warning against some of the threats to life or health found in the immediate external environment. Fourth, it concerns itself with those reactions which heighten the body's immunity to disease. And, finally, it is an organ of expression, of many disorders, both infectious and psychic, which may affect the body.

Bacterial resistance on the part of the skin is high. This applies also to the mucous membranes of the lips, mouth, and other parts of the body. So long as the skin is clean, it very quickly gets rid of unwelcome bacteria that may come to lodge upon it. The mechanism of this repellent action is not altogether clear. Unless the skin is cut, broken, punctured (as by an insect), or abraded, harmful bacteria have a difficult time getting through its horny layer. Of course some bacteria always lie on the surface of the skin, just as some are always to be found in the mouth.

Skin blemishes, such as blackheads, pimples, sores, and scabs, should not be picked at anywhere on the body, but this warning should be doubly observed concerning the area that is called "the danger triangle of the face." This area is bounded by the bridge of the nose and the corners of the mouth. Because of the peculiar arrangement of veins and arteries feeding this area, bacterial infections originating here may be carried directly into the brain and set up a possibly fatal inflammation.

Sun Tan. The protective mechanism of the skin is expressed in still another way, namely, the release of skin pigment (melanin) to protect against injury to the skin from strong doses of sunlight. In the white races, which have comparatively little skin pigmentation, exposure to sunlight increases the amount of pigment produced by the specialized Malpighian cells. The result is a coat of sun tan. The tanning is caused by the invisible ultraviolet rays from the sun. The coat of tan disappears as the more highly pigmented cells die and move toward the surface of the skin.

How to Avoid Sunburn. Actually, a good suntan has little or no physiological value, but there is a therapeutic result in the sense of well-being gained from basking in the warm sunshine. An overexposure to hot sun can cause burns. Less known is the fact that continued overexposure over a period of years can cause the skin to look weatherbeaten, wrinkled, leathery, and coarse in texture.

Human skins vary a great deal in the amount of sun they can stand. Redheads, blondes, brownettes, blue-eyed, fair-skinned (and literally thin-skinned) people need to be especially wary of direct hot sunlight. Dark-skinned, darkhaired, dark-eyed persons have more immunity—but not complete immunity—from sunburn.

The time of day of exposure is important. The burning ultraviolet is most intense from 11 A.M. to 2 P.M. No sunburn is likely before 8 A.M. and after 4 P.M. High noon is the hottest time of the day for sunburn. Rays reflected from sand or water can burn, even though you may not be directly exposed.

Since individual sensitivities differ, you must learn for yourself how much sun you can tolerate. A general guide for most persons, assuming that previously untanned white skin is exposed about noon, is:

First day, expose skin to sun for 15 to 20 minutes each on face and back. Second day, increase exposure by one-third, to a little less than half an hour. Third day, again increase exposure by one-third, to from 30 to 40 minutes.

By the fourth day, a new pigment should begin to darken your skin. In a week you should have enough skin thickening and pigmentation to give considerable protection against burning sunshine.

Most of the suntan lotions contain chemicals called sunscreens, which absorb various wave lengths of burning ultraviolet rays to various degrees. The better lotions allow you to stay in the sun longer with less risk of burning. They do not shut out all radiation, or else you would never tan at all. There's no really good way of telling which of the suntan lotions is most effective for you until you try them.

The suntan pills, used under medical supervision and obtained by prescription, can help "easy burners" be better protected against painful burn while acquiring a tan. They are not for self-dosage.

Freckles are produced by the same mechanism as skin tanning. In this case, however, the areas of increased pigmentation are spotty instead of consistent.

Cosmetics. Cosmetics are beauty aids. Since the search for beauty is a universal and perennial pastime, the history of cosmetics stretches back into antiquity and may be expected to be reformulated in all future generations. Today in the United States cosmetics are big business. Well over a billion dollars a year is now spent annually on *all* varieties of cosmetic preparations, including soaps, shampoos, hand lotions, and the like. The people in the cosmetics business say, "We don't sell merchandise, we sell illusion." The danger in this is that many cosmetic preparations are overenthusiastically promoted and overpriced. Women are repeatedly cozened to expect miracles from cosmetics.

From the standpoint of mental health, the increasing use of cosmetics is probably justified. Yet cosmetics can never be a substitute for good health, and no better cleansing agent than ordinary soap and water has been developed. There is no way to "nourish" the skin by creams or lotions or falsely labeled "skin foods" applied

from the outside. The skin is nourished, like all body tissues, through its own blood supply. There is no known substance or combination of substances that can live up to the promises suggested in any of the following names: contour cream, crow's-foot cream, deep pore cleaner, enlarged pore preparation, eye wrinkle cream, miracle oil, nourishing cream, pore paste, rejuvenating cream, scalp food, skin conditioner, skin firm, skin food, skin tonic, eyelash grower, wrinkle eradicator, spot reducer, bust developer, bust reducer.

The hundreds of skin disorders that have been named generally represent the response of the skin to some insult or assault from within or without the body.

The diagnosis and treatment of these disorders require expert medical judgement. The attempt to self-medicate often makes them worse, sometimes causing "overtreatment dermatitis."

Contact dermatitis, of which poison ivy is a typical example, is the most common skin disorder produced by outside agents. To fight against such agents, the skin pours forth lymph fluid, which forms blisters. Along with the blisters usually come a burning sensation, itching, redness, and swelling. A number of industrial chemicals produce contact dermatitis.

Skin inflammations, rashes, and pustules arise

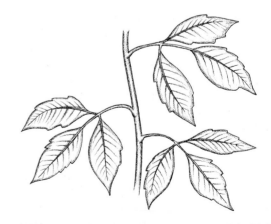

POISON IVY is one of the most common causes of the kind of skin trouble known as "contact dermatitis."

also from systemic infections of the body—the assault from the inside. Many diseases write their signature on the skin, for example, the permanent pock marks of smallpox and the temporary rashes of scarlet fever.

Welts, wheals, and bumps sometimes appear on the skin in protest, one might say, against something in the victim or his environment to which he is peculiarly sensitive. Hives (urticaria) is a sign of allergy. So, for example, is "strawberry rash."

Acne. Acne is often the bane of adolescent years. The skin appears greasy; it is covered with blackheads; pimples are numerous. The blackheads are the result of the clogging of the seborrheic ducts with oily plugs surrounding a dirt particle. An increased but sometimes excess secretion of sebum seems to be a normal event in the many body changes that occur with puberty. A clean face may well help prevent the development or aggravation of acne. Regular washing with soap and water is the important step. Avoidance of tampering with the facial skin will further help to ward off the risk of disfiguring secondary infection. However, the treatment of acne is not always quite so simple as this. The persistent case requires medical attention. New methods of treatment are constantly being devised. Some cases of acne respond to psychotherapy, just as others do to nutritional therapy. A lowered intake of fatty foods is sometimes helpful.

There is a gross, vulgar, and completely erroneous superstition that acne is "caused" by autoerotic practice or by "sexual experience" or, conversely, by the lack of it. This is pure nonsense.

Athlete's Foot. "Athlete's foot" is a type of fungus infection (epidermophytosis) on the feet and between the toes. The fungi grow from spores under favorable conditions of heat and moisture. That is why the "seed spores" tend to persist in swimming pools and gymnasium showers and locker rooms. Perspiring feet also favor their growth.

Most important on the individual's part in avoiding the itching scaling, and blistering of

"athlete's foot" is to make sure that his feet, socks, and shoes are kept thoroughly clean and *dry*.

Athlete's foot is sometimes a community problem. The use of a strong fungicide or detergent on premises where the spores are likely to be seeded should be undertaken at least twice a week. The ordinary footbath is not likely to have much effect on the fungi.

The Hair and Nails

Like the skin, the hair and nails are part of the tegumentary system of the body. They are not sense organs, although the hair is highly sensitive even to a light touch.

The distribution and growth of hair on the head and on the body are definitely linked to the endocrines. Hair growth is overt evidence of secondary sex characteristics. The Biblical story of Samson and Delilah demonstrates an ancient belief that hair means strength and cutting it loss of essential manhood or womanhood.

No "Cure" for Baldness or Gray Hair. There is no scientifically demonstrated "cure" for baldness (alopecia). The receding hairline is apparently an hereditary characteristic transmitted through mother to son. No hair tonic or "treatments" will restore hair to the head that is bald by reason of hereditary tendency. The loss of hair that occasionally follows acute diseases will, however, usually be made up. Hair cells are not "starved" through lack of circulation in the scalp, though stimulation of the scalp may possibly help to prevent premature baldness.

No "cure" for gray hair has yet been discovered either. The color of the hair is determined by the pigment in the cells of the central shaft of the hair, which is no longer living tissue when it emerges from the hair follicle. Gray hair, which lacks pigment, can be dyed to change its color, but there is no known and practicable way of stimulating the production of hair pigment.

One type of cosmetic preparation that must be used with special caution is the depilatory for removing unwanted hair. The only permanent way to remove unwanted hair is with the electric needle in the hands of a competent technician under medical supervision. The needle actually destroys the hair root.

Nails. The nails require little care except being cut and cleaned as dictated by social custom, which varies greatly. Nails grow out of a bed of skin beneath them and the cuticle in which they are imbedded. Infections at this margin sometimes occur. If serious, they require medical attention. "Hangnails" should be snipped, not pulled off. Ingrown toenails can usually be avoided by cutting the nails straight across.

SUMMARY

We have devoted this chapter to the crucial sense organs of the human being—eyes, ears, nose, mouth, and skin. We have also pointed out the numerous other bodily functions which these sense organs perform and discussed the special care and attention which each requires. A satisfactory feeling of personal fitness can hardly be achieved if these special sense organs are abused or neglected. The brain, of course interprets and gives meaning to the responses of the specialized end-plates of the sense organs.

SUMMARY REVIEW QUESTIONS

1. To what extent, if any, do you think the following objects or conditions are threats to eye health: television, sunglasses, snow blindness, artificial lighting, eyestrain, contact lenses, a cinder in the eye? Give reasons for your answer to each item.
2. What are the common defects in focus of the human eye? With what kinds of lenses can each of these defects be corrected? What part of the apparatus of the eye is primarily at fault when defects in focus are present?
3. What are the conditions of illumination which favor eye health and proper use of the eyes? To what extent do these conditions prevail in your own work and study quarters?
4. What are the principal parts of the human eye? Which part is chiefly affected by the disease conditions to which the eye is commonly subject? (Name at least four disease conditions—not counting defects in focus.)
5. What is the structure and function of the human ear? What are the most common causes of deafness?
6. How do the senses of smell and taste operate? Approximately how many odors can a human being distinguish? How many different tastes can a person distinguish? What are they?
7. What is the structure of the human skin? What precautions in the care of the skin are suggested by its structure?
8. What are the functions of the human skin? What suggestions for intelligent care of the skin (and complexion) does knowledge of these functions supply?
9. What are the common skin troubles to which a college student is subject? How can each of these be prevented? (Name at least four.)
10. What is the purpose of cosmetics? What are the dangers of their use? What cosmetic care is required by the human hair and nails?
11. Are the following statements sense or nonsense? Why? *Never read in bed. . . . "I feel positively undressed without my lipstick." . . . The only thing to put in your ear is your elbow. . . . Beauty*

is only skin deep. . . . It is just as good to squint as to wear glasses. . . . The way to treat gray hair is to dye it or forget it.

12. What do the following terms mean to you: optometrist, ophthalmologist, otologist, Malpighian layer, hyperopia, semicircular canals, olfactory chemoreceptors, alopecia, taste buds, "second sight."

Worth Consulting: *The Truth About Your Eyes* by Derrick Vail. *You and Your Skin* by Norman Goldsmith, M.D. *Cosmetic Science,* 1962, ed. by A. W. Middleton. For more complete references, see Appendix E.

10

NUTRITION, DIET, AND WEIGHT CONTROL

AMERICAN COLLEGE STUDENTS TODAY ARE probably the best nourished group of human beings who have ever lived. They have benefited physically by the startling advances that have been made in science and technology since the beginning of the twentieth century. These advances have included the sciences of nutrition and agronomy (scientific agriculture). Agronomy has given us such a plethora of foods in the United States of America that in the mid-1960's the government was still paying farmers *not* to grow certain plant and animal crops, and it held in storage around 8 billion dollars worth of excess agricultural products accumulated over the previous decade.

In the United States, well-stocked supermarkets lie within easy driving distance of practically any family, and packaged or refrigerated food delicacies from all parts of the world are available to any table. Much of our conversation about food concerns itself with how to diet and lose weight Eating places are the most common commercial enterprises in the country; cookbooks, next to Bibles, are the most staple items of the book publishing business.

We may sometimes forget that a vast number of the people in the world, and still some in the United States, are struggling just to get enough to eat.

An International Congress of Nutrition[1]

The Sixth International Congress of Nutrition convened in Edinburgh, Scotland, in August 1963. A review of this meeting by Krehl and Hodges will give a hint of the present breadth and complexity of the science of nutrition and also of the advanced subjects of research with which experts in the field are concerned. As the reviewers say, "The science of nutrition is a very diffuse subject, since it cuts across a number of basic disciplines. . . . The breadth and scope of nutrition is so great that it is impossible for one individual to encompass the entire field."

Two key themes at the nutrition congress were (1) the relationship of food supply to the world's present population explosion; and (2) the relationship of diet to disease, especially coronary heart disease—a relationship which implies a closer application of nutrition principles in medicine. But the congress also covered such topics as proteins and amino acids, vitamins, minerals and trace elements, lipids (fats), the

---

[1]"Sixth International Congress of Nutrition in Retrospect," reported by W. A. Krehl, M. D., and Robert E. Hodges, M. D., in Borden's *Review of Nutrition Research,* **24**: 4 (October–December, 1963).

nutrition of ruminant animals, animal production, plant genetics, endocrinology, nutrition in pregnancy, and early growth.

Later in this chapter we shall provide a simpler description of the fundamentals of nutritional science; but this early presentation of the jagged edges of front-line research should serve as a challenge to understanding the subject.

Food Supply. "The threat of hunger and malnutrition in a world undergoing a population explosion is the great threat and challenge to the future of man," affirmed Lord Boyd Orr, honorary president of the congress. He pointed out that the present world food supply would have to be nearly doubled to eliminate hunger and malnutrition, and that the chief increases would have to be in the expensive, protein-rich foods. If the world population actually reaches 6 billion by the year 2000, as sometimes predicted, the world food supply will have to be increased *fourfold,* Boyd Orr said. He believes that it would be possible to meet the demand by the extension of agricultural methods presently in use in the most technically developed countries, an optimistic point of view. Should these agricultural methods prove inadequate, however, he looks to biological and chemical methods applied to synthetic food production to provide a supplement to natural foodstuffs. Boyd Orr has long been an advocate of good nutrition and progressive agriculture as means of resolving key international problems.

Nutrition of the Preschool Child. The executive director of UNICEF told the congress what nutrition can do to better the lot of the world's children. He pointed out that the death rate of children from birth to one year in the technically underdeveloped areas of the globe is five times as high as in developed areas; and the death rate of preschool children, one through four years, in the developing countries sometimes 40 times as high as in the more fortunate areas. The quantity and quality of food available to the young child is a dominant factor in these statistics. To relieve the plight of children in many countries it is recommended that a "crash" preschool protection program be inaugurated—to supply protective foods within economic reach of the population.

Diet and Disease. The 1963 congress also debated dietary factors in causation of cardiovascular disease. There seemed little doubt in the minds of most nutritionists that diet in some elusive way is related to the etiology of coronary heart disease. But there were positive differences as to the degree of this relationship and the nutrients most responsible. For example, the Canadian Heart Foundation, accepting the premise that high levels of cholesterol in the blood significantly increase the risk of coronary heart disease, has recommended that people generally, and especially males, should consider the desirability of replacing about 50% of their intake of animal fats with unsaturated fats of vegetable origin. Other nutritionists questioned whether such a sweeping dietary change was justified.

A South African investigator reviewed the relationship of dietary protein to atherosclerosis (the accumulation of fat particles on the inner lining of the arteries), a presumed primary cause of coronary heart disease. One suggestion in his paper was that really long-term nutritional studies, beginning at birth and running 60 to 70 years, might have to be initiated to prove the debatable points in the relationship of diet to chronic and degenerative diseases. A Russian scientist, reporting animal (rabbit) experiments, claimed that vitamin C and nicotinic acid inhibit the development of atherosclerosis while vitamin D tends to increase it. Other nutritionists reported on changes in carbohydrate intake as a factor in reducing blood cholesterol. Among recommendations were (1) shifting the source of carbohydrate from readily available sugar to cereal starches, and (2) maintaining a larger intake of cereals (breadstuffs) in proportion to fat. A report on the milk and meat-eating Masai tribe of East Africa demonstrated that in this population, at least, a high intake of animal fat bore no relationship to increased blood cholesterol or atherosclerosis.

Proteins and Amino Acids (the building blocks of protein). Some points made and questions raised at the congress on this topic were the following:

A high-protein diet increases work capacity and favors increased productivity. For optimal growth, the diet must contain sufficient carbohydrate and fat so that the balanced protein is drawn on only minimally as a source of calories. At low protein intake levels the addition of certain amino acids may lead to amino acid imbalance and impaired growth. New research tools are needed to evaluate in a quantitative way the amino acid needs of different levels of calorie intake. More definitive measures of protein nutrition than determination of nitrogen balance are needed. What is the role of "protein reserve" in the body cells toward maintaining a nutritive balance?

Vitamins. The importance of vitamin B_6 (pyridoxine) in human nutrition was reported on by several investigators. After 21 days on a pyridoxine-deficient diet most of 11 healthy male subjects had abnormal electroencephalograms. On the characteristically high-protein American diet, a daily intake of about 2.0 milligrams of pyridoxine is recommended as optimum. Isotopes have proved valuable in nutritional studies. With radioactive vitamin D, it was possible to get a much more exact picture of its distribution in body tissues. Vitamin D is apparently destroyed in the liver. Isotopic techniques have also provided a clearer picture of calcium metabolism and recommendations for daily intake.

Minerals and Trace Elements. Several studies on mineral and trace element metabolism were reported at the congress. For example, the importance of metallic enzymes in cellular function was pointed out. These catalytic enzymes contain a metal atom firmly incorporated in their structure and essential to their activity. There is a *zinc*-containing enzyme which splits peptides. It was noted that the trace element, selenium, apparently exerts an activity comparable to that of fat-soluble vitamin E.

The brief summary of the Sixth International Congress on Nutrition presented above certainly does not cover all aspects of research in nutritional science now going on in the world. It should strongly suggest, however, the kinds of research upon which our present knowledge of nutrition is based. It is obvious, however, that a broad consideration of the subject of food and nutrition demands attention to social and psychological factors as well as to the findings made through physiology and biochemistry.

Food Prejudices

Unprejudiced normal appetite is the best guide to nutrition. Man and rat are omnivorous creatures; they eat everything. Even some of the things we call prejudices or superstitions about eating have a sensible basis, sometimes deep in folk-wisdom. For example: On a particular island in the South Pacific, it was observed that all food was liberally sprinkled with pepper made from a pepper tree that grew in front of every household. Indeed, the marriage ritual of people on this island absolutely required that the girl to be married must take shoots or seeds from the pepper tree in front of her mother's house, plant and grow them in front of her own. When a scientific analysis of the diet of these people was made, it was discovered that the pepper tree was the only source of vitamin C on the island.

Some personal food prejudices also have a reasonable basis in physiology and psychology. When a person says he doesn't like milk—or eggs, or chocolate, or onions—he may well know by personal experience that this particular food or beverage does not agree with him. He may indeed have a slight or pronounced allergy to it. Allergy to cow's milk, for instance, occurs both in infancy and later life.

Generally speaking, it is a good idea to avoid foods that you can still taste for several hours after eating—foods that "repeat on you," as the saying goes. It is also understandable that you may resist foods that were forced upon you at some time earlier in your life. You may secretly feel that you are swallowing your pride with every mouthful, and this masked resentment is a detriment to digestion. On the other hand you may learn to like foods that you formerly disliked—sometimes because you have discovered their nutritional value.

The child who cries for candy, ice cream, or

soda pop may sometimes be expressing a real need for the extra caloric values that they make quickly available or for the love and affection the giving of them represents. The disgruntled, crying child may also be lacking other nutrients —often minerals—in his diet.

We must also reconcile sex differences in attitudes toward food. Woman has traditionally played the role of food-giver in the household; indeed, this may be considered an extension of the mammary function. As food-giver, woman holds a position of power in the household and psychological implications of this fact should not be overlooked. To give (or withhold) food is in the final analysis to have the power of life or death, and even in subtler ways it is a means of controlling members of a family.

Food Fallacies. There remains, nevertheless, a vast amount of food prejudice and faulty eating habits arising from sheer ignorance, foolish fads and fashions, and from faulty and even fraudulent advice and advertising about food.

Some examples of nonsense preached in the name of nutrition are: "Eat raw foods only," "Don't mix carbohydrates and proteins at the same meal" (the stomach mixes them beautifully), "Molasses and yoghurt guarantee a ripe old age," and the like.

Half-truths and misstatements about food find millions of willing believers. This is a field in which the "big lie," told with a straight face, readily flourishes. People are more gullible about food nonsense than about almost anything else. They can be easily sold on the "magic" powers of one food or another. Here are some more of the lies about food that you are likely to encounter. *Don't believe them!*

"You are what you eat." Nonsense—you are also what you breathe and what your heredity determines you shall be.

"Fish is brain food." So is all other food.

"An apple a day keeps the doctor away." The apple-growers get sick and call physicians.

You may also hear such nonsense as: celery is a tonic, onions will cure a cold, garlic is good for heart disease, only "organic" foods supply proper nourishment, tomatoes are poisonous,

corn is hogfood. Don't believe it! You may also be urged to buy "health foods" (at fancy prices), daily vitamin pills (at even fancier charges), or "reducing foods." Save your money!

All pure foods are health foods when included in a scientifically sensible eating plan. A wide variety of common foods will supply all the vitamins you need. There are no "reducing foods." The amount not the kind of food is what counts in any diet safely designed to effect weight loss. Knowledge of the scientific facts about food and nutrition will fortify you against any of the food fallacies and myths you may henceforth encounter.

The Science of Nutrition

Nutrition is a comparatively young science. It dates back only to 1833, when a backwoods American army surgeon, William Beaumont, published at his own expense a thin classic volume entitled *Experiments and Observations on the Gastric Juice and the Physiology of Digestion.* The experiments were performed on a half-breed Indian, Alexis St. Martin. He had suffered a gunshot wound in the abdomen and it had never completely healed over. Beaumont tied different articles of diet to silk threads and introduced them into the Indian's stomach through the unclosed wound. He pulled the strings out again at suitable intervals of time and observed what had happened to the foodstuffs. He thus demonstrated that digestion was essentially a chemical process. (See pages 208 to 210.)

Intense research in nutrition since Beaumont, especially in the 1920's, has established some 50 to 60 chemical substances as essential to the nutrition of the human race. It is not necessary to know all their names, for the ingestion of a wide variety of common foods will deliver them all in adequate quantities.

Food and nutrition are not the same subject, although they are intimately related. Food does not become nutrient until it is eaten, digested, and absorbed through the alimentary system and delivered by way of the blood stream to the tissues and cells of the body which require these various nutrients for their function. A sick person can be "fed" by dripping purified essential nutrients into his veins (intravenous feeding). The more important use of the science of nutrition, however, is as a guide for selecting and eating foods which give the normally working organs of the body what they need for highest function.

The functions of food in the human body are obvious: to supply energy for muscle and other tissue function, which goes on all the time, to provide substance for the growth and repair of body tissues, and to insure a supply of all the nutrients, for example, vitamins and minerals, needed to regulate and control the complicated metabolic processes of the body. Water is equally essential. The energy requirements of the human being are provided by the combustion (oxidation) of the end products of carbohydrate, fat, and protein digestion.

When we are talking about proteins, carbohydrates, fats, and vitamins we are talking a chemist's language. These are not foods—like bread, meat, or butter—but rather chemical classifications of the ingredients in foodstuffs. Carbohydrates are so named because they contain definite proportions and arrangements of carbon, oxygen, and hydrogen. Proteins contain also nitrogen, which is their distinguishing chemical element, and sometimes other basic elements like sulfur or iron. By dealing with foodstuffs as organic chemical compounds we can better understand their function and effect in the human body.

The Digestive System and Process

The alimentary or digestive system of the human being is an extremely complicated apparatus and process. Fortunately, however, the process of digestion, turning food into nutrient, is practically automatic; man need be concerned only with getting food into his mouth and ejecting the waste products of that food—about 10% of the total—in a socially acceptable manner. The physiology of digestion is managed by the autonomic nervous system; it takes no conscious effort.

In its simplest terms the digestive system is a flexible mucus-lined muscular tube, 24 to 36 feet long, beginning in the mouth and ending at the anus. (See figure, page 180.) Along the tube lie a series of glands and cells which produce the chemical substances—such as saliva and gastric juice—that act upon foodstuffs taken into the mouth and break them down for absorption into the cells of the body.

Another process that takes place in the mouth is that of mastication, the chewing of food into small bits so that it can be efficiently handled by the rest of the digestive system. Mastication is the function of the teeth, which must be considered as part of the digestive system.

The Physiology of Digestion. The process of digestion begins in the mouth, where the teeth chew and grind food, and enzymes secreted by the salivary glands immediately go to work breaking down carbohydrates. About 7 seconds later—the time it takes for swallowed food to transverse the esophagus—the stomach takes over. Its 5 million tiny glands manufacture about 3 quarts of gastric juice a day. This includes hydrochloric acid, in a weak solution ranging from 0.2 to 0.5%, and the enzymes pepsin and rennin. The stomach itself is a pear-shaped distensible pouch, capable of holding 2 to 3 pints of food. Very few substances, notably honey and alcohol, are absorbed into the blood stream directly from the stomach.

Food stays in the stomach about 2 to 4 hours —sometimes longer. It is churned into a mushy, semi-solid mass, called chyme, and discharged into the duodenum. There it is acted on by more enzymes, arriving by way of a common duct (or channel) from the pancreas, and by bile. Bile is not an enzyme; it is essentially a solvent and emulsifier of fats. It is produced by the liver but stored and concentrated in the gall bladder. The pancreatic juices contain a great number of powerful and important enzymes. Some absorption of nutrients takes place in the duodenum, but to a far greater extent in the lower reaches of the small intestine.

Projecting from the inner lining of the small intestine are thousands of tiny absorptive organs

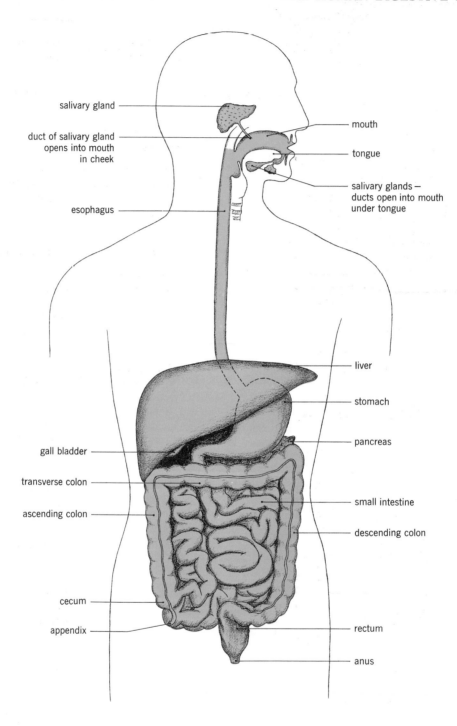

salivary gland

mouth

duct of salivary gland
opens into mouth
in cheek

tongue

salivary glands —
ducts open into mouth
under tongue

esophagus

liver

stomach

pancreas

gall bladder

transverse colon

ascending colon

small intestine

descending colon

cecum

appendix

rectum

anus

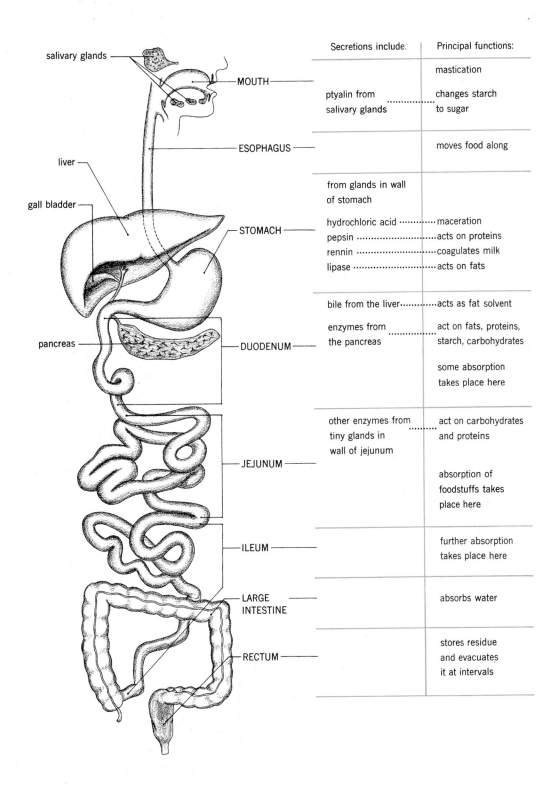

	Secretions include:	Principal functions:
MOUTH		mastication
	ptyalin from salivary glands	changes starch to sugar
ESOPHAGUS		moves food along
STOMACH	from glands in wall of stomach	
	hydrochloric acid	maceration
	pepsin	acts on proteins
	rennin	coagulates milk
	lipase	acts on fats
DUODENUM	bile from the liver	acts as fat solvent
	enzymes from the pancreas	act on fats, proteins, starch, carbohydrates
		some absorption takes place here
JEJUNUM	other enzymes from tiny glands in wall of jejunum	act on carbohydrates and proteins
		absorption of foodstuffs takes place here
ILEUM		further absorption takes place here
LARGE INTESTINE		absorbs water
RECTUM		stores residue and evacuates it at intervals

salivary glands

liver

gall bladder

pancreas

called intestinal villi (singular, villus). Finger-shaped projections, about $\frac{1}{25}$ inch long, the numerous villi give the lining of the small intestine the feel of velvet. Within each villus is a network of minute blood vessels, capillaries, surrounding a small tube called a lacteal.

When the broken down food particles are finally absorbed by the villi and conveyed to the blood stream for distribution to the rest of the body, the process of digestion is completed and the far more complicated processes of tissue nutrition and body metabolism may be said to begin.

About 90% of all nutrient substances in the food stream have been absorbed by the time it reaches the last 5 feet of the bowel, called the colon or large intestine. This is the drying portion of the bowel, which absorbs the remaining nutrients and water. The indigestible residue of food originally ingested remains in the large intestine about 24 to 30 hours before it is evacuated. Much, but not all, of the water is absorbed and returned to the blood stream. Swarms of bacteria, harmless to the individual for they are his own "bacterial flora," normally inhabit the colon. Approximately a third of the stool (feces) is composed of these bacterial swarms.

Eating and Bathing. During the process of digestion, special demands are made on the blood supply in the alimentary tract. The stimulation or rapid cooling of the skin by bathing also demands special functioning by the blood. Muscles engaged in heavy exercise draw heavily on the blood stream. Diversion of the blood supply from the digestive tract by bathing or exercise therefore tends to slow the process of digestion and may cause discomfort. Hence it is usually advisable to wait about an hour after eating before bathing. The great risk is that of swimming in cold water immediately after eating; cramps and drowning may result. Vigorous exercise soon before and after eating is inadvisable.

Peristalsis. The alimentary tract—the food tube—has walls containing smooth muscles capable of contraction. The particular arrangement of the muscle fibers of the food tube enable it to perform the unique type of muscular move-ment known as peristalsis. At intervals the tube contracts upon itself. A wave of contraction runs down the tube. The semi-liquid, partially digested food inside is thus squeezed bit by bit along the tube.

Peristaltic movements are most pronounced in the stomach and small intestine. The process is under the control of the autonomic nervous system. However, it can be stimulated by laxative drugs, by the sight and smell of food, by eating, and by the presence of irritating or bulky foods in the digestive tract. That is why the urge to defecate often occurs shortly after mealtimes.

The Chemistry of Digestion. A complex series of chemical processes, not all yet fully understood, breaks down the food we eat into ultra-microscopic particles, no longer than one twenty-five millionth of an inch in diameter.

The chemical processes of digestion are accomplished largely through the work of *enzymes* contained in the digestive juices. Enzymes are delicate chemical substances. Many are known to be simple proteins. Chemically, they act as catalysts; that is, they promote the chemical reactions going on about them but they are not themselves changed by the reaction. Most enzymes are powerful in their specific functions; for instance, the starch-splitting enzyme called amylase, if pure, will break down 20,000 times its own volume of starch in half an hour.

The end products of the digestive system proper are principally amino acids, simple sugars and neutral fats in very tiny globules. The amino acids are derived from proteins, usually animal proteins, taken into the human body. They are the building blocks of the cells that make up the human body; they are essential to tissue growth and repair and there is no substitute for them. There are some ten "nutritionally essential" amino acids. Given adequate supplies of these ten amino acids, the human body can manufacture others. A protein that contains all the essential amino acids is designated as a "complete" protein. All of these come from animal sources.

Simple or single sugars, primarily dextrose, are the end products of carbohydrate digestion. When absorbed through the intestinal walls and carried to the liver by the blood stream, these simple sugars are transformed into glycogen and later delivered to all body tissues as demanded in order to provide fuel or energy for their manifold activities. The end products of fat digestion are a number of fatty acids and glycerol. These are recombined into neutral fat. Some fat is quickly oxidized to provide energy for the body; some is stored in the adipose (fatty) tissues of the body.

Food Components

We now turn brief attention to "food components," that is, the specific needs for water, protein, carbohydrates, fats, vitamins, and minerals in the human diet.

Water. The human body is two-thirds water. We may readily conclude, therefore, that water is the prime requisite of the living person. Without it none of the other elements in food would be of any use. Water holds all the other elements in solution, both in and outside the body cells. The blood and lymph are principally water. The entire metabolism of the body requires water for its processes. A loss of 10% of the body's water is serious; a loss of 20% (as by extreme perspiration or bleeding) is scarcely tolerable.

The body excretes about 2 quarts of water a day. Most of it passes off through the kidneys as urine. However, sizable amounts of water are also lost through the skin by sweating and through the lungs in the process of breathing. Water is also expelled in the feces. The rate of water excretion is not constant. Hot weather, fever, or excessive exercise, for example, will increase the rate of water loss from the body, which strives, however, to maintain a water balance.

The powerful sensation of thirst is the mechanism by which the body makes known its water demands. Abnormal thirst, of course, may be a sign of disease (diabetes). If you follow your own sensations of thirst, your water intake will probably be adequate.

Various estimates have been cast up as to how much water a person should drink a day. The right answer to this question is simply,

"Enough"—as guided by your thirst. Additional water will be taken in as part of the foodstuffs eaten, and about a half pint will be created as a result of the oxidation of these foods in the body.

The water content of most foods is very high, especially in fruits and vegetables, many of which contain over 80% water. Fish foods are 75% water and many meats, such as beefsteak, are over 50% water. Ham and eggs are about half water; bread is more than a third water; butter contains comparatively little water (about 15%).

Under conditions of summer heat, where extreme sweating occurs, the replacement of fluids should be supplemented with the intake of salt (sodium chloride), which is intimately associated with the body's water metabolism. The extra salt may be taken in salt tablets or by generous salting of food.

Protein. Protein is the protoplasmic stuff of which living animal tissue is made. It is manufactured in and by the animal body. The building blocks of protein are the so-called amino acids, all of which contain nitrogen. Animals get their amino acids primarily from plants—through carnivores like lions and omnivores like rats and men get the largest share of their protein requirements by eating other animals. The corn-fed hog is the most efficient machine yet designed for the manufacture of protein.

Protein is essential to any human diet. No protein, no life! Indeed, the word, protein, adapted from the Greek by an early investigator, Mulder, means, "to take first place." The animal body uses the end-products of protein digestion to build and repair all of its essential cells and tissues.

Plants are capable of synthesizing amino acids by withdrawing nitrogen from the soil and the atmosphere. All animal proteins eventually derive from plant proteins. In the human diet it appears advantageous, however, that at least one-third of its protein requirements be met by animal proteins, for they are the complete proteins that contain all the essential amino acids. Plant proteins are incomplete.

The human diet is adequate in protein when

the combination of animal and vegetable proteins makes up about 10 to 12% of the diet.

There are many sources of protein in the mixed human diet. Among the richest sources of complete proteins are milk and liver. Other good sources of protein are meat (especially beef which has 50 to 90% protein exclusive of water), fish (which is 6 to 25% protein), eggs, cheese, nuts (especially Brazil nuts), and some vegetables like peas, beans (especially soy beans), and lentils. Cottage cheese is the least expensive protein food; lamb chops the most expensive—when figured in price per pound of protein.

There is a strong argument for including proteins in breakfast menus. They are digested more slowly than carbohydrates and most fats. Hence their presence in the digestive tract often prevents annoying midmorning hunger pangs.

The vegetarian gets some proteins from vegetables, if he is a strict vegetarian, or from animal-derivative products, such as milk and eggs, if he is not so strict. The need for some complete proteins cannot be obviated.

Amino Acids: How They Got Their Place in the Diet.[2] It took about a half a century of research to discover and demonstrate the essential amino acid requirements of man. German chemists, Kossel and Kutscher, at the turn of the twentieth century, found a quantitative method for separating the basic amino acids, arginine, histidine, and lysine. Emil Fischer at the same time discovered techniques which put in the hands of biochemists reasonably adequate tools for the study of proteins. Two distinguished American chemists, Thomas B. Osborne and Lafayette B. Mendel, then picked up the trail and proved, about 1914, that certain amino acids cannot be synthesized by living cells out of materials ordinarily present and must be supplied in a preformed state. This set the stage for thousands of animal experiments (largely rats) and eventually for the quantitative investigation of

human requirements. In 1949 W. C. Rose was able to publish a list of the eight amino acids essential, or indispensable, to man and define the minimum daily requirement of each. He set a recommended daily intake at twice the minimum daily requirement. The eight indispensable amino acids for man and their recommended daily intake in grams is as follows: tryptophan, 0.5; phenylalanine, 2.2; lysine, 1.6; threonine, 1.0; valine, 1.6; methionine, 2.2; leucine, 2.2; and isoleucine, 1.4.

Analyses of U.S. dietary habits, food purchases, and per capita consumption of proteins containing the eight essential amino acids reveal that the possibility of anyone in the United States experiencing an amino acid deficiency would be very remote indeed—except, of course, in extremely impoverished areas.

Carbohydrates. Carbohydrates are energy foods. They are the chief source of the fuel which the body burns to meet its energy requirements. In the average, normal American diet about half the requisite calories should be supplied by carbohydrates. Fats are also fuel foods, but much richer in energy, weight for weight. It should be pointed out that fats and carbohydrates play somewhat interchangeable roles in the body metabolism. Both contain the same basic chemical elements—carbon, hydrogen, and oxygen—though in greatly varying proportions and chemical structures. The carbohydrate requirement is the most elastic food need of the body. It is the easiest to cut down without losing nutritional essentials.

All human beings ingest a certain amount of cellulose, which is a tough plant fiber. In reasonable quantities this supplies "roughage" for the diet and aids the processes of digestion and excretion. Excessive amounts of "roughage," such as bran, act, however, to irritate the alimentary canal and should be avoided.

The common sources of carbohydrates are familiar: potatoes and other "starchy" vegetables (which may contain from 3 to 20% carbohydrate); bread, cake, spaghetti, macaroni and all other products made from cereal grains (of which

[2] "A Half Century of Amino Acid Investigations," W. C. Rose, *Chemical and Engineering News,* **30**: 23, 2385–2388 June 9, 1952.

wheat, containing about 70% carbohydrate is the most common); candy, sweetened drinks and all other forms of ingesting sugar.

Carbohydrates are in general the cheapest foods and can usually be produced at the least expenditure of land and labor. That is why the masses of most lands have taken some adaptable cereal grain as their staff of life. Even in the United States the price per pound of such staples as flour and sugar is substantially lower than that of meat or butter.

Fats. Like carbohydrates, fats play their principal role in human nutrition by helping to satisfy the energy requirements of the body. More than that, however, they are often the vehicle of other food substances, such as fat-soluble vitamins, needed by the body. In addition they form substances (lipids) which insulate nerve tissue. For optimum nutrition, approximately 25% of a person's total caloric needs should be derived from fats. Fed in excess, fat is neither appetizing nor assimilable and the body balks at it.

Fat-free diets are sometimes prescribed in the treatment of certain diseases, notably acne and heart disease. The fact remains, however, that the animal body can synthesize most if not all its needed fats out of carbohydrates and proteins. The cow, producing butter fat, does this lavishly every day.

The human dietary gets its fat supply from three principal sources: animal fats, dairy products, and plant oils. Among the plants the nuts and seeds are the richest sources of fats and oils. Peanut butter and peanut oil are vegetable fats. Olive oil is one of the most anciently used of vegetable fats. Margarine is hydrogenated vegetable oil; its nutritive qualities, if certain fortifiers are added, are equivalent to those of creamery butter. Claims have been made in recent years that "unsaturated" (soft) fats are to be preferred over "saturated" (hard) fats in the human dietary (for prevention of hardening of the arteries). These claims are not proved.

Fried and fat foods in the human diet often appear indigestible because the fats have been *overcooked*. It becomes difficult for the fat solvents in the digestive tract, such as bile, to break down these particles for full digestion.

Vitamins and Minerals

More nonsense has been written and spread about vitamins than about any of the other dietary essentials. The history of the discovery of vitamins provides a fascinating tale of scientific discovery and the commercial manufacture of synthetic vitamins literally by the ton was a triumph for modern industrial chemistry. However, diet which takes in a variety of common foods will supply all the necessary vitamins, since they are widely distributed in nature. Except in the case of clearly demonstrated vitamin deficiency, it is not necessary for the individual who eats a varied diet to get his daily vitamins from pills. The need for vitamin supplements in reducing diets or in the presence of illness or following surgical operation is something else again.

The recognition of a whole class of vitamin deficiency diseases must be chalked up as one of the major victories of twentieth century medical science. Many disease entities are now known to be caused by a lack of specific vitamins in the diet and to be curable by the administration of those vitamins in some item of food or in synthetic form. For example, lack of vitamin D causes rickets; of thiamin (vitamin B_1), beriberi (polyneuritis); of ascorbic acid (vitamin C), scurvy; of niacin, pellagra. All these are clearcut cases. The diseases were known and described long before vitamins were discovered and named.

Only when vitamin depletion or deficiency has gone a long way can the diagnostician put a sure finger on it. Physicians have sometimes prescribed vitamins in vague and obscure ailments because "they can't do any harm and they might do some good." People who prescribe vitamins for themselves are often taking only a "sophisticated faith cure." One general observation about vitamin deficiences now seems clear. The deficiency is rarely that of a single vitamin; it is much more likely to be a multiple vitamin deficiency. As they actually operate in the human body, we may now think of vitamins as components of its complicated enzyme system.

It is not enough simply to have vitamins in the diet; the body must be able to absorb and utilize them. For these reasons the official estimates of human vitamin needs—so far as they can be determined—are usually on the generous side. (See table of Recommended Daily Dietary Allowances on pages 192 and 193.)

In the history of science vitamins were employed on an empiric basis without any knowledge of their actual existence. The ancient Egyptians, for example, knew that eating liver would enable them to see better at night. We know that liver contains stores of vitamin A, whose absence from the diet tends to cause the condition of night-blindness (xerophthalmia). Again, the discovery that scurvy could be prevented by taking small amounts of lemon juice and cured by larger amounts was made as early as 1593 by the English sea dog, Captain Hawkins. Today we know that citrus fruits are very rich sources of ascorbic acid.

The word "vitamin," a misnomer, was invented in 1911. Casimir Funk, a Polish chemist, working in London, took great masses of rice hulls and endeavored to extract from them by chemical methods the substance that would cure beriberi. He got a white, crystalline compound that he christened—wrongly but luckily— "vitamine." His theory was that the compound contained "amines," a class of chemical compounds, and that it was vital to life. Neither of these facts turned out to be correct. Nor was Funk's compound a pure product. Nevertheless, the name caught on and stuck. (Later it lost the final "e.")

There was great value, however, in Funk's easily stated hypothesis that lack of vitamins was the cause of a number of deficiency diseases. It was on this assumption that a great volume of nutritional research was undertaken. The vitamin field turned out to be far more complicated than anyone had imagined. At first it seemed useful and possible to identify vitamins simply by the use of letters of the alphabet. Now we know that there are probably more vitamins than

there are letters of the alphabet, and it has become the general practice, except in a few instances, to refer to vitamins by their chemical names. Thus vitamin B_1 has become thiamin; vitamin B_2 or G, as it was variously designated, is now known as riboflavin; and vitamin C is ascorbic acid. There are at least a dozen vitamins in the B complex.

Important Vitamins. From the practical standpoint of human nutrition, only a few vitamins have to be seriously considered in diet planning, namely A, C, D, and three members of the B complex—thiamin, niacin, and riboflavin. Other known vitamins include: pyridoxine, pantothenic acid, choline, biotin, inositol, para-aminobenzoic acid, folic acid, vitamin B_{12} (probably concerned in blood formation), vitamin E (possibly concerned with the integrity of the neuromuscular system), and vitamin K, essential to normal blood clotting. Vitamins are distinguished as fat-soluble—vitamins A, D, E, and K—and water soluble—most of the others. Some are heat-labile and therefore easily destroyed by cooking; most are heat-stable. The functions and principal dietary sources of the more important vitamins are as follows.

Vitamin A was once known as the "anti-infective" vitamin. It appears to aid somewhat in resistance to infection by preserving the integrity of the epithelial tissues. The formation of "visual purple" in the retina of the eye requires vitamin A.

Excellent sources of vitamin A are fish oils (e.g., cod-liver oil), liver, milk, egg yolks, spinach, lettuce, broccoli, mustard and dandelion greens, green beans, carrots, yellow sweet potatoes, Hubbard squash, and such fruits as peaches and apricots.

Thiamin (vitamin B_1) is essential for carbohydrate utilization, normal appetite, and intestinal function. It is the lack of this vitamin which creates the disease beriberi. The body does not store thiamin as effectively as it does many other vitamin substances. By far the best single source of thiamin is dried brewer's yeast.

Riboflavin (vitamin B_2 or G) appears to be necessary for normal growth and for the integrity of mucous and epithelial tissues. Its absence from the diet is usually most evident in cracks in the skin, on the face, lips, tongue, and about the eyes.

Milk is the most common source of riboflavin in the human diet. Other rich sources are liver and kidneys, dried brewer's yeast, lean meats, fish, chicken, beet and turnip greens, carrots, eggs, and peanuts.

Niacin, also called nicotinic acid, was originally identified as the vitamin substance necessary for prevention of pellagra. This disease is characterized by digestive disturbances, usually diarrhea, skin eruptions, mental depression, loss of appetite, sore tongue, and loss of weight. The disease was once extensive among the poor of the southern part of the United States. The addition of fresh fruits and vegetables and milk to their diet, which had been rather strictly limited to "salt pork, hominy grits, and molasses," soon began to wipe out the pellagra belt.

The best sources of niacin in the human diet are liver, dried brewer's yeast, salmon, kidney, lean meats, poultry, peanuts, milk, spinach, lettuce, whole-wheat bread, enriched bread, green cabbage, and peas.

Ascorbic acid (vitamin C) is one of the most delicate of the important vitamins—that is, most easily destroyed by heat and oxidized by standing. Extremely water-soluble, it is often lost in cooking water. The body does not store this vitamin well, so it must be constantly replenished. Ascorbic acid prevents (and cures) scurvy and all the subclinical, mild manifestations of this disease, such as bleeding gums.

Citrus fruits—grapefruit, oranges, lemons, and limes—are the best sources of vitamin C. However, many other *fresh* fruits and vegetables, notably tomatoes, contain generous amounts.

Vitamin D, sometimes called the anti-rachitic vitamin or the "sunshine vitamin," prevents rickets in infants and children. It is essential to the proper absorption and utilization of calcium and phosphorus by the body. It is important to normal tooth formation. Without sufficient vitamin D, children are subject to bone deformities, pot bellies, restlessness—the syndrome of rickets.

Adult men and women, except pregnant women and nursing mothers, have little if any need of vitamin D supplements in their diet. The human body manufactures adequate supplies of vitamin D for itself when sufficiently exposed to the ultraviolet rays of the sun.

Overdosage with vitamins is not common, but it is possible and may have deleterious effects. Overdoses of vitamin D can cause hypercalcification (overhardening of bones), and too much vitamin A can stunt bone growth in a child. Vitamin C is perhaps the "safest" vitamin.

Minerals in the Body. About 4% of the total weight of the body is made up of inorganic or mineral elements, chiefly calcium and phosphorus. Still, there is enough iron to make a good size nail and enough sodium for a small shaker of table salt. In general, the minerals are regulators of metabolic processes. The fourteen so-called mineral elements deemed essential in human nutrition are calcium, phosphorus, iron, sodium, zinc, copper, potassium, sulfur, manganese, magnesium, cobalt, iodine, fluorine and chlorine. "Trace amounts" of other minerals, such as aluminum, silicon and nickel, are also present.

From the standpoint of human diet, however, we must give the most important consideration to the three mineral elements which are most likely to be lacking in the American diet—namely calcium, iron, and iodine. When these elements are supplied from natural food sources, the other mineral elements needed are also likely to be present. A good variety of common foods supplies required minerals in adequate quantities. The body stores and utilizes them well.

Calcium plays many roles. It is essential to the growth, development, and maintenance of bones and teeth. It is necessary to the clotting of the blood. It helps to regulate the heartbeat, to maintain the acid-base balance in the body, and to control the irritability of the neuromuscular system.

Calcium is needed throughout life, but is most important in the early years. The richest source of calcium in the human diet is milk—mother's, cow's, goat's, camel's, or mare's. Another good source is shellfish.

Phosphorus likewise is essential for the development of the bony structure of the body and the regulation of acid-base balance. In many respects calcium and phosphorus play complementary roles. Phosphorus plays an added role in carbohydrate and fat metabolism. Phosphorus is widely distributed in many foodstuffs, often in the form of phosphates. If calcium intake is adequate, phosphorus usually comes along with it.

Iron in the human body is concentrated largely in the blood and blood-forming organs, chiefly the bone marrow. It is an essential constituent of hemoglobin, the crucial element in the red blood cells. It is needed for the transport of oxygen by the red blood cells.

Actually, the amount of iron required by the body is small—only a few specks, equivalent to the daily intake of about 12 milligrams. Variety meats, like liver, are the best sources of iron.

Copper, as a dietary essential, usually goes along with iron, but only about one-quarter as much is needed. *Sodium* and *potassium* are another pair of minerals that complement each other's effects in cell and body metabolism; they are importantly concerned with water balance. Sodium is found in common table salt, along with chlorine that appears as hydrochloric acid in the stomach juices. *Iodine* is essential for the manufacture of thyroxin by the thyroid gland. Iodine is found in seafood and it is added to common table salt in the form of potassium iodide.

The Teeth

A presentation of the human digestive system and the processes of digestion could hardly be complete without an adequate discussion of the teeth. Necessary for chewing food, the teeth are an integral part of the digestive system in man and lower animals. A human being can lose all or most of his teeth and still remain alive; but for wild animals such a loss spells an early death. Many species of animals require tooth and fang both to obtain food and to keep from becoming prey themselves. In man, too, the teeth have functions beyond mastication. They have an important role in speech, assist in maintaining the position of the jaws, and affect the shape and appearance of the face.

A full set of adult teeth numbers 32; 16 each in the upper and lower jaws. The four sharp front teeth in each jaw are called incisors. Next to them on each side stands a cuspid tooth, followed by a first and a second bicuspid. Beyond these, stretching toward the back of the mouth, lie the molars or grinding teeth: the first, second, and third molars. The teeth grow from embryonic tooth buds.

First permanent molars, sometimes called sixth-year molars, are probably the most important teeth in the mouth. They erupt through the gum usually during the sixth year of life and take over much of the heavy work of chewing while the "baby," "primary," or deciduous, teeth are falling out.

The last of the permanent teeth to appear in the mouth are the third molars, or "wisdom teeth," which appear during the late teens and early twenties. Very often these molars come in at a wrong angle, or impacted against the second molar. It may then be necessary to have them extracted. However, they are not a serious loss to the business of mastication.

The part of a tooth that can actually be seen in the mouth is called its crown. This is only about one-third of the tooth. The other two-thirds, the roots, lie below the gum margin. The front teeth usually have only one root; the others have two or three roots. The crown of the tooth is covered with enamel, which is the hardest substance in the body. The roots are covered with a bonelike material called cementum.

Directly inside the cementum and enamel is a softer bonelike substance known as dentin. Inside this is a space called the pulp chamber, where the blood vessels and nerves of the tooth are located. The blood vessels and nerves reach the pulp chamber through narrow channels (root canals) which originate at the tip of each root. Exposure of the dentin through breaks in the enamel usually causes the nerves to register sensitivity to sweets and to temperature (hot and

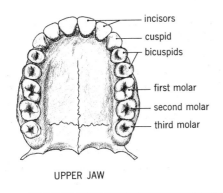

UPPER JAW

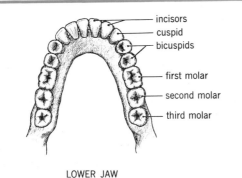

LOWER JAW

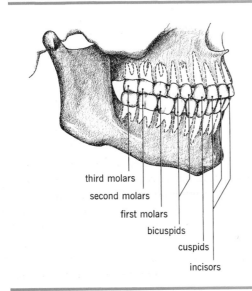

HUMAN TEETH. Top: The dental arch (adult upper jaw). Center: The dental arch (adult lower jaw). Bottom: A side view of the teeth in the upper and lower jaws. The dotted lines indicate how the roots of the teeth are set in the jawbones.

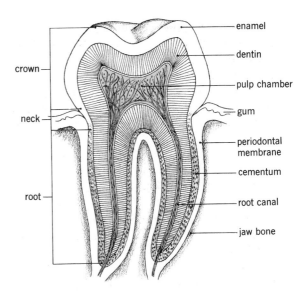

INNER STRUCTURE OF THE TOOTH. Only about one third of it—called the crown—is visible above the gum margin.

cold). Toothache occurs when the decay of the dentin goes deeper and comes closer to the pulp of the tooth.

Below the gum line the tooth is surrounded by a thin soft tissue called periodontal membrane. This membrane helps to take up the shock of chewing, and its presence helps to explain why the teeth can be moved slightly in the jaw. The teeth are not set directly in the jawbone, which lies outside the periodontal membrane.

Tooth Decay (Dental Caries). Along with the cold, dental caries is among the most common diseases of civilized man. Ninety-seven out of a hundred Americans suffer in some degree from tooth decay.

American dentistry is the best in the world, but statistics on the incidence of dental disease in the United States remain appalling. One explanation may be needless, childish fear of dentistry as a "necessary evil" instead of a positive health measure.

A high incidence of dental caries occurs during the late teens and early twenties, essentially the college years. By the time he has reached his thirties, the average American has only twelve healthy unfilled teeth in his mouth. Artificial dentures, so-called false teeth, are worn by fifteen out of a hundred Americans, and it is estimated that another twenty per hundred could profitably use them.

A great deal of research has gone into the attempt to find a satisfactory method for the control of dental caries. The mechanism of tooth decay—the steps by which it proceeds—is well known, but the real "causes" of dental caries remain as obscure, and possibly as complex, as the causes of cancer. The Council on Dental Health of the American Dental Association declares: "There is as yet no single factor which in itself will give complete control over tooth decay." The Council urges a four-part program including early and frequent examinations of the teeth, early treatment of small areas of decay found, attention to certain factors of diet and nutrition, and mouth hygiene.

For adolescents and adults it would seem that the only practical steps toward preventing caries are the practice of oral hygiene and possibly the reduction in the diet of fermentable carbohydrates, especially sugar, on which acid-forming bacilli flourish.

For young children, however, dental research has achieved an important chemical method of helping to prevent caries. The direct (topical) application of a fluoride solution to the surfaces of the teeth of children appears to reduce the caries attack rate as much as 40% on the average.

Fluorine and the Teeth. The story of fluorine in relation to the teeth is a fascinating example of controlled research and bears brief retelling. In the 1890's dentists began to observe that children and adults who had lived in the area of Colorado Springs for the first eight years of their lives had a strange kind of enamel on their teeth. It was mottled enamel, pocked with little brown or chalky-white patches.

Later this mottled enamel began turning up in other communities. Eventually it was traced to the drinking water of the community. About 1931, the specific element in the water which caused the mottled enamel was discovered. It was fluorine.

Then, in the 1930's, the dentists began to make a careful study of the people with mottled enamel. Contrary to previous assumption, it turned out that these people had about 60% fewer cavities than people who were brought up in areas where there were no fluorides in the water supply. In other words, the fluorides helped to protect teeth from decay.

The U.S. Public Health Service, whose dental division has conducted much of the fluoride research, then set out to determine how much fluorine added to the drinking water would cut down the caries rate and still not produce mottled enamel. The answer came out—about one part per million. This amount is perfectly safe and does not mottle the teeth.

On the basis of this research some ten cities in the United States and Canada began the mass public health experiment of adding fluoride (one part per million) to their drinking water (fluoridation). The results were so convincing that hundreds of communities have now added fluorides to their municipal water supplies, but not without public objection in many places.

Campaigns for fluoridation of public drinking water supplies as a strong line of defense against dental caries were pioneered by the U.S. Public Health Service and have been approved by virtually all important public health agencies including the American Dental Association. Nevertheless there are still some voices raised against it.

Oral Hygiene. The "father of modern dentistry," Pierre Fauchard, a Frenchman, wrote in the first great textbook of dentistry, published in 1728: "Little or no care as to the cleansing of the teeth is ordinarily the cause of all the maladies that destroy them." This half-truth has rung down the centuries. However, there is no such thing as a bacteriologically clean tooth. There are always some bacteria in the mouth. The Council on Dental Health scotched the old falsehood in these words:

Cleanliness of the mouth may aid in the control of tooth decay. The purpose of brushing the teeth, in this respect, is to remove fermentable food debris.

. . . Toothpastes, powders, and liquids are used only to aid the brush. As far as is known, there is no powder, paste, or liquid dentifrice which in itself will prevent tooth decay. . . . In most instances, the proper use of a satisfactory toothbrush, a safe dentifrice, and . . . thorough rinsing of the mouth with water immediately after eating will assure maximum benefits; but the effectiveness of this procedure in the control of tooth decay has not been established.

Your choice of a safe dentifrice may be made on the basis of taste or size of package as well as any other consideration. Otherwise powdered table salt and baking soda will provide you with as abrasive a dentifrice as you need. Too much abrasion of the teeth may harm them; too little, as with liquid dentifrices, may provide too little cleansing action. Plain water with a little salt added is as good a mouthwash as any.

Other Dental Disorders. Among the dental and oral disorders, other than caries, to which an individual may be subject are gingivitis (inflammation of the gums), root abscesses, "trench mouth" (Vincent's infection), and another periodontal disease, popularly called pyorrhea.

Though gingivitis is not uncommon in children, the condition often occurs in middle or later life partly as a result of failure to keep the gum line free of tartar deposits (dental calculus). Poorly fitted dental appliances may also cause irritation of the gums. One advantage of tooth brushing and having the teeth cleaned twice a year by a dentist is that cleaning will help prevent the development of gingivitis and periodontal disease.

Disease in the periodontal membranes that surround each tooth appears to be the greatest single cause of loss of teeth after age 35. The condition commonly arises from neglect of an earlier gingivitis. If this disease is not treated, it may spread to the tooth sockets so that the teeth become loosened and may eventually fall out. Adequate dental treatment can usually cure periodontal disease, but there is no simple "home remedy" for "pyorrhea." Complete and regular dental care, including the replacement of extracted teeth and correction of malocclusion (failure of teeth to come together properly), is important to the prevention and treatment of periodontal disease.

The Balanced Diet

If you eat a wide variety of common foods, the chances are that you will be eating wisely. Your nutritional needs can be as readily satisfied by the breadth of your taste for many kinds of food as by the sharpness of your arithmetic in calculating daily food allowances. Your weight will depend not on the kinds but rather on the amounts of food you eat.

Malnutrition, sometimes called "hidden hunger," is the outcome of prolonged failure to include essential food components in the diet. Except in the presence of disease conditions which warrant direct medical attention, malnutrition can easily be prevented by regularly (although not necessarily daily) eating so-called protective foods. These include tomato or citrus-fruit juices ($\frac{1}{2}$ cup a day), milk (at the rate of a pint a day), whole-grain cereals, one raw fruit or vegetable, and some inexpensive fat (for example, peanut butter).

Wise selection of a tasty, well-balanced diet of food and drink is a genuine aid to healthier living, improved personal appearance, and a better outlook on life. Furthermore, as research on the dietary needs of pregnant (and prepregnant) women is increasingly showing, proper choice of diet has an important bearing on the future of the human race.

The six essentials or components of the nutritionally adequate, or "balanced," human diet are water, protein, carbohydrates, fat, vitamins, and minerals. *A good variety of common foods supplies them all in adequate quantities.*

Food Selection: "The Essential 4"

Many valid systems of food selection, aimed at optimum nutrition, are based upon the scientific knowledge of human nutrition summed up in the Recommended Daily Dietary Allowances table on pages 192 and 193.

One such system, now designated as the "Es-

RECOMMENDED DAILY DIETARY ALLOWANCES,[a] REVISED 1968, FOOD AND

Designed for the maintenance of good nutrition of practically all healthy people in the U.S.A.

	Age[b] (years) From Up to	Weight (kg)	Weight (lbs)	Height cm	Height (in.)	Calories	Protein (gm)	Fat-Soluble Vitamins Vitamin A Activity (IU)	Vitamin D (IU)	Vitamin E Activity (IU)
Infants	0–1/6	4	9	55	22	kg × 120	kg × 2.2[e]	1,500	400	5
	1/6–1/2	7	15	63	25	kg × 110	kg × 2.0[e]	1,500	400	5
	1/2–1	9	20	72	28	kg × 100	kg × 1.8[e]	1,500	400	5
Children	1–2	12	26	81	32	1,100	25	2,000	400	10
	2–3	14	31	91	36	1,250	25	2,000	400	10
	3–4	16	35	100	39	1,400	30	2,500	400	10
	4–6	19	42	110	43	1,600	30	2,500	400	10
	6–8	23	51	121	48	2,000	35	3,500	400	15
	8–10	28	62	131	52	2,200	40	3,500	400	15
Males	10–12	35	77	140	55	2,500	45	4,500	400	20
	12–14	43	95	151	59	2,700	50	5,000	400	20
	14–18	59	130	170	67	3,000	60	5,000	400	25
	18–22	67	147	175	69	2,800	60	5,000	400	30
	22–35	70	154	175	69	2,800	65	5,000	—	30
	35–55	70	154	173	68	2,600	65	5,000	—	30
	55–75+	70	154	171	67	2,400	65	5,000	—	30
Females	10–12	35	77	142	56	2,250	50	4,500	400	20
	12–14	44	97	154	61	2,300	50	5,000	400	20
	14–16	52	114	157	62	2,400	55	5,000	400	25
	16–18	54	119	160	63	2,300	55	5,000	400	25
	18–22	58	128	163	64	2,000	55	5,000	400	25
	22–35	58	128	163	64	2,000	55	5,000	—	25
	35–55	58	128	160	63	1,850	55	5,000	—	25
	55–75+	58	128	157	62	1,700	55	5,000	—	25
Pregnancy						+200	65	6,000	400	30
Lactation						+1,000	75	8,000	400	30

[a] The allowance levels are intended to cover individual variations among most normal persons as they live in the United States under usual environmental stresses. The recommended allowances can be attained with a variety of common foods, providing other nutrients for which human requirements have been less well defined.

[b] Entries on lines for age range 22–35 years represent the reference man and woman at age 22. All other entries represent allowances for the midpoint of the specified age range.

Water-Soluble Vitamins							Minerals				
Ascorbic Acid (mg)	Folacin[c] (mg)	Niacin (mg equiv)[d]	Riboflavin (mg)	Thiamin (mg)	Vitamin B_6 (mg)	Vitamin B_{12} (μg)	Calcium (g)	Phosphorus (g)	Iodine (μg)	Iron (mg)	Magnesium (mg)
35	0.05	5	0.4	0.2	0.2	1.0	0.4	0.2	25	6	40
35	0.05	7	0.5	0.4	0.3	1.5	0.5	0.4	40	10	60
35	0.1	8	0.6	0.5	0.4	2.0	0.6	0.5	45	15	70
40	0.1	8	0.6	0.6	0.5	2.0	0.7	0.7	55	15	100
40	0.2	8	0.7	0.6	0.6	2.5	0.8	0.8	60	15	150
40	0.2	9	0.8	0.7	0.7	3	0.8	0.8	70	10	200
40	0.2	11	0.9	0.8	0.9	4	0.8	0.8	80	10	200
40	0.2	13	1.1	1.0	1.0	4	0.9	0.9	100	10	250
40	0.3	15	1.2	1.1	1.2	5	1.0	1.0	110	10	250
40	0.4	17	1.3	1.3	1.4	5	1.2	1.2	125	10	300
45	0.4	18	1.4	1.4	1.6	5	1.4	1.4	135	18	350
55	0.4	20	1.5	1.5	1.8	5	1.4	1.4	150	18	400
60	0.4	18	1.6	1.4	2.0	5	0.8	0.8	140	10	400
60	0.4	18	1.7	1.4	2.0	5	0.8	0.8	140	10	350
60	0.4	17	1.7	1.3	2.0	5	0.8	0.8	125	10	350
60	0.4	14	1.7	1.2	2.0	6	0.8	0.8	110	10	350
40	0.4	15	1.3	1.1	1.4	5	1.2	1.2	110	18	300
45	0.4	15	1.4	1.2	1.6	5	1.3	1.3	115	18	350
50	0.4	16	1.4	1.2	1.8	5	1.3	1.3	120	18	350
50	0.4	15	1.5	1.2	2.0	5	1.3	1.3	115	18	350
55	0.4	13	1.5	1.0	2.0	5	0.8	0.8	100	18	350
55	0.4	13	1.5	1.0	2.0	5	0.8	0.8	100	18	300
55	0.4	13	1.5	1.0	2.0	5	0.8	0.8	90	18	300
55	0.4	13	1.5	1.0	2.0	6	0.8	0.8	80	10	300
60	0.8	15	1.8	+0.1	2.5	8	+0.4	+0.4	125	18	450
60	0.5	20	2.0	+0.5	2.5	6	+0.5	+0.5	150	18	450

[c] The folacin allowances refer to dietary sources as determined by *Lactobacillus casei* assay. Pure forms of folacin may be effective in doses less than $\frac{1}{4}$ of the RDA.

[d] Niacin equivalents include dietary sources of the vitamin itself plus 1 mg equivalent for each 60 mg of dietary tryptophan.

[e] Assumes protein equivalent to human milk. For proteins not 100 percent utilized factors should be increased proportionately.

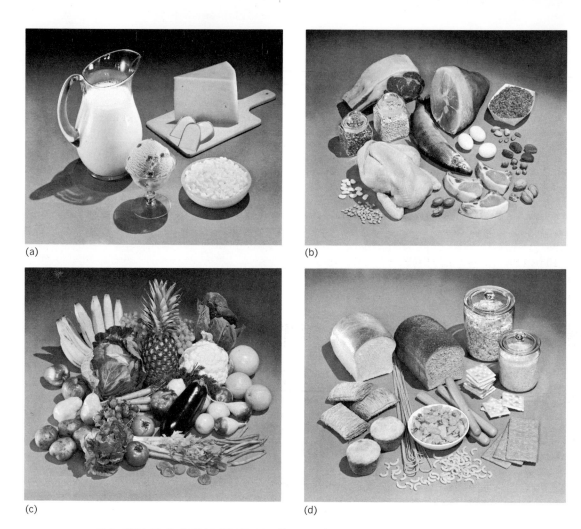

THE "ESSENTIAL 4" FOOD GUIDE: (a) Milk group; (b) Meat group; (c) Vegetable-fruit group; and (d) Bread-cereals group. (Photographs courtesy of National Dairy Council)

sential 4" food guide, is centered around protective foods and omits specific groupings for fats, oils, sugars, and syrups on the ground that these are usually eaten in combination with the "essential" foods and that their nutritional contribution is mainly in calories.

The "Essential 4" food guide suggests that *daily* food intake include "servings" from each of the four following food groups:

1. *Milk group*—milk, cheese, ice cream.

2. *Meat group*—meat, poultry, fish, eggs, dry beans and peas, nuts.

3. *Vegetable-fruit group.*
4. *Bread-cereals group.*

Let us apply these groupings to the matter of shopping for food or selecting meals at an eating place.

1. Milk Group (2 plus servings a day). This grouping might also be labeled "dairy products" or "milk and milk products."

Some milk or milk products should be taken daily. The "serving" is an 8 ounce cup or glass. In terms of fluid whole milk the recommended amounts are: children, 3 to 4 cups; teen-agers,

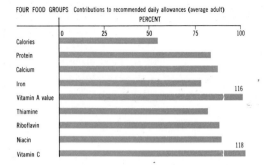

FOUR FOOD GROUPS Contributions to recommended daily allowances (average adult)

	PERCENT				
	0	25	50	75	100
Calories					
Protein					
Calcium					
Iron					
Vitamin A value					116
Thiamine					
Riboflavin					
Niacin					
Vitamin C					118

4 or more cups; adults, 2 or more cups; pregnant women, 4 or more cups; nursing mothers, 6 or more cups.

In place of fluid whole milk may be substituted fluid skim milk, buttermilk, evaporated or condensed milk, dry milk, cheese—cottage cheese, cream cheese, cheddar-type cheese, natural or processed—or ice cream. The milk equivalent of ice cream and cream cheese is about half that of fluid whole milk, volume for volume; that of cottage cheese, about two-thirds. A 1-inch cube of cheddar-type cheese is equivalent to $\frac{2}{3}$ cup of milk.

2. Meat Group (2 servings a day). This grouping might also be labeled "protein foods," for it contains many foods beyond meats which are valued for their protein content—notably poultry, fish, eggs, nuts, and some high-protein vegetables. Another label for this grouping might be the "main-course" dishes—for these are the foods which generally comprise the main course of a meal and establish its price or cost.

Two or more servings a day should be chosen from this group. Count as a serving: 2 to 3 ounces of lean, cooked meat, poultry or fish—all without bone; 2 eggs; 1 cup of cooked dry beans, dry peas, or lentils; 4 tablespoons of peanut butter.

3. Vegetable-Fruit Group (4 servings a day). These are usually the "side-dish," salad, appetizer, and sometimes dessert courses of a meal.

Four or more servings of fruits and/or vegetables a day are recommended. Count as a serving: $\frac{1}{2}$ cup of vegetables or fruits or such portions as are ordinarily served—i.e., one medium apple, orange, banana, or potato; half a medium grapefruit or cantaloupe. Fruits and vegetables

are reasonably interchangeable in this system. You could eat 4 servings of fruit and no vegetables; or vice versa; or 2 and 2; or 3 and 1 either way—provided, however, that you include 1 serving, every day, of a good source of *vitamin C* (ascorbic acid) or 2 servings of a fair source; and

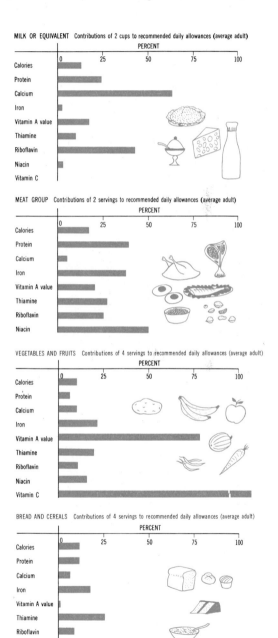

MILK OR EQUIVALENT Contributions of 2 cups to recommended daily allowances (average adult)

	PERCENT				
	0	25	50	75	100
Calories					
Protein					
Calcium					
Iron					
Vitamin A value					
Thiamine					
Riboflavin					
Niacin					
Vitamin C					

MEAT GROUP Contributions of 2 servings to recommended daily allowances (average adult)

	PERCENT				
	0	25	50	75	100
Calories					
Protein					
Calcium					
Iron					
Vitamin A value					
Thiamine					
Riboflavin					
Niacin					

VEGETABLES AND FRUITS Contributions of 4 servings to recommended daily allowances (average adult)

	PERCENT				
	0	25	50	75	100
Calories					
Protein					
Calcium					
Iron					
Vitamin A value					
Thiamine					
Riboflavin					
Niacin					
Vitamin C					

BREAD AND CEREALS Contributions of 4 servings to recommended daily allowances (average adult)

	PERCENT				
	0	25	50	75	100
Calories					
Protein					
Calcium					
Iron					
Vitamin A value					
Thiamine					
Riboflavin					
Niacin					

Nutrition, Diet, and Weight Control   195

1 serving, at least every other day, of a good source of *vitamin A*.

4. Bread-Cereals Group (4 servings a day). This grouping includes many items that are sometimes designated as "energy foods." It might also be called the "grain-food" group. It includes many low-cost carbohydrates which supply calories and satisfy hunger. However, if these breads and cereal foods are whole grain, enriched, or restored—as they should be and their *labels* will tell—they also furnish worthwhile amounts of thiamin, niacin, iron, and protein to the diet.

Four or more servings a day from the bread-cereals group should be taken. This means 3 slices of bread and 1 serving of cereal, or 5 slices of bread and no cereal. Count as a serving of cereal: 1 ounce of ready-to-eat cereal, ½ to ¾ cup of cooked cereal.

Included in this group are bread, crackers, ready-to-eat and cooked cereals—including rice, cornmeal, grits, and rolled oats—macaroni, spaghetti, noodles, and dumplings. Biscuits, muffins, cake, cookies, and other baked goods made with whole grain or enriched flour can also be counted.

Other Foods. You are not through eating when you have taken the indicated number of servings of the "Essential 4" foods. Depending upon the choices you have made among them, you will still be one-third to one-half short of the daily calorie allowance for an average adult. The deficit can be made up by additional servings of the "Essential 4" foods or by butter, margarine, other fats, unenriched refined cereal products, sugar, and sweets. This additional food will serve to round meals out and to provide additional nutrients. The "Essential 4" food guide is only the *foundation* for an adequate diet. Its minimum number of specified servings together provide most, but not all, of the nutrients needed for good nutrition.

Faulty Eating Habits. Faulty eating habits result not only from poverty and food prejudices but also from emotional stress or sheer carelessness. Skipping breakfast because you are in a hurry to get to class or to the office is a faulty eating habit. The digestive system is "at rest," actually in its normal condition, when it is working on food. Too long an interval between meals may put needless stress upon it. A certain regularity in mealtimes is desirable, though this does not have to be made a rigidly monotonous rule. Eating the same food—often at the same place—every day is another faulty eating habit; a one-track diet is usually a poor diet. Overspicing foods is another habit to be avoided. Here is a simple test for a food ignoramus: he puts salt on his food *before* he tastes it.

How Many Meals a Day? The common American meal pattern has been set at three meals a day, but this is simply a matter of custom and convenience. Other countries, peoples, and climes have evolved different patterns. On the European continent, for example, a "first" and "second" breakfast were once common. Natives of Liberia deem one meal a day sufficient. Industrial workers are more efficient when they have five meals a day instead of three. The midmorning and midafternoon "coffee break" for worker or student and the "late snack" before going to bed are now common and sensible American customs. Eat when you like provided that you get the same general balance of nutrients as given by the conventional three-meals-a-day pattern. The best time to eat is when you are hungry. It is a mistake to engorge a heavy meal when your appetite says "No." The great danger of eating outside of scheduled mealtimes is that it promotes a tendency to ingest far more calories than you need.

Weight Control

Almost everyone at some time would like to add or take off a few pounds. A young woman is usually interested in losing weight to improve or keep her figure. Many young men want to gain weight to step up their physical or athletic prowess. Older people strive to keep their weight down to help resist the degenerative diseases. Within limits one can control his weight. A certain amount of weight consciousness is a good thing, but constant worry about weight is unhealthy. For the most part you must accept a weight appropriate to your body frame just as you accept the color of your skin, hair, and eyes.

Body Build. Body weight is crucially determined by body build. You inherit your body build, whether it is tall and slim, short and stocky, or in between. The breadth of your shoulders, the thickness of your bones, your tendencies to slow or rapid fat metabolism, and possibly the peculiarities of your endocrine system descend to you from a long line of ancestors. Nutritional practices cannot change your "destined" body frame and organs, although lack of nutritional essentials may deform or disorder potential structure and function.

Although no amount of wishful thinking can change your body frame, it is possible, to control—within limits—the amount of flesh, and particularly the amount of body fat, that is suspended from that frame. Some of this control lies definitely within the scope of medical treatment; a lesser part may be achieved by personal effort.

Gradual increase in body weight from childhood through maturity is a normal and expected process. Long-continued *failure* to gain weight at this time of life demands medical investigation. Sudden or radical *change* in weight, whether up or down, is often a sign of disease.

So-called standard height, weight, and age tables have long been in vogue. These have their uses, but they do not tell you what is a normal or optimum weight for you. The tables are only averages, based on measurements of many thousands of people. Few people hit the mathematically calculated standard figure. The range of the normal is very wide. Your best weight may be as much as 10% under or 10% over the calculated standard for your height and age. Beyond that 10% limit, however, which is the common definition of overweight, a medical evaluation of your weight is called for. In terms of your body frame it may still be normal for you.

Overweight. Records of life-insurance companies indisputably show that death rates are

WHAT SHOULD YOU WEIGH?

Women[a]	Weight (Indoor Clothing)			Men	Weight (Indoor Clothing)		
Height with Shoes	Small	Medium	Large	Height with Shoes	Small	Medium	Large
4' 10"	92– 98	96–107	104–119	5' 2"	112–120	118–129	126–141
11"	94–101	98–110	106–122	3"	115–123	121–133	129–144
5' 0"	96–104	101–113	109–125	4"	118–126	124–136	132–148
1"	99–107	104–116	112–128	5"	121–129	127–139	135–152
2"	102–110	107–119	115–131	6"	124–133	130–143	138–156
3"	105–113	110–122	118–134	7"	128–137	134–147	142–161
4"	108–116	113–126	121–138	8"	132–141	138–152	147–166
5"	111–119	116–130	125–142	9"	136–145	142–156	151–170
6"	114–123	120–135	129–146	10"	140–150	146–160	155–174
7"	118–127	124–139	133–150	11"	144–154	150–165	159–179
8"	122–131	128–143	137–154	6' 0"	148–158	154–170	164–184
9"	126–135	132–147	141–158	1"	152–162	158–175	168–189
10"	130–140	136–151	145–163	2"	156–167	162–180	173–194
11"	134–144	140–155	149–168	3"	160–171	167–185	178–199
6' 0"	138–140	144–159	153–173	4"	164–175	172–190	182–204

[a]If you are a woman between 18 and 25 years of age, you should subtract one pound for each year under 25.

While these "new" desirable weight tables are "actuarially sound," and represent average normal patterns of weight, you may still be within a normal weight range for yourself if you are 10% over or 10% under the figures given above. Beyond that range you owe yourself a medical check-up for professional diagnosis and possible assistance in your personal weight-control program. (Tables from Metropolitan Life Insurance Company.)

higher than average among obese, overweight people. Doctors have long observed that obesity is associated with increased incidence of diabetes, gallstones, high blood pressure, some forms of heart disease (coronary artery disease), and their complications. But nobody has yet proved that overweight is a *cause* of these diseases.

Many overweight individuals can profit from losing weight. Some cannot and some may even be harmed by trying. The doctor treats the whole patient, not just his excess fat. Serious attempts at extensive weight reduction should not be started without a physician's advice.

A person becomes overweight when he takes in and holds on to more calories than he puts out. Technically, he has a positive caloric balance. The aim of any weight-reduction treatment or regimen is to achieve a negative caloric balance. To this end a reduction in food intake is usually the safest and most effective means. Any diet low in calories but adequate in proteins, vitamins, and minerals is a reducing diet. Vitamin and mineral pills may sometimes be necessary and prescribed; in themselves they do not take off any weight.

The use of thyroid substance to take off pounds is inadvisable and may be dangerous. Appetite-killing drugs are of doubtful value.

It is one thing to lose weight, quite another to keep it off. Most people who diet strenuously to lose weight regain poundage—return to what is perhaps their "normal weight"—soon after they stop dieting. The best way to keep from becoming overweight is to eat sensibly, exercise reasonably, and live happily from childhood on.

Few people achieve that way of life. A high percentage—probably 75%—of overweight people are anxious people. They use food as a tranquilizer to allay their anxiety. Quite often this anxiety can be traced to the development of unhealthy attitudes toward food and eating in earlier years of their lives. For example, some families regard eating as a chore—to be finished up as quickly as possible. In others, food is used as a reward or a punishment; children are given certain foods (candy, apples, oranges, popcorn, for example) if they are "good," or sent to bed without dinner because they have been "bad."

Some people have unhappily learned to turn to food as a substitute for love and acceptance or as a consolation prize in lives. (Prison riots are often touched off by a decline in the quality of meals.) Some people use their teeth on food as weapons of defense or offense. They overeat either to armor themselves with fat against a too-demanding world, or to become "big as a house" so they can't be pushed around. Some fat people refuse to admit they are overweight; they simply see themselves as big and strong.

Food is intimately connected with the emotional and social circumstances of life from birth. If the helpless infant is not fed by his mother, he dies. It is not surprising, therefore, that distorted attitudes about food and eating often arise early in life or that overweight from overeating is a common result. It is not the only possible outcome. Underweight and many disturbances of the digestive system result from distorted attitudes and emotions about food.

The problem of *weight control is more of a psychosomatic problem* than the "diet faddists" care to admit. The motivations for weight control must be strong and long continued. There are no quick miracles—no drugs, no pills, no salves, no baths, no electric belts or queer exercise machines—that can permanently "take off those pounds of unsightly fat." There is no royal road to the optimal weight. Even with the best of medical advice, the persistent cooperation of the individual is requisite.

Calories and What They Mean. In the simple mathematics of weight control the key is the calorie: the amount of heat required to raise 1 kilogram (2.2 pounds) of water 1 degree centigrade (from 15 to 16 degrees centigrade). This is the definition of the large calorie, as used in nutritional studies, and it was originally written with a capital "C." There is also a small calorie, used in other physical measurements, which is just one-thousandth ($1/1000$) as large as the nutritional calorie. The popular phrase, "Count your calories," simply suggests that you reckon the number of heat units that you pop into your mouth with your food.

The caloric value of any foodstuff can be easily determined. Experiments reveal that carbohydrates and proteins, weight for weight, yield the *same* number of calories. Fats produce $2\frac{1}{4}$ *times* as many calories as do equal weights of proteins and carbohydrates. In other words:

Fats produce   9 calories per gram
Carbohydrates produce   4 calories per gram
Proteins produce   4 calories per gram

Expressed in pounds, this set of figures means that 1 pound of protein or carbohydrate will yield 1814 calories while 1 pound of fat will yield 4082 calories.

If you want to calculate your own caloric intake, the following table of ratios will be helpful:

Fat: $2\frac{1}{4}$ Water ⎫
Carbohydrate: 1   Vitamins ⎬ :0
Protein: 1   Minerals ⎭

You must remember, however, that nutrient values of food cannot be judged by gross weight because different foodstuffs contain greater or lesser amounts of *water*.

What price water? It is a question that can be profitably asked when buying food. Butter, as noted, contains only about 15% water, but bread carries twice as much (30 to 35%) and beefsteak three times as much (45 to 50%). The differing percentages of water present explain why you will get the same amount of food energy from a $\frac{1}{2}$-ounce pat of butter as from a medium-sized potato (5 ounces), a large orange (10 ounces), or 33 large lettuce leaves.

The energy requirements of human beings, in terms of calories, are not constant. They vary with weight, age, sex, occupation, and presence or threat of disease. Many interesting calculations have been made concerning the daily caloric requirements of people doing different kinds of work or performing different kinds of exercise (See figure, page 126.) Thus we find that a male student—sitting at his books for ten hours a day—would consume merely 2500 calories. Moderately active, he would need an extra 500 calories. If he were a football player, he would use up 5000 calories a day on game and practice days. The woman student needs about 2100 calories a day. When she becomes a housewife doing her own work, she will need an extra 400 calories a day. If she takes a job as a waitress, her daily caloric requirement will rise to 3000. It must be recognized that all these figures are estimates and averages around which many individual factors play.

Basal Metabolism. Your body expends energy—uses up calories—even while you are asleep, for obviously there is a great deal of internal work that must be done. Energy must be found to keep up the body temperature—man being a warm-blooded animal—to perform the functions of breathing, circulation of the blood, digestion and other metabolic processes, and to keep up the muscle tonus.

The amount of energy that the body must expend to get all its internal work done is designated as its basal-metabolic energy or, more simply, as its basal metabolism. The basal-metabolic *rate* of an individual can be measured, and remains at a surprisingly constant level in adults. Endocrine-gland disorders, especially overactivity of the thyroid gland, can, however, greatly increase the basal-metabolic rate.

Basal metabolism is usually somewhat lower in women and in older people. In the sedentary man about three-fourths of his caloric intake goes to maintain his basal metabolism. The "average" (154-pound) man requires about 1775 calories a day just for this purpose.

How to Lose Weight

The sum and substance of all scientific advice on weight control is simply this: If your intake of calories is greater than your output of calories, you will gain weight. If the output is greater than the intake, you will lose weight.

In a general way you have a "natural weight," just as you have a "natural height," based in the main on your genetic inheritance, your constitutional diathesis, and the general state of your health. The big problem is not really to take off weight but to keep it off. Your emotional attitudes toward food may well stand in the way of maintaining your "natural weight."

Although you have probably heard or read of scores of reducing diets, there are really only three basic systems for safely reducing your daily caloric intake. Though they go under many names, we shall describe them as (1) the Essential Four System, (2) the Fraction System, and (3) the Caloric Number System. All of them require the exercise of some willpower for which there is no obtainable substitute.

1. *The Essential Four weight-reducing system* means restricting your daily food intake to the servings of the four essential food groups (dairy, meat [protein], fruits and vegetables, cereal grains) without supplementation of other servings. This system assures you all the protective foods you need and gives you (depending on your actual bodyweight) somewhere between 50% and 80% of daily caloric requirements necessary to maintain your current weight.

2. *The Fraction System for losing weight* means that you eat a balanced, low-calorie diet by cutting down normal servings, or portions, to a fraction ($\frac{1}{4}$, $\frac{1}{2}$, $\frac{3}{4}$) of their usual size. This is the theory behind most diets advertised as "eat what you want and get (or stay) slim."

3. *The Caloric Number System for weight loss* is operated as follows:

a. Pick the desirable weight for yourself from the tables "What Should You Weigh?" on page 197.

b. Multiply that number by 15, if you are moderately active; by 13, if you lead a very sedentary life; or by 17 if you are exceptionally active physically. This will give you your own caloric number; that is, the number of calories that you must ingest daily to maintain your desirable weight.

c. If you want to lose weight, deduct 20% to 25% from your caloric number and limit your daily caloric intake to that number of calories. Roughly speaking you will come out with a 1000, a 1200 or a 1500 calorie a day diet. Examples of such diets are on pages 201 and 202.

More drastic dieting than this should not be undertaken without medical supervision. If you reduce your calories by about 500 to 600 a day, you can expect to lose about a pound a week. It often takes a week or two of reduced food intake, however, before your dieting program begins to show effect on your weight. So don't be discouraged if you seem to be making slow progress during the first few weeks of your dieting regime.

Some Practical Hints for People on Weight-Reducing Diets.

¶ Avoid those high-fat, high-calorie "tempting treats" listed in the table of High-Calorie Foods on page 203.

¶ Eat slowly and in small bites. If you don't wolf down your food, small portions will seem bigger than they are and keep down hunger pangs.

¶ Drink water freely—before, during, and after meals. That will help to give you a "filled up" feeling.

¶ Go light on salt, which may tend to give you a "waterlogged" feeling, but be generous to yourself with other spices (which don't contain countable calories).

¶ Practice some appetite-killing habits: (1) take a cup of hot bouillon or half a cup of skim milk before dinner, (2) remove yourself from the smell as well as the sight of tempting foods; (3) stem hunger pangs at any time of the day by nibbling on low-calorie, high-bulk foods; for example, vegetables like raw carrots, celery, lettuce, and endive; fruits like watermelon, honeydew melon, apples, and grapefruit (unsweetened); breadstuffs like a slice of Melba toast or a rye wafer or two; no-calorie beverages like hot (or iced) coffee or tea (without sugar or cream); and high-protein, low-calorie foods like cottage cheese and fruit gelatin.

¶ Space your food intake generously through your waking hours. You don't have to stick to three meals a day. Eat midmorning, midafternoon, and bedtime snacks of the low-calorie variety as long as you don't exceed your desirable daily caloric intake for a "reducing" diet.

SAMPLE DIETS TO FIT YOUR CALORIC NUMBER

In all the sample diets and menus given in this series, count 1 cup as 8 ounces, 3 teaspoons as 1 tablespoon, 4 tablespoons as $\frac{1}{4}$ cup.

These diets can be varied by substituting foods of equal caloric value in the same Essential Four categories and can be moved up or down a few hundred calories a day by omissions or additions of a few items. Take a few double helpings to increase the caloric count; cut some servings in half to decrease the caloric count.

1000-CALORIE MENU

Breakfast
Grapefruit, medium size
Egg, one
Butter, one-half teaspoon*
Skim milk, one glass
Coffee without cream or sugar†

Lunch
Ham omelet, made with one egg and two tablespoons
   of lean, diced ham
Squash, three heaping tablespoons
Celery, one large heart
Radishes, four small ones
Apple sauce, three tablespoons
Skim milk, one glass
Tea without sugar

Dinner
Chicken, medium serving, two ounces
Mashed potatoes, two tablespoons
Beet greens, three heaping tablespoons
Salad, made with two lettuce leaves, twelve slices of
   cucumber, one slice of tomato, dressed with vinegar,
   lemon juice, and spices
Banana, medium, sliced if desired

*Use it either to fry or scramble the egg, or, if egg is boiled, on toast

† Some of the skim milk may be mixed with the coffee, giving you *café au lait*.

1200-CALORIE MENU

Breakfast
Orange juice, one-half glass or cup
Egg, boiled, scrambled, or fried[a]
Wholewheat or enriched bread, plain or toasted, one
   slice
Black coffee[b]
Butter or enriched margarine, one teaspoon or "pat"

Lunch
Roast beef, hot or cold, one two ounce serving, 4-inch
   square slice
Whole wheat or enriched bread, two slices[c]
Vegetable salad with one tablespoon of French
   dressing
Cherries, 10 to 12
Skim milk, one cup[d]

Dinner
Chicken, three ounces (one large thigh or leg or three
   slices of breast)
Green peas, one-half cup
Potato, small
Salad, with one teaspoon of salad oil
Butter or enriched margarine, one teaspoon or "pat"
Peach, medium
Skim milk, one cup[d]
Black coffee[b]

[a] Use half the butter to fry or scramble egg, other half on toast

[b] Chemical sweetener may be added

[c] Obviously the two slices of bread and the roast beef will make a hot or cold roast beef sandwich that can be conveniently ordered at a restaurant

[d] You can pour part of your skin milk on sliced peaches. You can also choose *buttermilk* in place of skim milk for lunch, dinner, or both.

See Calorie Counter of Common Foods, Appendix C, to construct other menus within your daily dietary allowance.

1500-CALORIE MENU

Breakfast

Orange juice, $\frac{1}{2}$ cup (4 ounces)

Breakfast cereal, enriched ($\frac{1}{2}$ cup)

Egg, boiled, fried, or scrambled

Butter, or fortified margarine, 1 teaspoon or "pat"[a]

Milk, whole fluid milk, 1 cup[b]

Toast or bread, enriched, 1 slice

Coffee[c]

Lunch

Cheese sandwich, made with 2 thin slices of Cheddar
    cheese, 4 inches square (2 ounces), and 2 slices bread
    or toast, enriched or whole wheat.

Butter, enriched margarine, mayonnaise, or peanut
    butter, 1 teaspoon, to add flavor to the sandwich

Watermelon, half a slice, 1 inch thick

Milk, whole fluid, 1 cup[b]

Coffee[c]

Dinner

Roast veal, 3 thin slices 4 inches square[d]

Mashed potatoes, $\frac{1}{2}$ cup

Green beans, sweet and sour (sauce made with vinegar
    and sugar equivalent to 1 teaspoon per cup of sauce)
    $\frac{1}{2}$ cup

Fresh tomato, sliced and salted, on 3 large lettuce
    leaves

French dressing, 1 tablespoon, on the lettuce and
    tomato salad

Dinner roll, enriched flour, 2 inches in diameter

Butter or fortified margarine, 1 teaspoon or "pat"

Grapes, $\frac{1}{2}$ cup

Tea with lemon[c]

[a] Use half, if desired, to scramble or fry egg, other half
on toast or bread.

[b] Use some of the milk on the breakfast cereal; put some
in the coffee, if you don't like it black

[c] Chemical sweetener may be added

[d] Liver may well be the principal meat dish at least once
a week.

3000-CALORIE MENU

(For a tall, husky, hardworking man, this menu might
still be part of a *reducing diet.* It might also serve as
a *balanced daily diet* for a big, moderately active man,
an exceptionally husky and physically active woman,
or a nursing mother. For most people, however, this
would be a *weight-gaining diet.*)

Breakfast

Orange juice, 1 full cup (8 ounces)

Enriched farina, 1 cup

Poached egg

Bacon, three strips, 4 inches long

Toast, 1 slice

Butter or fortified margarine, 1 teaspoon or "pat"

Milk, whole, fluid, 1 glass (8 ounces)

Coffee *with* sugar (2 teaspoons) and light cream (2
    tablespoons)

Lunch

Oyster stew, 1 cup

Chef's salad with 1 tablespoon French dressing

Bread, white, enriched, 1 slice

Butter or fortified margarine, 1 teaspoon or "pat"

Cantaloupe, $\frac{1}{2}$

Coffee *with* sugar (2 teaspoons) and light cream (2
    tablespoons)

Midafternoon snack

Malted milk, 10-ounce glass

Dinner

Black bean soup, one cup

Sirloin steak (cut 4″ x 3″ by 1″ thick)

Baked potato

Whole wheat bread, 2 slices

Eggplant, slice 4 inch diameter by 1 inch thick

Dill pickles

Butter or fortified margarine, 2 teaspoons

Chocolate eclair

Coffee *with* sugar (2 teaspoons) and light cream (2
    tablespoons)

Before bedtime

Milk, whole, 1 cup

Crackers, 2 graham or 3 soda crackers ($2\frac{1}{2}$ inches
    square)

NO-CALORIE AND LOW-CALORIE FOODS

Eat freely, even on a reducing diet.

Pickles (dill, sour, "bread-and-butter")

Cucumbers

Onions

Radishes

Watercress

Salad greens (e.g., lettuce, endive)

Soups (hot or jellied, such as consomme, bouillon, and chicken)

Parsley

Lemon or lime juice, slices, sections (without sugar)

Celery

Green peppers

Cranberries (unsweetened)

Gelatin (unsweetened)

Rennet tablets

Spices and flavoring agents (e.g., salt, pepper, paprika, vinegar, mustard, horseradish, celery and onion salt, mint, sage, cinnamon)

Chemical sweeteners (e.g. saccharin)

Black coffee, without sugar

Tea, hot or iced, without sugar

Lemon and lime drinks, without sugar

HIGH-CALORIE FOODS

Avoid these foods when you want to *lose* weight. Eat them freely when you want to *gain* weight.

	Number of calories
Malted milk (usual fountain size)	450 to 500
Fruit or chocolate sundae (large)	325 to 350
Fruit or chocolate ice cream soda	300 to 325
Lemon meringue pie (3-inch slice)	300
Mince, blueberry, cherry, and other rich and fancy pies (3-inch slices)	300
Beef hamburger on bun (3-inch patty)	300
Cheesecake (2½-inch slice)	250 to 300
Avocado pear (½ of a 4-inch pear)	250 to 275
Hot dog (frankfurter) on roll	250
Iced cupcake (medium)	250
Waffle (griddle cake, 6-inch diameter)	200
Candy bar (chocolate almond, 5-cent size)	200
Peanut butter (tablespoon)	100
"Hidden calorie" foods (depending on number or size of helping)	100 + or −

Potato chips	Olives
Potato salad	Nuts
Salad dressings (with oil)	Fried foods

Reducing Exercises. Contrary to popular opinion, vigorous exercise is not by itself an effective means of losing weight. Moderate exercise, in conjunction with careful dieting, may sometimes prove beneficial, but even this is not always the case, for exercise often sharpens appetite. So-called reducing exercises have more value in helping to redistribute body fat about the contours of a plump figure that they do in helping to get rid of the fat.

Swimming is probably the best of all recreational exercises for weight reduction. The reason is twofold: first, considerable energy is actually expended (about 125 calories in a fifteen-minute swim); and second, the metabolism of the body is forced to speed up in order to counteract the cooling effect of the water on the body temperature. Of course there are limits both to the length of time one should stay *in* the water (not over an hour) and to the temperature of water in which it is safe to swim.

If you actually want to lose weight, you will encourage yourself by keeping a record of your success. Weigh yourself twice a week under the same conditions (same time of day, same scale, same clothes) and make a chart of your progress. Do not expect miracles. You will gradually lose weight if you can resist excess food.

Gaining Weight. If you want to gain weight, you should reverse the processes suggested for losing weight. In other words, *eat more.* Underweight is generally considered a sign of ill health, and often it is. On the other hand, it must be remembered that some people may be naturally slim or even "skinny" as a result of their inherited body build. No matter how much they eat, they cannot put on weight.

The obvious causes of underweight are wasting illness—particularly hyperthyroidism, diabetes, or infections producing fever; overactivity—restlessness, lack of sleep, constant running around—in short, the "social whirl"; actual lack of food because of poverty or abnormal social conditions such as war and famine, and loss of appetite. These conditions must be corrected before weight gain can be expected as the result of consuming more calories. Lack of appetite may in itself be an expression of some underlying illness.

Psychology of Obesity

Many studies on the relationship of psychologic factors to obesity have been made. One of the best studies was made by Dr. Hilde Bruch, who noted that fat children were the ones who most often became obese adults. Dr. Bruch has written:

Deposition of fat is not a passive process; it is more than a mechanical sequel of positive energy balance. Storage of fats is regulated through the [autonomic] vegetative nervous system and is controlled through impulses from the midbrain.

Thus an individual can give material expression to the inner picture of his own self. Through accumulation of fat tissue the child [or child grown up adult size] aggrandizes his physical appearance . . . Overweight in the child is an active process, expressing the child's effort to achieve growth and self-realization, though in a distorted way.

Although every person, thin or fat, has his own unique personality pattern, there appear to be some common inner characteristics of people who are or grow fat.

The truly fat person, the chronic or compulsive eater, is rarely the happy-go-lucky, food-loving individual that he is often pictured to be. Almost always he is suffering from one or more inner emotional conflicts. He is making use of food in large quantities to overcome the discomfort of his inner struggles. He often employs the resultant obesity as a weapon of offense or in defense of his ego.

Fat children and fat adults may seem passive or submissive, but these appearances are usually deceptive. They have a stubborn determination to control their family environment by being helpless or dependent. They raise a fuss when there is any frustration or delay in meeting their incessant demands. When they meet rejection at school or in later life, they resort to overeating for comfort and compensation.

Many fat people are preoccupied with tales and incidents of crime and violence; their fantasies are engaged by these subjects. They may also have a secret fear of their own feelings of violence and aggression. Because they think of themselves as "big," many fat men have avoided fights all their lives because they imagine that they might kill someone. In retaliation, they attack their food.

Many fat people have a false image of their own bodies. They equate size and strength. To lose body substance—as by going on a reducing diet—means loss of strength or power and may give them a sense of emptiness. One patient put it this way: "I felt I had to eat a lot so my skin would be kept full; I didn't want it hanging loosely around my body."

The fat person frequently views himself as "something special." He does not want to give up this image of himself, even though it is a false and damaging image when viewed realistically. In secret he fantastically misinterprets and overrates his importance, and never is able to live up to his exaggerated expectations. He feels—falsely—that he suffers from one undeserved defeat after another. To him this is an intolerable condition. He seeks a primitive kind of solace through overeating. He turns even his realistic successes into failures because they do not come up to his overwrought expectations.

Fat people often fight back against the demands imposed on them from within or without by refusal to make any effort at all. This is an important reason for their lack of initiative and activity, especially physical activity. In some cases it is more difficult to change their established pattern of inactivity than to change their eating habits! This points up the value of exercise in many programs of weight reduction.

The fat person is certainly not the only one who has psychic conflicts and neurotic problems, but he is the one who seeks to resolve his problems through overeating. He uses food for psychological purposes in a number of ways—to regain comfort, to allay anxiety, to find reassurance, to serve as a symbol of security, and at the same time to express and keep down his hidden aggressive impulses, hostility, anger, and envy.

It is not surprising, therefore, that he should often view with alarm the prospect of giving up what has to him so many meanings and does so much for him.

In general we can say that people consistently overeat because they are satisfying hungers other than those for food. Their appetites are regulated by emotional—and, as we shall shortly see, by social—responses rather than by any strictly physiological need for food. Their unmet psychological needs have taproots in childhood, and they have become careless, impulsive, or compulsive eaters.

External Factors in Obesity. In a series of studies on obese and normal subjects, Dr. Stanley Schacter, of Columbia University, observed that internal and external cues to eating affected the eating behavior of obese persons differently from the way they affected normal people. He noted the following facts:

Obese and normal subjects do not refer to the same bodily state, as measured by gastric motility, when they use the word "hunger." The actual state of the stomach has nothing to do with the eating behavior of the obese. In one so-called "taste" experiment, the obese ate slightly more when their stomachs were full than when they were empty.

Fear markedly decreased the amount of food normal subjects ate but had no effect on the amount eaten by the obese. There is good reason to believe that the eating habits of the obese are relatively unrelated to any internal control (hunger pangs) but are in large part activated by external factors or cues (sight or smell of tasty foods). These external cues to eating affect the eating behavior in obese subjects considerably more than they do that of normal eaters.

In the choice of eating places, it seemed more plausible that obese persons would seek out good restaurants and avoid bad ones. This indeed proved to be the case when studied in Columbia University students.

In general, as variously tested, it turned out that the obese are relatively insensitive to variations in the physiological correlates of food (true hunger pangs) but highly sensitive to environmental food-related cues (the sight of someone else eating).

Nutrition Nonsense

It would be unfair to end this chapter without a warning to be continually on the alert for nonsense about nutrition.

In the 1960's nutrition nonsense in the amount of about $1 billion a year was being foisted upon the American public. At the 1962 annual meeting of the American Medical Association two experts on sound nutrition and good medical practice voiced warnings that are worth repeating and remembering:

Fredrick J. Stare, M.D., of the Harvard Medical School, called upon health and medical authorities to stop "pussyfooting" on problems of food quackery and speak out clearly against the nonsense that is issued in the name of nutrition. He pointed out that nutrition quacks display a curious ambivalence, seeking medical approval while at the same time condemning sound medical opinion.

Quacks exaggerate small symptoms and turn *normal* physiological events (such as everyday fatigue) into signs of illness. In other words, by using the power of suggestion they try to make people feel sick so that they can take credit for "curing" them.

Dr. Arthur M. Master, a distinguished New York cardiologist, went even further in his warnings, criticizing physicians for letting their medical judgment be swayed by fad diets that have captured the fancy of the public and their individual patients. Dr. Master said that several fads in treating heart disease had become so popular that physicians who were not convinced of, and even doubted, their value nevertheless felt constrained to prescribe them. In the "nutritional nonsense" surrounding the treatment (and theoretical prevention) of heart disease, he pointed a skeptical finger at popular concepts of cholesterol and fat in the diet and of salt restriction. (He also warned against the misuse of anticoagulant therapy.) Dr. Master said these diet fads are based on "data insufficiently tested and controlled" and may be of serious significance since they raise implications of considerable change in the dietary habits of the nation.

Many people are trying to avoid all cholesterol and fat in their diet. This may be dangerous nonsense because, as Dr. Master asserted:

There is no conclusive proof that the incidence of coronary disease and thrombosis is directly affected by the amount of cholesterol and fats in the diet. Although in general blood cholesterol is higher in coronary disease, a normal or even low figure is common in such persons. Actually no true standard of normal blood cholesterol has been established.

Dr. Master also designated as still "open to debate" the enthusiastic emphasis on polyunsaturated (soft) fats in the human diet. (It may be recalled that this was also the position taken at the Sixth International Congress on Nutrition.) That soft fats by themselves lower blood cholesterol, as once asserted, has been disproved.

Lowered cholesterol is the result of avoiding undue amounts of saturated (hard) fatty acid foods. Consuming larger amounts of soft fats may therefore be both unnecessary and harmful. On the cholesterol controversy Dr. Master offers this summary: "Surely in the present inadequate state of our knowledge it is essential to avoid the extreme anxiety so many people have been thrown into concerning blood cholesterol or foods containing a little fat." (Recent research findings have suggested that the increase in *triglycerides* in the blood serum may be a better index of disease than the cholesterol levels. Dietary fats are composed chiefly of triglycerides.)

In conclusion, when you hear nonsense about nutrition preached by quacks who draw threadbare robes of science about them, remember that the real experts are extremely skeptical about such unwarranted nutritional claims. The human body, when prejudices of appetite have been eliminated, remains the best of all indicators of human food needs.

SUMMARY

This chapter has served to introduce the subject of food and the science of nutrition, both on the American and the international scene. It has portrayed the human digestive system, including that important adjunct, the teeth. It has outlined the food components of the human diet: proteins, carbohydrates, fats, vitamins, minerals, and water and suggested their sources and functions. It has warned against food prejudices and food fallacies. It warrants the conclusion that good nutrition, following scientific knowledge and principles, underlies good health. With this background you will more quickly grasp, the reasons behind the practical selection of foods and diets that will help to keep you healthy at the weight you want to maintain.

SUMMARY REVIEW QUESTIONS

1. Is the food supply of the United States adequate? Why or why not? How does it compare with the food supplies of other nations? What are the principal lacks, if any, in the world's food supply?
2. What food prejudices, if any, do you have? How do you think they arose? What are some of the common myths about food (name at least four)?
3. What six vitamins and what three minerals are most apt to be lacking from the ordinary American diet? What role in nutrition do each of these elements play?

4. What was the origin and what is the present range of study and research in the science of nutrition?
5. What are the main component parts of the human digestive system and what is the principal function of each part?
6. What are the six essential food components? What role in nutrition does each one (or group) essentially play?
7. What are the functions of food?
8. What is the structure of the human jaws and teeth? What practical steps can an individual take to prevent (1) tooth decay and (2) periodontal disease.
9. What did you eat and drink in the last twenty-four hours? How many times did you eat? Do you think this one-day's food intake was adequate in quantity and quality? Why? Why not?
10. What ten foodstuffs do you like best? What is the principal or most significant food component or nutrient, exclusive of water, in each of these favorite foods of yours?
11. What specific foods or kinds of foods do you like least? How do you explain your prejudice, dislike, or avoidance of these foods?
12. What are the four categories of daily food selection in the "Essential 4" system?
13. Do you presently want to gain or lose weight? Why? How do you plan to go about it? How can you be sure your plan is a safe one? If you are fully satisfied with your present weight, state it and tell why.
14. What risks to health do you see in overweight? Underweight? Losing weight?
15. In the process of losing weight, which three of the following methods would you choose or recommend as the most sensible and effective and why? (*a*) Taking vitamin pills. (*b*) Exercising. (*c*) Reducing food intake. (*d*) Consulting a physician. (*e*) Taking drugs. (*f*) Talking out your problems.
16. Describe the essential features of the three basic systems for losing weight. (*a*) The Essential Four System. (*b*) The Fraction System. (*c*) The Caloric Number System. What do you consider to be the advantages and disadvantages of each?
17. Are the following statements sense or nonsense? Why? *Flouridation of public water supplies is a racket. . . . You are what you eat. . . . Never drink water with your meals. . . . Fish is brain food. . . . Ceremony is the sauce to meat. . . . Fat people are always jolly. . . . Americans run a great risk of amino acid deficiency in their diets.*
18. What do the following terms mean to you: villus, peristalsis, enzyme, complete protein, beriberi, malnutrition, balanced diet, basal metabolism, caloric number, obesity, overweight, cholesterol, triglycerides?

Worth Looking Into: *Recommended Dietary Allowances,* 7th revised edition, 1968, a report of the Food and Nutrition Board of the National Academy of Sciences, National Research Council. *Teeth, Health, and Appearance* by the American Dental Association. *Everybody's Book of Modern Diet and Nutrition* by Henrietta Fleck and Elizabeth Munves. *Essentials of an Adequate Diet* from the U.S. Dept. of Agriculture. *Reduce and Stay Reduced* by Norman Joliffe, M.D. *Your Emotions and Overweight* by Elizabeth M. Dach. *Mayo Clinic Diet Manual, 1961* from the Mayo Clinic. For more complete references, see Appendix E.

How We Digest Our Food: The Scientific Account

William Beaumont (1785–1853)

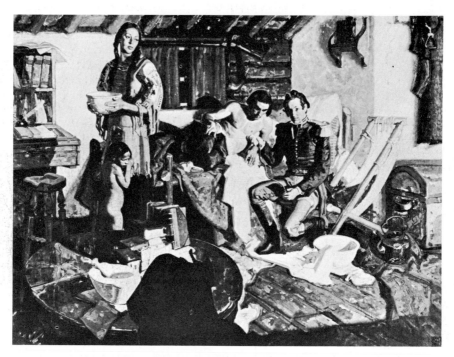

WILLIAM BEAUMONT, backwoods American army surgeon, and father of the modern science of nutrition, is shown here with Alexis St. Martin, a half-breed Indian with an unhealed gunshot wound in the abdomen, who served Beaumont as a "living laboratory." To observe the chemical action of the human gastric juice on carious foodstuffs, Beaumont inserted them on silk threads into the Indian's stomach. (The original picture, in full color, is by Dean Cornwell; it is reproduced here by courtesy of Wyeth Laboratories, Philadelphia.)

Abstract: Great laboratories are now to be found within every metropolis in the civilized world, but it is impossible to foretell where a great scientific mind will arise to discover and develop new truths. "Experiments and Observations on the Gastric Juice and the Physiology of Digestion," 1833, rated as the greatest single contribution to the knowledge of gastric digestion, was produced in the backwoods of America by a much harassed United States Army surgeon with no other laboratory than the gunshot-wounded body of an Indian.

SOURCE. From "Experiments and Observations on the Gastric Juice and the Physiology of Digestion," by William Beaumont, M.D. privately printed in 1833. Reprinted here from *The Autobiography of Science,* edited by Justus J. Schifferes and Forest R. Moulton, revised 2nd edition (New York: Doubleday and Co., 1960), p. 310.

Experiments and Observations on the Gastric Juice and the Physiology of Digestion

Alexis St. Martin, who is the subject of these experiments, was a Canadian, of French descent, at the above-mentioned time about eighteen years of age, of good constitution, robust and healthy. He had been engaged in the service of the American Fur Company, as a voyageur, and was accidentally wounded by the discharge of a musket, on the sixth of June 1822. . . . The whole mass of materials forced from the musket, together with fragments of clothing and pieces of fractured ribs, were driven into the muscles and cavity of the chest.

I saw him in twenty-five or thirty minutes after the accident occurred, and, on examination, found a portion of the lung, as large as a turkey's egg, protruding through the external wound, lacerated and burned; and immediately below this, another protrusion, which, on further examination, proved to be a portion of the stomach, lacerated through all its coats, and pouring out the food he had taken for his breakfast, through an orifice large enough to admit the forefinger. . . .

August 1, 1825. At 12 M., I introduced through the perforation, into the stomach, the following articles of diet, suspended by a silk string, and fastened at proper distances, so as to pass in without pain, viz., a piece of high-seasoned à la mode beef; a piece of raw, salted, fat pork; a piece of raw, salted, lean beef; a piece of boiled, salted beef; a piece of stale bread; and a bunch of raw, sliced cabbage; each piece weighing about two drachms; the lad continuing his usual employment about the house.

At 1:00 P.M., withdrew and examined them. Found the cabbage and bread about half digested; the pieces of meat unchanged. Returned them into the stomach.

At 2:00 P.M., withdrew them again. Found the cabbage, bread, pork, and boiled beef all cleanly digested and gone from the string; the other pieces of meat but very little affected. Returned them into the stomach again.

At 3:00 P.M. [sic], examined again. Found the à la mode beef partly digested; the raw beef was slightly macerated on the surface, but its general texture was firm and entire. The smell and taste of the fluids of the stomach were slightly rancid; and the boy complained of some pain and uneasiness at the breast. Returned them again.

The lad complaining of considerable distress and uneasiness at the stomach, general debility and lassitude, with some pain in his head, I withdrew the string and found the remaining portions of aliment nearly in the same condition as when last examined; the fluid more rancid and sharp. The boy still complaining, I did not return them any more.

August 2. The distress at the stomach and pain in the head continuing, accompanied with costiveness, a depressed pulse, dry skin, coated tongue, and numerous white spots, or pustules, resembling coagulated lymph, spread over the inner surface of the stomach, I thought it advisable to give medicine; and, accordingly, dropped into the stomach, through the aperture, half a dozen calomel pills, four or five grains each; which, in about three hours, had a thorough cathartic effect and removed all the foregoing symptoms, and the diseased appearance of the inner coat of the stomach. The effect of the medicine was the same as when administered in the usual way, by the mouth and esophagus, except the nausea commonly occasioned by swallowing pills.

This experiment cannot be considered a fair test of the powers of the gastric juice. The cabbage, one of the articles which was, in this instance, most speedily dissolved, was cut into small, fibrous pieces, very thin, and necessarily exposed on all its surfaces to the action of the gastric juice. The stale bread was porous, and of course admitted the juice into all its interstices; and probably fell from the string as soon as softened, and before it was completely dissolved. These circumstances will account for the more rapid disappearance of these substances than of the pieces of meat, which were in entire solid pieces when put in. To account for the disappearance of the fat pork, it is only necessary to remark that the fat meat is always resolved into oil by the warmth of the stomach before it is digested. I have generally observed that when he has fed on fat meat or butter the whole superior portion of the contents of the stomach, if examined a short time after eating, will be found covered with an oily pellicle. This fact may account for the disappearance of the pork from the string. I think, upon the whole, and subsequent experiments have confirmed the opinion, that fat meats are less easily digested than lean, when both have received the same advantages of comminution.

Generally speaking, the looser the texture and the more tender the fiber, of animal food, the easier it is of digestion.

This experiment is important in a pathological point of view. It confirms the opinion that undigested portions of food in the stomach produce all the phenomena of fever; and is calculated to warn us of the danger of all excesses, where that organ is concerned. It also admonishes us of the necessity of a perfect comminution of the articles of diet.

PART THREE   FAMILY LIVING

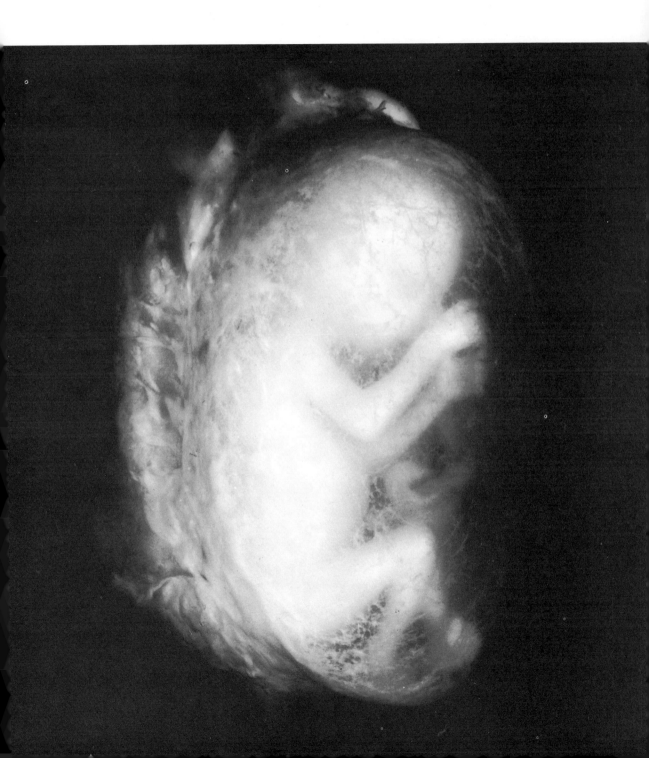

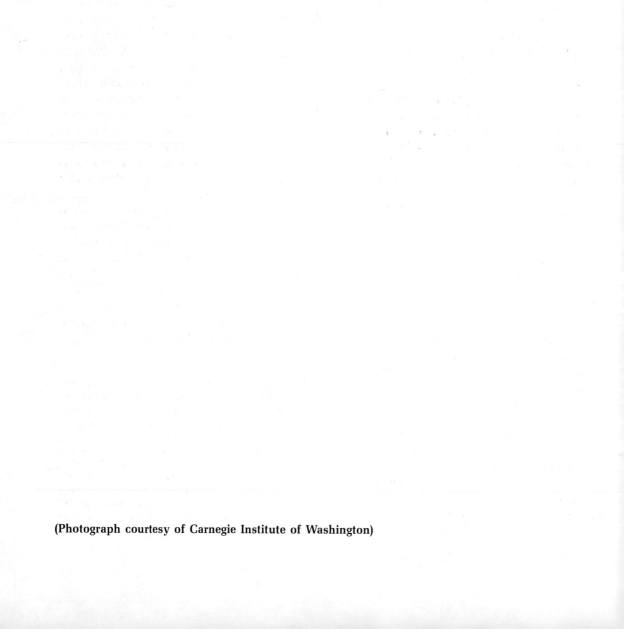

(Photograph courtesy of Carnegie Institute of Washington)

11

EDUCATION FOR FAMILY LIVING

A FAMILY CAN BE DESCRIBED IN MANY WAYS. First of all, it is a group. (We speak of families of nations and languages as well as of families composed of human beings.) A human family is a group of people tied together by physical factors, such as common ancestry, residence in the same household, or by legal bonds, such as marriage and adoption. The family is the tangible link between the generations of mankind, past, present, and future. In some cultures, such as the Chinese, little distinction in conversation is made between the living and the dead members of the family.

What Is a Family?

The family may also be viewed as a social entity, the fundamental unit of all stable human societies, a cultural pattern, a legal entity, an economic arrangement, a political fact, and a biological process. The relationship of the individual to the family is tinged with all these points of view. Since we have all grown up in families, we tend to take these complex relationships pretty much for granted. It is only when we analyze the functions and operations of the family that we begin to realize how one or more of these interrelationships may be out of joint and that disjointedness the root of discontent and personal unhappiness on the part of individual members of the family.

The pattern of family organization in the United States today is different from the patterns that appear in earlier times and in other cultures. Historians and anthropologists supply us with many other observed patterns of family organization. We have, for example, the matriarchy, common to certain primitive[1] tribes, in which the mother is the dominant and legally central figure. In the patriarchy, which reached a stage of classical development in ancient Hebrew, Greek, Roman and Germanic cultures, the father was the undisputed head of the household and often held absolute power of life and death over its members. There are still matriarchal and patriarchal features in many modern American families; but the ideal of romantic, monogamous marriage has tended to make the modern family more of an equal partnership between mates. Within the last century the rights of children have been increasingly recognized. We must not fall into the error, however, of believing that the family as we know it today is the final stage of its development. It is still evolving. Indeed, especially rapid changes in the patterns of family living have taken place in recent years along with the accelerated tempo of scientific and technological developments throughout the world.

---

[1] Primitive, as the anthropologists now use it, means nonliterate, possibly preliterate; or cultures that are transmitted through an oral rather than a written tradition. Primitive cultures differ greatly; they range from the Eskimos and Australian bushmen, with hunting and gathering techniques, through complex agricultural societies like the Inca and Aztec. Primitive peoples are not intellectually or "morally" inferior to residents of more advanced cultures; they are human beings (*Homo sapiens*) in the full sense of the word. We of the modern world are not the lineal descendants of primitive societies, some of which are contemporary, though we have inherited and borrowed from some of these cultures.

The Function of the Family

The family serves many functions essential to the survival both of the individuals who make it up and of the society of which it is a part. Broadly speaking, these functions can be placed under four general headings: satisfaction of personal drives and desires; perpetuation of the race; transmission of culture; and personality development of children.

The family satisfies the personal needs, aspirations, desires, and drives of the individuals who make up the family. This applies particularly to the man and woman who come together to create a family. Marriage may be described as the birth of a family. It is also the normative pattern of sexual adjustment within any society. However, providing a socially approved pattern for the fulfillment of sexual needs and desires is only one part of the much larger pattern of marriage and family living.

If sexual outlet were all there was to marriage, probably few people would be found willing to take all the risks of founding, rearing, and launching a family. There are a few people, of course, who look on marriage simply as a necessary evil; they seek only tolerance or safe-keeping from their spouses and expect little intimacy or response. In general, however, a time of marriage is a time of hope. The founders of a family look to the building of a home and the enlargement of the family circle through children as the surest means of satisfying their deepest emotional needs and their highest social aspirations.

The family perpetuates the race. It provides the physical and social environment through which the human infant can be protected and reared to a state of maturity so that he or she can continue the process of procreation.

There is one important biological fact that helps to explain why the institution of the human family has developed in its own particular way. The human infant has a longer period of helpless infancy and childhood than the young of any other species. The infant must be fed and protected from the elements by its parents or other adults for many months before it is capable even of locomotion. Years must pass before a child can get for himself the food necessary to his survival. Social and environmental factors of dependence also emerge.

The family is the mechanism or medium through which the culture (or way of living) of a society is transmitted from one generation to the next. In this sense the family is the first and most powerful of educational agencies. We get our basic ideas of "right" and "wrong" from observing and hearing in childhood what actions the older members of our families approve and disapprove. Later in life we often lose track of this simple connection and look to some abstract ethical concept to explain our behavior.

The patterns of speech, belief, feeling, and action that guide our conduct are learned from other human beings, and primarily from the members of our family. For example, there is no biologic instinct that teaches us to respect the person and property of other people. The concepts of private property and sanctity of person are ideas that have arisen historically in the minds of men; the newborn infant has to learn them. That teaching takes place primarily within the family circle. Soon, of course, playmates and unrelated adults also influence his conduct. As the child grows up, he is admonished not to take other people's things and not to strike other people without provocation. If he persistently fails to heed these admonitions, he is punished.

The culture of any community is a complex thing. It is a pattern of responses to a wide variety of specific symbols, rituals, and tools. Although we are impressed with tiny fragments of a culture, such as the Western custom of tipping the hat to women, or the Chinese habit of eating with chopsticks, a culture pervades the whole life of the individual reared in it. Folkways, customs, mores, taboos, and laws, both written and unwritten, subtly influence the individual's conduct every moment of his life. We see this more clearly, perhaps, through the study of the cultures of primitive and preliterate peoples, such as South Sea Islanders and American Indians. Yet the weight of our own culture continually bears down on us, creating the climate of opinion which dictates many of our actions.

Cultures change—but slowly. Part of the reason for this is that the "design for living" whose rightness or wrongness strikes closest to our hearts was inculcated in early childhood. In the broadest sense we have all picked up the pattern of our culture from our families.

Our ideals and our prejudices grow from a common stalk, the family in which we were brought up. The attack on the social problems that perennially challenge the conscience of the world—war, poverty, unemployment, vice, and crime—can probably best be made through sharper consideration of the problems of the family. The happy family is the model for the stable nation.

The family molds the personality of the child. To a lesser extent it also reshapes the personalities of all who are party to it. The influence of the family pattern upon the personality of the child begins almost at the instant of birth. Having become a part of the family, the infant must immediately begin to adjust to it. In this process his feelings will inevitably be involved; how he reacts to the process of being acclimatized to family life begins inexorably to set the mold for his future course of life and personal conduct.

From the very beginning of his life the baby is expected to do what the family, and especially the mother, thinks proper. Such demands do not coincide with the baby's drives and instincts. But he is compelled to accede to the family's wishes. Though "self-demand" is increasingly the rule, nevertheless the child must usually eat on mother's schedule, whatever it is. He will be weaned when mother decides it is time. He must go to the toilet when mother says so. Growing up immediately conflicts with the "physiological autonomy" of the child.

His aggressive emotional drives are also restrained. He is not allowed to grab, punch, and strike as he wishes. A strain of resentment against such thwarting is built up, and some hostility consequently takes root. If love is withheld from an infant, a feeling of insecurity takes over. The child's personality grows in a multitude of moments of deep feeling and inner reactions to those

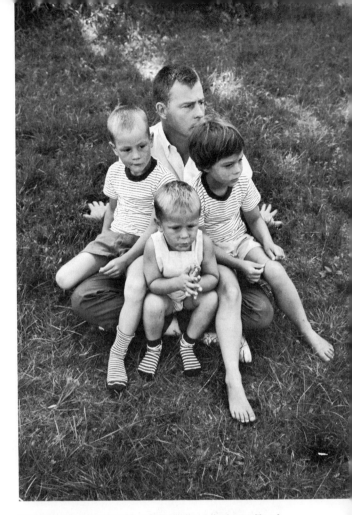

FATHER AND CHILDREN, U.S.A. 1970's . . . The profile of the American family has changed greatly since World War II. Young people marry earlier, and at a higher rate. Family chores, once considered "women's work," are more generally shared by husband and wife. (Photograph by Ken Heyman)

feelings. In adult life these childhood feelings are forgotten or repressed while the deep reaction patterns continue. The individual who has been severely compelled to conform to the family dictates laid upon him in early childhood often reacts with a warped pattern of conduct in later life.

Family Equilibrium

Every family has its own way of getting along. This applies both to the relationships between the members of the family and to their relationships with people outside the family. It is a common pattern, for example, that individuals within the family—such as husband and wife, brother and sister—may criticize one another devastatingly but will fall vehemently upon any outsider who disparages one of the group.

The family evolves; its relationships change as the members of the family grow older and as new members, infants or adults, are added to it. A family is never a static, finished thing like a cut flower or a fly in amber. It is always a growing, changing organism. We may properly speak of the dynamics of family living and seek to understand this process as it applies generally and to our own family constellations.

No matter how poorly a family gets along, it always moves in some direction. We can think of this as a family equilibrium—a balance of needs, hopes, interests, traditions, and interpersonal relationships—through which every family continues to operate. As seen from the outside, all families are in a state of equilibrium; the family is making some sort of adjustment, be it good or bad, to the society in which it is enmeshed. Inside the family circle, however, things may be in a sorry state with open or threatening hostilities between family members on every side. The results of such unresolved hostilities may be very serious and lead eventually to a "broken family."

It will be useful to understand the factors that keep a family in equilibrium, that permit it to make adjustments as it rolls along. The first of these is *imitation;* this takes place at all times within a family circle. It is easy to see how children imitate their parents and sometimes their older brothers and sisters in speech, gestures, eating habits, food preferences, sex prejudices and modesties, and even symptoms of illness. We are often astonished, for example, when a child answering a telephone speaks in a tone of voice that mimics and is mistaken for that of a parent.

A second factor that we encounter in observing the dynamics of family life is *identification.* This goes further than imitation in that it suggests a strong need, whether conscious or unconscious, on the part of the imitator to be like the family member with whom he identifies. A typical example is the tomboy girl, who wants to be like her brothers. The wish to identify one's hopes and aspirations with those of some other family member usually fastens upon the powerful or winning characteristics of that member, such as his or her appearance, position of authority, financial success ("the rich uncle"), or social triumph ("the sister who married so well"). However, there are also distorted identifications in which a weakness rather than a strength is imitated. A daughter, for example, may insist on having "sick headaches" just like her mother.

Profile of the American Family. The American family is flourishing, as the following brief statistical "profile" indicates:

In the United States today close to 95% of the population lives in families, with an average of $3\frac{1}{2}$ persons per household. However, something over 1 million married couples (out of a total of around 38 million) do not have their own households. These are mainly young newlyweds who share living quarters with their parents.

Almost one-half of American married couples have a child before the third year of marriage and about three-fourths start a family within the first five years. Around 3.5 million babies are now being born every year in the United States. This means a lower birth rate than in the fifties and early sixties.

Americans are marrying earlier than in any previous generations. The median age of American husbands at first marriage is just a little over 22 years and that of wives just under 20 years. Over 70% of the men and women in the United States are (or have been) married before they are 25.

Influence of Modern Family "Constellation." The shape and size—we might also say the constellation—of the family of which you are a part will both reflect and in a way create the population picture of the United States in the 1970's and later. By 1967 the U.S. population had passed the 200 million mark, and the Bureau of Census noted that it would continue to increase.

The composition (or proportion) of the American population is also constantly shifting, with significant effects on family living. During the 1960's, the population at ages 18 to 24—the college generation—and at ages 65 and over increased substantially. (This means, among other things, more difficulty in getting into college and fiercer competition for jobs from the older generation at the termination of your college career.) See the graph on page 16.

During the sixties, also, a slight decrease occurred in the early-adult, mostly high productive generation, aged 25 to 44, while the proportions of the population (and by inference, individual families) in the 45 to 64 age brackets—the "established" families—and the proportion of people under 18 (youth, children, and infants) remained about the same.

Marriage: The Normative Pattern of Sexual Behavior. Marriage is the name we give to the social institution which upholds the family and permits it to function to the best interests, as far as society can judge them, both of the individuals who make up families and of society as a whole. Marriage is defined by a cluster of laws, customs (mores), habits, and traditions, some written, some unwritten, with both civil and religious sanctions. In primitive societies they are enforced by strict taboos; in the United States they are upheld by public opinion. One must note that as societies and cultures change, laws (or at least the interpretation and enforcement of them) change.

In any society marriage is the normative pattern of sexual behavior. This behavior is condemned or condoned to the extent that it is judged to threaten or support the institutions of marriage and the family. Sexual function is universally regarded as going to the very root of the marriage relationship. Without it there would be no need for marriage.

Social Control of Sexual Behavior

It cannot be denied that the sexual drive in the human species is at times imperious and aggressive. Furthermore its consequences affect lives other than that of the individual involved.

From the earliest recorded times and among the most primitive peoples, therefore, sex has been regarded both as necessary and dangerous, and subject to social control.

The Historical Background. There are a few possible combinations of mating between male and female. These include *monogamy*, which is the exclusive right of one man and one woman to each other; *polygamy*, which means multiple or plural marriage, but is sometimes construed as the exclusive right of one man to several wives; *polygyny*, which is the right of one man to more than one woman—for example, to hold concubines in addition to a wife or wives; *polyandry*, which is the right of one woman to several husbands at the same time; *group marriage* (also called complex marriage), which defines the sexual rights of one group of men to a specific group of women. No society has ever tolerated complete sexual license, or the right of any man to any or as many women as he could get hold of.

Among primitive societies monogamy is exceptional and polygamy is often legitimate, sanctioned by law and custom. Marriage at the earliest possible time is the general rule; it is expected just as soon as biological readiness is established.

In antiquity the strong feelings surrounding the sexual drive caused many primitive tribes, groups, and nations to endow it with magic powers. Hence there arose a number of so-called "fertility cults," usually worshipping a female deity, a symbol of fecundity, who was implored to bring increase to fields, flocks, and families. Evidence of such fertility religions is found in studies of ancient Egypt, Crete, Persia, and parts of Asia Minor.

But there is also to be found in ancient history a tradition of asceticism—the idea that sexual abstinence creates special virtue, especially among those who perform holy offices. The concept of asceticism stood in opposition to the fertility cults of the ancient world. It made its way into Western culture through the Old Testament and the preaching of the prophets of ancient Israel against "the abomination of the heathen." Early Christianity also found itself in the position of opposing the fertility cults. Old Testament attitudes on asceticism were emphasized by St. Paul in the New Testament.

The ascetic ideal came to America in the seventeenth century with the Puritans, "the people of the Book," who left us the heritage of the "New England conscience." The Puritans followed the strictest interpretations of the Bible, even including the ancient Hebrew law prescribing the death penalty for adultery of women.

Over the centuries public opinion, however, seems to swing between what might be described as liberal and conservative poles of permissiveness toward different outlets of sexual behavior. Victorian society, both in England and the United States, generally tolerated segregated districts of prostitution, but would not permit a "nice" woman to show her ankle. Two generations later women were permitted to wear the briefest bathing suits, but most of the "red-light" districts had disappeared. In the United States today public opinion upholds romantic monogamous marriage both as the norm and the ideal.

There is a long history of individual and organized community rebellion against sex restrictions. But it is, on the whole, a history of failure, for society will not long tolerate threats to marriage and family structures.

The Inner Censor. The social control of sex expression is actually achieved in two ways: one open, one hidden. Laws, customs, taboos, and religions present open and obvious controls, intermingled with promises and threats, stated prohibitions, and generally known, even if unstated, permissions.

The real censor of sexual behavior, however, rests in the unconscious mind. Most frequently we obey laws, observe customs, and accept moral codes because something inside us tells us, often commands us, to do so. That something, hidden from other people and operative even when they are not around, is sometimes labeled "the still, small voice of conscience." More exactly, it is the *superego,* formed in childhood, which operates both in the conscious and unconscious minds.

Managing Sex Impulses

While there is at any time a consensus of public opinion about sexual conduct, there remains a wide range of individual attitudes and personal opinions within this consensus.

It must be recognized that every individual has his own particular attitudes toward sex. These attitudes arise from family background, from the total civilization or culture in which one is reared, from the stress of different historical eras, and from economics pressures.

The mid-Victorian (nineteenth century) attitudes toward sexual matters are certainly not the same as those of the mid-twentieth century. The economic stresses and dislocations of widespread military conflicts in the twentieth century have also had the effect of changing sex mores.

The codes of sexual morality set down in the Old and New Testaments, and forming the basis of the moral codes of Western Judaeo-Christian civilization cannot be held as the only possible codes for all peoples of the world—for example, the believers in the Koran, which permits polygamy, and the followers of some of the prominent religions of the Far East.

Even within the confines of Western civilization there are wide ranges of opinion concerning sexual morality and propriety. To some members of Western culture sex is "a joke"; to others, perhaps the majority, it is something "holy" or "heavenly." The divergences of opinion on this subject that you are likely to encounter are sharply illuminated in the two following quotations, each written and published by an eminent American physician.

1. [Sex] is the master joke of the universe. It is so magnificent a joke that the very stars rock with the echo of the laughter it arouses. That is just why it has attracted all those masters of the art of words from the beginning of time—the great comedians, Aristophanes and Rabelais and Cervantes and Shakespeare and Sterne and James Branch Cabell. It is because it is a joke that it is holy. It is because it is a joke, not because it is holy, that it keeps us fascinated even

after we have found out about it.—*Logan Clendening, M.D., in The Human Body.*

2. I shall make no apology for the way the world is made and for the process that brought us all into existence. If one person says that it was God, and another insists that it was Nature which developed it, who is to say?

The most important episodes in the life of a man or woman are those which have to do with marriage and the relations arising out of that marriage. Surely it would be better to fail in everything else and succeed in this, than to succeed in everything else and fail in this. If this is true—and it must be left to the reader to decide—it is rather surprising that information on this subject should be so frequently suppressed. . . .

The relations that exist between a husband and wife, who are deeply in love with each other, are good and clean and pure. . . . It is impossible to suppose that the source of all life is unclean or indecent. Therefore, *sex is good.* It is clean unless dragged in the dirt. Even then, usually it can be made clean again if the persons concerned are willing to get themselves out of the gutter and into a decent way of living.— *Thurman Rice, M.D., in Sex, Marriage, and Family.*

The great variety of individual opinions about sexual matters reflects the restless uncertainty, most intense among marriageable women and young bachelors, as to whether their current conduct will lead them to get the most out of their natural sexual instincts. It must be abundantly clear, however, to any thinking person that managing one's sexual drives cannot be divorced from the overall, continuing problem of living with one's whole armory of emotions.

Personal decisions concerning sexual conduct are and must always be intimate, individual decisions, unique in time, place, and personalities involved. In making your own decisions, however, it is always helpful to have a long perspective and wide range point of view on the possible outcomes of the actions you propose to take. The information presented here is for the purpose of helping you to appreciate the long view for yourself.

Marriage itself does not automatically solve all sex problems; the evidence is all to the contrary.

On the other hand, for *most* people, sex life in marriage represents the ideal way of handling the great, beautiful, and potentially dangerous sex drive of the individual.

It must be pointed out, however, that sex adjustment before marriage will inevitably have an effect upon sex life in marriage. This is an exceedingly complex topic with scanty scientific information on the subject. To what extent the use, nonuse, or abuse of one or more varieties of sexual outlet before marriage will affect the personalities involved and their interaction with one another in "building a marriage" is a question to which there is no single answer.

It has sometimes been suggested that early marriage is the solution for the common problem of sexual adjustment before marriage. However no one has seriously suggested lowering the legal age for marriage down to that of puberty or biological readiness for reproduction. Experience shows that very early marriage too often results in either unhappiness or divorce. There is a trend toward earlier marriage in the United States, but no one can pretend that this has eliminated the problem of premarital sexual adjustment.

It should also be pointed out that for *some* men and women sexual adjustment never was, is, or will be a problem. Of these some are secure in their moral tenets; others have a comparatively weak sex drive. For still others, the problem of sexual adjustment will not appear as a problem or be recognized as such. For some of this group, hidden and diverted sexual energy may operate capriciously in the unconscious mind.

How Physiological Factors Influence Sex Attitudes. Physiological factors also influence an individual's attitudes toward sex matters and the conduct stemming from such attitudes or feelings. This implies more than the drives associated with increase of sex hormones at the time of puberty. It relates also to the acceleration of growth in all dimensions that the present generation of young people have enjoyed. As was already pointed out (in Chapter 9) young men and women today are 3 to 4 inches taller than their immediate and remote ancestors. This acceleration in growth begins early; by the end of the first year of life babies are about $1\frac{1}{2}$ inches taller than year-old infants a century ago.

This early maturation and larger size of children and young men and women today (teenagers can literally "look down on" their parents) has widespread social and medical significance. As Dr. Harry Bakwin, of New York, put it in 1962:

The frustrating period between the time when drives for self-expression, social dominance, sex experience, economic independence appear and the time when these drives and desires can be satisfied is prolonged. Attitudes must be re-evaluated regarding the length of compulsory education, the proper age for military service, the age for marriage, the time to choose a career, the age of responsibility for criminal acts, inheritance laws and child labor.

That the problem is serious may be further attested by the fact that in the 1960's somewhere between 100,000 and 120,000 illegitimate births to teenage mothers were expected annually.

Biological Bases of Feeling. The intensity of sexual feeling and interest varies enormously with age, sex, condition of health, and other factors. A kind of imitative "puppy love" is occasionally observed between childhood sweethearts in elementary school, but sexual feelings—in the more specific and narrow sense of the term—do not really arise until biological readiness for reproduction occurs at puberty. This is accompanied, by significant changes in the endocrine gland secretions within the body ("leaping hormones" is the popular term) and is outwardly evident in the development of secondary sex characteristics—growth of pubic hair, change in body contours, menstruation (in women), change of voice (in men), and other changes. The physical factors underpin the psychological feelings and the social conduct. There is what we might call a biological rudder steering the course of life. Disease sometimes twists the rudder.

In addition to the obvious anatomical differences between male and female, it is also important to recognize that the biological patterns of sexual development differ between the sexes. In boys the physical changes of adolescence come on more or less abruptly, usually somewhere between the ages of 11 and 15. Their active sex interest begins at that time and is soon stepped up to the point where most males reach their maximum rate of sexual outlet in their middle teens.

It is also generally true that sexual feelings in men are more volatile; they are more quickly aroused and more speedily satisfied. Furthermore, men are often involuntarily subject to evident physical response to sexual stimuli of almost any kind, for example, the mere presence or picture of a woman.

In the human female, even after the onset of menstruation, sexual development occurs more gradually. Women generally reach their peak of sexual outlet a good many years later than men. Sexual feelings are reflex reactions of the human organism. Given adequate stimulus, a normal man or women cannot help having some sexual feelings any more than he or she can avoid feeling hungry, thirsty, or angry under the appropriate circumstances. The feeling itself cannot be wiped out, but the action based upon the feeling can be controlled and modified.

We must distinguish between the normal sexual reaction and more complex behavior patterns of which it is only a part, for example—lust, love, romance, and infatuation. Lust is an *excess* of feeling, often leading to selfish or violent action; its goal is as often power or money as sexual license. Love in its fullest sense is an emotion that pervades all of life. It need not be directed solely to sexual objects; nor should mere sexual desires be masked or disguised as love. Infatuation may be described as the temporary delusion that "love conquers all."

Self-Direction of Sexual Desires by a Guiding Philosophy. There is no harm in suppressing one's sexual desires. In fact, throughout life, they must be suppressed most of the time by the responsible individual. This suppression represents willing obedience to a personal code of ethics which stems from or includes the more formal religious, ethical, and moral codes.

Control of one's sexual feelings is possible and to a great extent inevitable; it is also desirable and valuable. The emotions centering in sexual desire are intertwined with all the other powerful emotions that energize and motivate the individual—love, hate, jealousy, anger, and fear. These too must be controlled, if one is to achieve a happy, well-balanced life.

Experience in self-control is not *denial* of oneself or one's demands and needs; it is *direction* of these desires and needs toward fulfilling the greater goals of the total personality. In this self-direction toward life goals, control of admitted sexual feelings has an important place.

The "trick" in controlling sexual desires is to accept them for what they are but not to overemphasize them either by indulgence or denial. Act need not follow feeling. An attitude may properly interpose between the stimulus and the response.

Sex-Releasing versus Sex-Stimulating Practices. In practice, this means thinking out a philosophy of sex for yourself in advance of possibly dangerous encounters with it. This may prevent many embarrassing situations. Sometimes it may mean deliberately choosing courses of action which are sex-releasing rather than sex-stimulating. Take social dancing, for example. You can dance for fun, attending to the rhythm of the music, the grace and conviviality of your dancing partner, and the whole pattern of social gaiety at the dance you are attending. On the other hand, you can concentrate exclusively on the physical contact and intimacy of the dancing posture. In the first case your activity is sex-releasing without being sex-denying. In the second instance it is sex-stimulating.

Reading as an avocation also plays this dual role. You can read the same book for the sexual stimulation you get out of its carnal passages, or you can read to achieve understanding of human personality under the stress of passion. The primary difference between sex-stimulating and sex-releasing activities is in the attitude with which you approach them.

The Conspiracy of Silence. The evidence is now overwhelming that the *problem* aspect of sexual adjustment in American society is being solved in large part by the conspiracy of silence,

or, as Hollingshead has described it, *the clandestine complex.* In a brilliant study of the impact of social classes on adolescent behavior (*Elmtown's Youth*), he wrote:

Young people . . . must repress their sexual desires or violate the mores. This perennial problem has been solved, in a way, in our culture by the development of a clandestine complex that enables individuals to release sex tensions secretly and simultaneously to maintain their "good name" and dignity publicly, but not without compromising the mores and creating serious personal and social problems. As a result, an adolescent who breaks the sex taboos does not talk about his "vices" even to his closest friends, for so long as the mores are adhered to outwardly no public embarrassment is experienced by youngsters who profess one thing and do another. It is only when accident or ill fortune brings secret violations into the open, and persons other than the participants in the experience learn what has happened, that delinquents are compromised by their conduct and condemned severely by the community. . . .

The strongest moral judgments in the culture are applied to the violations of the sex mores. Perhaps the clandestine complex has developed as a reaction to the severity of these judgments. . . . [It is] a conspiracy of silence.

The publication of the "Kinsey reports" on sexual behavior in the United States put numbers on the open secret of the conspiracy of silence. The shock of these reports arose more from surprise that the unofficial secrets of the conspiracy should be openly published than from the statistical facts they revealed. These well-known reports have limitations, admitted by the scientist-authors themselves and generously pointed out by their critics. Nevertheless the findings of these reports offer the largest and most significant statistical samples of sexual behavior in the United States. The Kinsey reports do not presume to tell what such behavior *should* be; they simply reveal what it is.

The following comments from a distinguished college president, Dr. Sarah Gibson Blanding, president of Vassar College, on the occasion of the publication of the third Kinsey report (1958), underline the importance of these reports from the standpoint of the college community:

The late Dr. Kinsey, and now his collaborators, have engaged in studies which are sincere, objective, and determined explorations into an area of human behavior which is manifestly important to educators. [These] volumes are a concise, sober, factual presentation of an aspect of life which is emotionally charged and which has not previously been regarded as within the province of the scientist. . . .

Like all new discoveries, these findings must be subjected to further scientific research to confirm or disprove the conclusions drawn from the available data. The three published studies indicate that sexual behavior and reproductive experience are at variance with the official moral code and traditional beliefs and values. Most of us find it hard to think of sexual behavior in purely objective terms. We defend ourselves against unwelcome truths by passionate denial. We try to interpret the facts in accordance with our own understanding of moral behavior. We protest the data not because it may be untrue but because of its social and moral significance. In our society sex is a dramatically exploited commodity. . . .

If the facts are what they seem to be on the basis of the studies to date, the problems of duplicity they imply cannot be solved by indignation or ostrichlike denial. Sensational exploitation can only exaggerate the discrepancy between what people do and what society sanctimoniously thinks they do or should do. Parents and educators, ministers and doctors, psychologists and sociologists are challenged to straightforward, openminded, courageous thinking. Concepts, beliefs, values and goals must be constantly re-examined in the light of scientific truth and intellectual honesty and with deep concern for human dignity and the integrity of society.

Some Premarital Adjustment Problems

Expectation and anticipation of marriage is very high among college men and women. Their basic sexual interest, therefore, lies in choosing (or refusing) a mate through the accepted processes of dating, "falling in love," courtship, engagement, and finally marriage. But this is often a turbulent course and may require along the way a fuller understanding of other problems of premarital sexual adjustment, which, if not properly understood and managed, might upset the more fundamental goals. The problems lie in the

areas of premarital intercourse, petting, autosexuality (masturbation) and homosexuality.

The Risks of Premarital Intercourse. The risks of premarital intercourse are well-known: venereal disease, unwanted pregnancy, illegitimate children, social stigma, psychic trauma, loss of self-respect, and others. Why, then, are so many found willing to run these risks? Some explanation is in order.

The risks are relative, what the military strategist calls "calculated risks." Those who take the risks are buoyed up by a false sense of optimism, fatalism, or, more rarely, responsibility. The optimists say, "Nothing can happen to *me*"; the fatalists, "Whatever happens, happens"; those who are responsible, "Whatever happens, I can take care of it."

Many who know the risks are temporarily blinded to them by love, hate, and other emotions, or by drugs like alcohol.

We need not stress the difficulties that those who gamble with premarital sexual intercourse sometimes encounter—for example, the boy trapped into marriage with a wife who will be a stone around his neck.

Fiction has made much of these tragedies. On the other hand, it must be admitted that these results are not the inevitable outcome of all sexual adventures.

While the sex drive is strong, it is not relentless. It does not begin as an overwhelming force; it has its rhythms. The motive which prompts sexual adventures in youth is not always love. Among the other common motives are to feel "grown up," search for adventure or romance, gang spirit, fear of not being "normal," rebellion against parents and other authority, and virtual seduction by older persons.

Young men take the risks of premarital intercourse generally for fear of "missing something"; young women often for fear of "losing someone."

Yet to divorce sex relationships from the total social context in which they take place is to denigrate their essential value. A few moments of sexual embrace in the back seat of an automobile or a night in a shady motel does not qualify as a sexual experience. The sense of "conquest" and the release of sexual tensions, if any, are only temporary and offer no positive, enduring satisfactions. To some degree such experience always engenders feelings of guilt or shame, overpowering and damaging to many people although lightly passed off in others.

There is a normal and natural tendency in any sex-tinged relationship to overvalue one's personal feelings. However, the lasting satisfactions to be derived from sexual experience depend upon social approval. Personal feelings are not entirely personal; they derive from the feelings of other people.

For some young people premarital intercourse has a negative value rather than a positive one. It is a symbol of rebellion and emancipation from parental control. The unconscious motives for doing something that parents have long forbidden are masked and unrecognized feelings of anger or hate against them, their ideas, and their guidance. Hence casual love affairs are often an expression of hate against one's parents rather than love for one's partner.

Petting. "Petting," a word that has many synonyms, describes a wide variety of bodily contacts and explorations undertaken both for the stimulation and satisfaction of sexual impulses. It represents a kind of sex play engaged in by many lower animals as well as human beings. Sometimes it is carried to climax.

The incidence of petting appears to have increased in recent years. The evidence seems to be that petting has become more accepted as a substitute for premarital intercourse, especially on the higher educational levels. There is little or no reason to suspect that petting *per se* causes any direct physical harm to those who engage in it. The psychological effects and social implications are something else again. Expert opinion is divided as to whether petting promotes or impedes later marital adjustment.

Certainly petting can invoke feelings of guilt, shame, disgust, and other uncomfortable emotions in young men and women who find a sharp conflict between what they are doing and what they think they ought to do. On the other hand it would be abnormal in modern society rigidly to refuse all physical contact with a person of the opposite sex, especially under conditions of a growing love relationship.

Some of the questions worth asking about the practice of petting are: "Is this getting me more deeply involved with someone than I want to be?" "Do I feel differently about the aftermath of this experience than I expected to feel?" "Am I getting a reputation for petting?" The question of "how far" one goes in petting is often a less important question than the question of under what circumstances one pets at all.

Petting and promiscuity are not the same thing. There are no good arguments in favor of promiscuity, which debases potentially valuable feelings to the level of a "cheap thrill." The Don Juan types, whether male or female, are basically unhappy people who sadly enhance their own feelings of insecurity by flitting from one person to another. They never really find the satisfactions they presumably seek.

Other Adjustment Problems. *Nocturnal Emissions.* Nocturnal or seminal emissions are spontaneous ejaculations of semen during sleep. They are often, but not necessarily, accompanied by dreams in which erotic fantasies occur. Over 99% of the men who enter college report nocturnal emissions at some time during their lives. Some individuals have many nocturnal emissions; others, very few. More imaginative individuals may have more erotic dreams, but these are not necessarily accompanied by ejaculations.

The incidence of nocturnal emissions is highest in the teens and gradually falls to very low levels. Very little is actually known about the physiological or psychological mechanisms involved. The semen ejected is, of course, exactly the same type of fluid released in all other types of ejaculations. No harm arises from nocturnal emissions, even when they are frequent, and most young men today simply accept them as a normal male experience.

Masturbation. Since very high percentages of both men and women report engaging, or having engaged in autoerotic practices (autosexuality, masturbation), the practice cannot be called abnormal. In the past great harm was done to emotional lives of young men and women by the false preachment that autosexuality had seriously damaging physical effects. Everything from pimples to insanity was blamed on it. There is *no* scientific evidence that any harmful physical effects result from autosexuality. The practice normally (and statistically) diminishes steadily with increasing age.

Homosexuality. In the normal course of psychosexual development, every individual goes through a stage of orientation to his own sex. This is the period of "gangs" and "crushes." However this is something quite different from overt homosexuality as an adult sex practice (in women referred to as Lesbianism). Any student who is genuinely bothered by homosexual feelings and longings is strongly advised to seek professional help for his problem. Attention should also be called to the fact that there are sophisticated and experienced homosexuals of both sexes who deliberately prey upon inexperienced young men and women.

A good marriage, conceived in affection and observed with fidelity, offers the best opportunity for successful resolution of problems of sexual adjustment. In the next chapter we shall discuss the factors involved in making a good marriage, particularly those concerned with choice of a mate.

SUMMARY REVIEW QUESTIONS

1. What are the functions of the family? Elaborate.
2. What do you consider to be the trends in family life in the United States today? How does this help create and how is this reflected in the total population pattern of the United States?
3. How do you interpret the statement: "Marriage is the normative pattern of sexual behavior"? Elaborate.
4. What is the historical background for the present American ideal of marriage?
5. How are private and personal attitudes toward sex formed? Why do you think they sometimes differ so greatly from person to person?
6. Do you think it is important to have a guiding personal philosophy for the management of sexual instincts? Why or why not? What is your personal philosophy of sexual behavior? Has it changed much in recent years? Why or why not?
7. What is the "conspiracy of silence" in the United States? How does it operate? What do you conceive to be its purpose? Its results?
8. What are the risks of premarital intercourse? Why do some young men and women take these risks?
9. Are the following statements sense or nonsense? Why? *The population of the United States will exceed 250,000,000 by 1980. . . . Love conquers all. . . . Early marriage is the best answer to all problems of sexual adjustment. . . . Men attain real sexual maturity years ahead of women. . . . The girl who will pet/Is a poor marriage bet.*
10. What do the following terms mean to you: matriarchy, birth rate, polygamy, polyandry, fertility cult, lust, infatuation, promiscuity, autosexuality, homosexuality?

Worth Looking Into: *Elmtown's Youth: The Impact of Social Classes on Adolescents* by August B. Hollingshead. *Love against Hate* by Karl Menninger. *Male and Female* by Margaret Mead. *Human Sex and Education: Perspectives and Problems* by W. R. Johnson. More complete references will be found in Appendix E.

FACTS FROM FICTION

Just as much can be learned about health from the study of disease, so much can be gleaned about the values in a successful marriage as a result of studying those which have failed. Many illuminating pictures of love and marriage relationships that have failed are to be found in fiction—novels, plays, and short stories. Dissect one or two of these, and see what evidence you can find *early in the story* to suggest that failure is being foreshadowed. Here are a few "classics" worth studying toward that end, but many others can be found: *Romeo and Juliet* (Shakespeare), *Madame Bovary* (Flaubert), *Craig's Wife* (George Kelly), *Vanity Fair* (Thackeray), *The Old Wives' Tale* (Arnold Bennett), *A Doll's House* (Ibsen), *Ethan Frome* (Edith Wharton), *Main Street* (Sinclair Lewis), *The Beautiful and the Damned* (F. Scott Fitzgerald), *Appointment in Samarra* (John O'Hara), *Back Street* (Fannie Hurst).

Sexuality: A Search for Perspective

Introduction

In the 1968–1969 college year, Michigan State University at East Lansing, Michigan, sponsored and arranged an Interdisciplinary Colloquy on "Sexuality: A Search for Perspective." Elaborate preparation was made for the colloquy proper, which was scheduled for two days each week for seven weeks during the Winter 1969 term. Many educational opportunities as well as specific lectures were made available to the student body and the general public.

In order to provide the necessary resources for the task at hand, 22 guest speakers, representing the disciplines of medicine, anthropology, law, literature, psychology, sociology, ethics, and theology, were engaged to present their viewpoints on different topics in the full colloquy. Press releases were issued by the Information Services of the University on each speaker. These releases gave the substance of the speaker's address and often some additional information gained from interviews. It is the gist of these releases, provided with "news headings" (which do not appear on the news releases proper), which are presented here. Arrangements for publication of the complete texts of the speeches is being arranged by Michigan State University.

In the prospectus for the col-loquy it was effectively stated, as follows:

"The topic of sexuality is of ultimate importance and it is timely. From the overall University standpoint the questions being raised regarding sexuality indicate clearly the importance of this topic to all members of society. They also suggest strongly the lack of adequate formal loci for obtaining information in this significant area. . . . Most collegians are sincerely searching for a *life style* which will give meaning to their actions, and concern with sexuality is necessarily an integral part of this search.

"If higher education is to take seriously the task of equipping the *whole man* for responsible participation in society, it is imperative that fundamental facts and principles regarding sexuality become a part of the educational process through course offerings, continuing educational opportunities, and informal dialogue."

The releases reprinted here follow the seven major topics originally outlined for the colloquy:

1. Physiological aspects of human sexuality.
2. Cultural perspectives.
3. Sexual roles in American society.
4. Sexuality and the law.
5. Premarital sexual standards and behavior.
6. Marriage and the family.
7. Value considerations for moral and ethical decision making.

A New Sex Morality

America needs "a new sex morality—one based on sense rather than mindless prejudice, on compassion rather than rigidity," a University of Houston psychologist, Dr. James L. McCary, said on January 7 at Michigan State University.

Opening a seven-week MSU series of talks, courses and discussions on "Sexuality: Search for Perspective," he called for a comprehensive, school-based program of sex education for everyone.

"We must educate," he said, "not indoctrinate; teach facts, not fallacies; be objective, not subjective; be democratic, not autocratic; aid the young in formulating a code of ethics, and avoid passing on to them our own irrelevant, guilt-producing, emotionally based opinions."

Dr. McCary said attitudes toward sex point up the need for sex education. He noted, for example, that women today are unwilling to accept a double standard of sexual conduct, that boys are propagandized to believe that their masculinity depends on their success in seduction, that girls are indoctrinated in the importance of being "sexy" but not promiscuous, and that little boys learn that tenderness and compassion is "sissy."

He also pointed out that the period of adolescence has been extended because young people become physically mature earlier and go to school longer.

"It must be apparent to each of us," Dr. McCary said, "that many of our rigid, outmoded, unrealistic, and guilt-laden attitudes must be changed. It should be equally apparent that the responsibility for these changes rests squarely upon the shoulders of the parents and other decent citizens of the community."

Sex education, said the clinical psychologist, can be approached in many ways ranging from an ostrich-like viewpoint to a very permissive one.

"The safest solution," Dr. McCary maintained, "would appear to be a course of compromise and selectiveness among the various philosophies of sex education.

"Certain sexual needs should be permitted expression; unadorned information about the physiological and psychological aspects of sex should be presented to all; and the Judeo-Christian traditions within which we live must be understood and dealt with sensibly in the framework of present-day society."

Dr. McCary said he believes that no sex revolution has taken place since about 1920, noting that studies show a significant increase in premarital sexual intercourse among women born after the turn of the century as compared with women born before then.

"Promiscuity," he declared, "is not rampant among college students. . . . There is, on the other hand, considerable evidence that today's young people —especially the college populations—are behaving responsibly. Indeed, they demonstrate considerable moral strength in their concern for the welfare and rights of others.

"There is more and more evidence," he added, "that sexual revolution looms on the horizon.

"One can hardly have escaped noticing a change in sexual attitudes in recent years, as evidenced by the growing freedom with which sexual attitudes are discussed in the various communication media, schools, synagogues, churches, and governmental circles—as well as at cocktail parties and by the man on the street.

"But attitudes (and the ease of discussing them) are not to be confused with behavior. Even those to whom a decision in the matter of a sexual ethic is most pertinent—today's college students—are bewildered and bedeviled by the dichotomy between prevailing sexual attitudes and sexual behavior.

"For example, although 75 percent of college girls express the belief that their classmates are sleeping around (attitude), surveys and research studies consistently point out that, actually, only 20 percent of all college girls experience premarital intercourse (behavior)."

The Sexual Revolution

Dr. Selig B. Neubardt, a practicing obstetrician and gynecologist of New Rochelle, N.Y., argued for contraception instruction, the right to abortion on demand, and long engagement periods in an address on (January 7).

But most important, said Dr. Neubardt, young people should strive for "self-affirmation in their sex lives" by not letting social pressures force them to do what they think is wrong or are not ready to do.

The real meaning of "the sexual revolution," Dr. Neubardt said, is that young people now reject the idea that sex is sin; they know that sex is healthy; they are not ashamed of their sexuality, and they do not hide it.

"Along with being proud of what you do," he said, "you must also be proud of what you don't do."

Dr. Neubardt called for a more rational approach to sexuality for all people at all levels.

Physicians, he stressed, are not well prepared to discuss sexual matters with their patients. Until recently, he explained, physicians studied the structure and function of sex organs but did not study "sexuality." He is now teaching a sexuality course at Albert Einstein College of Medicine and finds medical students very receptive.

Dr. Neubardt also said that, in spite of advice often dispensed by the press, doctors are often the worst rather than the best sexual counselors. He said physicians have their own hangups on sex and that many are "sexual cripples."

The three areas in which sex education is most strikingly needed, said Dr. Neubardt, are contraception, marriage and self-affirmation.

The threat of overpopulation makes contraception necessary, he said. While unplanned pregnancies are forgivable due to ignorance and some other special circumstances, he noted, there is usually no good reason for an intelligent American woman to have an unwanted pregnancy.

He derided the mysticism and "stork psychology" that surround teaching the facts of life to children. At the basis of this kind of approach, he said, is the assumption that sex is evil and that children should be spared the lurid details.

"The truth," he maintained, "is much easier for young children to comprehend than that bird myth."

A realistic concept of contraception should be a part of sex education, he said.

"When children are taught how babies are conceived, they should be taught how babies are not conceived."

If unwanted pregnancies do occur, Dr. Neubardt said, women should be able to legally demand an abortion, which he defined as a termination of a pregnancy during the first three months. He said that an abortion during the first three months of pregnancy is safer than a tonsillectomy or the delivery of a baby when done under hospital conditions by a qualified person.

Only the pregnant woman can make the decision, and the only moral course is to let her decide, he continued. For a Catholic, he acknowledged, abortion is immoral because he thinks of a human life as beginning at con-

ception. For Dr. Neubardt, however, the embryo is a mass of cells with a potential for human life. Both viewpoints should be acknowledged by the law, he argued.

"If I am forced to deny an abortion to a woman whom I honestly feel should not bear a child, I am demeaning the dignity of a human being and to me that is the height of immorality."

Dr. Neubardt said there is an overemphasis on sex in marriage and that it is immoral for a couple to enjoy themselves sexually when they fall out of love. He said that incompatibility and other factors outside of sex break up marriage and then sex deteriorates. Making a couple good sexual partners does not guarantee that the marriage will be happy, he explained.

He suggested long engagements as means of insuring better marriages.

"An engaged couple," he maintained, "should enjoy sex together, not as a barometer of what their marriage is going to be like—to enable them to predict anything—but to enjoy it as a healthy enjoyable thing."

After marriage, he believes, couples should not have children right away but should let the marriage stand the test of time before cementing it with their offspring.

Sex: An Invention of Society?

Human sexuality is not an inborn force; it is an invention of society and owes little to biology, a New York sociologist said on January 8.

John H. Gagnon, associate

professor of sociology from the State University of New York at Stony Brook, said man has a biological capacity for sex but that this capacity does not determine a person's overall behavior any more than any other biological capacity.

"If sex plays an important role in human affairs, it is exactly because societies historically have invented or created its importance."

Sexuality, Prof. Gagnon argued, attains the appearance of a basic drive because of the way that it is talked about—and not talked about.

Attitudes toward sex, he noted, have varied historically and between different cultures, even though man's biology has not varied.

"What does vary," he said, "is the talk about sex, the complex symbols and meanings that transform mute nature into sociosexual or psychosexual drama."

While adolescents and adults are potentially sexual, only a small percentage of their interpersonal encounters have sexual significance, and these occur only in a context which most persons have learned to regard as sexual, Prof. Gagnon pointed out.

A typical reaction, he said, is to not regard a married couple as "sexual," but a prostitute or a homosexual is considered so sexual that she or he can be thought of in no other context.

"Libido (the sex drive) does not create fantasy, but fantasy creates libido," he maintained. "Unless the social situation is proper, fantasy and hence sexual arousal will not occur."

The ways in which parents

and other persons talk—or do not talk—about sex plays a major role in shaping a child's sexuality. A child may learn that what he does innocently is regarded by adults as "dirty" and at the same time is made attractive by the mystery surrounding the act, Prof. Gagnon explained.

Adolescents, he continued, learn a little about sex through formal sexual education, but the mass media are more influential and peer group talk is most influential.

"Most parents," he added, "do not communicate sexual information as much as anxiety."

Boys, he said, learn from other boys to be concerned primarily with the physical aspects of sex while girls learn from other girls that romantic love is the important thing.

As courtship develops, an exchange takes place, he continued.

"For males, the movement will be from sex to love and for the females from love to sex.

"What one observes in this process," he added, "is a kind of underlying effort by which they both begin to understand."

Silence about sex also underlies sexual attitude. Most people, he said, lack the ability to talk about their own sexual activity, particularly with persons with whom they are having sex relations. "There is even major difficulty in talking to the self about sex most of the time.

"For most persons," he added, "the silence mounts and with it a sense of guilt, frustration and inadequacy. These in turn decline as sex itself declines in importance. And this decline is more easily managed than most would imagine.

"It is important to remember that people receive social recognition and support for many things, but—except for very special populations who pay different kinds of costs—there is no basis for the kind of recognition and support for sexual competence. Conversely, people may be judged a failure for many things, but rarely for failing sexually, as only their partners really know, and they are equally committed to silence."

Emergence of a New Sexuality

America's much-discussed "sexual revolution" might better be described as a continual "human revolution," characterized by:

—Current painful cultural changes in sexual attitudes and styles.

—Men and women struggling to "find a new way of understanding and experiencing each other."

—A blurring of the once-sharp distinctions between masculinity and femininity.

—The emergence of "a new sexuality."

These points were made in remarks by a theologian and an anthropologist who spoke on January 14.

Dr. Tom F. Driver, professor of theology and literature at Union Theological Seminary in New York, said that today's culture is in the midst of "a crisis in sexuality." What is needed, he added, is a "new sexuality" which is an expression of human values and relationships.

The anthropologist, Dr.

Weston La Barre of Duke University, told an MSU audience that revolution, sexual or otherwise, is constant in human culture. "Things change with geography and with time," he said, "and we're now in a period of great change."

The present younger generation, Dr. La Barre added, may simply be practicing what it has been told by past generations, with a freer and safer sexuality in sight—"and this shocks the older generation."

Dr. Driver, an ordained Methodist minister, said that the impact of the industrial revolution, together with improved communication techniques, has caused confusion in the area of sexuality.

He said, "The real reason for the (sexual) crisis is the family's loss of its economic function," which has caused less definition in the male and female roles.

"That loss has made it necessary for men and women to find a new way of understanding and experiencing each other," he added. "No longer defined by economic collaboration within the family, their relation has had to be thought out and lived anew."

He observed that modern men and women "have had to ask about the human meaning of their being male and female. Neither the family, the state, the church nor the cultural tradition has been able to answer this question for them. They have had to try to work it out on their own.

"There could be no more telling sign of cultural crisis."

Dr. Driver said that "a new sexuality is not only possible, but it is urgently necessary." To a large extent, it is already here, he added.

But those who follow the new sexuality, he warned, face two branches of the road "that lead nowhere good."

"Down one of these roads have gone the cultists of homosexuality," he said. "What I have against them is not their homosexuality but their cultism." He added that the cultism has been marked by "mockery and sham."

Dr. Driver said the other false road is an "imaginary curve. . . . where there is neither male nor female, the body is not flesh and there is no more division to overcome.

"To hear of paradise is one thing," he noted. "To try to rent a house there is another."

Dr. La Barre, author of "The Human Animal," pointed out that sexuality "goes through historical changes in style.

"In the Renaissance," he noted, "long-haired Florentine youngsters may have had more sexual experience than their modern equivalents in age. . . . Louis XIV wore silks and powdered hair—but he was then probably the most powerful man alive.

"In every generation," he said, "we set up rigid norms and stereotypes and then are unhappy that only statistically few individuals can actualize them."

Dr. La Barre emphasized that each generation also fosters its own "largely unconscious" stereotypes about male and female, and these stereotypes change rapidly from generation to generation.

He noted that not too many years ago the late Dr. Alfred Kinsey proclaimed first that "the human male is extremely oversexed" and, later, that the "human female is greviously undersexed."

"Plainly, what Kinsey has discovered is not the sexual nature of the human male and female," Dr. La Barre said. "He discovered the folklore about sex in this society and in that generation."

Dr. La Barre pointed out that each generation is made up of "a mosaic of traits taken from both father and mother, just as genetic physical traits are."

But he added that generations vary in primary identification with either the father image ("authoritarian, restrictive") or the mother image ("libertarian, democratic").

The former is a "patrist" and the latter is a "matrist."

He said America today may be leaning toward a "patrist" period of control, partly in reaction to the new generation's extreme alienation from "patrist authority, whether that authority be the demeaned and ridiculed father, the recent President-reject, the Papal authority, the police or the college administration."

He said there is a need for both the "patrist" and "matrist" characteristics, to avert chaos and to insure against rigid conformity.

The Fear of
Four-Letter Words

Fear of the body and a fear to use words that refer to sexual parts of the anatomy characterize the American attitude toward sexuality, according to the president of the American Association of Marriage Counselors.

In an address on January 15 Dr. Gerhard Neubeck explored this and other cultural aspects of "The Universality of Sex." Dr. Neubeck is professor and chairman of family studies at the University of Minnesota.

"You have been brainwashed," he told a predominantly student audience, "with the idea that by even looking at your own body you are already committing a sin.

"This being afraid of the body, this wondering about how bad I am, has brought with it our fear to use words that signify certain parts of the anatomy."

Using the argot of the college crowd, Dr. Neubeck called this inhibited attitude "a typical middle-class hangup."

This hangup, he explained, results not only from our feeling guilty about being sexual or from ignorance, but, "to a large degree, it has been the result of language difficulties."

In the area of sexuality, he explained, words that were meant to be used to convey meaning accurately have become loaded.

"We say relations when what we really mean is sexual intercourse."

Other cultures express their attitudes toward sexuality in many different ways, he said, relating anecdotes that characterized Greek, Israeli, German, French, Japanese and Scandinavian attitudes.

His focus, however, was primarily on the contrast between Scandinavian and American attitudes about sexuality.

Dr. Neubeck spent a year in

Scandinavia in 1960–61 as a Fulbright lecturer, and in Minnesota had studied attitudes of children of Scandinavian descent.

He cautioned his audience against believing that the kind of liberalness toward sexuality that characterizes Swedish culture is a panacea for all social ills.

"These people have achieved a degree of personal sexual satisfaction," he said, but indicated that other personal problems in Sweden remain unsolved.

In his research at the University of Minnesota, Dr. Neubeck found that Americans are generally more affectionate (in terms of familial affection) than Scandinavians. But he found no difference among Americans and the second and third generations of American-born Scandinavians.

In terms of expression of sexuality, American culture has been much more "inhibitive" and "prohibitive," he said.

Women: Separate But Not So Equal

America has failed to match other nations in freeing women from the effects of prejudice and its accompanying social apartheid, a philosophy professor said on January 27. Mrs. Violette S. Lindbeck, an assistant professor of philosophy at Southern Connecticut State College in New Haven, discussed "The Other American Dilemma: Sexual Apartheid—Women, Separate But Not So Equal."

"The other American dilemma," she explained, "is not just a 'women problem' but the problem of what constitutes a proper understanding of masculine and feminine being."

The problem, she continued, is one of how men and women are to confront and relate to one another in personally and socially constructive ways.

"New demands on men and women now blur the lines which formerly defined their relationship, but as the old notions have not been easily surrendered, the result has been personal conflict and social confusion, individual and social wastage of lives."

There is a great similarity between racial and sexual prejudices, she said.

"Prejudice is everywhere the same in its nature and its fruits."

It feeds upon stereotyped images, rationalizing restrictions upon the full cultural participation of the suppressed group, imposing a necessary measure of apartheid, of separation, between the alleged social superior and inferior.

It develops in its victims, she continued, a pervasively crippling minority psychology and in its exploiters a blind, delusionary, yet socially powerful, self-image of vicarious superiority.

"The comparison between the social status and fate of the Negro and that of the woman remains an illuminating one for Americans in particular," she emphasized.

"It could be argued," Mrs. Lindbeck asserted, "that the over-all sociopolitical and economic conservatism that marked the American way of life in the '60s. . . . is one factor in our seeming inability to undertake the radical surgery needed to cure the ills of our minority and marginal groups, left so far out of the new American abundance. . . .

"The ideology of 'separate but equal'. . . . between maleness and femaleness is used, as in the parallel case of Negro-White alleged differences, to rationalize the continued social subordination of women and their relegation to marriage and family."

She said, "As with the Negro, women's personality traits and tendencies, developed by virtue of the restricted life-pattern which society permitted her, are taken as the evidence of innate differences between feminine and maculine types of humanity."

During the Victorian age, America saw the emergence of two, new distinct classes of women—a new female proletariat, whose labor was exploited in factories, and a new middle-class woman who became a symbol of the conspicuous consumption made possible by the rise of the new commercial class.

She said it was here that the "my wife doesn't have to work" pride of the American middle-class male was born.

Economic interests and policies have thus in large part influenced the narrowing of man's role to breadwinner and that of woman's to the domestic sphere. In the process, she said, man's economic role has become the prime determinant of his masculine identity and woman's role as glamour girl and home manager the determinant for her sense of feminity.

"Governmental and educational agencies have only recently become concerned about the loss and wastage of women's talents and training," she said.

Sweden, she said, has granted women almost complete social and economic equality, and in the Soviet Union, there are more women doctors than men.

The pressure on women of being isolated in the home, caring for children during the early years of marriage, is felt and articulated mostly by educated women whose training and previous occupations had prepared them for other roles.

This pressure, she said, is also felt by a large group of working-class women whose jobs prior to marriage gave them wider social contacts.

It is only slowly coming to public attention that once women's child-rearing responsibilities are over, "many women have 25 to 30 years of prime left in them," she pointed out.

How much better off women would be, she said, if society had informed them of this eventuality and had taught the majority who do marry and rear children that this is but one stage of their lives.

In conclusion, she asked: "Is not the recognition of common humanity, of equality, of co-responsibility the answer to both American dilemmas and all forms of apartheid?"

The Clamor of Sex

Twentieth-century enlightenment has erased sexual repressions of the Victorian era, but iy has created a modern age with "so much sex and so little meaning or even fun to it," a noted psychotherapist said on January 27. Dr. Rollo May told students that "in an amazingly short period following World

War I, we shifted from acting as though sex did not exist at all to being obsessed with it."

Dr. May, a practicing psychotherapist in New York City, said that the current obsession with sex "serves to cover up contemporary man's fear of death."

Americans repress death as the Victorians repressed sex, he observed. They consider death to be "obscene, unmentionable and pornographic."

Dr. May said that "the clamor of sex all about us drowns out the ever-waiting presence of death."

"Repression of death equals obsession with sex," he said. "Sex is the easiest way to prove our vitality, to demonstrate that we are attractive and virile, to prove we are not dead yet."

He pointed out that this obsession has a biological explanation: "Sexuality and procreation are the only ways of carrying on our name and our genes in our children who live beyond our own death."

In the course of bringing sex into the open, Dr. May said, modern man now faces three paradoxes:

(1) Anxiety and guilt associated with sex have been internalized, not removed.

He said that "couples can, without guilt and generally without squeamishness, discuss their sexual relationship and undertake to make it more mutually gratifying and meaningful."

But at the same time, he noted, men and women are now being subjected to tests of their sexual performance, where their sense of "adequacy and self-esteem is called immediately into question" and the "whole

weight of the encounter is shifted inward" to how they meet the test.

(2) There is a "new emphasis on technique in sex and love-making" that backfires.

Dr. May noted that a preoccupation with sexual technique, indicated by reliance on "how-to-do-it" books, creates "a mechanistic attitude toward lovemaking, and goes along with alienation, feelings of loneliness and depersonalization."

(3) America's "highly vaunted sexual freedom" has turned into "a new form of Puritanism."

He defined the new Puritanism as "a state of alienation from the body, separation of emotion from reason and use of the body as a machine."

What this means, he noted, is that people try to perform sexually "without letting themselves go in passion or unseemly commitment . . . which might be interpreted as exerting an unhealthy demand on the partner."

Too often sexual relations involve no commitment by the partners, he said. "The Victorian person sought to have love without falling into sex; the modern person seeks to have sex without falling in love."

Dr. May also chided what he termed a "great emphasis on bookkeeping and timetable" in modern lovemaking.

If a couple falls behind schedule, he noted, "they become anxious and feel impelled to go to bed whether they want to or not. Elaborate accounting and ledger-book lists . . . make one wonder how the spontaneity of this most spontaneous act can possibly survive."

The differences between men and women have been placed

into "wrong and misleading" stereotypes, he said. But he warned that in our zeal to erase these stereotypes, we have decreed that "everybody feels the same, and both sexes were to react the same way to the same things."

He added: "But we found, to our horror, that we had thrown out the delight-giving differences along with the unfair suppression."

Sexuality should provide human beings with the means to affirm one another in terms of differences, Dr. May said. "We must value difference and appreciate unique capabilities in each human being."

The Status of the Fetus

A "spectacular" revolution in legal opinion regarding the status of the fetus is largely responsible for the current controversy over legalizing abortion, says a professor of law from the University of California at Berkeley.

Dr. John T. Noonan Jr., discussed this revolution on February 11 in a talk entitled "The Protection of the Person in Laws Regarding Sexual Behavior."

Since the end of World War II, said Dr. Noonan, "a slight majority of judges have ruled that the fetus who is killed is entitled to the protections of civil law."

This trend marks "a most spectacular reversal," he explained, in historical tradition. Since Roman times, the fetus had been regarded as a part of the mother.

The findings of science, Dr.

Noonan explained, are responsible for the recent reversal. Today, the fetus is considered as an individual, and as such, entitled to the protections of law.

Data from the study of the fetus and from child psychology have led to this conclusion, he said.

In essence, the drive to legalize abortion conflicts with the womb-bound child's right to life by taking advantage of its weakness, Dr. Noonan contended.

Before legal opinion changed, he pointed out, "doctors had been saying for a century that once a child is conceived there is no point drawing any lines about whether the fetus is a person."

Until the 19th century, canon law treated killing the fetus as criminal after the fortieth day of life. But canon law changed, Dr. Noonan said, and the Catholic church now imposes the social sanction of excommunication on any abortion.

The arguments people are using to convince legislators of the necessity for legalizing abortion, says Dr. Noonan, are "unmitigated nonsense."

Several arguments are used, he said, but the most effective with legislators to date has been one emphasizing the number of abortions in the United States and the number of maternal deaths from abortions.

"We do not actually know how many abortions are committed annually," he said.

"The probable figure for the U.S. may be 50,000 criminal abortions a year. But even if doubled," he said, "the number would be only one-tenth of the figure being used to persuade

legislators of the immensity of the crime."

Legislators are often asked to consider the hardship of the woman who conceives in cases of rape or incest.

The big question, says Dr. Noonan, is "Are you going to make the law for the exceptional cases of rape and incest? If so, you destroy the right to life."

How Effective Are Sex Laws?

Sex laws do more harm than good.

This was the position presented by Dr. Ralph Slovenko, a New Orleans attorney, speaking on the topic of "Sexuality and the Law." Dr. Slovenko said on February 11 that other criminal laws can better deal with sexual crimes than so-called sex laws.

"We often think of sex as giving pleasure," he explained, "but for many people—too many people—sex is a source of pain. Freud opened sex up to discussion, but the law on sex remains the same."

The emphasis of the law, he adds, ought to be on deterring aggressive activity, gross public indecency and seductiveness of minors. The law ought not to be concerned, he continued, with sexual activities performed in private and between consenting adults.

"The laws needed to regulate intolerable sexual behavior," he pointed out, "can actually be accomplished more effectively, and with less emotional stigma, by nonsex criminal laws."

Speaking out against current

laws concerned with rape, he said that these laws are self-defeating. A rape victim, he explained, would be more likely to assist law enforcement officials if the court proceedings were less humiliating.

"The crime of indecent assault or assault and battery," he said, "with adjustment in the penalty, could take the place of a rape charge."

Discussing "crime against nature" or homosexual crimes, Dr. Slovenko said that the typical arrests made on this charge are limited to sex acts committed in public.

He added, "The community has a need to control against and to express its feelings about gross violations of established social codes, but it can do this without sex laws."

The crimes of public disorder, disturbing the peace, and assault and battery, he pointed out, while protecting the public, are at the same time less stigmatizing than "crime against nature" or "sodomy" laws.

"Sexual deviation," Dr. Slovenko explained, "should be recognized as an attempt at adaptation—at problem solving. The homosexual, frightened by the opposite sex, turns to the same sex to satisfy his dependency, sexual and other human needs. He at least has not withdrawn from the human race."

Concerning sexual psychopath legislation and special institutions for sexual offenders, Dr. Slovenko noted that the "sorry" experience of states that have enacted such laws furnishes ample evidence that this approach is not to be followed. Rather, he added, we should proceed in the opposite direc-tion and utilize nonsex legislation.

In discussing current divorce laws, he stated that the law is not very helpful to persons going through the breaking up of a marriage. The parties, he explained, are forced by the law to go through a procedure that is degrading and which widens even more the gap between them.

"Apart from property matters," Dr. Slovenko explained, "the process of divorce ought to be taken out of the courts."

The courts, he maintained, are set up to decide issues and there is really no issue in a divorce case for courts to decide. Divorce, he explained, is really an administrative matter.

The Battle Over Fertility

The individual is winning in the world battle over the ownership of human fertility, Dr. Alan F. Guttmacher, president of Planned Parenthood-World Population, told his audience on February 12. Dr. Guttmacher said there has been a contest over who owns fertility: the individual, the state or the church.

"There is no doubt in my mind over who owns fertility," he said, "the individual does."

Why does the state have such a vested interest in one's fertility?

"Before the nuclear age," Dr. Guttmacher said, "the nation needed cannon fodder: the big nation was the powerful nation.

"Now that has changed. Technological power outweighs muscle power. Now, the country is losing interest in increasing its numbers. Nations are now interested in contraception.

"For example," he said, "the Office of Economic Opportunity budget for birth control jumped from $2.5 million in 1968 to $13 million in 1969."

Dr. Guttmacher said, the nation has come to realize that the most effective dollar in the war on poverty is the birth control dollar. And the most effective way to reduce infant mortality is effective contraception.

For instance, he explained, the death rate for the first year among children born after a family has reached the size of four children, is much higher than when the family is smaller.

What do parents do now to limit their families?

"About 10 percent of the marriages are made sterile by the time the wife reaches 40 years of age," said Dr. Guttmacher.

Sterilization, that is, cutting and tying the tubes that carry the sperm in the male or the eggs in the female, is a very useful method of birth control, Dr. Guttmacher said. The operation is relatively simple, especially in the male.

The main drag in the progress of sterilization in this country is the conservatism of the medical profession, according to Dr. Guttmacher.

"The doctor does not know his law," he said. "He is a very conservative person at best. The doctor's social conscience is of a rather small order."

Women go to doctors for several different services. Besides sterilization, another commonly used service is abortion, Dr. Guttmacher said.

He pointed out that for every 125 million children born every year in the world there are about 25 million illegal abortions.

"Some day, in America," he said, "we shall have abortion by demand. The decision of abortion will be up to the pregnant woman."

Sex Without Guilt

Dr. Albert Ellis, the author of more than two dozen controversial but widely read books on human sexuality, brought his crusade for "sex without guilt" to a campus setting on February 18.

Addressing an audience of students, Dr. Ellis said: "Literally millions of Americans, including untold numbers of college students, are still exceptionally guilty in regard to sex in general and to premarital affairs in particular."

Such feeling is not healthy, he said, because "guilt, when accurately defined, is virtually always irrational, self-defeating and evil. In relation to sex behavior, it is particularly idiotic."

Dr. Ellis said he found no fault with the rational element of guilt: that "I have done a wrong, erroneous, mistaken or unethical act, and it is unfortunate that I have committed this act."

But he strongly rejected what he termed the "irrational element" in guilt, which is the conclusion that "because I unfortunately committed a wrong act, I am a pretty bad person."

The latter feeling, he said, usually encourages a person to "put himself into a hell on earth and to stop progressive change."

Dr. Ellis, a practicing New York City psychotherapist and executive director of the Institute for Advanced Study in Rational Living, listed and then challenged a host of objections to premarital sexual relations:

—That premarital sex overemphasizes sex apart from interpersonal relations.

Assuming that college students do emphasize sex at the expense of interpersonal relations, Dr. Ellis asked, "What is so awful about that?"

He pointed out that students already engage in a variety of activities—eating, politicking, picketing, dancing, fishing, skiing, studying and others— "without really relating to each other interpersonally, and no one seems to think anything of this.

"Why, then, should they have to engage in intense, depth-level interpersonal relations just because the activity they are engaging in happens to be sexual?"

—That premarital relations indicate a person is "exploiting" a member of the opposite sex and is therefore immoral.

He said that "humans are simply not the kind of beings who always love the people they lust after; and to demand that they should do so is to help make them guilty and self-hating."

Not only do sexual feelings often result from love, he added, but often "sex also begets love, particularly in the male of the species."

Dr. Ellis contended that anyone who downgrades a premarital affair on the grounds that it is not totally unexploitative is "quite unrealistic and perfectionistic."

—That premarital sex "leads to unbridled freedom and to undisciplined behavior."

He pointed out that nearly everyone now advocating premarital freedom wants "man's so-called sex insincts to be solidly embedded in a context of honesty, considerateness, mutual consent and even love."

"What we sexual libertarians invariably fight for is the removal of arbitrary, needless, foolish, anxiety-abetting and hostility-fomenting fetters on sex relations. . . . We do not want complete sex freedom, any more than we want removal of all restrictions on business transactions, on automobile driving or on using murderous weapons."

—That premarital intercourse is only good "when it is part of a meaningful or worthwhile relationship," and that otherwise it is a form of "moral nihilism."

He defended the concept of "secular humanism," which means that a sex act is immoral "only when it needlessly and definitely harms oneself or another human being."

Sex acts, he added, "are not in themselves wrong and may be quite good and proper when they are engaged in by consenting adults."

—That premarital acts are antispiritual.

He challenged the notion that loveless sex is a contradiction. "If anything, the reverse is often true: since some sex partners love their mates so much, and themselves so little, they fail to concentrate adequately on their own sexual arousal and satisfaction, and, consequently, miss out on considerable gratification.

—That to desire someone else

solely for physical satisfaction is "of the lowest animal nature."

Dr. Ellis listed several rebuttals to this argument: sexual enjoyment is hardly lower than the pleasures of "eating, watching a sunset, hearing a symphony or smelling a rose;" man's ability to think rationally makes it virtually impossible for him to be purely "animalistic" in any act; knowing oneself and loving are animalistic pursuits necessary to happiness and mental health.

He acknowledged that premarital intercourse has "distinct limitations and disadvantages," but so do all human relations, including love.

"Premarital sex, again like every other imaginable human act, can definitely be performed stupidly, self-defeatingly and antisocially," he said.

Commitment to Chastity

A commitment to chastity and marital fidelity may well characterize a return to idealism, said Sidney Cornelia Callahan a noted author, speaking on "The Emancipation of Women and the Sexual Revolution," on February 18.

"A sexual renaissance is dependent upon our changing both our ideals of sexuality, and our stereotypes of men and women," she said.

After all, in order to have an interpersonal relationship, she said, you must first have two persons. In any refined idea of love, there must be freedom for the beloved to choose his or her lover.

As a consequence of greater emancipation of women, the New York author and lecturer believes that American mar-

riages have the potential of being the best marriages the world has ever seen.

"It is now possible to combine friendship in marriage, in ways impossible in the past," she explained.

Freedom in marriage, she added, should include ability to divorce, the control of fertility, acceptance of feminine sexuality, and civil equality in marriage and in the outside society.

After exploring changes in the modern view of marriage, Mrs. Callahan discussed premarital behavior.

"The emancipation of women will make a huge difference in the premarital picture," she said.

Today, women are no longer objects to be purchased "intact," she said, while men are no longer the purchasers. Women have become more equally responsible for their own premarital years.

The author of "The Illusion of Eve" and "Beyond Birth Control" suggested three models representing current premarital and marital ideals.

The first advocates total permissiveness in both premarital and marital behavior, she pointed out. Adherents of this philosophy may think of sex either as a tension which demands relief, or as an exalted, spiritual form of communication which should be shared with every human being.

This total permissiveness conflicts with society and with man's innate aggressiveness and possessiveness, she said. Man has always found sexual limits and limits to aggressions necessary for common life.

A second model, she explained, condones premarital

permissiveness, leading to fidelity in marriage. The premarital state is regarded as a learning experience, where young people live with their partners, in relationships of deep affection and responsibility.

However, she said, the emphasis is always on individual fulfillment, so that even marriage may be easily dissolved if one member feels confined. Serial monogamy is often the result of this concept of marriage.

Mrs. Callahan preferred yet a third model—that of premarital chastity and marital fidelity. She believes that youthful control leads to greater social stability, and sensitivity to others.

Early experimentation may make young people unable to keep deep, lasting commitments, she explained. Without the ability to keep promises, they may never find, or maintain their own identity.

"Too much sexual permissiveness without commitment will corrode our basic trust in one another," she added.

Although she sees a sexual renaissance approaching, with permissiveness as the keystone, she hopes that once our reaction against the past has been played out we might see a cultural return to idealism."

"In the meantime," she concluded, "I feel the minority's commitment to chastity and fidelity can serve the community very well."

Premarital Sexual Standards

Popular beliefs about human sexuality are fast falling by the wayside.

Among the folk myths that fell

this year, cut down by the research of a distinguished Iowan sociologist, were these:

—"There is no sexual revolution, no runaway sexual permissiveness.

—"A gadget, like the pill, doesn't change the values of society.

—"There is no generation gap of any significance in sexual standards between this generation and the last.

—"The 'New Morality' is not really new."

And Dr. Ira L. Reiss, researcher, author and professor of sociology at the University of Iowa, has data to support his assertions.

He has held three grants from the National Institute of Mental Health for studies which focused on the development of scales to measure premarital sexual permissiveness.

From his findings he has authored two books: "Premarital Sexual Standards in America" and "The Social Context of Premarital Sexual Permissiveness."

His findings, were that sexual behavior has changed very little in the 20th century, and for that matter since the so-called "Puritan" and "Victorian" periods.

According to his research, Dr. Reiss says that the divorce rate is the same as it was 30 years ago; the age at which women marry hasn't changed in 20 years; and, as in the 1920s, about half the women entering marriage today are virgins.

"What has changed," Dr. Reiss said, "are attitudes about sex."

There is more open discussion and less guilt about sex, he says.

In fact, "this generation, more than any other," he contends, "has made its peace with its sexuality—probably because of its willingness to discuss it."

But the basic difference between today and the past is this:

"Freedom to choose a sexual code has been legitimized for the individual, much like choosing a religion or a political affiliation," Dr. Reiss contends.

"And that is why we talk about it more, why we find more young people living together, and why we can expect sex to be even more public in the future."

With that freedom, and the freedom built into the social system of dating and courtship today, says Dr. Reiss, "the really amazing thing is how little premarital sex there is.

"Only 25 to 30 percent of college girls are nonvirginal," he says.

As for the future, according to Dr. Reiss, the next decade will bring American sex codes closer to those in Scandinavia.

Culture, Class, and Color

Many of the problems of our central cities are directly attributable to the dislocations of Southern agriculture, contends a leading Negro sociologist who grew up in rural Mississippi.

According to Dr. Charles R. Lawrence, chairman of the department of sociology at Brooklyn College of the City University of New York, "the workers who are least suited to contemporary farming in the Deep South are precisely those workers who lack the literacy and work discipline needed in the urban labor force."

Dr. Lawrence made his remarks in a talk entitled "Culture, Class and Color: A Mi-

nority View." Dr. Lawrence focused on the origins of black nationalism, ghetto pathology, and contemporary Negro family patterns.

"Family life among Negro Americans," he said, "is peculiarly a product of the American experience. Chattel slavery involved a systematic elimination of the African cultural past."

Because American slavocrats were unwilling to tolerate the patriarchal, frequently polygamous families of Black Africa, Dr. Lawrence explained, a variety of new family styles emerged during the slave era.

At the very bottom of the evolving slave structure were the field hands. Because the males in this group constituted a large part of the masters' liquid assets and were the most likely to flee, the field-hand household became matricentric.

The role of the grandmother became the most important source of nurture and continuity—a still-common phenomenon among lower-status Negro families, Dr. Lawrence noted.

"House servants and Negro artisans tended to assimilate European values regarding families and 'monogamous-cum-concubinage' marriages," he says, "and a quasi-patriarchal family life developed."

Among the free Negroes in this period, who provided much of the antislavery leadership, the family organization was often strongly patriarchal, according to Dr. Lawrence.

"The development of this intraracial system of social stratification, he pointed out, "was highly correlated with pigmentation."

There was concrete evidence,

he said, that the blacker one's skin was, the further down he was found in the social heirarchy.

Field hands, for example, were predominantly of unmixed African ancestry, he noted, while a very high proportion of the free population was made up of mulattoes.

Even today, said Dr. Lawrence, "color and class continue to be the most important parameters for consideration of family life among Negro Americans."

The uppermost stratum within America's black population is roughly comparable to the general American upper-middle class, he noted, and had its origin among the predominantly mulatto-free families and domestics of the pre-Civil War era.

Among black families of middle-class standing, there is a high incidence of home ownership and wives are likely to be employed. But, he said, even when Negroes have worked hard and saved their money, it is almost impossible to escape the confines of the ghetto.

In the working class Negro families the importance of education is realized and the extended family continues to function despite the ravages of urbanization.

It is through the extended family, he explained, that matricentrality is maintained within working class black families.

"Working class blacks," Dr. Lawrence said, "have always been more attracted to black nationalism than have their highly situated brethren."

Lower-class families consti-tute about 40 percent of America's black families and more than half of her black children.

Dr. Lawrence questioned those sociologists who are emphasizing the breakdown of the black underclass family.

"Though a father is present more often than absent in black underclass families," he contended, "the pattern is clearly matrifocal. The stability and continuity of the nuclear family is mainly dependent on the mother or the grandmother."

The historical powerlessness of the black male in American society, Dr. Lawrence explained, has been a source of weakness and rage.

"An important element of the contemporary black mood," he said, "is the elevation of the black male to a position of dominance—even if this means that the black female must feign weakness."

Marital and Sexual Health

Married couples fight most at the time they love themselves least, Dr. Clark E. Vincent, director of the Behavioral Sciences Center at Wake Forest University, told his audience on February 24.

If our self-love is strong, we are happy and easy-going, Dr. Vincent said. If our self-love is weak, we are sad and critical.

For example, when the husband comes home "shot down" he is critical.

"He points out all sorts of mistakes," Dr. Vincent said, "that on another day, he would have overlooked."

His attack leads to his wife's retaliatory attack; they are both "right."

"Each of us," Dr. Vincent said, "were brought up in families where we've had a mother and father arguing as to who is right and who is wrong.

"The beauty of the marital argument is that they will never run out of ammunition."

If it's not what they said that morning, it is what was said yesterday, last week, last year, ten years ago, or before they were married. And then there are each other's parents to attack.

"People should learn to recognize these attacks for what they really are," Dr. Vincent said. "The attacks are signals that say, 'I do not love myself enough.'"

This misunderstanding carries through to the sexual realm, Dr. Vincent said.

For example, many people do not understand that men and women have different sexual needs. The wife wants sexual relations at the height of her self-esteem, whereas the husband often wants "sex" at the depths of his self-esteem.

The husband does not understand that what works once will not necessarily work again. The same approach may get different results.

Dr. Vincent said, "She keeps changing."

Woman is a very complex creature, he said. But the husband was not told this when he was a boy. He was conditioned to prove himself.

"As an adult," Dr. Vincent said, "he spends most of his productive hours continuing to prove himself with more education, more money, better church relations. It will never end: Prove, prove, prove . . ."

The proving goes even into the bedroom, the marriage counselor said.

"Everytime the male wants to make love, he has to prove it. First, he has to provide physical evidence of sexual capability."

The husband is so busy proving himself in an endless array of projects that the wife's attractive powers are not enough to give her the attention she needs.

The wife, as a girl, was conditioned to be pretty. Beauty is her primary concern. She must attract and be noticed.

Dr. Vincent pointed out:

"The girl is literally brainwashed with the aid of a multi-billion-dollar cosmetic and clothing industry. If she is worth her salt as a woman, she can attract attention."

The solution to the problem of misunderstanding in marriage is improved communication.

The Family as a Teacher of Sex

Differences between the sexes can contribute to an increased sense of aliveness, or to a destructive competitiveness Virginia Satir, counselor, author and lecturer, said on February 25. Miss Satir spoke on "The Family as a Teacher of Sex."

"We have long accepted the fact that men and women are anatomically different," she said. "But it is terribly difficult for many families to appreciate personality differences in each other."

Often one parent simply withdraws, she explained, leaving the business of running the family to the other. This "solution" can cause serious trouble for their children.

A little boy learns from his father what it is like to be a male, she said. However, he must also learn from his mother what it is like to be in the presence of a male—how a man relates to women, as well as to other men.

If one parent gives all the messages, the child is deprived of half his sexuality, she said.

Parents should be willing to fight in front of their child, she stated, so that he can see that the sexes are different, and become aware that this difference can be a tool for growth and awareness, not just a source of contention and hate.

"In my experience as a family counselor," she said, "I have found that most parents want the best for their children, and for themselves.

"When I see severe problems and failures," she said, "I can be sure they are not the outcome of design, but of confusion, ignorance, and lack of awareness."

Sex and Human Wholeness

The attitude which regards human sexuality with both fear and disgust is a perversion perpetrated by the whole culture and must be corrected, contends a professor of family life.

"Our culture has torn man's sexuality out of context and in the past has done its utmost to deny its existence," says Lester A. Kirkendall, professor of family life at Oregon State University.

Dr. Kirkendall made his re-marks during a colloquy focused on "Value Considerations for Moral and Ethical Decision-making."

Dr. Kirkendall's topic was "Sex and Human Wholeness."

In describing ideas about sex which are responsible for the attitude of fear or disgust, he said: "The male's role in reproduction was carefully bypassed and children were regarded and treated as nonsexual beings. So were youth to the extent that their behavior permitted this pretense to exist."

Recently a kind of counter-reaction point of view was developed, he noted, in which sex is regarded as an aspect of life subject to no restrictions.

However, what is urgently needed, Dr. Kirkendall contends, is an approach that is concerned neither with promoting or repressing sexual activity and interest.

Answering the question "How can human sexuality be used at all stages and circumstances of life so that it becomes an integral, meaningful, purposeful part of living?" should be our concern, he says.

"The concern would be to understand how and under what circumstances sexuality could be used to establish confidence, trust, warmth and understanding in relationships.

"We would ask how and if expressions of sexuality and sexual attitudes could counter expressions of hostility and aggression," explains Dr. Kirkendall.

Dr. Kirkendall is the author of six books, the most acclaimed being "Premarital Intercourse and Interpersonal Relationships." He is cofounder of the

Sex Information and Education Council of the U.S. and belongs to the Society for the Scientific Study of Sex and the American Society of Marriage Counselors.

He believes that in order to answer the major questions about sexuality we must concentrate on the processes and meanings of interaction rather than on acts and episodes.

He said, "We must be done with our preoccupation with counting and census-taking for the purpose of determining how many have violated the conventional standards."

What people ought to consider instead, he contends, is the relationship of sexual expression to love and responsibility; ways in which the generations can help each other in understanding the meaning of sexuality; the shifting sex roles; and the ways in which values which govern behavior are established.

Better Marriages
to Come

Permanent marriage in the future—built on the fulfillment of human needs including but not limited to sexuality—will be better than the marriage of today, a noted counselor-theologian predicted on March 3.

Dr. Otis A. Maxfield, director of training for the American Foundation of Religion and Psychiatry in New York City, said that marriage partners of the future "will be more demanding of the relationship than many are today."

But at the same time, he added, "the attitude of possessiveness—of owning other persons, which has historically

dominated sexual unions—is likely to be greatly diminished."

"While it is true that marriage can be 'wholly wedlock' or 'unholy deadlock,'" he said, "it is equally true for me that the ultimate fulfillment of sexuality comes best within a context of the marriage situation.

"It is also increasingly clear to me that a man-woman relationship will have permanence only in the degree to which it satisfies the emotional, psychological, intellectual, spiritual and physical needs of the partner."

Dr. Maxfield outlined several characteristics of marriage in the future:

—"There will be the feeling of commitment as opposed to the idea of contract.

"Marriage at its best is not a bargain but a commitment where each through a lifetime seeks to give all that he has and then some to the other."

—Future marriage will affirm "the free acceptance of a bond, something which limits the undisciplined type of self-expression which is natural to man.

"Self-expression means nothing unless put within a framework. A man who understands marriage is not blind to the physical attractiveness of women other than his wife, but the possibility of making love to them is ruled out. . . . Living on the basis of inclination robs life and relationship of its richness.

—"Marriage in the future will positively vote in favor of the vocation of motherhood and fatherhood." Each partner "will accept the obligation involved in having and rearing children."

—Marriage will become a career for men as well as for women.

There is hope that "for a man the vocation of fatherhood will be enriched and enhanced in the future. . . . Father has a place in the home and a responsibility of authority which he should neither avoid nor abdicate."

Dr. Maxfield, a senior Congregational minister in Greenwich, Conn., observed that "a considerable amount of the sex behavior of the American people is of a social, pathological nature—a by-product of our failure to integrate sex with the rest of life."

He said, "Until a man relates to the feminine principle and a woman comes to terms with the masculine principle, the unconscious will keep provoking disastrous, destructive and essentially tragic experiences."

Dr. Maxfield suggested that "behind much of our sexual dilemma lies the longing for the soul," which he described as "the last four-letter word that is not 'in.'"

While soul has "an old-fashioned ring," he said, it still seems to be the goal of every man "who longs with heart and soul, or who puts his whole soul into anything."

Sex Masquerading
as Love

Prescription for sexual hang-ups—talk.

Psychiatrist Roy W. Menninger, president of the Menninger Foundation, Topeka, Kansas, said on March 4 that the prescription may not seem satisfactory but "talking with the right people about the right things" seems to be the best way of resolving mental conflicts.

Pressures from within and without, Dr. Menninger noted, mean that conflict and accompanying anxiety, guilt and doubt will always be the lot of man. "The issue," he said, "is not how we avoid conflict, but how we manage it."

Dr. Menninger said sexual activity often becomes a means of resolving common emotional conflicts and concerns. Sex, he explained, masquerades as love, as an antidote for loneliness, as evidence of worthwhileness, and as a demonstration of potency.

"In the context of a loving relationship, sex does all of these things," he said. "The difficulty comes when the sexual act is preeminently serving needs which are unrecognized.

"The difficulty, therefore, is identifying and becoming aware of these kinds of illegitimate or inappropriate needs which are piggybacking their way to solution through sexual activity."

As an example, he cited the need for a person to prove his worth by means of sex, believing that "if someone wishes to love me, then I must be worth something."

Sexual fulfillment of this need, he continued, leads to feelings of guilt about the sex act, and thus to greater feelings of unworthiness.

"To treat this guilt, they move on to another liaison and hope that true love will win through

and that feelings of guilt and unworthiness will be washed away, only to find the cycle reinforced and made worse," he explained.

Part of the reason that many people fulfill their needs through sexual acts is that modern American culture perpetuates numerous myths stressing the importance of satisfying sex acts, Dr. Menninger said. In particular he noted:

"There is a myth that a successful marriage depends on a successful sex life. The implication is that without the one, you will never have the other."

"Nonsense. In point of fact," he said, "the situation is the other way around. Those of us who are involved in treating and dealing with marriages are very much aware that the best barometer we have about the health of a marriage is the sex life. People who are in love do not complain of difficulties.

"Those who do complain about sexual difficulties do not do so because they lack training in college, but because they lack the warm qualities that hold marriages together."

Dr. Menninger urged his audience to attempt to analyze and understand the decision-making processes that lead to sexual and other emotional problems.

"What needs to follow is a process of talking about the things which are deeply personal to you, the kinds of issues

that bear on one's ego, the kinds of pressures to which one is subjected.

"Without the opportunity to review, to examine, to consider, to think about the questions and pressures which one is experiencing, one really is no better than victimized by the forces operating on us."

He said a person could talk to himself ("admittedly a hazardous course") or to a friend, but he recommended talking in groups or to "trusted elders."

"Talking to groups," he noted, "runs counter to the high premium put on isolation in America's individualistic society. This premium," he explained, "says in effect 'It's your bag; you solve it.' For better or for worse, that is what most of us do until we hit the breaking point."

He defined "trusted elders" as "wise men over 30 who have not lost the capacity to talk to and to understand those who are younger. Whether they be faculty members or psychologists, or counselors, or even resident advisors (in the dormitories), they constitute a resource that I suspect is not being adequately or sufficiently used."

"The trusted elders," he added, "should not give advice, but should ask such questions as, 'Are you sure that you are being honest with yourself?' and 'Is this what you really want to do?'"

12

PREPARING FOR MARRIAGE

THE TRANSITION FROM CHILDHOOD TO MAN-hood in modern American culture often seems to be particularly turbulent. One paradoxical reason for this is the comparatively high degree of independence enjoyed by young people, since parental authority wanes early. The formal landmarks of growing up have been erased; there are no traditional initiation ceremonies to mark acceptance into adult status. In youth the underlying theme of conduct is independence and the goal is maturity.

In early adolescence the physical changes wrought by new hormone patterns and differential growth rates of different body parts create problems of adjustment; adolescent awkwardness must be mastered. In the late teens and into college years the need for making new kinds of social and emotional adjustments becomes more intense. The relationship of college students with their parents and other members of their family changes and sometimes becomes strained.

More important, the need for establishing new kinds of attitudes and relationships with members of the opposite sex becomes paramount. A feeling for adventure is gradually modified by a desire for permanence in man-woman relationships. The drive toward growing up is slowly integrated with the feeling for settling down in marriage. But interposed and imposed on these feelings is the demand for love, that is, the need to love and be loved by a particular mate. The choice of a marriage partner becomes an expedition for discovering the sensation of "falling in love." This predominantly American way of arranging for marriage has both its advantages

and disadvantages, its successes and its failures.

In this chapter we shall give particular consideration to the factors in choosing or refusing a mate that enhance the chances of success in marriage and minimize its risks. We shall also discuss briefly the social processes of dating, courtship, and engagement through which marriages in the United States occur.

Taboos on Choice of Mate

Prohibitions and taboos on one or another kind of sexual conduct are as universal as marriage itself. Most elaborate and complicated rules exist among many primitive tribes to say whom a man or woman may or may not marry. Most of these rules prescribe *exogamy*, that is, selection of a mate outside one's own family, tribe, clan, "totem," or village. More rarely, but with equal insistence, they demand *endogamy*, which means that the marriage partner must be found within a particular group.

Endogamy is generally practiced, if not enforced, among higher social class and caste groups and sometimes along religious lines, for the preservation of that particular social group within the larger social structure. The peak of endogamy was reached among the Pharaohs of ancient Egypt and the Incas of Peru, where brother-sister marriages were prescribed. But endogamy is still subtly enforced in old, upper-class society in the United States. Utmost family and social pressure, sometimes including the threat of disinheritance, is brought against many a socially elite young man or woman who proposes to contract a marriage with a mate of dissimilar background. Fiction has made much of this dilemma; *Kitty Foyle* by Christopher Morley and *Back Street* by Fannie Hurst are good examples.

Exogamy is fundamentally a bar to marriage rather than a ban on sexual relationships. As observed in primitive tribes and enforced by its social and religious taboos, the practice of exogamy forbids marriage between members of the same "clan" or "totem." This does not, however, exclude marriages between rather close blood relatives. Indeed, in some tribes cross-cousins are the preferred marriage partners; this means that it is considered an exceptionally good match if a young man marries his mother's brother's or his father's sister's daughter. This comes close to the practice of *homogamy,* or like marrying like. Homogamy is actually the practice in most modern civilized societies. Contrary to the opinion that "opposites attract," they do not often marry; most individuals choose and marry someone with a background very much like their own.

Universal Incest Taboo. The taboo on primary incest is almost absolutely universal. Primary incest may be defined as sexual congress or marriage between mother and son, father and daughter, brother and sister. Among thousands of societies studied by anthropologists, none —even the most primitive and culturally backward—fails to impose the strongest kind of prohibitions and punishments on incest. Primitive people explain their system of exogamy as an extension of incest taboo; their extensive kinship acknowledgements therefore provide for different "degrees" of incest which must be prohibited. In some places the risk of incest is held to be so great, and regarded with such awe, that no contact between brother and sister is permitted from infancy onward. In extreme cases all the children of one or the other sex are removed to different households for rearing.

A completely satisfactory explanation for the incest taboo has not yet been formulated. Malinowski and others hold the opinion that incest taboos are rigidly enforced and universally accepted because of their high social utility in keeping family and clan together. Without them, the family might too easily be torn apart by sexual rivalries and jealousies, and hence fail to fulfill its other functions. The so-called eugenic argument for prohibitions on incest has never been proved; "first-cousin" marriages do not commonly engender defective children.

Whatever their origin, incest taboos have a great social usefulness in safeguarding the family. They are rooted in the deepest folk wisdom of the human race. Even if there is no agreement on a rational basis for them, any scientific study of society would warn against relaxing them.

Taboos on Adultery. Almost as universal as incest taboos are those against adultery. In a world-wide study of 250 societies, Yale anthropologist Murdock found only five, a mere 2% in which adultery was socially condoned. Social utility again is probably the reason for this stricture. Extramarital affairs generally threaten the stability and function of the family. Scientific study does not justify the position that fidelity in marriage is an "outmoded superstition." Indeed, it is just the contrary.

The definition of adultery, however, is more flexible than that of incest. In most primitive tribes adultery means only sexual intercourse with a married woman. This was the Biblical definition of the word on which the Seventh Commandment rests. In some societies adultery is considered a theft. The property rights of the husband have been infringed, and his recourse is against the offender.

Adultery on the part of the husband has almost universally been more lightly regarded than on the part of the wife. In some tribes, for example, it is frequently expected when the wife is under a taboo of sexual continence—as when she is still nursing an infant.

In many societies the taboos against adultery have been circumvented by other legally permissible customs, for example concubinage and polygamy. In our culture "serial polygamy," frequent divorce and remarriage, has been attempted as a solution to the taboos on extramarital affairs.

Few Primitive Taboos on Sexual Experimen-

tation. In contrast to their strong and almost universal taboos against incest and adultery (and also against rape and child seduction) most primitive societies are more permissive than our own about premarital sexual experience. Murdock found that 70% (of 250 societies) permitted varying degrees of sexual experimentation before marriage. In the remaining 30%, the taboos were directed mainly against females. Premarital pregnancy is often severely castigated, though sometimes it is considered desirable. The basic premise seems to be concern for the status of the child without a "legal" father. Who will be responsible for it?

Dating and Courtship

Where do you find the person you marry? Practically all studies made on this subject by sociologists show that most people find their marriage partners within a few blocks of their own homes, and the nearer they live, the more likely they are to marry. Young people tend to choose mates whose backgrounds are substantially like their own. In some communities, however, the number of marriageable men or women may be smaller than the number of persons of the opposite sex seeking marriage. The moral is plain: if you seek marriage, go where the sex ratio is favorable.

A unique factor in the American social scene is the amount of casual contact between young men and women before marriage. "Dates" and "dating" as practiced in the United States are not characteristically found in other cultures. Dating is certainly a preliminary to courtship and always includes the possibility of "falling in love," but it has other values. It is a social experience, of which young people today may acquire more in a few years than their grandparents did in a lifetime.

On every college campus we know that there is a "dating and rating" pattern whose object is not necessarily matrimony. The crucial point here is that a good "date" is not necessarily a good mate. The relationship of dating to marriage is very indirect, even though each individ-

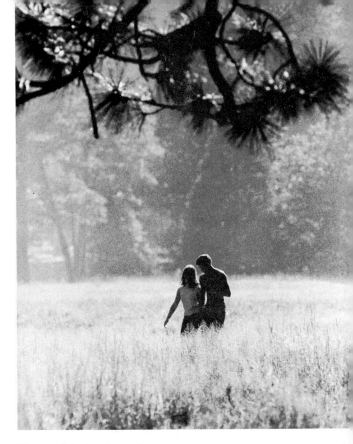

(Photograph by Ken Heyman)

ual meets or gets to know the person eventually married on some sort of dating or social occasion.

The social process leading toward marriage, a pattern which American young people have evolved for themselves in the past few decades, usually moves in the following sequence: group dating (parties), double dating, single dating, going steady, courtship, engagement, and marriage.

The values of courtship are not the same as the values of marriage. During courtship individuals tend to be on their best behavior toward their prospective spouses and often wittingly, or unwittingly, conceal their true personalities and mask their flaws from each other.

Courtship is a time of psychological exploration. Couples already in love, or on the verge of it, may properly raise questions about the suitability of a particular marriage and the probable compatibility of a particular partner.

Engagement. Engagement is a trial period in which the engaged couple has the time and freedom to discover each other. It is not and should not be mock marriage. It is a time when many subjects previously avoided, such as sex, children, money, and relatives, can be realistically discussed. It is a time when fundamental character and emotional reactions can be carefully scrutinized and evaluated.

How long should an engagement be? Long enough to begin to learn much about one's intended marriage partner, but not so long as to put both man and woman under needless stress. There are no figures in weeks or months that apply to all cases. Every couple must decide this for themselves.

Love

In the 1950's around 1,700,000 weddings a year took place in the United States. By the mid-sixties this number had decreased somewhat but a higher marriage rate was forecast. The vast majority of these marriages, it may be assumed, were conceived in romantic love.

Marriage for love is the accepted American pattern of mating; romantic, monogamous marriage is both the ideal and the norm. Yet it is necessary to draw a sharp distinction between romantic love and other manifestations of this "profound and complicated sentiment."

The poet Shelley has given as scientific a definition of love as you are likely to find, thus: "That profound and complicated sentiment which we call love is the universal thirst for a communion not merely of the senses, but of our whole nature, intellectual, imaginative and sensitive. . . . The sexual impulse, which is only one, and often a small part of those claims, serves, from its obvious and external nature, as a kind of type of expression of the rest, a common basis, an acknowledged and visible link."

There persists among young people a zealous but naive curiosity for the answer to the question, "How can you tell you're in love?" The only sensible answer that can be given is the standard one: "When you are, you'll know it yourself and

you will stop asking how you can tell." You may also encounter some cynical answers, such as Voltaire's. "If one were to judge love solely by its effects, it would seem a great deal more like hate than like friendship."

The phenomenon of love at first sight does occur. More commonly there is a gradual intensification of interest in and feeling for another person which, when it reaches a certain pitch, can be dignified with the name of love. There are three simple tests that can be applied: the test of time, the test of absence, and the test of companionship. If your interest in and feeling for the other person rapidly pass away, are easily diverted, quickly submerged, or casually overridden by other interests, don't dream that you are in love. If reasonable absence or separation makes your heart grow emptier not fonder, if you find yourself more and more forgetting the person you suspected you might be in love with, drop the suspicion. If you are increasingly bored with your companion, you are not likely to be in love with that person.

Psychologically speaking, a human being has no greater single need than that of giving and receiving love. We must "love or perish." But there is no law which says that all valid love must be romantic love.

The great fallacies in the American pursuit of romantic love are the beliefs that it will "last forever," that with it everything can be conquered, and that without it nothing else counts much. This is nonsense; there are many kinds of love beyond the romantic that yield superb life satisfactions. Romantic love may spark a wedding, but unless it ripens into a deeper conjugal love, it may later burn itself out. It is easier to fall in love than to stay there.

The gospel of the supreme value of romantic love has left far too many people so busy being "in love with love" that they cannot establish firm and genuine love relationships with other people; others who spend their whole adult lives trying to recapture the rapture of their first romantic love.

This emphasis and overvaluation of romantic love on the American scene may be viewed as the outcome of a number of factors, some long in the making, for example, urbanization, social mobility, economic emancipation of women, and global war. Against the casual impersonality of the big city, or the threat of atomic annihilation, romantic love shines as a protest and a last opportunity for happiness. Progress in transportation has brought about greater mobility and the automobile has supplanted the family parlor as the scene of courtship. Since women have won a high degree of economic emancipation, they do not have to accept marriage as their only road to economic security. Against the "soulless organization" for which one works and the stark objectivity of modern science, romantic love often stands out as a bright (and therefore presumably valuable) personal possession.

The ancient Greeks thought of romantic love as a kind of madness visited upon men and women by the caprice or malevolence of the gods. Certainly the socially acceptable conduct of many eager young lovers is such as would be considered symptomatic of mental illness in other people. Yet we accept the fact that people in love should "go around in a trance"; lose appetite and weight; suffer from illusions, delusions, compulsions, and the alternating heights of joy and depths of despair that mark a manic-depressive cycle.

Romantic love has had the effect of bulwarking the American ideal of monogamous marriage. The reason is simply that romantic love demands an *exclusive possession* of the beloved, and this is the essense of monogamy. The token of

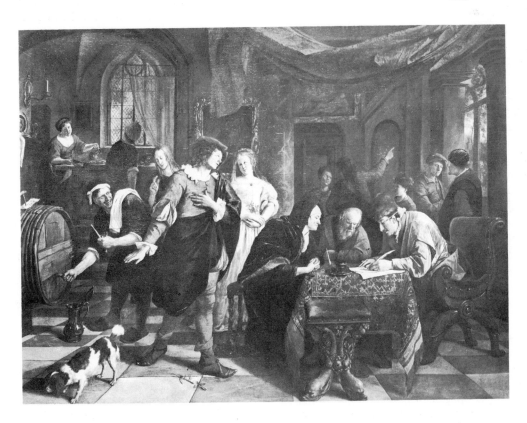

PERSONAL CHOICE OF MATE by young lovers was never so free as it is in mid-twentieth-century America. This painting—the original is by the Old Dutch master Jan Steen—shows a young girl being sold into marriage at a marriage broker's establishment in seventeenth-century Holland. Wives and daughters were legally considered as chattels up to the nineteenth century.

the engagement ring should be understood in this connection. When the young man places it on his sweetheart's finger, he is not only saying to her, "I love you." He is also jealously asserting to all other men, "She's mine. Stay away."

Romantic love probably will govern American marriage practices throughout the foreseeable future. Yet it is wise to understand it for what it really is—the prelude, not the whole feast of marriage.

Marriage

If marriages are "made in heaven," they nevertheless have to be lived out on earth. The simple determination to make a marriage succeed is one of the most important factors in its success. There are no marriages completely without crises, just as there are no lives without problems. The words of the wedding ceremony are full of truth: "for better or worse, in sickness and in health. . . ."

Children who have had the advantage of observing "good marriages" in their own homes often enjoy a greater chance of success in their own marital adventure. They have had the benefit of seeing how "normal" marital quarrels and difficulties can be compromised and happily resolved.

Nature of Marriage. Marriage provides an opportunity for two people in love to live, work, play, and worship together. Living together obviously requires readjustments in personal habits on the part both of man and wife, and demands emotional realignments. Because of serious flaws in their own personality structures some individuals cannot properly adjust to the needs and demands of their mates. This is the real source of marital unhappiness.

Marriage may in many ways be regarded as a *sublimation*, in which primitive emotional energies, including sexual drives, are directed to higher social ends. A certain amount of immediate renunciation of self is required to discover a greater self. In a happy marriage one no longer thinks in terms of "What am I doing for *you*" but rather "What can I do for *us*." The marriage becomes a third entity, above and beyond the partners to it—a deep well from which the whole family, mother, father, and children, draw strength, sustenance, and love.

Divorce. One in every three or four marriages in the United States ends in divorce. In addition, probably another one in six ends in annulment, informal separation, or desertion ("the poor man's divorce"). This situation, though distressing, is probably not so socially alarming as it is sometimes depicted. The general pattern is early marriage and early divorce, with a high rate of remarriage. Because so many people whose marriages are broken by divorce or annulment tend to remarry, the number of "broken homes" actually existing in the United States is nowhere near so great as the number of divorces on the statistical records.

Despite so-called "legal grounds" for divorce, the real source of wrecked marriages lies in incompatibility of temperament (immaturity usually) of the partners. Sexual maladjustment, though often mentioned, is not really a very common cause of divorce.

In possibly 50 to 75% of current American divorces, no children are involved. A sensitive discussion of "children of divorce," of whom there are about 1.5 million under eighteen, has been provided by Dr. J. Louise Despert. It is her opinion that children are more likely to suffer when "emotional divorce" between parents is *not* followed by legal divorce.

Marriage on the Campus. Marriage has been woven pretty firmly into the fabric of campus life since World War II. Undergraduate marriage is taboo today only in very few collegiate institutions—primarily the armed service academies. In the graduating classes of June 1964, almost one-fourth of all graduates were already married and a high percentage already had children. Approximately 38% of this "class of '64" were women; they received 40% of the 490,000 bachelor's and first-professional degrees and one-third of the 90,000 master's degrees.

Within 20 years, since 1949, the number of

women graduating from college nearly doubled, increasing from 117,000 to 224,000. Within this same time, as for 35 years earlier, there has also been a decline in the average age at marriage in the United States. In the present decade the modal age at marriage—the most frequent age at which women get married—is 18. The modal age for men is 21. However, it is 2 to 3 years lower for women who did not attend high school, and it averages 4 years higher—age 22—for women college graduates.

Why girls who attend college tend to marry considerably later than those who do not, is a subject for speculation. It may seem paradoxical that college education delays marriage for a girl since she is constantly in contact with boys her own age. It may be imagined that familiarity with many young men may evoke a more critical and choosey attitude. Furthermore, while a good many young men marry while they are still in college, the majority do not.

Many married coeds manage to continue their studies on a part-time basis: 44% of all part-time coeds are married. In 3% of all American families, both husbands and wives have college degrees. However, four out of every ten men graduates choose wives who have had no college training.

There have been variations in the overall marriage rates in the United States in the past few decades. For instance, in 1950, when the population was 151 million, the marriage rate was 11.0 per thousand; and there were 1.7 million marriages that year. In 1963 the marriage rate was only 8.8 per thousand and only 1.65 million marriages took place. In 1964 the rate was between 9 and 9.5 per thousand, producing slightly more marriages than in immediately previous years.

It may come as a surprise that brides and grooms in the United States are younger and closer in age at first marriage than are those in any other major urban-industrial country in the world. Indeed the American age-at-marriage pattern is now closer to the Asian than the European.

Choosing or Refusing a Mate

We all speak glibly about selecting a mate. The real question is *on what grounds to reject as a mate—* before marriage—an individual of the opposite sex toward whom you have feelings that already are or may unmistakably become classified as love. This is a difficult decision for the simple reason that few, if any, unmarried young people really know what to expect of marriage or of each other in marriage.

Young men and women in the United States enjoy exceptionally free choice of marriage partners. In far too many cases, however, they do not really exercise this choice. They plunge, jump, fall, leap, drift, stumble, rebound, march, or amble into a particular marriage partly because of outside pressures from family or friends or sometimes because of inner fears or drives.

Some young women, approach the grave responsibility of marriage as if it were a game of musical chairs in which the sole object is not to be left out. Some bachelors stalk wives as if they considered a wife a trophy of the chase, like a stuffed moosehead. Many accept husband or wife because they are weary, afraid, or ashamed to look further. Some couples marry hastily because, as they put it, "We're in love and that's all that matters." Some are eventually nagged into apparently unattractive marriages by family pressure or conversation, including one or another variation of that most infuriating remark: "Such a nice girl! Why isn't she married?"

A very high percentage of marriages contracted on trivial grounds nevertheless turn out remarkably well. On the other hand, even the most plausible matches fail. The attempt to select a mate on completely reasonable grounds is ludicrous. Marriages made by computers which attempt to match mutual compatibilities and traits are among the most foolish of all. A wedding is a commencement, not a termination. It is also a gamble, never a sure bet.

Let us review briefly the areas in which questions about the suitability of a particular marriage partner commonly fall.

What probable effect on the outcome of a marriage shall we assess for each of the following factors?

Physical Attractiveness? This factor is often overrated. It may be enough to get a marriage started, but not enough to hold it together.

Physical Size? Matching for size is a trivial consideration. Incompatibility on account of disproportions in physical size can be considered negligible.

Age? There are two questions here. Are the parties individually too young to be married (no one is ever really too old) and is the discrepancy in their ages so great as to suggest difficulties?

Mature, well-adjusted adults are more likely to make a success of marriage than adolescents. Society acknowledges this by laws establishing minimum ages for marriage. In about three-fifths of the states in the United States the age is 21 years for men, 18 for women, without parental consent; 18 years and 16 years, respectively, with consent. Biological readiness for reproduction, of course, occurs much earlier.

Marriages with great discrepancies in age between husband and wife are comparatively rare, about one marriage in twenty. The much older husband usually assumes a predominantly father role toward his wife, the older wife a strong mother role toward her spouse. If the psychological demands of *both* parties to the marriage are thus fulfilled, who can object?

Health? A medical certificate of physical fitness for marriage is required in three-fourths of the states of the United States before a marriage license is issued. In too many cases this requirement is purely perfunctory and means only that the applicants have passed a laboratory test which certifies them to be free of syphilis. A complete premarital physical examination by a physician is an excellent idea for both men and women. Such examinations should not be approached with the fear of finding something wrong, or as a bar to marriage, but rather as an opportunity for discussing and preventing specific health problems that might later complicate the marriage.

Heredity? When a person contemplating marriage knows for certain that one of the rare diseases (e.g. hemophilia or "bleeder's disease," or Huntington's chorea) transmitted by defective genes runs in his family, he should surely reveal this fact to his intended partner. Other worries about heredity should be discussed frankly with a physician.

Religious Faith? All organized religions frown on intermarriage, but all permit it under specific conditions and provisions. The circumstances surrounding a given or proposed intermarriage are always unique and highly individualized. Some succeed, some fail completely; many are maintained at uncertain medium levels of happiness. Young men and women contemplating intermarriage may well inquire into *all* their psychological motives at such a time and ask themselves such questions as: How strong are my deepest religious convictions? Do I secretly resent and *want* to hurt my parents and family by marrying out of their faith? Am I doing this because I want to be different and thus attract attention, concern, and even sympathy to myself? Have I the maturity and strength of character to make this marriage work? Will I feel truly at home in the new household I am helping to create?

Intelligence? The ability to think clearly is an asset in any human undertaking. What passes for intelligence (or the lack of it) is often only a reflection of different interests and motivations. A wife does not have to understand the intricacies of her husband's business or profession. She only has to be intelligent enough to appreciate him.

Education? The mere possession of an academic degree per se has no bearing on suitability for marriage or on the outcome of marriage. Insofar as degrees reflect intelligence, the promise of professional competence, a record of personal development, and opportunity for employment and advancement they do have value on the marriage market.

The present generation of college students in the United States is not quite so troubled by the dilemmas that acutely plagued their parents and grandparents. They often had to choose sharply between college or marriage, between marriage or a career. Since World War II, and the GI Bill, which provided educational benefits for veterans, the choice between going to college or getting married is no longer an either/or proposition. Young people today can have both, provided they have the strength and courage to accept both challenges. Married students do as well academically as unmarried students, often better.

Personal Abilities? This is a factor that can be grossly overrated. You don't marry a man because he is a good dancer or a woman because she is a good bridge player. You don't dismiss potential marriage partners on such trivial grounds as not liking the way they dress or comb their hair. Extreme fanaticism in any direction, however, may be a warning signal.

Money? The relationship of money to marriage has more ramifications than we can deal with here. Historically the relationship of wealth to marriage was more important than the relationship of love to marriage. For centuries marriages were arranged by families, and the marriage contract was a legal document that dealt largely with exchanges of property. Wives were chattels.

The question, "Can we afford to get married?" does not bother the present generation of young people so much or as often as it bothered earlier generations. One reason for this is the simple calculation that if both husband and wife work full or part time, they can make enough money together to support a small apartment or household. Prejudice against the working wife, once strong, has largely disappeared. The modern young woman does not expect her husband to support her immediately in the style to which she was or would like to have been accustomed. She frequently wants to share the financial responsibility of establishing and maintaining a household.

Any young couple insistent on marriage can scrape up enough money to get married and "get by" on what they make for some length of time. They are buoyed up, and properly, by hope for the future. But when financial hopes are disappointed, when family expenses rise, when the wife has to stop working to stay home with the children, crisis and test of the marriage occur. This is when strength of character and compatibility of temperament become important, when wise choice of a mate becomes more clearly apparent, when the power of personal love and true understanding of the meaning of marriage is revealed.

Millions of married couples weather their money troubles and build firmer, happier marriages out of their times of financial and other crises.

Money has many meanings to different people. It is not just a simple commodity or means of exchange. Attitudes toward money and the handling of money reflect some of our deepest psychological needs and basic philosophical outlooks on life. Money values reflect life values, and these change with age. When married, engaged, or even "dating" couples disagree about money, it is usually symptomatic of significant cultural and psychological differences in their total views of life.

Compatibility? The ability of two people to get along with each other is not a predictable factor and can be tested only by the experience of marriage itself. Strong youthful differences of opinion on political issues of the day are not an indication of incompatibility for marriage. A practical test is the ability to disagree on questions or problems, then compromise and agree on solutions.

Personality Structure in Marriage. Each man and woman brings to marriage the personality structures that they have developed through all their previous life experiences from infancy onward. Though marriage itself exerts a strong stabilizing influence on later personality development, it cannot undo traits and characteristics already ingrained. These normal emotional reactions are firmly established long before the individual is thinking of marriage.

As a guide to studying reactions we have formulated a list of twenty questions for testing a potential mate. These questions, which you ask yourself, may aid you in interpreting the real significance of the behavior of the person you intend to marry. Asking them will give you a better insight into the kind of person you are taking or have taken for a marriage partner.

In one way these questions are tests of social and psychological readiness for marriage. They add up to one big question, "Is this person mature enough to manage the real responsibility of marriage?" Taken one at a time, each question seeks to indicate whether the individual under observation makes excessive use of the so-called "mental mechanisms" stemming from the unconscious mind. If he excessively employs a considerable number of them, you should perhaps go slow in setting a date for your marriage.

If you must conscientiously answer *yes* to a considerable number of the following "twenty questions," you have good reason to doubt whether the person you are observing is really the mate for you (the word *she* can be used for *he* when the male is asking himself the following questions):

1. *Does he frequently fail to keep definite appointments with me?*

This can be a form of purposeful forgetting, a symptom of repression of deepest and partly unpleasant feelings about you.

2. *Does he make me feel very much like a rank outsider when I am with his family and friends?*

He may be overidentified with his family.

3. *Does he constantly compare me, favorably or unfavorably, with his mother?*

He may have overidealized his mother, fantasizing her as a superwoman and expecting you to fit this impossible picture.

4. *Is he always hurrying me off from one round of activity to another when we are together?*

He may be too much of an extrovert.

5. *Is he afraid to be alone?*

Such conduct may betoken a lack of inner resources, common among extroverts. The extrovert often substitutes the trappings of excitement for genuine inner feelings.

6. *Is he extremely indecisive?*
Many introverts are.

7. *Is he too withdrawn, shunning even my company on many occasions?*

This also may indicate a high degree of introversion which will make it difficult to enter into normal, realistic give-and-take of married life.

8. *Does he repeatedly talk big plans for the future while failing to carry through small everyday obligations?*

No marriage can succeed where fantasy is constantly substituted for fact.

9. *Is he always presenting plausible excuses for bad behavior?*

He may have fallen into the habit of rationalization and be unwilling or unable to face marriage problems as they occur in real life.

10. *Does he always blame me when things go wrong?*

The greater insight you have into the personality structure of another person, the better you can get along with him or her. Nowhere does this obvious rule of trying to understand one another apply with greater force than between mates, actual or intended. During a period of courtship, engagement, or "going steady," you should, if possible, observe the *emotional reaction* of your intended husband or wife to a variety of life problems.

The things to watch out for are overreaction, excessive reaction, rigid reactions, and "clang reactions" (like a firehorse at the clang of a firebell). Such reactions will give you quite valuable

TESTING A POTENTIAL MATE

This is the bad habit of projection.

11. *Does he usually call his own failures the other fellow's fault?*

It is hard to live with a person who does not take responsibility for the outcome of his own acts.

12. *Does he feel and express many strong prejudices—against people, ideas, and even food?*

You too may some day offend his unreasoning prejudices.

13. *Is he abnormally superstitious?*

14. *Does he have to do things in a certain way to feel comfortable about them?*

This rigidity of conduct can make you decidedly uncomfortable.

15. *Is he abnormally afraid of things that don't bother most people—such as cats or bridges?*

Such an attitude betrays a phobia. Like superstition and prejudice it is often a cloak for guilt, shame, and anxiety feelings that encourage a neurotic personality.

16. *Does he tend to "take it out" on me when things go wrong for him?*

This displacement of feeling can have serious repercussions. Marriage on the rebound is a not uncommon outcome. The jilted partner seeks marriage not for love of a new personality but rather to hurt and take revenge on the one who jilted him.

17. *Does he get sick whenever he runs into difficulties, obstacles, or even "lovers quarrels"?*

The habit of retreat into illness when things go wrong, the conversion of emotional problems into physical symptoms, can produce a whining, hypochondriacal spouse.

18. *Does he expect marrying me to make up for everything he feels he has missed or been deprived of so far in life?*

This is asking too much. Successful marriage can compensate for failures and inadequacies in many other areas of life, but to look deliberately to a specific marriage as complete compensation for all one's own deficiencies is to woo disappointment. Each partner must bring his entire personality, its weaknesses and strengths, to a marriage.

19. *Does he repeatedly express in word and action feelings of inferiority?*

Everyone needs some bolstering of the ego, and this is one of the happiest opportunities arising out of the marriage relationship. But there is a limit to what one spouse can give or bear. Husband and wife must mutually support and give confidence to each other.

20. *Does he react in a decidedly childish manner whenever he doesn't get his own way?*

Repeated regression into childish behavior when one's immediate wishes cannot be met is perhaps the most overt sign that a person is not yet mature enough to make a successful marriage.

You have probably guessed that the "Twenty Questions for Testing a Potential Mate" represent specific applications of the mental mechanisms (or dynamisms)—regression, projection, and the like—discussed in Chapter 3, "The Unconscious Mind."

clues to the underlying personality of your intended.

Sex and Religion

"The ancient religious codes are still the prime sources of the attitudes, the ideas, the ideals, and the rationalizations by which most individuals pattern their sexual lives. The apparent conflicts between the religious codes and the patterns of sexual behavior may lead one to overlook the religious origins of the social patterns."

The author of this forthright statement is the late Dr. Alfred C. Kinsey, professor of zoology at Indiana University, presenting a scientific study of sexual behavior in the United States. He says further: "For the individual who is particularly concerned with the moral values of sexual behavior, none of these scientific issues are, of course, of any moment. For such individuals, moral issues are a very real part of life. . . . They should not be overlooked by the scientist who attempts to make an objective measure of the outcome of [sexual practices, such as] premarital intercourse."

In discussing the social and psychological aspects of sexual adjustment, especially as it affects the lives of young men and women in American colleges, we have chosen to examine the moral and religious issues in depth and detail.

"Why have religions generally failed to help the individual with his life problems by not admitting the force of the sex drive?" is a question commonly asked by college students during discussions of the religious and moral point of view toward sexual adjustment. Other common questions are: "Why have organized religions placed so much emphasis on wedding ceremonies and so little on personal adjustment in marriage?" "Dare I have premarital intercourse with a clear conscience?" and "Are there religions which today condone premarital intercourse?" These questions demand information, discussion, and decision on the part of every student who poses them out loud or to himself. They are central to American college life today, and they cannot be ignored.

The questions themselves betray an ignorance, not by any means limited to college students, about the present and true interest of the great modern religions in sex behavior and their authoritative statements on the subject. There is a widely held, flippant, and cynical attitude that this interest is limited to enforcing the Seventh Commandment: "Thou shalt not commit adultery." There is an appalling lack of knowledge concerning the stress placed today by all the major religions of Western culture on the positive and happy aspects of sex and marriage relationships. It seems to be generally overlooked that organized religions stemming from the Judaeo-

Christian tradition take their primary warrant for concern with the sexual life of mankind from the first words of God to man. As anyone who opens the Bible to the first chapter of Genesis can rediscover, these words (in English) are, "Be fruitful and multiply."

Organized religion in all societies has taken this Biblical commandment most seriously and attempted only to stipulate conditions, coordinate with the rest of the culture, under which it can be most effectively carried out. In American society, the right to accept or deny these codes remains an individual right and responsibility. Obedience cannot be commanded, but the consequences of disobedience, however light or grave, cannot be avoided. Choice is free, but ignorance is no excuse for a poor choice.

Fundamental to any personal decision or to any real understanding of the social and psychological aspects of sexual adjustment in modern American society is an awareness of what religions actually have to say on the subject. We are fortunate in being able to present verbatim quotations from official documents and authorized statements emanating from the three major religious denominations in the United States.

In presenting this material we have sought for the common ground in these three points of view; but we have not neglected to point out significant differences where they occur. We have not and we do not imply any criticism, nor do we concern ourselves with any of the properly theological questions on which these statements ultimately rely. Space limitations prevent giving the statements in full, and some students may wish recourse to the complete texts.

The Protestant Point of View

The following statements are direct quotations from the document *Christian Marriage,* issued in 1952 by the National Council of Churches of Christ in the United States of America:

This is an attempt to state unofficially the Christian view of marriage as generally held by the great body of Christians constituting the

National Council of the Churches of Christ in the United States of America. These include a majority of non-Roman [Catholic] Christians in North America. While these bodies represent a wide range of opinion on many debated points, they hold strongly to the ideal of chastity, of reverence for personality, and the sacredness of family ties. . . .

While there have been times when the efforts of the church seemed more defensive than constructive, in the long run great progress has been made. Gradually the inherent democracy of the Gospel has helped to emancipate women from the disabilities and handicaps of patriarchal culture, and young people have been defended in their rights to select marriage partners according to their own ideals and preferences.

On the Christian Conception of Marriage. Stated by Christ Himself in beautiful and sensitive words, He speaks of how "He who made them from the beginning made them male and female," and quotes the words, "for this reason shall a man leave his father and mother, and be joined to his wife." The man and woman in marriage become one flesh, that is to say, the union is organic, and it is God who unites them, which means that it is a profound biological-spiritual experience which comes out of the depths of life. The union is permanent: "What therefore God hath joined together, let no man put asunder." The Mosaic law which permitted a man to divorce his wife with no recourse for her is abrogated. . . .

In this sort of marriage the two become not merely "one flesh" but one in spirit, for the highest values of marriage are in the realms of personality. In Christian marriage the meeting of all the needs of personality and the enhancement of delicate mutual regard must be sought. At the same time the welfare of society must be loyally promoted through the home. . . .

On Freedom of Personality. The home calls for a fine combination of responsibility and freedom. The fullest freedom is not gained in isolation but in a set of well-chosen loyalties. . . . Yet a certain amount of restlessness in the home and of irritation between husbands and wives is due to unnecessary limitations of freedom. . . . Differences

may be handled successfully . . . if each through kindly interest in activities and tastes which are different from his own gives encouragement to the full self-expression of the other.

But beyond this there is also great reward in transforming as many one-sided interests as possible into common interests mutually shared. In fact this process of the sharing of life is the very essence of marriage on its inner side.

On Tensions in Marriage. A measure of tension in making adjustments in marriage is almost inevitable. . . . The romantic emotions of the early period must grow into something hardier and more discerning. . . . Success results from meeting these difficulties with patience, with resourcefulness, and especially with great mutual consideration. People must win their happiness and sometimes wrest it from hard conditions.

On Love. Love, however, has an incalculable power to transmute life. Married people by continuing as lovers can create a home atmosphere in which the little difficulties can be absorbed and all obstacles to full success can be put in a setting of endeavor to reach the higher levels of personal fellowship. . . .

On Children. Although a man comes of age at twenty-one, he becomes more fully a citizen when he is married. When his first child is born he enters more consciously into relationships which are universal and eternal. . . . The high calling of parenthood is one of the supreme fulfillments of personality at the same time that it enables the parents to make their contributions to the future as well as to the present life of the church and the community. . . .

On Rearing Children. Parents should be encouraged to give full personal attention to children and to share sympathetically in their daily lives. Other persons, capable as their service may be, can never take the place of mother and father. . . . The home needs much of the presence of the father as well as of the mother. . . . Children need the contribution which their father is in a position to make to their training. . . .

On Economic Resources Adjusted to Family Needs. [A nation] must be concerned to give every family its fair access to economic opportunity and to its share of national production. . . .

Abnormal deferring of marriage on economic grounds is a serious problem for some young people and their families. This fact challenges society to create an order more favorable to family life. For the young people concerned it requires emphasis on the fact that a home may be begun on a modest basis. . . .

On Attitudes toward Sex. Mistaken attitudes make sex a serious problem. . . . Christianity regards sex as God-given in its origin and purpose, not to be disdained but rather to be fitted into a Christian way of life. Sex union, however, when it occurs outside of marriage is a menace to the welfare of the individual, the family, and society.

Sex desire, if no more than desire, passes with satisfaction. Therefore this desire must always be in subjection to a plan of living which safeguards all the values of the personality. It can never be put first and expressed irresponsibly. To do so is to degrade not only the mind but sex itself.

Sex experience is elevating and wholesome to body and mind only when it is under moral control and when it is transmuted into a spiritual experience by love and devotion. Love includes but transforms desire and lifts it to a spiritual plane.

The Christian ideal of marriage can therefore make no compromise with laxity in sex relations. No matter how great the compassion of the church, or how swift its sympathy and its redemptive action, it must always speak to sex delinquents as did Christ to the woman whom He refused to condemn to a shocking death, but to whom He said, "Go, and sin no more."

What people need is purposeful restraint, not greater freedom in the form of sex indulgence. . . . Young people are in the difficult situation. . . . The problem of sexual self-control often becomes aggravated under such circumstances. Moreover, the situation is affected by the widespread and increasing knowledge of the use of contraceptives. However, the solution is in the correction of the social and economic maladjustments and not in the violation of our sex ethics. The convictions of religion based on long experi-

ence and the findings of modern research studies agree in indicating that the forward path is not in the direction of laxity.

On Divorce. Differences of conviction as to divorce, and freedom of divorced persons to marry again, must be recognized. Civil divorce and remarriage are now provided in all nations, even in those predominantly Catholic. The state exercises wider latitude as to permissible grounds of divorce than the church, as a teacher of ideals, can allow itself to recognize. All churches, however, either recognize divorce and remarriage on one or more grounds, or, as in the Roman Catholic Church, grant annulment of marriage. . . .

The most beautiful and satisfying experiences are for those who, having chosen wisely their life partners, achieve a life-long marriage with ever deepening love and loyalty. . . . [However] divorce or separation may seem preferable to the enforced continuance of a relation which has no true basis in mutual respect and affection as far as the two individuals concerned are involved; but the effect on the children, the family, and society must never be ignored or minimized. Moreover, it is evidence of failure, always to be deplored, and to be avoided if by any means success can be achieved even over what may appear insurmountable obstacles.[1]

On Family Planning. Marriage should provide for the fullest development of personality, and at the same time homes should carry on and continually reinvigorate all traditions which aid fine family living. . . . [Under such circumstance] family planning takes greater prominence, both in respect to size of the family and to the genuine quality of family life.

*   *   *

The likenesses between the Protestant, Roman Catholic, and Jewish points of view on marriage and family life deserve to be emphasized. Despite some traditional and historic differences, they all point to the same goal. These statements which present the Roman Catholic and Jewish attitudes

[1] This paragraph is from *Social Ideals of the Churches,* published by the Federal Council of the Churches of Christ in America.

toward sex, marriage, home, and children, may be profitably compared with the Protestant attitudes already delineated.

The Roman Catholic Position

The following statements are direct quotations from the Encyclical Letter on Chaste Wedlock (*Casti Connubii*) given at Rome, in St. Peter's, on December 31, 1930, by Pope Pius XI:

How great is the dignity of chaste wedlock, Venerable Brethren, may be judged best from this—that Christ . . . not only ordained it in an especial manner as the principle and foundation of domestic society and therefore of all human intercourse, but also raised it to the rank of a truly and great sacrament of the New Law, restored it to the original purity of its divine institution, and accordingly entrusted all its discipline and care to His spouse the Church. . . .

On the Divine Institution of Matrimony. Let it be repeated as an immutable and inviolable fundamental doctrine that matrimony was not instituted or restored by man but by God; not by man were the laws made to strengthen and confirm and elevate it, but by God. . . . Hence these laws cannot be subject to any human decrees or to any contrary pact even of the spouses themselves. . . .

On the Nature of the Marriage Contract. Yet, although matrimony is of its very nature of divine institution, the human will, too, enters into it and performs a most noble part. For each individual marriage, inasmuch as it is a conjugal union of a particular man and woman, arises only from the free consent of each of the spouses; and this free act of the will, by which each party hands over and accepts those rights proper to the state of marriage, is so necessary to constitute true marriage that it cannot be supplied by any human power. This freedom, however, regards only the question whether the contracting parties really wish to enter upon matrimony or to marry this particular person; but the nature of matrimony is entirely independent of the free will of man, so that if one has once contracted matri-

mony, he is thereby subject to its divinely made laws and its essential properties. . . .

By matrimony, therefore, the souls of the contracting parties are joined and knit together more directly and more intimately than are their bodies, and that not by any passing affection of sense or spirit, but by a deliberate and firm act of the will; and from this union of souls by God's decree, a sacred and inviolable bond arises. Hence the nature of this contract . . . makes it entirely different both from the union of animals . . . and also from the haphazard unions of men, which are far removed from all true and honorable unions of will and enjoy none of the rights of family life. . . . The sacred partnership of true marriage is constituted both by the will of God and the will of man. . . .

On the Blessings of Matrimony. "These," says St. Augustine, "are all the blessings of matrimony on account of which matrimony is itself a blessing; offspring, conjugal faith, and the sacrament." And how under these three heads is contained a splendid summary of the whole doctrine of Christian marriage. . . .

On Children. Amongst the blessings of marriage, the child holds first place. . . . The blessing of offspring, however, is not completed by the mere begetting of them, but something else must be added, namely the proper education of the offspring. . . . This is also expressed succinctly in the Code of Canon Law: "The primary end of marriage is the procreation and the education of children." . . .

On Conjugal Fidelity. Nor did Christ our Lord wish only to condemn any form of polygamy or polyandry, as they are called, whether successive or simultaneous, and every other external dishonorable act, but, in order that the sacred bonds of marriage may be guarded absolutely inviolate, He forbade also even willful thoughts and desires of such like things: "But I say to you, that whosoever shall look on a women to lust after her hath already committed adultery with her in his heart." . . .

On Mutual Love. This conjugal faith, which is most aptly called by St. Augustine the "faith of chastity," blooms more freely, more beautifully, and more nobly when it is rooted in that more excellent soil, the love of husband and wife. . . . For if man is the head, woman is the heart, and as he occupies the chief place in ruling, so she may and ought to claim for herself the chief place in love. . . . If the husband neglect his duty, it falls to the wife to take his place in directing the family. . . .

On Marriage as a Sacrament. Since the valid matrimonial consent among the faithful was constituted by Christ as a sign of grace, the sacramental nature is so intimately bound up with Christian wedlock that there can be no true marriage between baptized persons "without it being by that very fact a sacrament" . . . from which they draw supernatural power. . . .

On Modern Fallacies. When we consider the great excellence of chaste wedlock, Venerable Brethren, it appears all the more regrettable that particularly in our day we should witness this divine institution often scorned and on every side degraded.

For now, alas, not secretly nor under cover, but openly, with all sense of shame put aside, now by word, again by writings, by theatrical productions of every kind, by romantic fiction, by amorous and frivolous novels, by cinematographs portraying in vivid scene, in addresses broadcast by radio telephony, in short by all the inventions of modern science, the sanctity of marriage is trampled upon and derided; divorce, adultery, all the basest vices either are extolled or at least are depicted in such colors as to appear to be free of all reproach and infamy. . . .

Not all the sponsors of these new doctrines are carried to the extremes of unbridled lust; there are those who, striving as it were to ride a middle course, believe nevertheless that something should be conceded to our times as regards certain precepts of the divine and natural law. But these likewise, more or less wittingly, are emissaries of the great enemy who is ever seeking to sow cockle among the wheat. . . .

To begin at the very source of these evils, their basic principle lies in this: that matrimony is repeatedly declared to be . . . invented by man.

Some confidently assert that they have found no evidence for the existence of matrimony in nature or in her laws, but regard it merely as the means of producing life and of gratifying in one way or another a vehement impulse. . . . How grievously all these err! . . .

On Family Planning. First consideration is due to the offspring, which many have the boldness to call the disagreeable burden of matrimony. . . . But no reason, however grave, may be put forward by which anything intrinsically against nature may become conformable to nature and morally good. Since, therefore, the conjugal act is destined primarily by nature for the begetting of children, those who in exercising it deliberately frustrate its natural power and purpose sin against nature. . . . Holy Mother Church very well understands and clearly appreciates all that is said regarding the health of the mother and the danger to her life. And who would not grieve to think of these things? . . . Holy Church knows well that not infrequently one of the parties is sinned against rather than sinning. . . .

Secondary Ends of Matrimony. In matrimony . . . there are also secondary ends, such as mutual aid, the cultivating of mutual love, and the quieting of concupiscence, which husband and wife are not forbidden to consider so long as they are subordinated to the primary end. . . .

On Mixed Marriages. The maternal love and providence of the Church dissuades her children . . . [from] mixed marriages. This attitude is . . . summed up in the Code of Canon Law. . . .

On Divorce. The advocates of neopaganism . . . continue by legislation to attack the indissolubility of the marriage bond. . . . Opposed to all these reckless opinions, Venerable Brethren, stands the unalterable law of God, fully confirmed by Christ, a law that can never be deprived of its force by decrees of men, the ideas of a people or the will of any legislator: "What God hath joined, let no man put asunder." . . .

If, therefore, the Church has not erred and does not err in teaching this, and consequently it is certain that the bond of marriage cannot be loosed even on account of the sin of adultery, it is evident that all the other weaker excuses that can be, and usually are, brought forward are of no value whatsoever. . . .

In certain circumstances the imperfect separation of the parties is allowed, the bond not being severed. This separation, which the Church herself permits . . . removes all the alleged inconveniences and dangers. . . .

On Due Preparation for Marriage. The basis of a happy wedlock, and the ruin of an unhappy one, is prepared and set . . . during childhood and adolescence. There is the danger that those who before marriage sought in all things what is theirs, who indulged even their impure desires, will be in the married state what they were before, that they will reap that which they have sown. . . . Worst of all, such parties will find themselves left alone with their own unconquered passions. . . . For the preservation of the moral order . . . religious authority must enter in to enlighten the mind, to direct the will, and to strengthen human frailty by the assistance of divine grace.

The Roman Catholic View on Moral Questions Affecting Married Life. The following statements are direct quotations from a discourse by Pope Pius XII delivered on October 29, 1951, under the title of "The Apostolate of the Midwife—Moral Questions Affecting Married Life," and these statements may be regarded as further explanation of the text set forth by Pope Pius XI, his predecessor, already quoted:

Nature puts at man's disposal the whole chain of causes giving rise to new human life. . . . Once man has performed his part and put into motion this wondrous evolution of life, his duty is to respect its progress religiously, and this is a duty that forbids his halting the work of nature or hindering its natural development.

The child formed in the womb of its mother is a gift of God, Who entrusts it to the parents. . . . Unfortunately there are many cases where speaking, even cautiously, of children as a "blessing" is sufficient to provoke contradiction or even derision. Very often the idea and remarks

about the great "burden" of children dominate. . . .

On Acceptance of Motherhood. It is one of the fundamental demands of the right moral order that sincere inner acceptance of the office and duties of motherhood corresponds to the use of conjugal rights. . . .

Unfortunately, it is not always thus. Often the child is not wanted. Worse, it is feared. Under such conditions, how can people be ready to carry out their duty? . . .

On Periods of Natural Sterility. There is the serious question today as to whether and how far the obligation of ready disposition to serve motherhood can be reconciled with the ever more widely diffused recourse to periods of natural sterility (the so-called agenetic periods of the woman) which seems to be a clear expression of the will contrary to that disposition. . . . The medical point of view about this theory and of the progress that is likely to be made in it . . . [should be] founded on scientific objectivity and the authoritative judgment of specialists in medicine and biology. It is the office [of the obstetric professions, e.g., physicians, midwives], not that of the priest, to instruct married people, either when they come for private consultations or through serious publication, on the biological and technical aspects of the theory. . . .

[But on] the norms of morality to which the application of this theory is subordinated, here it is the Church that is the competent judge. . . .

There are serious motives, such as those often mentioned in the so-called medical, eugenic, economic, and social "indications," that can exempt for a long time, perhaps even the whole duration of the marriage, from the positive and obligatory carrying out of the [conjugal] act. From this it follows that observing the non-fertile periods alone can be lawful only under a moral aspect. . . .

If, according to a rational and just judgment, there are no similar grave reasons of a personal nature or deriving from external circumstances, then the determination habitually to avoid the fecundity of the union, while at the same time to continue fully satisfying their sensuality, can be derived only from a false appreciation of life and from reasons having nothing to do with proper ethical laws. . . .

On Attitudes toward Sexual Pleasure. The Creator, Who, in His goodness and wisdom, has willed to conserve and propagate the human race through the instrumentality of man and woman by uniting them in marriage, has ordained also that, in performing this function, husband and wife should experience pleasure and happiness both in body and soul.

In seeking and enjoying this pleasure, therefore, couples do nothing wrong. They accept what the Creator has given them. Nevertheless, even here, couples must know how to contain themselves within the limits of moderation. As in eating and drinking, so in the sexual act, they must not abandon themselves without restraint to the impulse of the senses. The right norm, therefore, is this:

The use of the natural inclination to generate is lawful only in matrimony, in the service of and according to the ends of matrimony.

Transgression of this rule is as old as original sin. But in our times there is risk of losing sight of the basic principle. . . . At present it is the custom to maintain in word and writing (and some Catholics do it too) the necessary autonomy, the proper end and the proper value of sexuality and its performance independently of the object of procreation. . . .

If nature had aimed exclusively or even primarily at a mutual gift and mutual possession of couples for pleasure, if it had ordained that act solely to make their personal experience happy in the highest degree and not to stimulate them in the service of life, then the Creator would have adopted another plan in the formation and constitution of the natural act. . . .

A Further Statement on Family Planning. The following passages are excerpts directly quoted from an address to the Cardinals of the Roman Catholic Church given in Rome on July 23, 1964, by Pope Paul VI. These remarks may be considered as an extension of the affirmations on this subject made by his predecessors in the papal office:

Thus our speech takes us from looking at the present and the past to the future. And here also we face a wide panorama, full of formidable problems and great events for us.

We will talk, in conclusion, about only one of these problems, and about only one of the events which the future prepares for us. The problem [which], everyone talks about, is that of birth control, as it is called; namely, of population increases on one hand and family morality on the other.

It is an extremely grave problem. It touches on the mainsprings of human life. It touches on the feelings and interests most close to the experience of man and woman. It is an extremely complex and delicate problem.

The Church recognizes the multiple aspects of it; that is to say, the multiple competences, among which certainly are in the forefront those of married people, [including considerations] of their freedom, of their conscience, of their love, of their duty.

But the Church must also affirm her own [competence]; namely, that of God's law, by her interpreted, taught, favored, and defended. And the Church will have to proclaim this law of God in the light of the scientific, social, and psychological truths which in these times have undergone new and very ample study and documentation. . . .

The question [of birth control] is being subjected to study, as wide and profound as possible, as grave and honest as it must be on a subject of such importance. It is under study which, we may say, we hope will soon be concluded with the cooperation of many and outstanding experts. We will, therefore, soon give the conclusions of [this study] in the form which will be considered most adapted to the subject and to the aim to be achieved.

But, in the meantime, we say frankly that up to now we do not have sufficient motive to consider out of date, and therefore not binding, the norms given by Pope Pius XII in this regard. These must, therefore, be considered valid, at least until we feel obliged in conscience to change them.

In a matter of such gravity it seems well that Catholics should wish to follow one law—that which the Church authoritatively puts forward—and . . . that no one, for the present, takes it on himself to make pronouncements in terms different from the prevailing norms.

Jewish Attitudes

The Jewish ideal of marriage and family life is reflected in many of the already stated Christian ideals of marriage stemming from the same Old Testament tradition. The following statements are direct quotations from materials issued over the signature of the Synagogue Council of America, an organization representative of the three major divisions of American Judaism: Reform [Liberal], Conservative, and Orthodox:

Judaism has always looked upon the home as the posit of religious life and sought to manifest religious teachings in family relationships. . . . Jews have always been aware of the unique value of the family, not only for the development of human personality but also for the survival of the individual within the framework of the group. Judaism has nourished the family by traditions and customs . . . rites and institutions. . . .

The Jewish family has a special function. The Jewish people owe their survival in large part to three institutions: the school, the synagogue, and the family. Of the three the family is the most important. ("One may even sell a scroll of the Torah [the Law] if he needs money for the purpose of getting married.")

The Jewish family becomes through the cultivation of its own genius a sacred circle in which members are bound together in a spirit of common understanding, mutual sympathy, and unremitting sacrifice. . . . Judaism has always stressed the integrity of the family . . . [and with it] such values as love, sanctity, purity, stability,

responsibility of parents and children, companionship, familial happiness. . . .

At the present time the family is passing into a new stage of development . . . reorganizing itself under the spell of the spirit of our age, the spirit of democracy. . . . The failure to recognize this change that is taking place results in many conflicts. An autocratic form of family organization can never train men and women for a democratic social order. . . . It is necessary, therefore, to combine every possible skill to deal with the complexities that go into the process of marriage, the rearing of children, the creating of a home, the conserving of a family.

The following statements are direct quotations from the pamphlet, *Judaism and Marriage,* by Felix Levy, Ph.D., issued by the Commission on Information about Judaism, representing the Reform [Liberal] position:

On Monogamy. Monogamy was probably the prevailing mode even in earliest Biblical times. That this was the Jewish ideal can be inferred from the creation legend, where one human couple are parents to the race. Though polygamy occurred among the ancient Hebrews from Adam onward, and was sanctioned, this can hardly be said to have been the norm. Moses and Job have each one wife; the prophets take for granted single partnership as the proper state; the spiritual relationship between God and Israel is conceived as an ideal marriage between the one divine husband and the single people Israel.

On the Position of Women. Proverbs and Ecclesiastes exalt the character and the position of the wife in the home and in society. ("Her children rise up and call her blessed,/Her husband also, and he praiseth her"—Proverbs 31. . . . "The joy of the heart is a wife"—Ecclesiastes 10:7). . . . The very part that women played throughout Jewish history takes the edge off the assertion that woman was man's property to dispose of at his will. . . . Even though admittedly woman was not man's equal before the law, the teachers assert that the unmarried man's existence is incomplete. . . .

On the Marriage State. Marriage is the most exalted state in the eyes of the Jew, and if the wife is good and virtuous, the greatest blessing has come to the home. The idea that marriage is more than a union of the flesh or nature's arrangement for insuring the continuity of the race lies behind the Hebrew term for marriage, "Kiddushin" ("Consecration"). . . . For the Jew it meant holiness and was symbolic of the sacred relationship between husband and wife, of a hallowed state in which they were to live. They were to be one flesh, but more, one spirit.

Marriage for the Jew never became a sacrament, with its mystery, or a concession merely to the weakness of the flesh; for the Jew believed in the satisfaction of all legitimate appetites as a duty, the condition imposed being that desire, including that of sex, should be directed into proper channels for the good of the person and the group. Hence marriage became obligatory, so that a man might build a home, rear a family, and grow in personality thereby.

On Children. Man became creator when he begat children, and the intimate physical relation between man and woman was only for the sake of founding a family. Celibacy was unnatural, and hence abhorrent, particularly in those of marriageable age. . . .

On Family Life. The family life of the Jew with its wifely purity and its husbandly fidelity, the counsel of prenuptial chastity for both sexes, are more eloquent testimony to the Jewish idea and ideal of marriage than all the codes and decisions of [its] courts. The beautiful service in the home that welcomes the Sabbath, itself poetically conceived as a bride, . . . reflects actualities.

On Attitudes toward Sex. A considerable body of statute and lore is discoverable in Jewish literature which attempts to protect the group against physical or moral taint—by insisting on sexual purity for man and woman before and after marriage, by discountenancing any union except in marriage, by advising early matings . . . by regulation of intercourse to safeguard the woman and the possible child, by the high esteem in which parenthood, especially motherhood, is held . . . by insistence on caring for bodily health,

even to the extent of regulation of diet. . . .

[Judaism teaches that the expression of sexual love is the exclusive right of husband and wife—for whom it is altogether normal, wholesome, and desirable. Such expression for any couples not joined in marriage is immeasurably damaging to them, is sinful before God, and is antisocial in the eyes of man. Judaism expects the daughters of Israel to remain virgins until their marriage and Jewish men to be chaste and continent until they are wed.] [2]

On Marriage Laws. Reform [Liberal] Judaism . . . has recognized the right of the state to supervise and control marriage . . . and though it does not encourage civil ceremonies, it does, unlike orthodoxy, recognize their validity. . . . In short, Reform Judaism looks upon marriage as a purely religious act, the contractual part involving property and dower rights governed by the civil regulations of the state, while orthodoxy still acts in the double capacity of "state and religion." Reform Judaism . . . waives the right to perform the old contractual marriage as documented in the "Ketubah" ("marriage contract") with its property stipulations. [3] . . .

On Mixed Marriages. Mixed marriages, or unions between Jews and non-Jews, are discouraged by Judaism, the chief reasons being that differing religious views in the household are not conducive to the peace and harmony, love and understanding, that an intimate relationship such as marriage must foster. . . . Judaism is the religion of a small minority, which can ill afford to weaken itself by loss of any of its members. . . . If, however, the stranger embraces Judaism wholeheartedly and willingly joins the Jewish people, he or she is made welcome and an inter-

[2] From *Wife of Thy Youth*, by Stanley R. Brav, Chairman, Committee on Marriage, the Family, and the Home of the Central Conference of American Rabbis. Published by the Union of American Hebrew Congregations, 1946 (Reform Judaism).

[3] In understanding Jewish marriage law, two facts should be kept in mind: (1) from the time of Abraham until less than a century ago almost all Jewish marriages were arranged by parents with the help of a professional matchmaker or marriage broker ("shadchon"); and (2) marriages were made when couples were still in their teens.

marriage may take place. [Cf. The Book of Ruth.]

On Divorce. Divorce has a history as old as marriage, though less is known about its beginnings. In the Bible we find the simplest procedure, viz., that a man could send his wife away at will. . . . Rabbinic legislation . . . made it increasingly difficult for the husband to get rid of his wife, by safeguarding her dower rights, far more so than did the Bible. . . .

Chief among the grounds for divorce was adultery . . . [which] then meant something else from what it did in the New Testament or does now. It was unfaithfulness on the part of a wife, and the guilty parties were punished by death. A married man who erred with an unmarried woman was a sinner but not an adulterer. . . .

Modern Jews try to follow the spirit of the Jewish law even though they may not agree with all its prescriptions. Reform Jews have yielded to the state as possessing exclusive rights in the question of divorce . . . and no Reform rabbi grants the "Get" ("divorce") or recognizes one other than that issued by the courts of the country. . . .

Religion then must reluctantly recognize the need of divorce and bewail it whenever it occurs. . . . Divorce is a remedy of last resort . . . and the means to lessen it must be those which invest marriage, as does religion, with sacredness and solemnity.

SUMMARY

This chapter has outlined the normal social processes of dating, courtship and engagement leading toward a successful marriage. It has presented the worldwide taboos, which surround the marriage process. In particular, however, it has stressed the role of romantic love in developing the American ideal of romantic, monogamous marriage. Romantic love, however, it was pointed out, carries the seeds of its own destruction. Grounds for choosing or refusing a potential mate have been thoroughly discussed—even to the extent of providing twenty questions for testing a possible marriage partner. Young people today do not have to choose between college and marriage; they can have both.

A key and often decisive point in choosing (or refusing) a possible husband or wife is his or her religious faith and background.

Sex, marriage, home, and family are all part of one pattern, which religion reflects and fosters.

Marriage may be considered a sacrament, divinely instituted (Catholic); a consecration, holy before God (Jewish); a blessing and a covenant, a "profound biological-spiritual union" (Protestant). It envisages a permanent bond of matrimony.

SUMMARY REVIEW QUESTIONS

1. What is the normal social process or pattern leading to marriage among young people in the United States? How does this differ from the patterns in other nations and cultures?
2. Where do you usually find the person you marry? Why should this be so?
3. What taboos on choice of mate are commonly found within primitive cultures? What are two almost universal taboos with regard to marriage practices?
4. What are the values of "dating" as practiced in the United States? What is the fundamental rule for behavior on a date?
5. How do you interpret the statement, "The values of courtship are not the same as the values of marriage"? What is the function of engagement?
6. How would you define love? How many different kinds of love can you think of?
7. What is romantic love? Why does it often carry the seeds of its own destruction? In what ways does it support the American ideal of romantic, monogamous marriage?

8. What do you expect of marriage? What personal attitudes toward marriage on the part of husband and wife can help to make it more successful?

9. What significant changes in attitudes toward marriage among college students have occurred since World War II? Why?

10. How would you personally assess each one of the following factors in accepting or rejecting a prospective marriage partner: physical attractiveness, physical size, age, health, heredity, religious faith, race, intelligence, education, social status, personal habits, wealth, compatibility? Which factors do you consider more important? Which least important?

11. How would you attempt to determine before marriage whether a particular person was a good marriage risk for you? What kind of questions about him (or her) would you ask yourself?

12. What is the relationship of love to marriage? Expound.

13. Are the following statements sense or nonsense? Why? *A good date makes a good mate. . . . Marriages are made in heaven. . . . When poverty comes in the door, love flies out the window. . . . College spoils a girl's chances of getting married. . . . When you're in love, you'll know it. . . . Every marriage is a gamble.*

14. On the basis of the texts presented in abridged form in this chapter, and any other documented information you may have, what would you say was the "common ground" of present-day Protestantism, Roman Catholicism, and Reform (Liberal) Judaism on the following points:
    a. The conditions that make for a happy marriage.
    b. The role of parents toward their children.
    c. Religious symbolism drawn from family life.
    d. Attitude toward sex in marriage.
    e. Attitude toward sexual relationships outside of marriage.
    f. The relationship of love and marriage.
    g. Monogamy.
    h. On the *value* of permanence in marriage relationships.
    i. Intermarriage.
    j. The *desirability* of parenthood.

15. In what ways, if any, have these official statements of present-day attitudes toward sex, marriage, and the family on the part of Protestant, Jewish, and Catholic faiths changed or corrected the ideas and beliefs that you formerly held?

16. Why should a discussion of moral and religious values be given a place of primary consideration in any presentation of the topic of "sex education"?

17. Do you think that the goals and aims of marriage, as defined in the official statements in this chapter, would be significantly different in cultures and societies not so strongly influenced as the United States by Judaeo-Christian traditions? If so, why? If not, why not?

18. Discuss the implications of the statement: "Children are a gift of God."

19. What do the following terms mean to you: endogamy, monogamy, homogamy, "falling in love," engagement ring, "poor man's divorce," "going steady," sublimation, compatibility, overreaction, chastity, celibacy, adultery, divorce, annulment, prenuptial, canon law, Judaeo-Christian tradition, *Kiddushin, Casti Connubii?*

Worth Looking At: *Love: A Garland of Prose and Poetry Woven Together* by Walter de la Mare. *Facts of Love and Marriage for Young People* edited by Aron Krich. *How To Understand the Opposite Sex* by William C. Menninger and others. *Marriage* by Herman R. Lantz and Eloise C. Snyder. *Christian Marriage* by the National Council of Churches of Christ in the United States of America. *Casti Connubii: Encyclical Letter on Christian Marriage* by Pope Pius XI. *Judaism and Marriage* by Felix A. Levy, from the Union of American Hebrew (Reform) Congregations. For more complete references, see Appendix E.

A Selected Reading

Dating Patterns of Harvard Men

Rebecca S. Vreeland, Ph.D.

About Thirty years ago, Willard Waller wrote an article about the "rating and dating complex" among the coeds at Penn State. In that article he argued that modern dating is not a prelude to courtship, but is rather what he called "a period of dalliance" in which the object of dating is to display one's catch. The winner of the dating game has the most popular girl as a date. The qualities desired in such a date are primarily physical attractiveness, possession of cars and clothes, and popularity with the peer group. Waller concluded that this sort of competitive dating, because it is exploitive, is injurious to the personalities of young people.[1]

Since the publication of Waller's article, a contradictory theory about the function of dating has been advanced by Burgess and Locke who contend that dating is not different in purpose from courtship.[2] Dating is an extension of coeducation used to find a companionable mate. It also serves to educate a person about the opposite sex. Burgess and Locke agree with Waller that dating does not involve a commitment to the partner. They contend, however, that dating leads naturally to courtship when the search for a companion is concluded, whereas Waller feels that dating and courtship are contradictory patterns of heterosexual relations. One is not naturally a prelude to the other.

Riesman subscribes to the latter theory and in a recent article has said that the rating and dating complex is no longer characteristic of modern youth. Today's young people are seeking more subdued and sincere relationships. They are preoccupied with the capacity to love as well as to be loved.[3]

Skipper and his associates, in a current article on dating functions speak of instrumental and expressive approaches to dating. By instrumental they mean dating which uses the relationship to further a person's own goals, for example, gaining sexual satisfaction or enhancing one's reputation.[4] This instrumental dating orientation is what Waller called the rating and dating complex. Skipper uses the term expressive dating to include the companionable relationships described by Burgess and Locke.

The evidence from the few studies that have been concerned with dating motives and qualities desired in dates suggests that it is an oversimplification to speak of American youth or even the students at one college as either instrumental or expressive in their dating motives. Both approaches to dating are found among contemporary college students. For

SOURCE. Rebecca S. Vreeland, Ph.D. is a research sociologist in the University Health Service at Harvard University, Cambridge, Mass. She originally presented this paper before the Section on Public Health and the 45th annual meeting of American College Health Association, in Washington, D. C. on March 30, 1967.

This article is reprinted with permission from the *Journal of the American College Health Association, 16*: 4, 335–338 (April 1968).

[1] W. Waller, The Rating and Dating Complex, *Amer. Sociol. Rev.,* 2: 727–734, 1937.

[2] S. H. Lowrie, Dating Theories and Student Responses, *Amer. Sociol. Rev.,* 16: 334–340; and, E. W. Burgess and H. J. Locke, *Amer. Sociol. Rev.,* 16: 843–844, 1957.

[3] D. Riesman, Permissiveness in Sex Roles, *J. Marriage and the Family,* 21: 211–217, 1959.

[4] J. Skipper, et al., Dating Behavior, *J. Marriage and the Family,* 28: 412–416, 1966.

example, a recent study by Hewitt shows that the most important qualities desired in a date by both sexes are sense of humor, consideration for others, emotional stability, and ambition.[5] Robert Blood finds at the University of Michigan, however, that fraternity and sorority members still support popularity and possessions as important attributes of good dates, although there is nearly unanimous approval of dates who are pleasant, cheerful, and who have a sense of humor.[6]

There is almost no evidence concerning the types of men who have different dating orientations. Smith and Monane show that at the University of Colorado the graduate students are more interested in the academic interests rather than in the companionability of their dates, the better students desiring more intelligence and fewer social graces. This survey, however, is too limited in scope to be a definitive study of dating orientations. It neither discusses general approaches to dating nor takes into account relevant characteristics of daters other than age, academic and financial standing.[7]

This paper will present data from the Harvard Student Study* concerned with the dating patterns of a sample of students from the class of 1964 as freshman and seniors. Three major topics will be discussed:

1. The general changes in dating orientations which occur between freshman and senior years
2. The different characteristics of persons who have instrumental and expressive dating orientations
3. The characteristics of students who have no particular dating orientations—the non-daters

General Changes in Dating Orientations

During their senior year Harvard students date significantly more often and spend twice as much money on dates as they did in their freshman year. They also date fewer girls, and are much more likely to make serious professions of love and express intentions of marriage. They are more sexually intimate with their dates than they were as freshmen. The mean moves from petting to attempting intercourse at least once. At the same time, they express more verbal and physical aggression toward dates.

During their four years at Harvard the students move toward a more expressive type of dating. For example, more students report having friends of the opposite sex and asking their advice about career and personal problems. The seniors also take more walks with their dates, participate in sports with them more often, take them to lectures and house meals instead of to dances and concerts, and study with them more. They more frequently list their primary dating activity as just having coffee and conversation. In general, the range of dating activities in which the students engage increases. The girls become companions and friends rather than objects of sexual conquests. The physical intimacy that the seniors have with their dates appears to be an extension of this companionship. For example, finding a wife and listener is more important than using dates to build their own reputation. In addition, as a student becomes more interested in a girl's intellectual, conversational, and artistic qualities, he becomes less interested in her reputation and religion.

This pattern of change in the qualities desired in dates and in dating activities reflects the changing interest of the students toward the opposite sex. In Skipper's terms, their dating orientation is changing from instrumental to expressive.[8]

Even though the general trend in the Harvard data shows a movement toward expressive dating, some seniors still have an instrumental orientation to-

[5]L. Hewitt, Student Perceptions of Traits Desired in Themselves as Dating and Marriage Partners, *J. Marriage and the Family, 20*: 344–348, 1958.

[6]R. Blood, Uniformities and Diversities in Campus Dating Preference, *J. Marriage and the Family, 18*: 37–45, 1956.

[7]E. Smith and J. H. Monane, Courtship Values in a Youth Sample, *Amer. Sociol. Rev., 18*: 635–639, 1953.

*The Harvard Student Study is supported by a grant from the National Institute of Mental Health, No. 5 R12 MH 09151.

[8]Skipper, et al., *op. cit.*

ward dating, and a few seniors have both.

Characteristics of Persons with Different Dating Orientations

Although only two major types of dating orientation were described in the literature, a factor analysis of the questions concerning dating activities, motivations, and desired characteristics in a date reveals three distinct dating orientations.

The first type of dating is expressive—wanting a companion date. Students who score high on this orientation have recreation as their primary motive for dating. Their dating activities are the informal ones mentioned above. These students don't consider any particular personality characteristics as essential in a date.

The second type of dating orientation is instrumental—wanting a chic date. Students who score high on this orientation want a date who is their social equal, who does not show her intelligence, is well dressed, effervescent, and uninhibited. Students take this sort of date to night clubs, private parties, spectator sports, and dances. The primary motivation these students have for such instrumental dating is sex and enhancement of their reputation.

By the senior year, a third dating orientation is quite distinguishable—finding a wife. (The elements are the same as during the freshman year, but the pattern is unclear.) This orientation can be considered both expressive and instrumental. Students who score high on this orientation want a date who is intelligent, religious, a good conversationalist, and who has similar academic interests. The major motivation of these students is finding either a wife or a good listener. These students do not participate in any particular type of dating activity.

Freshmen with expressive dating orientations date more frequently and are more sexually intimate with their dates than the other students, perhaps because they dated more frequently and intimately in secondary school. These freshmen are also more extroverted and have more friends than students with other dating orientations.

On the other hand, the freshmen who have a more instrumental dating orientation are very traditional and orthodox in their opinions and attitudes. They do not like Harvard students, feeling that they are cold, aloof, emotionally immature and caught up in intellectual fads. These students are also culturally unsophisticated, conservative in their political opinions, and traditionally religious. They subscribe to traditional middle-class values in their ideas of the future. For them the most important characteristics of their prospective career are its income, prestige, and security. That these students subscribe to conservative values is not surprising since their parents are also conservative, both religiously and politically. These instrumental daters also participate in athletics more often than students with other dating orientations.

The final group of freshmen which is both expressively and instrumentally oriented—the wife hunters—is not distinguished by either a pattern of values or experience. The only characteristic these students have in common is that they are almost all going steady, more often with girls from their home town.

By senior year, the characteristics of the students with different dating orientations have not changed substantially. However, those students who are looking for wives have some distinguishing characteristics by their senior year. For example, they are religious and very interested in making a career of helping people. Besides wanting a companion, they also want someone to share their academic and altruistic interests.

The Harvard Student Study also asked seniors what characteristics they prefer in a wife. A factor analysis of these questions reveals two distinct types of wife: the modern wife who works outside the home, is intelligent, sophisticated, uninhibited, and a good conversationalist. The traditional wife, on the other hand, must be a housewife, a good cook, and housekeeper. She must also be well dressed, religious, a virgin, and the student's social equal. The chic daters prefer a traditional wife, the companion daters want a modern wife, and the students who are "wife hunters" do not have a distinct preference.

The data presented above suggest that the kind of orientation Harvard students have toward their dates is part of a more general value orientation. For example, the instrumental orientation seems to be part of a traditional collegiate syndrome explaining, perhaps, why

Blood found this type of dating more often among sorority and fraternity members than among independents.[9]

The Nondaters

In the analysis of the Harvard Student Study material, certain characteristics of the students are associated with all three types of dating orientation. For example, all the dating orientations are associated with low scholastic ability. This finding suggests that we have overlooked an important group of students who have no particular dating orientation—the nondaters.

There are interesting differences between the dating and nondating students (those who date less often than once a month). The freshmen nondaters are men whose high school experience included neither participation in extracurricular activities nor frequent dating. The nondaters also have few extracurricular activities at Harvard. Instead, they are tied to their home town, communicating with parents and friends from home more frequently than the other students. They also have high scholastic ability.

By senior year, these nondaters are even more distinguished from the rest of the class in that they are a smaller and more select group. The characteristics that differentiated this group as freshmen still differentiate them as seniors. In addition, nondaters are different from daters in that they derive most of their satisfaction from the academic side of life at Harvard. They are also more sure of their career plans, and are much less satisfied with Harvard than are the other students. Finally, they are very concerned with themselves and anxious about their own personalities. These students come very close to fitting the traditional stereotype of the "grind."

From the data that have been presented in this paper, it is possible to draw some tentative conclusions about the dating patterns of Harvard men, which can be used as hypotheses in future research in other colleges.

1. In general, Harvard men become more expressive in their dating approach during their undergraduate years. By their senior year their orientation is much closer to the Burgess and Locke interpretation of the dating function as educational and expressive.[10]

2. These data also make it clear that there are several distinct types of dating patterns present in the Harvard population. Although the expressive, companion type of dating is the dominant orientation of the students, a sizable minority has a strictly instrumental orientation toward dating. By their senior year an additional group of students combines these two orientations, using dating primarily to find a wife.

These dating patterns are part of the student's general values. For example, the men who are instrumentally oriented in their dating and want traditional wives are more conventional and conservative in their opinions and attitudes. This idea that dating orientation is a part of a more general value system is contrary to the treatment of dating in the literature where it has been thought of as a sexual phenomenon quite separate from other values.

3. Finally, this paper suggests that there is a definite group of the brightest, most academically oriented students who do not date to any extent even as seniors. These men are certain of their future careers and avidly pursue them to the exclusion of all kinds of extracurricular activity including dating. It is interesting to note, however, that these men are plagued much more than other students by self-doubt and anxiety. Perhaps it is not one's dating orientation that is injurious to the personality but one's not dating at all.

[9] Blood, *op. cit.*

[10] Lowrie, *op. cit.*

The Beige Epoch:
Depolarization of Sex Roles in America

Charles Winick

Abstract: One of the most pervasive features of our cultural landscape is the depolarization of sex roles and a concomitant blurring of many other differences. The appearance, given names, and play of boys and girls have become less gender-specific since World War II. Young girls appear to be demonstrating the sexual precocity and aggressiveness once associated with boys. Clothing and appearance are steadily becoming increasingly ambisexual, along with recreational activities, work, and family roles. Extremes of taste in food and drink are less common. Blandness also characterizes the color and shape of home interiors and the exteriors of many buildings. Opera, theatre, musical theatre, and movies have been dominated by women in recent decades although male stars once were the major audience attractions. Our rapid industrialization and World War II are among the contributors to depolarization, and the trend may have some ominous implications for the future.

Perhaps the most significant and visible aspect of the contemporary American sexual scene is the tremendous decline, since World War II, in sexual dimorphism. Sex roles have become substantially neutered and environmental differences, increasingly blurred.

Our Age of the Neuter begins to leave its mark on young people in their very tender years. Gender-linked colors like pink and blue for children's clothing are yielding to green, yellow, and other colors which can be used for either Dick or Jane. Such names, however, are less likely nowadays. A study of a large sample of given names reported in birth announcements in the *New York Times* from 1948 to 1963 concluded that almost one-fifth of them were not gender-specific, for example, Leslie, Robin, Tracy, Dana, Lynn, although the 1923–1938 period had few such names.[1] Since the name helps to position a person in his culture, many young people are starting out with an ambisexual given name.

The hair of little girls is shorter and that of little boys is longer, and such blurring is given fashionable designations, that is, the Oliver or Beatle haircut. Other kinds of his-hers appearances are chic for young people. Boys and girls may have similar toys, and the last few years have witnessed the popularity of dolls for boys (G.I. Joe and his many imitators).

Reading habits of young people are less related to gender than they were a generation ago. Both sexes are likely to enjoy the same books, for example, *The Moon Spinners* and *Island of the Blue Dolphins,* and there is less interest in books which are clearly sex-linked, like the *Nancy Drew* series for girls or the *Hardy Boys* for boys. School curricula are offering fewer subjects which are unique to each sex, and both sexes learn some subjects, for example, typing.

SOURCE. Charles Winick, Ph.D. is Professor of Sociology in the Department of Sociology and Anthropology at The City College of the City University of New York. The article abridged here was published in the *Annals of the American Academy of Political and Social Science* for March 1968. This was a special issue on "Sex and the Contemporary American Scene."

[1] Charles Winick, *The New People: Desexualization in American Life* (New York: Pegasus, 1968), chap. vi.

The Teen-ager

Dating behavior of teen-agers reflects the crossing over of sex roles which pervades so much of the preadolescent years. The teen-age girl increasingly is looking for her own satisfaction and may want to be even more equal than her date. Such tendencies have become more important since the 1950's, which experienced the first movie about a sexually aggressive teenager (*Susan Slept Here,* 1954), an extraordinarily successful novel about a sexually sophisticated girl (*Lolita,* 1958), and, perhaps most important, a series of very popular mannequin dolls, beginning with Betsy McCall in 1954 and culminating in Barbie in 1959. Barbie is a sexy teen-ager, and playing with her involves changing costumes and thereby preparing for dates. During the last decade, an average of more than 6,000,000 mannequin dolls was sold each year.

The rehearsal for dating provided by Barbie and her imitators may even further accelerate the social development of their owners. By the time an owner is ready to engage in actual dating, she could be much more forward than her male companion. Studies of teen dating suggest that, not too long ago, the aggressiveness displayed by many contemporary teen-age girls was once found primarily in young men.[2]

So much time separated the nine-year-old with an old-fashioned baby doll from her role as mother that she could enjoy fantasies about motherhood and not be concerned about doing something about them. But the distance in years that separates a Barbie fan from a socially active ten- or eleven-year-old girl is slight, and she can easily translate doll-play fantasies into real social life. Barbie owners may be more ready than any previous generation to take the traditional male role in teen-age courtship behavior.

[2] Ira L. Reiss, "Sexual Codes in Teen-Age Culture," *The Annals, of the American Academy of Political and Social Science,* Vol. 338 (November 1961). pp. 53–62.

A Selected Reading

The Decline and Fall of the Double Standard

Erwin O. Smigel and Rita Seiden

Abstract: The limited available information on premarital, heterosexual behavior of young people in the United States reveals that the changes in sexual behavior which took place in the 1920's have changed only slightly in the 1960's, and that this slow change is continuing. The belief that a gradual transformation is taking place (except in overtness) rests on a comparison of the early studies on sexual behavior, the data from attitudinal studies, researched from 1940 to 1963, and observations of the current scene. Conclusion: the double standard is declining but has not yet fallen.

We know that sexual attitudes have changed and that sexual standards appear to be in a period of transition. "What was done by a female in 1925 acting as a rebel and a deviant can be done by a female in 1965 as a conformist." [1]

Data based on a large sample are available on sex behavior up to 1949 and on attitudes up to 1963. We do not know what has happened during the last five years or what is happening now. The general public impression is that there has been a very recent sexual revolution and that it is still going on. Most researchers do not believe that this is the case. The authors of this article, as social observers and recent reviewers of the literature on sexual behavior and attitudes toward sex, will attempt to "crystal ball" what has occurred during the last five years and what is occurring now. What follows, then, is not fact, but guess.

Past trends in social change, in behavior, and in attitudes toward sex are continuing. What seems to be taking place (except for pockets of our society) is a growing tendency toward more sexual permissiveness among the young unmarried. Sex with affection appears to be increasingly accepted. More and more this norm is based on personal choice, and it manifests itself for middle-class college youth in the form of trial marriage, for the girl, and for the boy at least as a stable, monogamous relationship, to the point of setting up housekeeping. Increasingly, this happens with parental knowledge though not necessarily with parental approval. If Kinsey repeated his study today, he would probably find premarital virginity slightly lower and figures for those who have had premarital intercourse only with their spouse, a circumstance which was already on the increase in 1947 (born before 1900, 10.4 per cent; born 1920–1929, 27.3 per cent),[2] somewhat higher.

Promiscuity, a word objected to by many young people, probably has lessened. Certainly the use of prostitutes has diminished. If we are correct in believing that more young people are living monogamously together, and if marriage for both men and women (the figures are: median age of first marriages in

SOURCE. Erwin O. Smigel, Ph.D., is head of the Department of Sociology of the Graduate School of Arts and Science at New York University. Rita Seiden is also associated with this Department. The article reprinted here was published in the *Annals of the American Academy of Political and Social Science,* March 1968. This was a special issue on "Sex and the Contemporary American Scene."

[1]Reiss, "The Sexual Renaissance: A Summary and Analysis," *Journal of Social Issues,* Vol. 22 (1966), p. 126.

[2]Reiss, "Standards of Sexual Behavior," *loc. cit.*

1890 for brides was 22.0 and for grooms was 26.1;[3] for 1966, the median age for brides was 20.5 and for grooms 22.8[4]) is occurring at earlier ages, then the statistical probabilities of premarital promiscuity have lessened, except when it is a reflection of mental illness. Today, except for the "hippies," who, according to the press, indulge in group sex, promiscuity as a form of rebellion is significantly on the decline.

We are living in a much more permissive society, and we are much more vocal about sex. As Walter Lippman put it, even as early as 1929: "It was impossible to know whether increased openness about sex reflected more promiscuity or less hypocrisy."[5] While we do not have much new evidence concerning sexual behavior, we do have nonsystematic overt indications about attitudes. It is seen in advertisements which are much more suggestive than they used to be. At one time, an advertiser would indicate to a male reader that, if he used a certain product, a pretty girl would kiss him. Now the ads suggest that she will have intercourse with him: "When an Avis girl winks at you she means business," and as Chateau Martin asks, leering only slightly, "Had any lately?" Movies have become less suggestive and more obvious; nudity as well as intercourse have become not uncommon sights. The Scandinavian picture, I, A Woman, for example, consists of a number of seductions with a number of different men. Perhaps what is more significant is that censorship boards, the courts, and power groups in this country have sharply amended their definitions of obscenity. The theater has, for some time, been more open about sex and its various ramifications, and four-letter words are becoming a theatrical cliché.

Another indicator of this generation's expressed attitudes toward sex are the omnipresent buttons, which express not only political, but also sexual opinions. The buttons are designed for fun and shock, and for public declaration for sexual freedom. Sold in large cities all over this country, they range from simple position-statements such as "Make Love Not War," "I'm For Sexual Freedom," or "Equality for Homosexuals," to invitations which read "Roommate Wanted," "Join the Sexual Revolution—Come Home With Me Tonight," to such shock jokes as "Phallic Symbols Arise," "Stand Up For S-X," and "Come Together."

More sophisticated young people feel that the dirty-word movements or the shock words no longer have any impact. In the October 26, 1967, Washington Square Journal, a New York University publication, the student reviewer of an off-Broadway production, The Beard, which freely uses four-letter words . . . , says: "Unfortunately the force of the play rests on the anticipated violation of social taboo, and violating social taboos just isn't what it used to be."

Except for the rediscovered poor, the United States is a society of unprecedented abundance. Upper- and middle-class white Americans pamper their children, give them cars and money, send them to college and abroad, and set them up in their own apartments while they are going to school. These young people have leisure and the wherewithal to use it in amusing themselves—only the war is real, which gives a special significance to college as a way of avoiding the war. This abundance means that college-age men and women can travel together, live together, and have a sex life encouraged by their peers, whose opinions they have now come to value more than those of their elders.

Abundance for the young unmarried in the city has made it possible to meet other young unmarrieds in new ways. Apartment houses are being built for them; clubs are formed for them,

[3]U.S., Department of Health, Education, and Welfare, Vital Statistics: National Summaries, Vol. 50, 28 (November 1959). Source: U.S., Department of Commerce, Bureau of the Census, "Population Characteristics," Current Population Reports, Series P–20, 105–3.

[4]U.S., Bureau of the Census, Statistical Abstracts of the United States, 1967 (88th ed.; Washington, D.C.: U.S. Government Printing Office, 1967), Table 75: "Median Age at First Marriage, by Sex: 1920–1966." Source: U.S., Department of Commerce, Bureau of the Census, Current Population Reports, Series P–20, No. 159.

[5]Walter Lippman, A Preface to Morals (New York: The Macmillan Company, 1939; originally published in 1929; Beacon edition, 1960), p. 228.

but perhaps the most significant of all the developments is the use of bars, now often called pubs, which serve as meeting places where singles can meet without prejudice. A girl who visits the pub is under no obligation to "go to bed" with the man whom she meets and with whom she may leave. These pubs (and they begin to specialize in different kinds of singles), in a sense, institutionalize a system of bringing together like-minded people; they speed the dating and the trial-and-error process, for they offer this particular group of affluent young people a wide variety of partners to choose from, and they can choose quickly, independently, and frequently.[6]

Many observers of the current scene consider the "pill" the most significant single force for increased sexual freedom. A count of the articles listed in the *Reader's Guide to Periodical Literature* reveals that more articles were published about birth control in the period March 1965 to February 1966 than were listed in a ten-year sampling starting with 1925 and ending with 1957. The sampling yielded 89 titles. But we doubt that the pill has added materially to the increase in the numbers of young adults or adolescents who have had premarital sex. Effective techniques of birth control existed, and were used, before the pill. True, the pill makes birth control easier to manage (except for the memory requirement), but romantic love is still important; it makes taking the pill, when no definite partner is available, undesirable. What the pill does is to give sexual freedom to those who are having steady sexual relationships, for then the use of the pill adds to romantic love by making elaborate preparations unnecessary.

According to our crystal ball, which, of course, may be clouded, we have not had a recent or current sexual revolution in terms of behavior. However, there probably has been some increase in the proportion of women who have had premarital intercourse. It is our guess that the increase has occurred largely among women who have had premarital sex only with their spouses-to-be. If there has been a sexual revolution (similar to the 1920's but ideologically different[7]), it is in terms of frankness about sex and the freedom to discuss it. Women have demanded and have achieved more education, more independence, and more social rights; one of these is the right to choose a partner for sex. Men are accepting many of these changes in the status of women and are tempering their insistence on what have generally been considered male prerogatives, for example, the right to demand that a bride be a virgin. Young men today are probably less promiscuous and more monogamous, and their relationships tend to be more stable. Both sexes are approaching a single standard based on sex with affection. We are still in a stage of transition. Despite the title of this article, the only indisputable conclusion which we can draw from the current scene is that we are witnessing the decline, but not yet the fall, of the double standard.

[6]For an interesting comment on this phenomenon see "The Pleasures and Pain of the Single Life," *Time,* September 15, 1967, pp. 26–27.

[7]See Bennett M. Berger, "The New Morality," Unpublished paper, read at the Plenary Session of the Society for the Study of Social Problems, August 27, 1967.

13

HEREDITY AND THE NEW GENETICS

MINENCE, LIKE DISEASE, APPEARS TO RUN
in families. It has been calculated, for example, that, if one of your so-called blood relatives achieved the eminence of being listed in
Who's Who, the chances are 1 in 4 that you too
will achieve this measure of eminence. However,
if none of your blood relatives achieved such
distinction, your chances of doing so are only 1
in 500.

Many families have arrogated "eminence" to
themselves, sometimes on the rather flimsy premise that their ancestors were present at the Battle
of Hastings (1066)—on the Norman side, of
course—or came over to America on the *Mayflower* (1620). Such appeals to heredity for personal distinction have little, if any, validity. Yet
eminent families do persist. Why this is so we
shall shortly discover. One of the first careful,
scientific students of the subject was Sir Francis
Galton, an English gentleman related to the
eminent Darwin and Wedgwood families. He is
usually remembered for introducing the concept
of "eugenics," which is in effect the good fortune
of being well born.

Galton was interested in finding out what each
parent, grandparent, great-grandparent, and so
on, contributed to the heritage of the individual.
By taking the pedigree records from a stud book
of hounds, whose colors were known for many
generations, he was able to work out mathematically a kind of law of ancestral heredity.
This law describes *statistical probabilities;* that is,
it tells what happens, not in individuals, but in
groups, classes, and types, as in fact do all the
so-called laws of genetics.

The Law of Ancestral Heredity

The law of ancestral heredity says that on the
average the contribution of *each* parent to the
individual's hereditary qualities, characteristics,
traits, or tendencies is just one-quarter of the
total. The contribution of each grandparent is
one-sixteenth, and so on. In other words, you can
thank both your parents together for just *half* of
what you are, speaking in terms solely of your
biological inheritance. You can thank your four
grandparents for another one-quarter of this inheritance. Your great-grandparents must be
credited with one-eighth of your inheritance; and
so on, mathematically, down the line. By the time
you get back to the *Mayflower* or the Norman
Conquest, there is not much left. Your remote
ancestors, for all their sins or virtues, have left
very little imprint on you. It is possible that they
left none at all.

You cannot explain your own "inborn" qualities in terms of the success or failure of any single
ancestor, not even your immediate parents. How
then do we account for "eminent families"?

Cultural and Physical Heredity

Before we can answer this question, we must
make a clear distinction between cultural and
physical heredity or inheritance. Cultural inheritance is the effect of the culture of a given society, or a level within the society, first impressed
upon the individual through the medium of the
family. The newborn infant becomes heir to the
culture that envelops his family. This culture

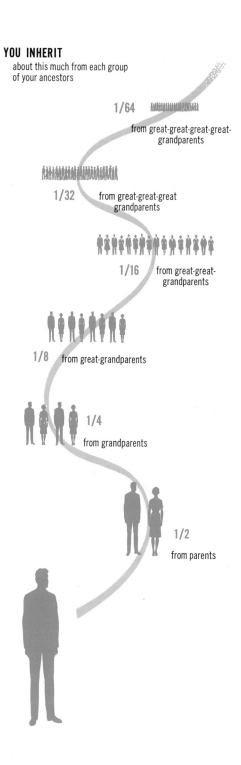

YOU INHERIT

about this much from each group
of your ancestors

1/64 from great-great-great-great-
grandparents

1/32 from great-great-great
grandparents

1/16 from great-great-
grandparents

1/8 from great-grandparents

1/4 from grandparents

1/2 from parents

**HEREDITY. Galton's law of ancestral heredity indicates where
your individual traits come from.**

includes both the social and physical environment into which the infant is born and that in which he is reared. We shall therefore speak herein of social inheritance and environmental inheritance as almost synonymous with cultural inheritance. In a broad sense a child's cultural inheritance is the whole state of the world at the time he is ushered into it, though obviously only a minute fragment of this whole pattern directly impinges on him.

Physical heredity, or inheritance, which is a term we shall use here almost synonymously with biological and genetic heredity or inheritance, is a process by which living organisms, including man, transmit their own intrinsic characteristics to their offspring. It is a complex process whose mechanisms have been brilliantly delineated in the twentieth century but whose final mysteries are still a long way from being unraveled. We shall discuss these mechanisms later in this chapter.

When we discuss the mechanisms of heredity, we shall be dealing with the new genetics, a fresh and brilliant area of scientific research. There are two keys to this stronghold: (1) the recognition that genes are molecules—a particular kind of molecules; and (2) the role of the nucleic acids, DNA and RNA, in "blueprinting" the growth and development of cells.

The processes of biological heredity apply to all living things; they are part of the commonly observed but fundamentally inexplicable ability of living things to reproduce their own kind.

Now let us return to our "eminent families." The question is not how they achieved eminence in the first place but why they tend to maintain it. The answer lies in both their cultural and their physical inheritances. Opportunities for eminence, including education, social position, and wealth, are passed along from parents to children in the cultural heritage of the family. Relatives other than parents are also often in a position to make opportunities for children and other relatives. Furthermore the chances of a favorable physical heredity, including intelligence, are enhanced both because the original founder of the family probably had to be above average to attain eminence and because the subsequent members of the family have been in an advantageous position to seek and select above-average mates for themselves.

What Is Heredity? It is difficult to give a sharp and concise definition of the process of heredity. Spencer said: "Heredity is the study of the likenesses and differences between parents and children and the way these are transmitted." Dunn and Dobzhansky describe heredity as "the way an individual reacts or responds to his particular environment." The inference here is that we designate as heredity all those characteristics of the individual that no known environment can change. We can also say that heredity is a natural force which prescribes, defines, and delimits all the individual's potentialities for development. In the human being this would mean setting limits on physical, mental, and emotional development. Potentialities for development, of course, are often hidden.

The things that most people want out of life are not often importantly controlled by biological heredity. Heredity is not destiny. When philosophers say, "A man's character is his fate," they are not speaking of physical heredity. Since culture is subject to change by human effort, man's fate on earth cannot be said to be predestined solely by his genetic heredity.

Heredity and Environment

Genetic heredity sets limits on potentialities of development, but it does not solely determine what the actual characteristics of a given individual will be. Here environment comes into play. This too is a complex of many obvious and concealed factors. To be exact, we should never describe any characteristic or trait of an organism as hereditary unless we specify the environmental conditions under which it will appear. In the nineteenth century, before the mechanisms of heredity were well understood, great debates raged over the question, "Which is more important to the development of the individual—heredity or environment?" Sometimes this last phrase was changed to "nature or nurture?" We

have not yet heard the end of this debate, but we recognize it as a nonsense question.

The individual inherits both his environment and his nature. He can escape neither; both influence his growth and development. Food comes from the environment, but the capacity to utilize it resides in the organism. If a human infant, for example, fails to get enough food, he will not gain the weight that normal hereditary patterns of maturation would indicate he ought to reach. Again, if abnormal hereditary patterns have invested the infant with constitutional disabilities which make it difficult or impossible for him to digest and utilize food which is plentifully available to him, the infant will not gain the stature to which he would seem entitled. The average height and weight of American college students have increased significantly since 1900. The explanation lies not in changed heredity but in improved environment, primarily better nutrition.

Congenital Defects. Environment can be favorable or unfavorable to normal development, and increasing attention is being given to the effects of *prenatal environment*. It is now recognized that many defects in development which were once thought to be hereditary are actually the result of conditions that the growing human organism encounters during intra-uterine life. Such defects are called congenital. It is now quite definitely known that if a mother suffers from a mild virus disease, such as German measles, during the early months of her pregnancy, her child may be born with congenital defects, for example, cataracts of the eye. Congenital syphilis also occurs but this disease is not hereditary.

It was once fashionable to attribute to "bad heredity" a great number of the diseases, "moral weaknesses" (e.g., drunkenness), and abnormalities to which human beings are subject. This is not the modern view. There are only a relatively few and generally uncommon diseases and constitutional disabilities—for example, "bleeder's disease" (hemophilia), red-green color blindness, Huntington's chorea, and PKU—for which an hereditary pattern can be clearly demonstrated. It is now recognized that many developmental abnormalities are probably the result of conditions encountered by the growing human organism during intra-uterine life.

There is no truth, however, in the ancient superstitions that an infant will be "marked" if the mother is subject to shocking experiences during pregnancy. Nor that favorable maternal impressions will have an effect.

The Study of Heredity. As human beings we are most interested in the operation of heredity among human beings. Often, however, this interest centers on superficial traits, such as eye and hair color. The scientific study of heredity has come to its surest knowledge through observations and experiments on plants, insects, and animals other than man. The rapid-breeding fruit fly (*Drosophila melanogaster*) has turned out to be an exceptionally useful subject for genetic investigations. In the laboratory this fruit fly produces 40 generations in a year, and a single pair of parents may have 200 to 300 offspring.

The direct study of human inheritance has been hampered by the fact that man is a long-lived creature. A single investigator cannot follow more than three generations. Furthermore scientific data about the traits and characteristics of previous generations of a family are difficult to obtain. Even when obtained, data about one's ancestors are usually incomplete, unreliable, and worthless from the standpoint of genetic study. An exception to this general statement must be made where gross physical abnormalities, such as extra fingers or webbed toes, run through several generations of a family. Some of the most valuable scientific information about human inheritance has been obtained from the studies of identical twins. But even twin studies have brought careful scientific investigators, like Newman, Freeman, and Holzinger at the University of Chicago, to the conclusion that human inheritance is even more complex than they had previously imagined it to be.

Mendelian Laws of Inheritance

Probably the most important scientific clues to the mechanisms of heredity as we now understand them were supplied by the Austrian monk, Gregor Mendel. The rediscovery in 1900 of his so-called lost paper, originally presented in 1865, marks the beginning of the modern science of genetics, which has flourished brilliantly since. The central fact of Mendel's contributions to the understanding of heredity was the demonstration, through experiments on sweet peas which grew in his monastery garden, that there actually existed *independent units* of hereditary influence. He called them simply hereditary factors; we now call them genes. The location of genes in body cells was made after Mendel's time. Genes can be said to stand for hereditary traits, qualities, or characteristics that appear in a living organism.

Mendel's work first suggested and demonstrated that these traits, and hence the genes that stand for them, might be either *dominant* or *recessive*. In hybrid stock, that is, in crossed breeds of plants or animals, including man, the dominant trait of a pair of traits *appears* to cover up the recessive trait. It does not blend with the recessive trait, nor does it eliminate it. The genes for the recessive trait remain in the sex cells of the organism and, as we shall trace, may appear in later generations.

An important question, obviously, is *how often* are recessive and *how often* are dominant traits likely to appear in the offspring of hybrids. There are simple and complicated cases. Mendel started with a simple case and came out with simple numerical formulas or ratios. When patterns of inheritance follow these ratios, we speak of Mendelian inheritance.

Genetic experiments such as Mendel performed must begin with true breeds, that is, parent stock which is known by observation over a number of generations to "breed true" with respect to the trait or quality under observation in the experiment. We can use Mendel's peas by way of example. One of the parent stocks is known always to produce purple flowers; the other stock always produces white flowers.

The true-bred purple and the true-bred white flowers are crossed. Careful scientific techniques of pollination must be observed. The offspring of this crossing will be hybrids. All of them will be purple, indicating that purple is the dominant color in this experiment. Now a pair of the hybrid-purple peas are crossed. Let us say that they have four offspring. Then three of the offspring of the hybrid-purple crossing will be purple and one will be white.

The following simple diagram will illustrate the case.

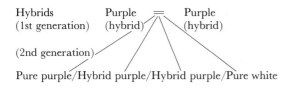

True breeds   Pure purple=Pure white

Hybrids   Purple   =   Purple
(1st generation) (hybrid)   (hybrid)

(2nd generation)

Pure purple/Hybrid purple/Hybrid purple/Pure white

This diagram gives you one of the fundamental Mendelian ratios: 3 to 1. This means that, when a pair of hybrids like the peas are crossed, the dominant trait will appear three times as often as the recessive trait. To the naked eye the pure purple and the hybrid purple flowers look alike. The hybrids can be sorted out only by another experiment in which all three apparent purples are crossed with another pure white. All the first-generation offspring of the pure purple and the pure white will be purple (as we have noted above). However, half of the first generation of the hybrid purple crossed with the pure white will show up as white.

The recessive trait continues to be carried in the genes of the hybrids. We may refer to hybrids as carriers of both dominant and recessive genes.

It is not always so easy to tell dominant and recessive genes or traits as this simple experiment may suggest. The color of human eyes appears to follow the Mendelian law, with brown (dark) eyes being dominant over light (blue) eyes. However, there are so many mixtures of hazel, green, and gray eyes that one cannot always carefully classify light and dark.

The Mendelian ratios for tracing (and predicting) the occurrence of dominant and recessive traits sum up the law of independent segregation of the genes. It should be pointed out that all the Mendelian "laws" of genetics are based on inferences drawn from statistical probabilities. This implies that the experimenter has a large population and true random sampling in his genetic materials.

A second Mendelian law, whose proof remains completely dependent on statistical probabilities, is that known as the law of the independent assortment of the genes. It states that, when double hybrids (that is, hybrids different in two genes) are crossed, all possible combinations in the offspring will appear by pure chance. In other words, each set of genes is inherited quite independently of other sets.

What Does the Individual Inherit?

Cultural inheritance aside, the individual can inherit from his parents, and through them from his more remote ancestors, only those physical and psychic characteristics that are transmitted to him through his parents' germ cells: specifically, the single egg and single sperm cell which united to begin the development of the new individual. The individual can pass on to his offspring only those traits that he carries in his own germ plasm. Most assuredly he cannot transmit those traits or characteristics that he has acquired in the course of his lifetime.

These would be the most obvious and self-evident of statements if it were not sometimes so difficult to determine which are the inherited and which are the acquired characteristics of the individual. The genetic constitution of a given individual can often be determined only by a progeny test, that is, by observing the actual progeny (descendants) of the individual over several generations and noting what traits are consistently duplicated. The geneticists distinguish carefully between visible or apparent types, called *phenotypes,* and truly hereditary types, called *genotypes.* The phenotype is the joint product of the genotype *and* the environment. Different genotypes can be hidden in the same phenotypes.

All the work of reputable modern geneticists points to the conclusion that acquired characteristics are not inherited. Cut off the tails of twenty generations of mice (a pointless experiment which was actually tried) and every newborn mouse still has a tail. Let a soldier who has lost an arm in battle sire a dozen children; all of them will be born with two arms. The Jews have been practicing circumcision for more than 2500 years, but Jewish boys are still born with foreskins. The physical characteristics, whether of strength or weakness, that are acquired by an individual during his lifetime cannot be transmitted to his offspring. Why this must be so we shall learn as we continue to trace the mechanism of heredity.

When acquired characteristics and environmental factors are eliminated, the question still persists, "What do human beings inherit from their parents?" The question can be answered broadly by saying all those traits and characteristics which make a human being a human being and not, for example, a monkey. Again in broad terms this is to say that we inherit our genetic constitutions. When it comes to breaking down and sorting out the specific factors in this complex whole, the question becomes much more difficult to answer. We know definitely about the human inheritance of only such traits and characteristics as happen to have been adequately studied.

There has been a great tendency to use heredity as a scientific waste basket and attribute to it all those human traits and characteristics, including a tendency toward certain diseases, for which no other satisfactory explanations could be found. The accumulation both of popular superstition and of scientific trash still makes it difficult definitely to specify all the hereditary traits in the human constitution. Nevertheless the factor of heredity does appear to play an important role in determining the following constitutional traits:

Longevity—the children of long-lived parents and grandparents do seem to have a better chance of living to an advanced age themselves.

Body build, whether slender or stocky, and including such characteristics as over-all body size, the arrangement or structure of specific muscles, the form and number of specific bones (such as length of the thigh bone and number of fingers or toes).

Shape of the skull, whether long or round, and such other traits in its vicinity as the form of the forehead, the nose, and the jaw and also the number and arrangement of the teeth.

Color of the skin, eyes, and hair.

Composition of the blood, the circumstance on which tests for paternity are based.

The Rh factor, originally identified in Rhesus monkeys, describes a human blood type which can be inherited. Approximately 87% of white and 92% of Negro Americans are Rh-positive; the balance, Rh-negative. The blood of an unborn infant with an Rh-positive father and an Rh-negative mother is sometimes affected by this discrepancy. This blood factor is the explanation of the highly jaundiced "yellow babies" that are occasionally born. In only 1 in about 150 pregnancies is Rh incompatability anything of a problem, and it is a matter of concern for obstetricians, not parents or parents-to-be.

There is also some evidence that heredity is a determining factor in the human tendencies to be nearsighted, to have twins, to be bald, to be left-handed, to be taste-blind to certain tastes, to be diabetic, and to have certain other abnormalities or deficiencies. The establishment of the importance of hereditary influences on the human constitution is clearest for those characteristics known to be sex-linked, such as bleeder's disease (hemophilia) and red-green color blindness (Daltonism), and for those that can be unequivocally observed and measured.

There are obvious differences in intelligence in any group of people. Yet it has turned out, despite earlier confidence, to be a complex problem to determine the influence of heredity upon intelligence. Part of the difficulty, of course, lies in the technique of measuring intelligence and validating tests for it. A Zulu child, for example, who might know his way around his own settlements would probably not score very high on an intelligence test validated upon the experience of French and American school children. Although it is still probable that heredity does play a crucial role in determining degrees of intelligence, we are less certain than we used to be about how this factor operates. This is a matter of particular social importance at the low end of the intelligence scale. About 2.5% of the population of the United States is judged to be feeble-minded. But the relationship of heredity to feeble-mindedness is no longer the open-and-shut case that earlier students considered it to be.

When it comes to evaluating the effect of heredity upon personality development, the evidence grows still cloudier. The best we can say here is that factors other than heredity, particularly early family influences, have been quite positively shown to be responsible for life conduct formerly assigned to heredity.

Heredity and Disease

On the old premise that "diseases run in families" there are still prevalent many misconceptions about the relationship of heredity and disease. The fact is that it has proved exceedingly difficult, if not impossible, to sort out the hereditary factors in the development of most diseases. It should also be pointed out that for a long time physicians tended to ascribe importance to hereditary factors in specific diseases to the extent that other causes could not be demonstrated.

Most of the physical defects, abnormalities, diseases, or deficiencies that can be transmitted from parent to child by physical heredity are apparent at birth or shortly thereafter. Such conditions include dwarfism (achondroplasia), albinism (lack of skin coloring pigments), extra fingers, webbed toes, and bleeder's disease. Such clearly demonstrable physical or psychic abnormalities as an individual is likely to have derived from his physical inheritance are almost certain to have become apparent by college age, if not much earlier. However, this fact does not preclude the possibility that an individual might still be a carrier of abnormalities, recessed and hidden in his or her genes.

Popular misconceptions about the possibility of inheriting or transmitting disease center largely about cancer and mental illness. It can be categorically stated that personal fears in these directions are needless and unjustified. Dr. Clarence C. Little, an outstanding authority on the subject of heredity in cancer, has declared: "The

role which heredity plays is so complex, so well concealed, and so difficult of evaluation that it is both unnecessary and unwise for individuals to consider it a personal problem."

Neither is there convincing evidence that either mild disturbances of the mind and emotions (neuroses) or serious aberrations (psychoses) are carried along inescapably in the physical inheritance of the individual. Dr. D. B. Klein[1] says of schizophrenia, one of the most prevalent of mental illnesses: "Some people seem to inherit something—exactly what is unknown—which renders them more likely to become schizophrenic than people who are born without this unknown something. However, this unknown something is neither necessary nor sufficient to produce schizophrenia; the psychosis may fail to develop despite its presence or schizophrenia may develop despite its absence." Dr. Jules H. Masserman[2] asserts: "While there might be a tendency to inherit feeble-mindedness and possibly epilepsy, there is no reliable evidence for definite hereditary factors in behavioral aberrations less directly dependent on organic or neurologic functions. Rather, controlled genetic-environmental studies indicate strongly that parents influence their children's patterns of behavior less by genes than by the nature of parental care, precept and example."

The Mechanisms of Heredity: Genes and Chromosomes

Before the twentieth century the exact mechanisms of heredity, including human heredity, were not known. Even scientists as distinguished as Charles Darwin, enunciator of the theory of organic evolution, made some rather bad guesses about it. Popularly the myth persisted, and still persists in many uninformed quarters, that heredity had something to do with blood. Common figures of speech, "blood relatives," "new blood in the family," and "blood will tell," still embody

[1] D. B. Klein, *Mental Hygiene* (New York: Henry Holt & Co., 1944), p. 151 (cited by Herbert A. Carroll).

[2] J. H. Masserman, *Principles of Dynamic Psychiatry* (Philadelphia: W. B. Saunders & Co., 1946), p. 11 (cited by Herbert A. Carroll).

this erroneous belief. Blood has nothing to do with the transmission or inheritance of truly hereditary traits.

The ultimate units of heredity, as we have pointed out, are genes. For practical purposes we may further describe a gene as a minutely small particle of matter located in and carried by a somewhat larger, but still microscopically small, bit of protoplasm called a chromosome. The word chromosome is from the Greek: *chromo* meaning color, and *soma* meaning body. When thinly sliced tissues are stained with dyes and examined under the microscope, the chromosomes appear as colored bodies. Chromosomes vary greatly in size and shape. At times, however, they appear through the microscope in a shape that we might aptly designate as a thread, rod, or chain. We can then picture the genes as comprising pieces of the thread, segments of the rod, or links of the chain. The chromosomes are at the very least the vehicles or carriers of the genes. In many cases that have been thoroughly studied, such as the fruit fly, it is possible to specify the location (locus) of different and separate sets of genes upon the chromosomes. The locale, or habitat, of the chromosomes is the nucleus of the living cell.

We know what genes do, of course, only by observing their effects upon the living organisms in which they occur. The genes alone determine the genetic constitution and the genetic inheritance of the individual. It is important to realize that in this sense *inheritance and constitution are the same thing*. Genetically, we are what our genes make us, and we cannot be anything else.

Although it is true that the genes in the living organism "work together," just as the organism itself is one piece despite the fact that it can be dissected into separate parts, it is also true that the effects of particular sets of genes, occurring at specific places in their chromosomes, can be specified. In this sense we can say that there is one *set* of genes (a set of several genes) that controls eye color, another set that controls hair color, still another set that controls stature and so on.

It is common to identify genes by the qualities they control. We can speak, for example, of "genes for longevity" or "blond-hair genes." Scientifically, of course, the genes are identified and specified by their position on the chromosome, if that is known. When we discuss genes as the ultimate units of heredity, it is often convenient to speak of a single set of genes controlling a specific hereditary trait as if the set were a single gene. The actual number of genes in a given chromosome cannot be positively stated. The number, however, is undoubtedly large, running into the thousands where human beings are concerned.

Concerning the number of chromosomes in the nucleus of each cell, there is no doubt. Chromosomes are plainly visible under high-power microscopes. Each living species has an exact, constant, and characteristic number of chromosomes, each of definite size and form. The chromosome number in man is 46. In a certain parasitic worm the number of chromosomes is 2; in sugar cane it is over 200.

Within the past decade, however, a phenomenal expansion in research devoted to human genetics, including cytogenetics (or the genetic study of the cell) and nuclear genetics (dealing with the molecular structure of genes), has shaken earlier concepts concerning the constancy of the number of chromosomes involved in human reproduction. At least half a dozen important abnormalities among human chromosomes have been revealed. This in turn has led to further understanding of the X and Y chromosomes with which sex-linked abnormalities are associated. For example, the condition of *mongolism* (in which an infant is born with slanted eyes and usually other developmental deficiencies) has been shown to occur in two forms, one form with 47 chromosomes and the other with a translocation among the usual 46 chromosomes.[3]

Sex of Infant. When a baby is born, two questions most commonly asked are, "Is it a boy or a girl?" and "Who does it look like?" It is a little late for these questions, because they were

[3]"Human Genetics," edited by A. C. Stevenson, *British Medical Bulletin,* 12:3, September 1961, London, British Council Medical Department (65 Davies St.).

in fact determined at the time of conception, an ineradicable part of the infant's physical heredity.

The sex of the forthcoming child is determined by its father: by the chance of whether the single sperm that penetrates the egg happens to be carrying in its *chromosomes* a male-making or a female-making *gene*. In this sex-determining chromosome, there are also other genes. These carry sex-linked human characteristics, for example, the tendency to red-green color blindness.

Cell Division. Cells multiply by dividing—an operation contrary to the rules of arithmetic. Cell division, called mitosis, is normally an orderly process though extremely complex. The important events in cell division take place in the nucleus.

When cell division begins, the chromosomes stretch out and arrange themselves in rod formations at about the center, or equator, of the nucleus. At the same time, two little bodies, called centrioles, just outside the nucleus, begin to move apart toward the opposite poles of the cell. These centrioles appear to act like powerful little magnets attracting the chromosomes. At a certain point in the process each chromosome rod seems to split down the middle. When the chromosomes thus duplicate themselves, the process can be pictured, figuratively speaking, as if two toothpicks were made out of one toothpick by splitting it down the middle with a razor blade. One set of the split or duplicated chromosomes appears drawn toward and moves toward one centriole; the second set moves to the other centriole. When this occurs the original, or mother, cell becomes elongated and thinner in the middle. Finally it separates, forming two cells. Each new daughter cell now has its own nucleus with exactly the same number of chromosomes as the mother cell.

In the adult body, cell division is a comparatively rare occurrence. In the fertilized egg cell, the embryo, the fetus, and the growing child it occurs with astonishing rapidity. Not all the differentiated cells of the human body retain the power of regeneration or self-reproduction. Yet every cut finger and broken leg reminds us that

HUMAN CHROMOSOMES

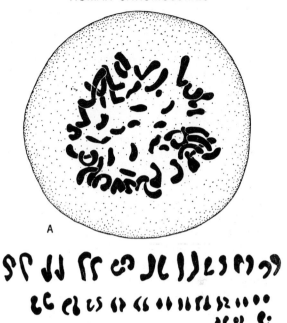

CHROMOSOMES CONTROL HUMAN HEREDITY, since they carry the genes (molecules) that will control it. In A of the illustration here, which has been redrawn from Patten's *Human Embryology,* are human chromosomes as they appear in an early division of the cells that will become sperm cells. In B are shown 22 well-matched pairs of human chromosomes. The 23rd pair is composed of the unmatched X and Y sex-determining chromosomes.

the adult body remains capable of cell division. Otherwise wounds and fractures would never heal.

DNA and RNA: The New Genetics.[4]

The orderly process of cell division does not just happen. It is directed by DNA and RNA—nucleic acids in the nucleus of the cell. The discovery of their importance and the many other new findings in genetics, especially in the last decade, permit scientists to write "a recipe for man." This biochemical recipe is made possible because we now know that genes are molecules

[4]See Chapter 8, page 136.

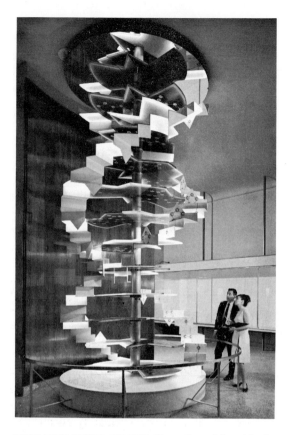

MAMMOTH MODEL OF DNA (deoxyribonucleic acid), the complex molecule that determines hereditary characteristics is shown here. Each nucleotide in this model is identified by chemical content. The white spirally ascending steps in the molecule represent DNA's sugar-phosphate chains. The horizontal pieces represent the nitrogeneous bases. (Photograph by Maris. Copyright Ezra Stoller)

and can therefore be dealt with by physical and chemical processes as well as in their normal biological way.

There may be as many as 10,000 to 100,000 kinds of genes in the nucleus of a human ovum. Each gene will control some specific property—like the structure of blood cells—in the living individual. An immense amount of information is packed into each gene in the form of a fairly simple four-letter code. The four letters are A, T, C, and G, standing for four nucleotides (nucleoprotein molecules which include nitrogen), *a*denine, *t*hymine, *c*ytosine, and *g*uanine, respectively.

The development of a human being (or any other living creature for that matter) from a fertilized egg is in principle something like baking a cake. As George Beadle has put it, "The genetic material is the recipe. It says what ingredients are necessary and how to put them together. The environment required for the right end result is the oven. If it is not right—if the temperature is too high or too low—the final product is something less useful than it should be. . . .

"The hereditary information, or recipe, is precise at the molecular level. How much so is illustrated by the red blood cell pigment, hemoglobin. This is a protein built up of 600 amino acid building blocks—of which there are twenty varieties—strung together end-to-end in a long chain, like dominoes. Their precise order determines that the protein will be hemoglobin rather than any other one of almost unlimited other kinds of protein (nerve, muscle, or skin cells, for example)."

The Code Letters of Living Things. The code letters A, T, C, and G of the genes that create the shape and form of all living things have a particular location in the nucleic acids which are part of the nucleus ("the brain and the heart") of every living cell. They are sometimes, therefore, called nucleoproteins. Nucleic acid was originally found by the chemist Miescher sometime before 1900 in cell nuclei isolated from white cells of pus; but it has required generations of patient scientific research to discover the overwhelming importance of nucleic acids. They are, we now know, the very "stuff of life," the key to growth and reproduction of living cells and all organisms made up of cells.

In the simplest terms, the nucleic acids provide the patterns, or templates, of growth for all other cells. They give the rest of the proteins in the living organisms "blueprints" of where they are supposed to be in the structure of the cell, and "traveling orders" on how to get there.

Again in very simple terms we can say that the nucleic acids are the brains of the cell. They tell it how to grow and how to divide into new cells. They provide the pattern for its future. The two most important nucleic acids yet known are *deoxynucleic acid,* usually abbreviated DNA, and *ribonucleic acid,* usually abbreviated RNA. Several forms of both DNA and RNA are known to exist, and these forms perform different functions in the "blueprinting" of cell growth, development, division, and decay. "Messenger RNA" carries to the new cell the pattern for reproduction set down by DNA in the original cell. Both DNA and RNA are long-chain (polymer) molecules wound in a double-helix (coiled spring) fashion.

Genes, Viruses, Molecules. Many strands of research are woven into our present knowledge of the importance of nucleic acids. (Within recent years nearly a dozen Nobel prizes have been given for research in this field.) Skillful research in biology, genetics, chemistry, and virology have all spun our present tapestry of knowledge about DNA and RNA and their unusual functions.

In particular the study of viruses (virology)— the smallest known entities that reproduce themselves—substances that are on the borderline between animate (living) and inanimate (non-living) matter, has led toward a deeper understanding of the chemical basis of life. Predictions of the possibility of producing "life in a test tube" (that is, from supposedly "inanimate" matter) have been freely made by Nobel prize-winning scientists. On this point chemist Wendell M. Stanley spoke very acutely when he said, "Perhaps it is true, as Aristotle suggested 2000 years ago (in his "Ladder of Nature"), that Nature makes so gradual a transition from the living to the non-living that the boundary line is doubtful, possibly nonexistent."

Practical Applications of the New Genetics. The unexpected new discoveries in genetics, a field which now has its own subdivisions (e.g. biogenetics, chemical genetics), have some immediate practical and some hopefully longer-range applications. These discoveries have made possible the concept of "molecular disease" in place of the older explanation of "inborn errors of metabolism." This means that disease can now be understood and attacked at the molecular rather than the cellular level. (Molecules are smaller and more precise than cells). Some relatively rare diseases of man can now be better managed by an understanding of their molecular nature; but the great hope for the breakthrough of this new knowledge into clinical usefulness lies of course in a better understanding and management of the "big killers," heart disease and cancer.

On the rare disease side we may cite the example of galactosemia in man—an inherited inability to use galactose, which is a component of milk sugar. This is a serious and often fatal disease in infants. If diagnosed early enough—in which diagnosis the new knowledge of molecular disease is a great help—a synthetic milk, free from galactose, can be substituted in the infant's diet; recovery is usually rapid and complete. It must be pointed out, however, that while the individual infant is "cured," his defective genes (with reference to galactosemia) are not repaired and can be passed on to his offspring.

Through increasing genetic knowledge and application of this knowledge to management of the "big killers," we can confidently expect new triumphs in both the control and prevention of disease in the decades immediately ahead. The idea of looking at cancer as a "molecular disease" is in itself a great stride forward.

A unifying concept regarding the cause of cancer emerged late in 1961: Cancer, no matter what the cause, is the result of a change in the chromosomal nucleic acid (DNA) of the affected cells. DNA is the chemical substance of the chromosome that plays a key role in both heredity and vital functions of the cell. The arrangement of subcomponents of DNA forms a code in which all the heritable information needed by the cell is stored. Apparently cancer is caused by a particular, though as yet undefined, change in DNA structure which alters this information code.

Methods have been developed for the isolation of DNA from the cancer-inducing polyoma virus. The purified DNA, like the intact virus, will initiate the development of cancer in laboratory animals. The DNA may be "tagged" with radioactive hydrogen so that it can be traced as it penetrates both normal and cancerous cells.

SUMMARY

The laws of human heredity have been operating inexorably since the beginning of mankind; but it is only within the last century that we have begun to understand exactly how hereditary characteristics are transmitted. Many scientists contributed to this knowledge: Sir Francis Galton, with his law of ancestral heredity; Gregor Mendel, with his experiments in plant (sweet peas) hybridization; Thomas Hunt Morgan, with his research on genes and chromosomes; numerous others, including many recent Nobel prize winners, who worked out the new genetics.

We now know that genes are molecules and that the orderly process of cell growth and division, on which heredity depends, is directed by the nucleic acids, DNA and RNA. We have also begun to understand the "amino acid code." Yet it must be stressed that heredity is not destiny and that environment ("cultural heredity") also plays a crucial role in determining how a given individual, regardless of his physical heredity, will eventually turn out. The complicated process of the transmission of human heredity is in fact carried out by the equally mysterious process of human reproduction, the subject of our next chapter.

SUMMARY REVIEW QUESTIONS

1. What does the following statement mean to you: "Heredity is not destiny"?
2. What is the "law of ancestral heredity"? Who discovered it?
3. What distinctions do you make between cultural and physical heredity?
4. What is the relationship between heredity and environment in determining the character of a living organism, including man? What is meant by *prenatal* environment?
5. What are the Mendelian laws of inheritance? How were they derived and established?
6. Cultural inheritance aside, what are some of the things (name at least six) that an individual inherits from his immediate and more remote ancestors?
7. What is the role of the chromosomes in the transmission of physical heredity? What is the normal process of cell division in human body cells?
8. When and how is the sex, whether male or female, of a human being determined?
9. How do the discoveries in "the new genetics" add to previous knowledge of the mechanism of transmission of human heredity? What practical value does this new knowledge have?
10. What are the connections, if any, between genes, molecules and viruses?
11. Are the following statements sense or nonsense? Why? *Man's character is his fate. . . . Environment is more important than heredity in shaping the character of the individual. . . . The number of chromosomes in human beings never changes. . . . Genes are molecules. . . . Chronic alcoholism is an inherited disease.*
12. What do the following terms mean to you: DNA, nuclear genetics, phenotype, genotype, hybrid, congenital defect, galactosemia, eugenics, recessive characteristic, Rh factor?

Worth Looking Into: *Experiments in Plant Hybridization* [the famous "lost paper"] by Gregor Mendel. *Memories of My Life* by Francis Galton. *Heredity, Race and Society* by L. C. Dunn and Th. Dobzhansky. *Understanding Heredity: An Introduction to Genetics* by Richard B. Goldschmidt. *Blueprint for Life: the Story of Modern Genetics* by Julius Fast. *The Genetic Code* by Isaac Asimov. *The Double Helix* by James Watson. For more complete references, see Appendix E.

14

HUMAN REPRODUCTION

THE URGE OR NECESSITY TO REPRODUCE one's kind is the mark, and one of the fundamental mysteries, of life itself. On the shadowy borderline between animate and inanimate objects, in the field of virus research, the ability to reproduce (or replicate) remains the basic test for classifying a *living* virus as against an inert chemical.

Among many living species reproduction appears to be the aim of life. Salmon swim upstream, leaping impossible falls, to return to their spawning grounds. Eels at maturity swim downstream to go back to their own place of birth in the black depths of the ocean, reproduce a new crop of elvers, and disappear. Among higher animals, the dog and the horse, for example, the instinct for reproduction is equally powerful, and involuntary. It is controlled by seasons of "heat" or "rut," which can be correlated with the activity of endocrine glands, especially in the female.

The human reproductive process has different rhythms of its own. After puberty, the time of attaining biological maturity, human beings are capable of reproduction at any time of the year. In fact, however, this capacity is physiologically limited in the female to certain times of the month and is controlled over the years by powerful social pressures.

It is profitless to ask why mankind desires to reproduce itself. Or why the overtones of the reproductive process, sexual pleasure, sound so sweet to the human race. It has proved equally futile to debate the question of bisexuality, to ask why in the course of evolution the union of male and female elements became necessary to initiate new life.

We may profitably consider, however, the observable processes by which a "gleam in the eye" may eventually become a full-fledged living infant which itself grows up to repeat the cycle of human reproduction. We shall deal here with the biological facts of human reproduction since we have already dealt with their social and psychological implications. Such information is properly described as education for family living, because it is for the sake of creating a happy family of one's own that one seeks fuller knowledge of the phenomenon of human reproduction along with perspective on risks and opportunities surrounding it.

No intelligent man or woman can afford to play ostrich with the facts about and surrounding human reproduction. The most elementary activities of our daily lives and our most fundamental feelings and attitudes are largely controlled by these facts. We are educated for and in family living, as male or female, from infancy onward. The attempts on the part of some individuals and groups to veil the facts of life behind prudish attitudes are responsible for much needless human doubt, guilt, suffering, and misery. "Nice-Nellyism" is out of key with our modern, science-oriented civilization.

The Reproductive Process

A human life begins with the penetration at the proper time and place of a single, ripe human ovum (egg) by a single, viable human sperm.

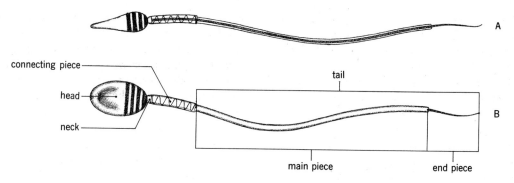

HUMAN SPERM CELL. Here are two diagrammatic views of a human sperm cell, magnified approximately 2000 times actual life size. A. Side view (profile). B. Top view (looking down).

This is the critical moment of conception, but it is in fact a "microscopically small and unfelt event." It occurs, normally, in one uterine tube of the female some hours after the deposit of semen in the vagina. The ovum arrives at this rendezvous by maturing and bursting out of a follicle in the nearby ovary. The sperm originates in the male testis, but the whole reproductive apparatus of the male, and some of that of the female, is required to get the sperm to the place of conception.

Sperm. Sperm[1] are microscopically small, measuring only 50 to 60 microns (thousandths of a millimeter) in length. You could pick up on the head of a pin all the sperm necessary to sire the next generation in North America.

Each normal human sperm can be seen in profile to have a spear-shaped head, a neck, and a threadlike tail. The tail is about ten times as long as the head and gives the sperm a whiplike power of locomotion. As observed under the microscope, it wriggles along by lashing its tail. Sperm move ahead, or "swim," at the rate of about an inch in twenty minutes. Comparatively speaking, this is roughly the speed of a good human swimmer. Sperm moving at approximately this rate, and normally shaped and proportioned, are considered *viable,* that is, living and capable of fertilizing a human ovum.

Sperm leave the male body in an ejaculate of

[1] The singular form of the word sperm is sometimes written as spermatozoon; the plural, spermatozoa.

semen, a white, viscous fluid, whose function appears to be exactly that of serving as a vehicle for the sperm. A normal ejaculate contains from 2 to 5 cubic centimeters of semen, each cubic centimeter carrying on the average about 100 million spermatozoa. When an ejaculate of semen is deposited in the female vagina, its huge swarm of sperm, numbering perhaps from 200 million to 500 million, begin to move under their own power toward that site in the female genital tract where a mature ovum is likely to be encountered. If encountered, however, one and only one sperm cell actually punctures, penetrates, and fertilizes the egg.

The sperm which do not fertilize the egg simply perish, like any seeds scattered on barren ground. Some of the sperm deposited in the female genitalia appear to remain viable up to seventy-two hours if they have entered the uterus. Most of those left in the vagina perish within an hour or two. Under controlled laboratory conditions the hardiest of ejaculated sperm can be kept alive in a test tube for one or two days. At least they retain some motility.

Beginning at puberty and continuing to old age, though at a slower rate in later years, the normal human male produces literally billions of sperm in the course of his lifetime. There is not ground for the belief that, if men "waste" their sperm early in life, the supply will run out. Nature's prodigality with sperm perhaps reflects the high degree of hazard that any single one will succeed in reaching a mature egg cell.

Ovum. Timing is a crucial factor in human conception. The mature or ripened human ovum has a comparatively short life span, probably not more than forty-eight hours and possibly less. Unless fertilized in the uterine tube during these crucial hours, the egg dies, disintegrates, and is discharged from the body in the course of menstruation.

A ripe (mature) human egg cell is about $\frac{1}{100}$ of an inch in diameter, just about visible to the naked eye.

The two female ovaries contain altogether about 50,000 egg cells, but these are immature cells laid down during embryonic life. These egg cells do not ripen or become mature until puberty. Then, with the onset of menstruation and ovulation, a small number of the ova eventually mature at about the rate of one a month. The outside limit would be about 500 in a lifetime. Each egg cell matures in its own pocket, called a *Graafian follicle*. This process continues until the menopause, which usually comes in the late forties.

Twins. On some occasions more than one mature ovum may happen to be released from the ovaries at about the same time. The proof that this occurs is the birth of so-called *fraternal twins* or triplets. Each separate egg cell is under these circumstances fertilized by a different sperm cell. Fraternal twins, therefore, are no more alike than any other brothers and sisters. *Identical twins,* however, come from the same egg and sperm cell; the egg splits after being fertilized. Identical twins are always of the same sex; they usually look almost exactly alike. About one pair of twins in every four is made up of identical twins.

Twins are born about once in every 80 pregnancies; triplets, once in every 6000 to 7000—roughly 80 times 80; quadruplets, once in approximately a half-million—roughly 80 times 80 times 80. Quintuplets occur once in about 50 million to 60 million pregnancies. There is some evidence that the tendency to multiple births runs in families.

The Male Reproductive System

The purpose and design of the male reproductive system is to deliver viable sperm for the impregnation of the ovum. Its essential anatomical apparatus includes the testes, also called male gonads; a series of sperm ducts, the prostate gland and seminal vesicles for elaborating and storing semen; and the penis, urethra, and accessory glands.

Testes. Two testes, or testicles, each about the size of a walnut, are enclosed in a sac of skin, called the scrotum, suspended from the groin.

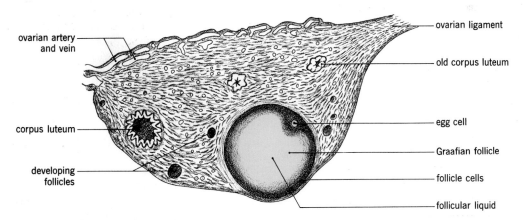

INSIDE THE OVARY. An ovary cut across looks like this. The Graafian follicles, in which the ova mature, are shown in various stages of development. Note also the corpus luteum, containing the old follicles whose eggs have been discharged. The egg cell itself is about as big as the period at the end of this sentence.

Hanging outside the body, between the legs, the scrotum has a temperature slightly lower than the rest of the body; this appears to be an essential condition for production of sperm. The testes normally descend from the abdomen into the cooler scrotum just before or shortly after birth. If they fail to descend (undescended testes, cryptorchidism), medical or surgical treatment may be needed.

The first important function of the testes is to manufacture sperm. This takes place, so far as is known, in a series of little twisted (convoluted) tubules, where the sperm develop from immature sex cells laid down in these membranes early in the life of the embryo. Mature sperm, capable of fertilizing an ovum, do not appear until puberty. The testes may continue producing sperm well into old age, as is evidenced by the not infrequent birth of children to aged fathers. From collecting tubes in the testes, the sperm move on to a series of ducts, beginning with the epididymes, through which they are eventually conveyed outside the body.

The second important task of the testes is to manufacture the male sex hormone, *testosterone,* which brings about development of secondary sex characteristics at puberty: growth of beard and pubic hair, deeper voice, comparatively rapid increase in size of the male sex organs, and general muscular development. The male sex hormone is produced in a set of specialized cells located in the tissues that support the tubules making sperm; a lesser amount is elaborated by the *adrenal glands.* Testes are part of the *endocrine* system (pages 146 to 149).

Epididymes. These are coiled-up tubes, several feet long but looking like a twisted ball of string, attached like a hood or pouch to the outer surface of each testicle. They collect and store sperm. In them the sperm become mature and motile, that is, capable of moving under their own power. However, they do not do this until they are discharged from the body. They are propelled through spermatic ducts by contractions of the tubes and tubules.

Spermatic cords, or ducts, convey sperm from the epididymes up to the seminal vesicles. They are winding tubes, about a foot long, including the *vas deferens* and other structures. The spermatic cords, one from each testicle, issue from the scrotum into the abdomen by way of the inguinal canal. Spermatic cords can be felt where they pass over the pubic bone near the base of the penis. Cutting the cords near this point is the simplest operation for *sterilization* of the male.

Seminal vesicles are the upper outlets of the spermatic cord. They are two small pouches or sacs located in the abdomen just behind the bladder. They secrete a large part of the thick, white, alkaline fluid, *semen,* in which the sperm float. Like the rubber bulb on an eye dropper, they can contract vigorously and spurt or squirt semen out into the *urethra,* the mucus-lined tube that traverses the penis and carries urine as well as semen. Because some of the same bodily organs are used for the discharge of urine as well as semen, the entire system is sometimes called *genito-urinary.*

Ejaculation of semen from the seminal vesicles is a nerve-reflex act, associated with the sensation called *orgasm.* The motor nerves that control orgasm respond to both physiological and psychic stimuli. The stimulating impulses usually arise in the head (glans) of the penis. The distention of the seminal vesicles with an accumulation of semen may also prompt the discharge of semen as a nocturnal emission.

The prostate gland, normally about the size and shape of a chestnut, is situated just below the bladder and seminal vesicles and surrounds the urethra where it emerges from the bladder. It is involved with secreting fluids which make up part of the semen. Anatomically it is the homologue of the uterus in women: its function as a genital organ, however, is still poorly understood.

Accessory glands among the male sex organs include a pair called *Cowper's glands.* They are about the size of a pea, are located near the base of the penis, and open into the urethra. They secrete a clear, oily lubricating fluid. A few drops of this fluid may come out of the penis following sexual excitation not carried to the point of orgasm.

The *penis,* a cylindrical organ suspended from

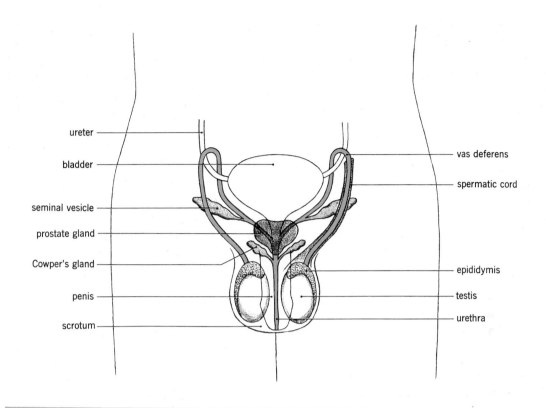

ureter

bladder

seminal vesicle

prostate gland

Cowper's gland

penis

scrotum

vas deferens

spermatic cord

epididymis

testis

urethra

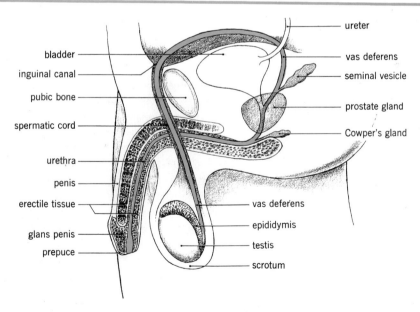

bladder

inguinal canal

pubic bone

spermatic cord

urethra

penis

erectile tissue

glans penis

prepuce

ureter

vas deferens

seminal vesicle

prostate gland

Cowper's gland

vas deferens

epididymis

testis

scrotum

THE MALE REPRODUCTIVE SYSTEM. The upper diagram is a straight front view. The lower diagram is a side view shown as if a section had been made a little to one side of the center of the body, from front to back.

the front and sides of the groin, is the male organ of intercourse, designed for delivery of semen into the vagina. Enlargement, or erection, of the penis is normally necessary for this function. This occurs when the usually retracted and flaccid organ becomes engorged with blood. The shaft and head of the penis are composed of a spongy, cavernous, erectile tissue, traversed by many blood channels. When stimulated, these channels become filled with blood, whose immediate return to the rest of the circulation is temporarily cut off by constriction of the veins leading away from the penis. Under conditions of adequate sexual excitation, erection of the penis is a normal and natural reaction of the male animal— part of nature's design to assure perpetuation of the species.[2]

Circumcision. The penis is covered with loose folds of skin, allowing for enlargement. The extra skin at the tip, or glans, is called the *foreskin* or *prepuce.* The operation for its removal is known as circumcision. Among Jews, Mohammedans, and some other peoples, the operation is performed as a ritualistic measure. Among Orthodox Jews it is always performed on the eighth day of life. In the Bible it is stated that the "tribe of Abraham" is to affirm its "covenant" (*bris*) with the Lord by this measure.

[2] At puberty the size of the penis usually increases markedly. The length of the organ is sometimes falsely taken as a measure of manliness. This is nonsense. Except in rare individuals in whom the sex organs fail to develop normally, usually as a result of some disease requiring definite medical attention, the size of the penis has no relationship to fertility, or marital adjustment. Despite the bawdy jokes that are brought to bear on the topic, fears on the part of the male that he will be unable to give or receive satisfaction in the marital act because of the size of his penis are completely unwarranted. The psychological satisfactions surrounding the act, the tenderness, warmth, affection, and love brought to it, are of far greater moment than the physiological mechanics. Furthermore, the innervation of the female genital tract—the comparative paucity of nerve endings in the distensible vaginal tissue itself—is such that actual penile dimensions are of insignificant import in the totality of sensations and satisfactions involved. To think otherwise is to retreat to a level of phallic worship found in primitive tribes. (The male organ and representations of it in model or symbol are designated by the word phallus.)

The origin of circumcision is lost in the history of antiquity. In modern times it is performed for both its ritualistic and sanitary values. It keeps "cheesy" secretions (smegma) of the foreskin from accumulating and irritating the penis, and it prevents cancer of the penis. Circumcision does not alter sexual satisfaction.

The Female Reproductive System

The female reproductive system consists of a pair of *ovaries,* a pair of tubes, the uterus or womb, the vagina, external genitals, and some accessory glands. The mammary glands (breasts) are sometimes considered part of this system.

All the important female sex organs are located inside the body. The whole system is greatly influenced at all times by hormones produced both in the ovaries and in other endcrine glands.

The female sex organs have at least three functions: to produce and yield mature ova for union with viable sperm, to shelter and nourish the fertilized egg cell until it has developed into a newborn baby, and to elaborate female sex hormones.

Ovaries. The ovaries, or female gonads, are two small glands, each about the size and shape of an almond, set in the pelvic cavity (lower abdomen). One is about 3 inches to the right and the other the same distance to the left of the midline of the body. The ovaries do two jobs: they bring ova to a point of readiness for impregnation and they secrete hormones.

The hormones released by the ovaries have several functions. They help to govern the monthly rhythm of ovulation and menstruation. They do this partially by their effect on other endocrine glands. Furthermore, these hormones spur the development and maintenance of secondary sex characteristics, for example, deposition of fat under the skin to give the characteristic feminine curves, enlargement of the breasts, growth of pubic hair.

Fallopian Tubes. When the matured egg cell escapes from its follicle, it is caught or picked up by one or the other of the two uterine tubes, or oviducts. Each of the two uterine tubes is about

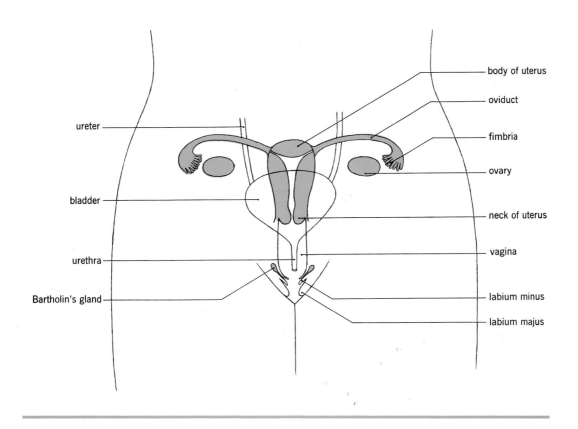

ureter ———
body of uterus
oviduct
fimbria
ovary
bladder ———
neck of uterus
vagina
urethra ———
labium minus
Bartholin's gland ———
labium majus

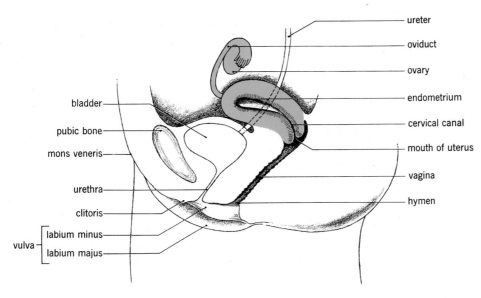

ureter
oviduct
ovary
bladder ———
endometrium
pubic bone ———
cervical canal
mons veneris ———
mouth of uterus
vagina
urethra ———
hymen
clitoris ———
vulva ⎰ labium minus ———
      ⎱ labium majus ———

THE FEMALE REPRODUCTIVE SYSTEM. The upper diagram is a straight front view. The lower diagram is a front-to-back section through the center of the body.

Human Reproduction   293

3 to 5 inches long. Its lower end clearly opens into the uterus. Its trumpet-shaped far end, however, is not really attached to the ovary. It just lies close to it and holds out fingerlike projections (called fimbria) toward it, reaching for the ripened egg.

The upper, inner lining of the tubes has little hairlike organs, called *cilia,* which by waving back and forth carry the egg down the tube. This action is essential because the egg itself has no power of locomotion. The journey down the tubes takes 3 to 6 days. This is the time and place at which the egg must meet and be penetrated by a viable sperm if pregnancy is to occur.

The fertilized egg normally completes its journey to the uterus. About once in 500 times, however, it implants itself in the tube, causing a *tubal,* or *ectopic, pregnancy.* This usually becomes a serious emergency, demanding surgery.

If both uterine tubes are blocked, usually as a result of inflammatory disease, pregnancy cannot occur. A common test to tell whether the tubes are open (patent) is to blow carbon dioxide gas into them with a special apparatus for this purpose.

The uterus, or womb, is the central organ of the female reproductive system. Non-pregnant, it lies just above and slightly behind the urinary bladder, in the center of the pelvic cavity. Enlarged with pregnancy, the womb fills a large part of the lower abdomen, displacing other organs as it rises.

The non-pregnant womb is a hollow, pear-shaped pouch of muscle, about 3 inches long and 2 inches wide. The stem of the pear points down. This narrower, lower end is called the *cervix,* or neck, of the womb. The upper, round portion, where the embryo actually grows, is called the body, or fundus, of the womb. The uterus is held in place, loosely, by a number of ligaments. This looseness of attachment is essential because it permits the changes in shape, size, and position of the womb that occur during pregnancy.

The uterine muscle is one of the strongest in the body. It has to be to expel a full-grown, newborn infant when the time of labor comes.

The inner lining (endometrium) of the womb is one of the most unusual tissues in the body. A soft, velvety tissue, greatly influenced by hormones, heavily interlaced with blood vessels, it grows and disintegrates in the monthly cycle of ovulation and menstruation.

The lower end of the cervix, called its os or mouth, extends into the upper vault of the vagina. A short cervical canal passes through the cervix. Male sperm must get through this canal to reach the uterus and the uterine tubes above it. If this canal is plugged with mucus, or otherwise blocked, conception cannot occur.

The vagina serves both as the female organ of intercourse and the birth canal through which the newborn infant enters the world. It is a tubular cavity about 3 or 4 inches long, extending from the cleft of the legs to and beyond the mouth of the womb. It is set at an angle of about 45 degrees to the front of the abdomen, and just below the bladder. The muscles that make up the vaginal tube can be greatly stretched without harm. The inner lining is soft membrane.

Accessory glands secrete some fluids during sexual excitation, which lubricate the vagina. These are *Bartholin's glands,* two small oval glands located on each side of the vagina, near its external opening, and *Skene's glands,* multiple small secreting glands located near the opening of the urethra into the vaginal vestibule.

The external genitalia of the female, found adjacent to the vaginal orifice, are the vulva and clitoris. The vulva consists of two pairs of "lips": the *labia majora,* elongated folds of skin covered with hair in the adult woman, and, underneath these, the *labia minora,* thinner folds of tissue covered with mucoid membrane. The clitoris appears at the far forward fold of the labia minora. It is a small, rudimentary structure, consisting, like the penis, of erectile tissue responding to stimulation.

Across the opening of the vagina appears the thin, perforated mucous membrane called the *hymen* (or maidenhead). This structure, whose biological purpose is not known, varies greatly in size, thickness, and extent. In many women it is merely rudimentary. Its absence is of no significance. It is usually broken by the first sexual intercourse, but may otherwise be reft. Being perforate, it does not block menstrual flow. Superstition notwithstanding, its presence is not an absolute sign of virginity, nor is its absence proof to the contrary.

Above the external genitalia, in front of the pubic bone in the area covered by pubic hair, is often found a thick mound of subcutaneous fatty tissue—the *mons Veneris* (hill of Venus).

Menstruation

Menstruation is a characteristic bodily function common to all healthy, adult, nonpregnant women. A menstrual period need not interfere with a woman's regular schedule of activities.

Myth, mystery, and superstition have long enveloped the facts about menstruation, the periodic issuance of blood from the female genital tract "at the waxing or waning of the moon." To the ancient Hebrews, Greeks, Romans, and early Christians the menstruating woman was "unclean." The American Indians, believing the moon to be the First Woman, saw in her waning the periodic "sickness" of the female. The Koran forbade the menstruating woman to pray or enter a mosque. Practically the only fact in the great cluster of erroneous superstitions was that menstruation occurred in cycles corresponding approximately with lunar months. The lunar (moon) calendar has 13 months of 28 days each. The word menstruation derives from the Latin word *mens*, meaning month.

Myths and Misconceptions about Menstruation. While we, fortified by scientific knowledge, tend to laugh at primitive myths about menstruation, nevertheless certain modern misconceptions of the hygiene of menstruation continue to crop up. Mark down as myths and misconceptions, entirely incorrect, such statements as the following:

"Don't take a bath or a shower—don't go swimming or wash your hair when you are menstruating." "Menstruation is a sickness—it's naturally painful." "Any exercise during a menstrual period is harmful—the best policy is to stay in bed." "Your hair won't take a curl or a wave when you are menstruating." "If you have your teeth filled at this time, the fillings will fall out." Nonsense!

The hygiene of menstruation can be summed up in one phrase, "Take it in your stride." Extremes, of course, are wisely avoided. Although some physicians would still interdict it, there are many others who accept evidence[3] that even such an activity as swimming, except in very cold water, can be safely permitted during the menstrual period. (Internal protection—a tampon—is worn.)

There is no objection whatsoever to ordinary bathing, showering, or shampooing or setting of the hair during the menstrual period. Going to bed when a menstrual period arrives is sometimes evidence of an unhealthy attitude not only toward the menstrual function itself, but also toward normal sexuality. Mild exercise will probably tend to relieve rather than promote menstrual discomfort.

Some women nourish the myth that they are as "regular as clockwork" in their menstrual function. This is rarely, if ever, so, as carefully kept calendar records for large groups of women reveal. A few days' so-called irregularity is perfectly normal. Extreme irregularities may be considered signals for a medical check-up. It is to be remembered, however, that many severe diseases, such as pneumonia, and even some mild ones, like a common cold, can upset the regularity of the menstrual cycle. So too can sudden change of altitude or climate, physical shock or emotional excitement, like an airplane trip, an auto accident, or an engagement. Irregularities are also to be expected at the beginning and toward the close of the childbearing years.

On the *average*, the length of the menstrual cycle is twenty-eight days. But every woman has her own rhythmic cycle of ovulatory and therefore menstrual function. For some women cyclic periods of twenty-one or thirty-five days, and occasionally even longer or shorter periods, if reasonably regular, are quite normal.

[3]Grace Thwing, "Swimming during the Menstrual Period," *Journal of Health and Physical Education,* (March 1943).

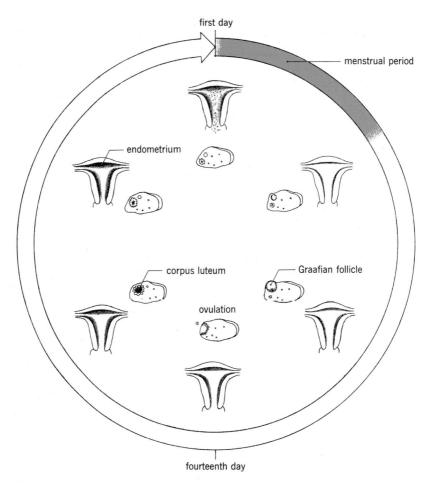

first day

menstrual period

endometrium

corpus luteum

Graafian follicle

ovulation

fourteenth day

THE MENSTRUAL OR OVULATORY CYCLE. This diagram of the menstrual or ovulatory cycle is based on an average (theoretical) 28-day cycle in the human female.

The total amount of blood lost in a normal menstrual period is usually only about three ounces and is quickly regenerated by the blood-forming organs (bone marrow).

A checkup is indicated for the woman who finds herself staining between regular periods, who skips one or more periods, who finds her periods extremely painful, or whose menstrual flow continues much more than a week. The *average* menstrual period is three to five days, but two to seven days are within normal range.

It is not to be denied that painful menstruation (dysmenorrhea) occurs. Yet this is far more commonly—by a ratio of at least 4 to 1 among normal college women—the exception rather than the rule. As Boynton has pointed out, this condi-

tion can often be relieved and prevented by a change in attitude toward the menstrual process.[4] Self-imposed invalidism or unconscious resentment can magnify slight cramps into apparently intolerable pain. When indicated, the physician can prescribe medication for relief of menstrual pain and tension.

The Menstrual or Ovulatory Cycle. Though we commonly speak of the menstrual cycle, dating from the first day of menstrual flow, we can also designate it as the ovulatory cycle, guided and controlled primarily by the time of ovulation. There is no completely accurate way of

[4]Ruth Boynton, "A Study of the Menstrual Histories of 2282 University Students," *American Journal of Obstetrics and Gynecology,* **23**:516 (April 1932).

determining the day of ovulation, although there is evidence that there occurs at this time a slight decrease, by fractions of a degree, in body temperature, following which a relatively sharp rise occurs.

Ovulation occurs at about the midpoint of the menstrual cycle. This is the time when a ripened egg cell bursts out of the tiny sac, or Graafian follicle, in which it has been maturing. This follicle manufactures ovarian hormones; it is a kind of "temporary endocrine gland." Most amazing, it makes one kind of hormone before the egg erupts, another kind afterward. The emptied follicle is called *corpus luteum* (literally, yellow body). Its hormone influences the endometrial lining to disintegrate. But it also influences the pituitary gland to issue hormones that speed another egg cell to maturity and another Graafian follicle to open up, thus starting the whole cycle of events over again.

The menstrual or ovulatory cycle is a complex process that involves the uterus, ovaries, and endocrine glands. However, the most evident changes during the cycle occur in the inner lining (endometrium) of the uterus.

During the menstrual flow this lining is being shed, torn away from the underlying uterine tissues to which it is attached. Small blood vessels (capillaries) are broken as this takes place, and this is the source of the menstrual blood. But even as this old lining is being shed, a new lining is commencing to grow. It gets thicker and thicker, soft and velvety, and enlaced with blood vessels, for the next 3 weeks.

The function of this lining is to receive a fertilized ovum, if one should appear. If none appears, which is usually the case, the lining is again shed, with bleeding, and still another begins to grow. If a fertilized ovum *is* present to embed itself in endometrium, the menstrual cycle comes to an abrupt halt, to resume after childbirth.

The Menopause

The menopause, sometimes called the "climacteric" or "change of life," marks the end of the potential child-bearing period that begins with the onset of menstruation (menarche). The menopause usually comes anywhere from the early forties to the late fifties, occuring on the average at about forty-seven. Just as the onset of the menses was marked with a sudden increase in ovarian hormones, so the menopause occurs when there is a gradual decrease in these hormones. The elaboration of ovarian hormones (by the ovaries) finally ceases. No more ova are matured. The menstrual flow becomes scanty and irregular or stops abruptly. That is all there need be to the menopause, and in about 85 out of 100 cases there are no other changes. Childbearing is no longer possible, but sexual feeling is not necessarily decreased (in some women it is heightened).

The outward physical symptoms of the change of life are usually mild and transient, if they occur at all: a few "hot flashes," lasting a minute or two; a feeling of fatigue at times; an occasional pain in the joints. It should be noted that many of the symptoms often associated with the menopause are today amenable to much relief with hormone and psychological treatment.

Some attempts have been made to define a "male climacteric," similar to the menopause. It may occur in a few men, but the cessation of function of the male sex hormones usually tapers off so gradually that no well-defined symptoms can be definitely associated with it.

Contraception

Despite the marvel of human reproduction, it must be admitted that there are millions of married couples (and others) who do not want to run the risk of pregnancy occurring with every incident of sexual intercourse. These people are more interested in contraception than in conception. Contraception is known by other names: birth control, birth prevention, family planning, child spacing, and planned parenthood.

A number of methods of contraception are now available, some more reliable than others, some very new, others very ancient. With one exception—surgical sterilization in the male—they are all reversible. That is to say, conception can be expected to occur when the particular technique(s) of contraception are no longer employed. Among the popular methods of contraception now employed are (1) "the pill," (2) intra-uterine devices, abbreviated to IUD's, (3) rubber diaphragm with or without spermicidal creams or jellies, (4) the rubber condom or male sheath, and (5) "the rhythm" or "safe period" system.

"The Pill". It is a hormonal stimulant and depressant, whose basic ingredients are related to the female sex hormones. The pill, taken orally, contains some synthetic progesterone and a little estrogen. These hormones suppress the follicle-stimulating hormone of the anterior pituitary gland. As a result, the ripening of an ovum in the ovary fails to occur. Without the presence of a ripe ovum in the uterine tubes or cavity, pregnancy cannot occur.

The woman who wishes to avoid pregnancy takes one pill a day for about 20 or 21 days, beginning on the fourth or fifth day after the beginning of her menstrual period.

Properly used, the pill can offer close to 100% protection against pregnancy. When discontinued for a month or two, normal pregnancy can be expected to occur following intercourse. It must be taken regularly, for even if one day is missed, ovulation and pregnancy might occur. Furthermore, investigations now under way indicate possible relationships between thromboembolism and other diseases and the taking of the pill. The risk, however, appears to be within permissible limits.

Intrauterine Devices—IUD's. These are usually made of a flexible plastic in the shape of loops, rings, spirals, "butterflies," etc. and can be folded down to small size for insertion through the narrow cervical canal of the uterus. Once inserted, they snap back to their original expanded state. This method has the advantages of low cost and relative permanence. Under the best conditions, it is from 97 to 98.9% effective in preventing unwanted pregnancies. The method has some disadvantages. In some women the device causes extreme menstrual flow and uterine cramps. In perhaps one woman in seven there is a tendency toward spontaneous expulsion of the device. It

must then be replaced with a different shape or size.

Diaphragm with or without Spermicidal Creams or Jellies. Until recent years this was the form of contraceptive most commonly recommended by physicians and birth control centers. The diaphragm is a rubber cap, shaped like a shallow dish, with a flexible metal spring or coil forming its outer edge. The diaphragm is fitted over the mouth of the uterus, and prevents viable sperm from entering. The diaphragm has to be anchored firmly between the back of the vagina and, in front, the pubic bone. This distance varies from woman to woman. Hence the diaphragm has first to be fitted precisely by a physician skilled in this work. It must be inserted by the woman each time sexual intercourse is anticipated. There has been some complaint that this method takes too much of the spontaneity out of sexual intercourse. However, it is a highly reliable method, especially when used as recommended with a spermicidal cream or jelly, which provides a chemical barrier to the diaphragm's mechanical barrier between sperm and egg.

Newlywed couples may have to use some other form of contraception (e.g., the condom) on their honeymoon because it is not easy, and sometimes not possible, to fit a diaphragm to a woman with an intact maidenhead (hymen).

Condom (male sheath). The condom is a thin rubber sheath, shaped like the finger of a glove, which rolls down to fit over the erect penis. It is probably the most popular form of contraceptive and has the added advantage of helping to guard against the risk of venereal disease. It is freely sold in drugstores as a "prophylactic."

"The Rhythm" or "Safe Period" System. This method depends upon the fact that there exists in most women of child-bearing age a reasonably regular menstrual or ovulatory cycle. Menstruation and ovulation are generally about halfway apart in the cycle. Pregnancy can occur only in the ovulatory phase of the cycle, that is, the time when a ripened ovum is present in the uterine tube. Hence the days that surround the menstrual period are "safe" from pregnancy, while those immediately before and immediately fol-

lowing the time of ovulation are the "fertile" period. In a woman with a regular menstrual cycle, the tenth to the eighteenth days following the onset of menstruation are the time when the fertile period occurs. A viable sperm may remain in the female genital tract for three days (72 hours) or possibly longer. The life span of the unfertilized ovum is less than one day (24 hours).

To prevent conception the couple must practice abstinence during the fertile period of the menstrual cycle. Illness, shock, emotional storms, and other events may influence the time of ovulation and throw the menstrual cycle out of kilter. The difficulty with the method lies in knowing exactly when ovulation occurs. A daily temperature record can help to determine this. If taken daily, the first thing in the morning, the body temperature will tend to rise a half to a whole degree about the day that ovulation occurs. The Roman Catholic Church has permitted birth control by the rhythm method (also by prolonged abstinence and celibacy).

Among other contraceptive methods are douching, withdrawal, and surgical sterilization.

Douche. This is a common but highly unsatisfactory method of contraception. It calls for cleansing the vaginal tract with water (sometimes with something added) immediately after sexual intercourse. Speed is the key to practicing this method. Within 90 seconds after intercourse some sperm are already within the uterine cervix, where they cannot be reached by the douche fluid.

Withdrawal. The essence of this method is that the male withdraws the penis from the vagina just before he reaches his climax or orgasm. However, there may be a leakage of semen into the vaginal tract even before orgasm. Though it has the advantage of requiring no apparatus, it cannot be depended upon for safety against the risk of pregnancy.

Surgical Sterilization. Sterilization in the female is accomplished by tying off the uterine tubes; in the male, by cutting through the spermatic cord as it emerges under the skin at the groin. In women, at any rate, the procedure is reversible and tubal potency can be reestablished by surgery. About 5% to 6% of white U.S. couples with three or more children have undergone the simple operation of surgical sterilization for contraceptive purposes.

There is still objection to birth control—on moral, religious, political, and other grounds. However, with the rapidly increasing population of the globe, some effective form of birth control will be necessary to curb the population explosion.

SUMMARY

A new human life is created when a viable sperm penetrates a mature ovum at an appropriate locale within the female genital tract (usually the oviduct). The male reproductive tract is designed for the production of the male sex hormone and the delivery of viable sperm to the female genital tract. The female reproductive system has wider scope. In addition to providing female sex hormones and ripened mature ova, it must provide nourishment and protection (in the womb) for the unborn infant. When the ovum, ripened as part of the normal ovulatory-menstrual cycle of the female, is not fertilized, the phenomenon of menstruation occurs—until the menopause in the late forties.

There is now a widespread interest in the methods of contraception (birth control, planned parenthood and the like), such as "the pill", "IUD's" and others. This is partly a response to increased sexual permissiveness, and partly a reflection of the need for curbing a population explosion.

SUMMARY REVIEW QUESTIONS

1. Why should an educated man or woman know the facts about human reproduction? Why do some supposedly mature adults fail to get the facts straight?
2. What is "conception"? Where does it occur? What are the crucial factors that make it possible? What sharp contrasts can you point out between human sperm and human ova with relation to size, shape, number, life span and mode of travel?
3. What is the difference between fraternal and identical twins? Approximately how often do multiple births occur?
4. What are the essential parts and functions of the male reproductive system?
5. What are the essential parts and functions of the female reproductive apparatus?
6. What myths and misconceptions, ancient and modern, about menstruation can you cite? How could you combat such misconceptions?
7. What is the menstrual cycle? The ovulatory cycle? How are they interrelated and how are they regulated?
8. What are the most effective means of contraception now employed? What are the objections to contraception?
9. Are the following statements sense or nonsense? Why? *Barrenness is always a woman's fault. . . . The menopause is usually a painful process. . . . Never wash your hair when you are menstruating. . . . If a man "wastes" his sperm when he is young, the supply will soon run out. . . . Shocking experiences during pregnancy can put marks on the unborn child.*
10. What do the following terms mean to you: bisexuality, Graafian follicle, Fallopian tube, circumcision, dysmenorrhea, ovulation, ectopic pregnancy, seminal vesicles, IUD, "The pill," diaphragm, accessory glands?

Worth Looking At: *Sex Anatomy* by Robert L. Dickinson. *Essentials of Human Reproduction* by Velardo. *Sex in Marriage* by Baruch and Miller. *Planning Your Family* by Alan F. Guttmacher. For more complete references, see Appendix E.

Evaluation of Developments in Contraceptive Technology

Howard C. Taylor, Jr., M.D.

The knowledge of the so-called new birth control methods has been shared with the public with a haste that seems almost unparalleled in medical history. The daily press, the weekly news periodicals, the romantic magazines of the newsstands, even staid financial journals have published articles in their own particular styles or from their own particular points of view. It will be a little difficult then to present to this professional group any startling developments that you may not have already picked up, if not in scientific journals, then over your breakfast coffee.

Yet an opportunity remains to correct some of the optimism, or at least the oversimplification, which seems an essential part of most introductory articles for the lay reader. The new methods of birth control have brought with them special problems of application, of acceptability, of reliability, and sometimes of unwanted side effects. Much work on evaluation remains to be done and much research is required for the perfection of technics which are perhaps still in the early stages of their development. It is, then, the subject of the more pressing problems which still need to be solved that will be discussed in this presentation.

A number of contraceptive technics which have been practiced widely for several decades, or indeed perhaps for several centuries, have recently acquired the slightly amusing, but still honorable, title of "traditional methods." These, as social and economic conditions change, continue to create their own new aspects of interest, but there is no space for them here. This presentation must be limited to four methods, none perhaps very new but each currently somewhat controversial: the safe period; the pill which suppresses ovulation; the intrauterine device; and, I would like to add, surgical sterilization.

The Rhythm

The effectiveness of the "rhythm" method, that of abstinence during the days when ovulation is expected to occur, remains somewhat of a mystery. Physiologists swear that it should be a success; statisticians doubt somewhat that it has been.

The resolution of this apparent contradiction is to be found, of course, in the number of days a month abstinence must be practiced if "safety" is to be assured. Using the Ogino formula, which is somewhat stricter than that of Knaus, a statistical model has been worked out by Tietze and Potter[11] which emphasizes the severe restrictions that must be imposed if real dependability is to be derived from the safe period method. Noting that even the most regular menstrual pattern has a variability of three days, these authors conclude that with the Ogino formula the days of abstinence must be 11 each month. For women with less regular cycles this figure may increase to as much as 15 or 18 days a month. Yet they point out that the observation of the rules implied by this theoretical model should give a 90 percent chance of avoiding pregnancy for five to ten years.

Data derived from actual use

SOURCE. Howard C. Taylor, Jr., is director of the International Institute of Human Reproduction at the College of Physicians and Surgeons of Columbia University, New York, N.Y. This article originally appeared in the January 1966, supplement to the *American Journal of Public Health*. It is here reproduced with permission of the *American Journal of Public Health*.

of the method is not numerous but that which exists indicates a high failure rate, apparently several times that cited for the usual traditional methods.[13] The conclusion seems inevitable that the use of the rhythm method gives only relative protection unless there is strict adherence to the Spartan regime required for real effectiveness.

Yet the physiological facts seem sound and the method is potentially an effective one. Success might be attained by a fundamental revision of current concepts of sexual behavior in marriage and, indeed, the standard frequencies of intercourse may be related more to fashion and custom than to physiological necessity. Alternately, the method must apparently await the discovery of a test, easily applied, which would indicate when ovulation was about to occur, or a simple medication which would precipitate ovulation on a convenient date. Such possibilities are indeed being worked upon in a number of laboratories and are quite within the realm of possible development.

The Ovulation Suppressing Pill

The general facts about the so-called "pill" are now widely known. The basic substance, a synthetic progesterone-like steroid, such as Norethynodrel or Norethindrone, taken daily from the fourth to the 25th day of each cycle, prevents ovulation and permits the regular recurrence of uterine bleeding at about 28-day intervals. Its mechanism of action is probably chiefly through an inhibition of the gonadotrophic function of the anterior pituitary and a consequent failure of the normal stimulus to ovulation. If taken in the prescribed manner, the protection afforded against pregnancy approaches 100 percent.

On account of the action of these substances on such a fundamental aspect of the reproductive function, it was to be expected that the method would have to defend itself against numerous apprehensive allegations. This it seems to have accomplished successfully. It was at first feared that fertility, after long use of the progestins, might be permanently impaired, but it has been shown that conception will occur within one or two cycles after discontinuation of the medication, and indeed there is some evidence for even a temporarily heightened fertility. The specter of a carcinogenetic effect has of course also been raised and apparently been excluded, at least so far as the cervix of the uterus is concerned, by the finding of an actually smaller number of positive Papanicolaou smears among the users of this method than was to be expected. Because the progestins are said to produce a physiologic state somewhat resembling that of pregnancy, and since thrombophlebitis is of slightly increased frequency in pregnancy, the observation of a few cases of thrombo-embolic disease among women taking Norethynodrel led to new anxiety. A careful study by an ad hoc committee of the Food and Drug Administration[3] led, however, to the conclusion that no significant increase in the risk of thrombo-embolic deaths had been demonstrated.

At the moment, then, there are no well-founded accusations pending against the progestins as health hazards. They have now been in use for [a decade] and reservations are still held by some as to the possible results of 20 years of use. Such concern, taking the form of worry about effects on any subsequently conceived offspring, or about possible carcinogenic effects on breast and endometrium, especially from the estrogen usually combined in the "pill," is largely theoretical. It is troublesome in that it cannot possibly be excluded completely until another decade has come and gone.

There remain a certain number of so-called "side effects," annoying symptoms, which cause a certain number of women to discard the method. These consist in nausea, some intermenstrual, so-called "breakthrough," bleeding, and gain in weight due principally to the retention of electrolytes and water. Consequently, a small number of users, possibly 5 or 10 percent, abandon the method for reasons other than the decision to have another child.[4]

Nearly ideal as this method appears to be, there are a number of improvements that are needed before it can be considered perfect. The price is still high, about $2.50 a month, if the 21 tablets are purchased at retail, and this, though far less than the cost of maintaining an average cigarette habit, is still out of the financial or psychological reach of a large segment of the world's population. Further, the taking of even one tablet a day may be hard to remember, and research is under way to produce longer acting compounds which might require only a single dose for a whole cycle. The discovery of such a substance and provisions for its distribution might give a final solution to the population problem.

The Intra-uterine Device

Interest in the last year, while continuing to be devoted to pharmacological contraception, has turned also to the intra-uterine device, a modern version of the once rather widely used, as well as maligned, Gräfenberg ring. The new devices, of many shapes, are for the most part made of a flexible plastic. They have the common property of adjusting their shape to permit insertion through the narrow cervical canal and returning to their original form when reaching the endometrial cavity.

These devices have been subject to a most carefully designed program of clinical research carried out under the direction of the Population Council and the National Committee on Maternal Health. An international conference devoted to intra-uterine contraceptive devices was held in 1962,[10] and a second conference of a similar but more comprehensive nature took place in 1964. Data compiled by Dr. Christopher Tietze[12] for those conferences will supply the few figures now needed for comment. The statistics of Dr. Tietze's report were derived from impressive material col-

lected from 38 institutions. The combined data yield percentage figures based on 16,734 cases and 132,460 months of use of the intra-uterine device.

First of all it is clear that the effectiveness of the intra-uterine device is very high, the cumulative pregnancy rate during the first year after insertion, for all devices combined, being 2.6 per 100 patients. For certain forms and sizes of the device the figure was as low as 1.1 or 1.3 per 100 patients. An additional small figure must be added for pregnancies occurring after spontaneous expulsion of the ring when this occurrence is unnoticed by the patient. Even with this addition the protection offered is substantially better than that from the traditional methods of birth control when used by the average clinic patient. If the undetected expulsions can be eliminated, the degree of security would approach, although perhaps never quite reach, the perfect safety afforded by the pharmacological technic.

The point of superiority of the intra-uterine device is of course its relative permanence, since only a single decision is required. Once the device is inserted, there is no need for further responsible action. This feature, coupled with the low cost, has given the device great promise for use by the less educated, less motivated, and less self-controlled.

Certain disadvantages of the intra-uterine devices must still be faced. In a proportion of women wearing the ring, menorrhagia and uterine cramps develop, requiring removal of the

device in about seven percent. The tendency to spontaneous expulsion of the device is a further problem. In perhaps 13.8 percent, the figure varying considerably with the shape of the device, the first one tried is expelled and must be replaced, or a new type or size tried. Finally, there is the possibility that the ring predisposes to infection. The old Gräfenberg ring was held responsible for pelvic inflammatory disease and instances of such inflammation have certainly occurred among the women in the present investigation. However, an incidence of 1.7 cases per 100 women using the device for 12 months is perhaps not very different from that to be found among a similar group of women not using the device.

Future work with the intra-uterine device must still be somewhat concerned with health hazards. The possibility of slight predisposition to pelvic inflammatory disease needs to be somewhat further considered. The hazard of carcinogenic action from a long retained foreign body has of course been thought of, and although this effect seems improbable, the question can finally be answered only by the passage of time. Studies of changes in the cervical epithelium, as measured by successive Papanicolaou tests, have been inconclusive. . . .

The technical developments that are needed include the development of shapes and sizes that will not be expelled, and, hopefully, such that will cause a minimum of cramps and bleeding. The need of a simple method by which the continued presence of the device in the uterus can be detected has given rise to some electronic thinking leading to some interesting and some frivolous proposals. In summary, the intra-uterine device like the pharmacological method, given the proper means of public information and application, could also solve the problem of overpopulation.

Sterilization

Among the technics of birth control, one which seems to be gaining in importance, but which has received relatively little attention, is surgical sterilization. Since this procedure is rarely undertaken until after there are three or more children in the family, its effect on birth rates may not be considerable. Nevertheless, the frequency with which sterilization is now carried out makes it a factor to be noted.

In a recently published article, Campbell[2] has reported that of 2,414 white couples, between the ages of 18 and 39 who were interviewed, six percent had been sterilized for contraceptive purposes. The average number of children born to couples having such an operation had been 3.6. Beside the operations undertaken specifically for contraceptive purposes, an additional four percent of couples had had an operation, with respect either to the husband or wife, incidentally producing infertility, to remedy some physical defect. The author estimates that some 200,000 operations preventing pregnancy were performed in the United States annually from 1955 to 1960 and of these 110,000 were contraceptive in intent.

The majority of contraceptive sterilizations in women consist in a tubal ligation carried out during the first week after delivery, an operation first reported by Adair and Brown in 1939.[1] The frequency of this procedure among 177,433 live births collected by questionnaire (Starr and Kosasky[9]) proved to be 3.2 percent of all deliveries.

Puerperal sterilization is an almost completely safe procedure and requires so small an incision that little discomfort follows it and the patient's postpartum hospital stay is scarcely prolonged.[6] Psychological and even physiological disturbances have been alleged to follow it, but these have not been proved or checked against unsterilized controls. A small percentage, perhaps half of one percent, of failures to prevent pregnancy have been reported. A very few sterilized women regret their decision, but here there is evidence that the surgical reestablishment of tubal continuity will be successful in a considerable percentage of patients. The freedom from concern and the absence of need for any continuously applied method of contraception are the great assets of this method.

The obstacles to the still wider application of surgical sterilization are two. One is the nagging fear in each case that the operation once done will be regretted. The other is the prevailing feeling in the medical profession, not at all limited to those of the Catholic faith, that the operation of sterilization is a special one, interfering with a provision of nature and not to be lightly undertaken.

Birth Control and Obstetrics

In approaching the conclusion, I should like to overstep slightly the bounds of my title and discuss briefly the way in which information on the technics just discussed is to be disseminated. In brief, I want to stress the extreme importance of the antepartum and postpartum visits of the obstetrical patient, whether these take place in the hospital of the woman's delivery or in a public health clinic.

The first pregnancy and delivery are major emotional and educational experiences. These include many weeks during which a reorientation toward a new set of values and responsibilities is taking place. It is this time above any other than the woman is ready for a consideration of her role as a family planner.

The women delivered by private physicians have at least the opportunity to ask about birth control methods and the majority probably have some advice actually given to them.[8] With the ward patients the story is quite different. Although a complicated series of antepartum visits are carefully organized, for the early detection of tuberculosis, syphilis, incipient cancer of the cervix or the beginning of toxemia of pregnancy, no mention is apt to be made of the most important point of all, the question of the next pregnancy.

Conditions seem to be rapidly changing in the United States and it appears that in a few years some consideration of family planning will be as integral a part of pre- and postpartum care as is the detection of physical illness. In such a program, the subject of birth control should certainly be introduced during the mother's classes in the antepartum period. Reference to the subject and a stress on the importance of the postpartum visit should be given at the bedside while the patient is still in the hospital.

Finally, at the postpartum visit birth control should again be discussed and the patient given a chance to select a method satisfactory to her taste and conscience.

Conclusion

There are thus two aspects to the birth control problem, one concerned with technics and the other with education. Although my subject has been specifically concerned with technics, it is the educational aspect which still seems to be the more important and the one that is furthest behind the needs.

REFERENCES

1. Adair, F. L., and Brown, I. Puerperal Sterilization. *Am. J. Obst. and Gynec.* 37: 472–476, 1939.

2. Campbell, Arthur A. The Incidence of Operations that Prevent Conception. *Ibid.* 89: 694–700, 1964.

3. Food and Drug Administration Report (Ad Hoc Advisory Committee for the Evaluation of a Possible Etiology Relation with Thromboembolic conditions). A Special Report, *J.A.M.A.* 185: 776–777 (September, 7), 1964.

4. Goldzieher, Joseph W.; Becerra, Carmen; Gual, Carlos; Livingston, N. B., Jr.; Maqueo, Manuel; Moses, Louis E.; and Tietze, Christopher. A New Oral Contraceptive. *Am. J. Obst. and Gynec.*

5. Pincus, Gregory, and Garcia, Celso-Ramon. Preliminary Findings on Hormonal Steroids and Vaginal, Cervical and Endometrial Histology. Symposium de Cancer del Utero (February), 1964. *Rev. Inst. Nacional de Cancerologia,* Mexico City.

6. Prystowsky, H., and Eastman, N.J. Puerperal Tubal Sterilization. *J.A.M.A.* 158: 463–467, 1955.

7. Rice-Wray, E.; Goldzieher, J. W.; and Arando-Rosell, A. Oral Progestins in Fertility Control: A Comparative Study. *Fertil. and Steril.* 14: 402–409, 1963.

8. Spivack, Sidney S. The Doctor's Role in Family Planning. *J.A.M.A.* 188: 152–156, 1964.

9. Starr, Silas H., and Kosasky, Harold J. Puerperal Sterilization. *Am. J. Obst. and Gynec.* 88: 944–951, 1964.

10. Tietze, C., and Lewit, S. (Editors). Intra-uterine Contraceptive Devices. *Excerpta Medica Internat. Congress* Ser. No. 54, Amsterdam, 1962.

11. Tietze, Christopher, and Potter, Robert G., Jr. Statistical Evaluation of the Rhythm Method. *Am. J. Obst. and Gynec.* 84: 692–698, 1962.

12. Tietze, Christopher, *Cooperative Statistical Program for the Evaluation of Intra-uterine Contraceptive Devices.* Fourth Progress Report, National Committee on Maternal Health, Inc., New York City (June 30), 1964.

13. Westoff, Charles F.; Potter, Robert G., Jr.; Sagi, Philip C.; and Mishler, Elliot G. *Family Growth in Metropolitan America.* Princeton, N.J.: Princeton University Press, 1961.

15

BIRTH OF A BABY

CHILDBIRTH HAS LONG BEEN SHROUDED IN secrecy, as a reaction to the pain and risk it entailed in earlier generations. Scientific progress in medicine, obstetrics, surgery, and anesthesiology has now reduced these hazards to the barest minimum. Women today can have their babies safely and relatively easily if they take advantage of the modern safeguards of adequate prenatal care and hospital delivery. In the United States today better than 3099 out of 3100 mothers come through childbirth safely.

Twentieth-century changes in the social and economic relationships between the sexes have also operated to make present-day attitudes toward pregnancy and childbirth quite different from those of our Victorian grandparents. Proper Victorians never "talked obstetrics." To the present day "organization man" and his wife, living in suburbia and exurbia, obstetrics is the grist of everyday conversation.

Modern fathers are no more directly engaged in childbearing than was Prince Albert, the consort of Queen Victoria. But it is the rare father today, among educated people, who can or wants to escape the responsibilities of child-rearing. He will be concerned with his children and children-to-be from the very moment that a diagnosis of pregnancy is established in his wife. Pregnancy is a family affair.

The gist of the modern enlightened attitudes toward pregnancy and childbirth is that these are normal, *natural* events of human life; there is no need to conceal them. The risks, as always, lie in ignorance and suppression of the facts.

Life Before Birth (Embryology)

When you were one month old, you were one-quarter of an inch long; at two months, an inch long; at three months, three inches long; at six months, a little over a foot long; and at nine months, when you were actually born, about twenty inches long. We are counting, of course, from the date of conception, not the date of birth.

Your weight increased as astonishingly as your length. The human embryo, growing in its mother's womb, weighs less than an ounce until the end of its first three months of life. At four months, on the average, it weighs six ounces; at five months, one pound; at six months nearly two pounds; at term, after nine months of intra-uterine life, about seven and a half pounds, more or less.

These facts are known to us through the science of embryology, characterized by Margaret Shea Gilbert, as writing "the biography of the unborn." Scientific inferences about human growth are based in part on microscopic examination of the embryological development of other mammals, for example, the monkey, the rabbit, and the cat.

From Egg to Embryo. Conception of the new individual occurs at the moment when sperm and ovum unite in the uterine tubes, leading from the uterus to the ovaries. The fertilized egg cell (zygote) quickly divides into two cells, the two into four, the four into eight, and so on. This process is called subdivision or cleavage. It continues while the zygote makes its way down the

LIFE BEFORE BIRTH
DEVELOPMENT OF HUMAN EMBRYO—COMPARATIVE SIZES

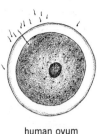

AT
CONCEPTION

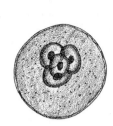

human ovum
impregnated

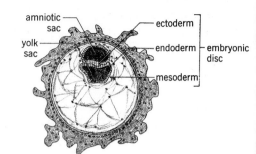

amniotic sac — — ectoderm
yolk sac — — endoderm — embryonic disc
— mesoderm

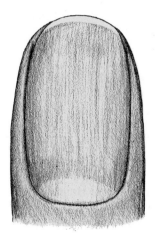

ONE-TWO
MONTHS

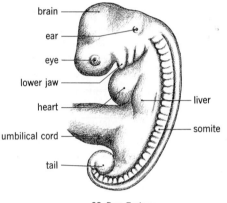

brain
ear
eye
lower jaw
heart
umbilical cord
tail
liver
somite

28-Day Embryo
(the human tadpole)

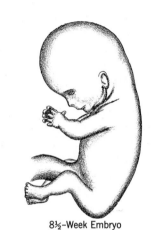

¾″

8½-Week Embryo

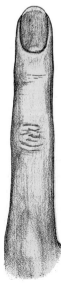

AT
FOUR MONTHS

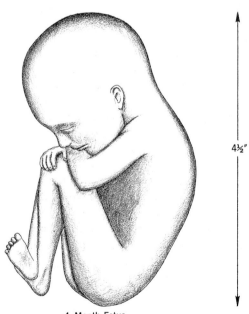

4½″

4-Month Fetus

uterine tube, about a three-day journey, and while it floats, so to speak, for a week to ten days in the cavity of the uterus. During this period is uses up the food substances contained in the human egg itself. Then it attaches or embeds itself in the uterine wall prepared for its reception. By this time the subdivision of cells has advanced to a point where the single fertilized egg cell has become a hollow ball with several layers of cells. At this point it is called a morula, from the Latin word for mulberry.

Not all the cells in the morula become the embryo out of which the individual develops. Some of them are in a sense shunted off to become accessory structures necessary to the growth and development of the embryo, for example, the placenta, the umbilical cord, and the amniotic sac ("bag of waters"). The placenta, embedded in the uterus, and the umbilical cord, running from the placenta to the developing embryo, function primarily as food supply lines, for the human embryo, a true parasite on its mother, must get from her body all the nourishment it requires. The amniotic sac forms in effect an elastic bottle of fluid within which intra-uterine growth of the embryo actually takes place.

The *placenta,* called the *afterbirth* following delivery of the child, is a flat disc of tissue by which the infant is attached to the mother's womb and through which it is nourished. It grows along with the embryo and fetus. At term it is a pancake-shaped tissue, an inch or two thick, 6 to 9 inches in diameter.

The placenta interlocks with the tissues of the uterus. The nourishment for the growing child in the womb seeps through the membranes of the placenta from the maternal blood stream. These membranes filter out many things that might harm the infant. But some things, like the spirochete of syphilis, certain viruses (like that of German measles), blood elements like the Rh factor, and some drugs (including anesthetics), can get through this membrane. The growing fetus has its own blood supply and circulatory system. The mother's blood does not circulate through the infant in the womb.

The *umbilical cord* runs from the middle of the placenta to the navel (umbilicus) of the developing infant. The cord increases in size as the placenta and the infant grow. At birth the cord is usually about 2 feet long, $\frac{1}{2}$ to 1 inch in diameter. It is usually twisted, and on rare occasion a loop of it may snare the neck or limbs of the fetus.

The *amniotic sac* or "bag of waters," is a kind of elastic bottle in which the growing infant develops, floating in amniotic fluid. This fluid is secreted by the inner lining of the bag of waters (amnion). It protects the child from pressures on the mother's body and helps regulate the infant's temperature. Just before the bag of waters breaks at term, it carries between 1 and 2 pints of fluid.

The embryo proper arises from a spot on the inner layer of cells of the morula. This spot is called the embryonic disc. The disc comprises two tiny layers of cells. In very crude terms, you can imagine the shape of the disc as that of two round pancakes rolled up. For the sake of convenience we call the outside layer of cells the ectoderm and the inside layer the endoderm. Almost immediately another layer of cells begins to form between these two. This middle layer is called the mesoderm. These events occur not only in human but in all embryos. The ectoderm layer, for example, always turns out to form the outer covering—skin, scales, or feathers—as well as the nervous system and sensory organs of the creature-to-be.

We shall now trace the growth of the strictly human embryo.

The First Month of Life. The human body, as we know, is made up of a myriad of cells. The first specialized cells to appear in the embryo are young blood cells. They are found in the mesoderm layer in patches called "blood islands," and show up about seventeen days after conception. With their appearance begins the formation of the body's blood and circulatory systems. Soon thereafter, the young blood cells take predictable shape. Tiny tubules, that is, blood vessels which are forerunners of the veins and arteries, begin to form, and the blood flows through them to initiate a kind of circulation. These tiny blood vessels gradually fuse to form a "heart tube." On about the twenty-fifth day after conception this tiny heart tube, precursor of the human heart, begins pulsating or beating. It will continue beating until the creature dies. The embryo heart beats much faster than the adult's or even the child's heart.

The human nervous system takes its origin in the embryo just about the same time that the heart tube is forming. The first step in the development of the nervous system is the appearance of a "neural plate" on the ectoderm layer of tissue. This plate then "rolls up" to form a "neural tube." This tube takes position right straight down the middle of what will later take shape as the human backbone or spinal column. The front end of the neural tube eventually becomes the human brain; the tail end becomes the spinal cord.

Heart and brain begun, the embryo next goes about forming its food (alimentary) canal. In its earliest stage this structure is called the "embryonic gut." It has two parts: a foregut and a hindgut. At the head end of the foregut, tissues from the ectoderm join it to form what will be the human mouth and lips.

The Human Tadpole. A month after conception the fertilized egg cell has grown into something that resembles a tadpole. It is a soft creature, about one-quarter of an inch long; and it has a head and a tail, but scarcely a face. Yet most of the essential human organs are already in the process of formation.

The head end of the "human tadpole" is approximately one-third its total length. Its heart is so large that it bulges out against the wall of the chest-to-be. Its lungs are scarcely more than little sacs.

At four "corners" of the embryo, where arms and legs will later appear, are to be found four little nubbins of flesh described as "arm buds" and "leg buds." Along the back of the tiny human tadpole are to be discovered 38 little bundles of tissue, called "somites," from which the strong muscles of the human frame will eventually take shape.

The Second Month of Life. In the second month of life, dating here always from concep-

tion, the "tadpole" that was changes into something that can be identified as being human. We may summarize the changes during the second month of intra-uterine existence by saying that it begins with a tail and ends with a face. The human tail at its longest measures only 1 to 2 millimeters; it reaches its maximum length during the fifth week of life. Then it disappears. On very rare occasions the tail fails to regress and an infant may be born with a tail.

By the end of the second month the embryo has a face, queer looking to be sure; a neck supporting a large head that is mostly brain; four limbs, the arms budding faster than the legs; five digits already in the process of formation on each limb; a trunk that houses the internal organs; some muscles; the beginnings of many bones; and internal sex organs which can often be identified as male or female.

The face is gradually put together around the head end of the foregut, where the preliminary structures of the mouth appear. The eyes, originally placed on the sides of the head, like those of a bird, converge toward their proper forward-looking position above the mouth and nose. Skin, that is, ectoderm, tissue above the eyes forms eyelids which seal the eyes shut for at least the next three months. The chin, mostly bony tissue, remains small.

The skeletal system, including bones and connective tissue, get properly under way during the second month. The "tadpole's" somites commence to swell out and form all the typical human muscles, which gradually insert themselves between the skin and the internal organs. The pattern of the bones-to-be is first laid down in a softer kind of connective tissue which we call cartilage (or "gristle"). The cartilage forms models for the bones in somewhat the same way that a sculptor forms in soft clay what he will later cast in harder stone or metal.

The process of exchanging cartilage for bone is called "ossification." The harder bone tissue contains minerals like calcium and phosphorus.

The bones of the skull and the face are an exception to the general rule for the ossification of ribs, backbone, long bones of the legs and arms, and other bones. The skull and face bones, some seventeen in all, are not first modeled in cartilage. They do not become completely and finally fused into one another to form a solid skull until the embryo has grown into an adult. The newborn infant normally has certain soft spots, called fontanelles, on his skull where the bones have not yet fused.

Beginning of Sex Differentiation. The sex of the person-to-be, is determined at the time of conception. During the second month of life those embryonic organs which will eventually be parts of the finished sexual apparatus of the adult man or woman begin to develop. By the end of the seventh week of life the internal sex organs of the embryo can usually be identified by an embryologist as either male or female.

The first internal sex organs developed in the embryo are the same for both sexes. Later they differentiate.

The sex-organs-to-be take their origin and make their first appearance on the embryo's middle kidney. There during the second month of life appears a little ridge of flesh, which embryologists call either a "genital" or a "sexual" ridge. Within it develop the individual's first "primitive" sex organs.

On the surface of the ridge are to be found growing little cords of cells, called "genital cords." The cords push or infiltrate their way down below the surface of the ridge. They make a place for themselves in the interior of the ridge which is then properly described as a sex gland or gonad.

If the embryo is to be a male, the genital cords continue growing as they started. They become the tubules of the testicles (seminiferous tubules), where the male in part manufactures his sperm.

However, if the embryo is to be a female, the genital cords stop growing and a new process takes place. Now from the surface, not the interior, of the tiny gonad (later to be a true ovary) a new set of cells start to grow. These surface cells are the forerunners of what will later be the female's egg cells.

The remarkable thing to be observed here is that inside every female ovary there is the undeveloped (embryonic) testis of the male.

The external sex organs in the male or female embryo do not become visible and apparent until the third month of life, though they start out in the same way during the second month. At this earlier time just in front of the "human tadpole's" tail can be located a little protuberance which the embryologists describe as the "genital tubercle." It appears the same in both sexes. Later it will develop into the penis in the male and its homologue (similar structure), the clitoris, in the female.

The Third Month of Life. By the time the embryo begins its third month of life, its internal organs have been pretty well laid down. We have now the recognizable sketch of a human being. It is all out of proportion, like a child's crude drawing of the human figure. Here are some of the important details in the development of the living creature that are filled in during the third month of life:

Sex emerges, more rapidly evident in the male than in the female. The teeth begin to sprout, though they will not become visible above the gum margins for years. Arms, legs, hands, and feet become more fully formed. Fingernails and toenails appear. The ears are formed. Liver, stomach, and kidneys commence functioning.

The stomach begins tentatively to pour out mucus; and other parts of the alimentary tract stir vaguely toward functioning. The liver starts its life-long job of manufacturing bile and takes on the temporary task of making red blood cells. The manufacture of mature red blood cells is eventually taken over by the bone marrow.

Mouth and jaws, nose and throat, including vocal cords, become more fully fashioned during this third month. On the rudimentary framework of the upper and lower jaws-to-be there now appears a dental ridge. Beneath it are soon to be found small cones of cells which turn out to be the "tooth buds" for the child's first set of baby (deciduous) teeth. There are normally ten sockets for baby teeth in each jaw. The dental ridge then sinks deeper into the jawbone, where it sets out buds for the thirty-two adult (permanent) teeth that will make their appearance above the gums anywhere from six to twenty years later.

After the third month the embryo is usually called a fetus. This change in name is a purely arbitrary matter, for which there is no special reason.

Fourth, Fifth, and Sixth Months of Life. During the fourth, fifth, and sixth months of life, the normal fetus makes rapid strides toward physiological maturity. As it leaps in weight from an ounce at the end of the third month to about two pounds at the end of the sixth, its presence generally becomes evident to the outside world in the rounding contour of its mother's abdomen.

The fourth month usually marks the time when the mother first feels a "quickening in the womb." This means that the fetus has grown to a stage where it can begin to move about.

Another interesting development in the fourth month is the increase in the volume and intensity of the fetal heart beat. With the use of a stethoscope, which conducts sound, the physician can often hear this minuscule heart beating through the mother's abdomen.

The forging of the human brain also makes significant progress at this time. The growth of the brain, which commenced in the "neural groove," is gradual. At first the hindbrain is most conspicuous. The midbrain appears less important. Most slowly developed of all is the forebrain. This is the part of the brain which gives rise to the large cerebral hemispheres of the adult where, it is commonly held, the real "thinking" part of the brain is located.

During the fourth month convolutions ("wrinkles") appear in the cerebral hemispheres of the fetus. From then on the brain develops with astonishing rapidity. Soon it outruns every other mammal's brain in complexity and capacity for ideation.

Beginning in the fourth month many changes occur in the external appearance of the fetus. The external sex organs for both sexes become more specifically delineated. Eyebrows and eyelashes may appear. A fine, soft, down-like hair, called "lanugo," covers the gnome-like body. Often it

is especially prominent on the face. The dark-wine color of the skin, which is produced by the blood vessels showing through it, becomes slightly less pronounced as the skin adds a few layers of thickness. The whorls and ridges on the skin of the toes and fingers are more or less fully patterned at this time; the four-month-old fetus already has the fingerprints by which he can be identified for the rest of his life.

In the fifth month real hair, something more than lanugo, shows up on the head of the fetus. Fingernails and toenails are also to be found, growing out beyond the tips of fingers and toes. Sweat glands and sebaceous (oil-secreting) glands come into being.

By the fifth month the internal organs are all present but they have not yet assumed the size, position, and function that they will have at birth. Heart and liver, for example, are still comparatively large and high up in the body framework. As the fetus continues to grow, its back straightens, its trunk lengthens, and its internal organs settle into their proper places.

During the sixth month of intra-uterine life the fetus begins to open its eyes, previously sealed shut. The eyes at birth usually appear an indeterminate gray-blue color.

The Final Months of Intra-Uterine Life. During the seventh, eighth, and ninth months of normal intra-uterine life the fetus fills out and develops in many ways. It gains much weight and strength. It waxes fat; its skin loses its wrinkles and improves in color. In the male an especially important event normally occurs during the seventh month, namely, the testes descend from their place of origin in the abdomen to the scrotal sac appended outside the body trunk.

During its sojourn in the uterus, the human fetus can theoretically assume any position and it certainly does move around. However, it rarely assumes strange or abnormal positions. About 95% of the time it grows head down.

The normal gestation period of the human infant is about forty weeks or nine months. Some infants, born prematurely[1], are not fully enough

[1]Technically speaking, any newborn infant weighing less than 2500 grams (5½ pounds) is considered premature.

developed to withstand the shock of birth and of facing survival outside their intra-uterine homes. The less the premature infant weighs at birth, the lower are his chances of survival, yet many can be saved and continue their development to full maturity.

Pregnancy

Pregnancy begins with conception and ends with childbirth (labor) or abortion (miscarriage).

In the very early stages of pregnancy even the wisest doctor may find it difficult to make a positive diagnosis. False pregnancies, with many of the classic symptoms of pregnancy, are sometimes discovered in women who have an overwhelming fear or desire of having a child. Tumors sometimes mimic pregnancy.

A delayed or missed menstrual period may raise a *suspicion* of pregnancy, but it should not be taken as a certainty that pregnancy has occurred. If *two* periods are missed, the woman should consult her doctor.

Starting about two weeks after a missed period, the condition of pregnancy can usually be confirmed by a laboratory test, the "mouse" or "rabbit test." These tests are about 98% accurate, but they do give a few false positives and false

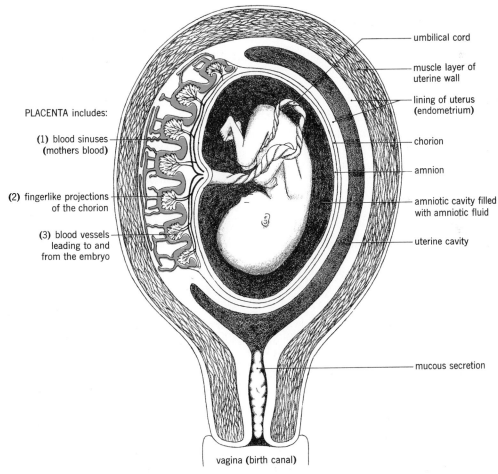

PLACENTA includes:

(1) blood sinuses (mothers blood)

(2) fingerlike projections of the chorion

(3) blood vessels leading to and from the embryo

umbilical cord

muscle layer of uterine wall

lining of uterus (endometrium)

chorion

amnion

amniotic cavity filled with amniotic fluid

uterine cavity

mucous secretion

vagina (birth canal)

THE UTERUS IN PREGNANCY. This is a diagrammatic cross section of the uterus containing a fetus about three months old. The cross section of the placenta is very much simplified.

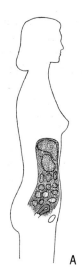

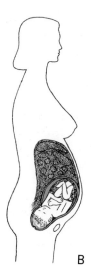

THE FIGURE IN PREGNANCY. A. This is a diagrammatic cross section of the mother's body at the beginning of pregnancy. B. This is the same figure at full term, just before the child is to be born. The figure returns to normal shortly after childbirth. Many women have better figures after bearing one or more (but not an excessive number of) children.

negatives. In the rabbit (Friedman) test, a sample of the woman's urine is injected into the ear of a virgin rabbit. If the woman is pregnant, changes in the rabbit's ovaries can be detected within 24 to 48 hours.

The rabbit and mouse tests, and all others depending on reactions in test animals (for example, toads and fish), are based on this fact: when pregnancy occurs, there is a drastic change in the hormone and endocrine balance of the body. This, incidentally, explains in part why many women feel different during pregnancy. Some may feel wonderful, others melancholy.

In particular, large quantities of gonad-stimulating hormones are made and released into the blood stream in early pregnancy. The kidneys extract hormones from the blood stream and release them into the urine. It is these hormones that stimulate the changes in the sex organs of the test animals, such as the virgin rabbit.

Timetable of Pregnancy. The following timetable suggests what a woman going through a normal, uneventful pregnancy may anticipate although, needless to say, not all women have the same experience.

1st Month. Within 2 to 3 weeks after concep-tion, the suspicion of missing a period must arise. Some of the early symptoms of pregnancy, described below, may appear at this time, but they usually come on somewhat later.

2nd Month. Morning sickness—nausea and vomiting—may develop; it is not inevitable. Easy fatigue, extreme sleepiness, full and sensitive breasts, frequent urination often appear—but not all these symptoms in all women.

3rd Month. The breasts begin to enlarge; the ring around the nipples may darken. The abdomen is not yet noticeably extended, but the uterus can be felt either as a small hard ball or softening and enlarging. The feeling of fatigue may be tremendous. An appetite for "strange foods" may begin. Neither symptom is essential.

4th Month. The pregnancy usually begins to show on the abdomen, unless concealed by obesity or artful dressing. Gain in weight commences. This usually continues at the rate of about *3 pounds a month*, with considerable variation in different women.

5th and 6th Months. The quickening of the baby is definitely felt by the mother; these at first are light, fluttery movements. Later they can be felt as definite kicks against the wall of the enlarged abdomen. The baby's rapid heartbeat can be definitely heard by the doctor.

7th and 8th Months. The rapidly growing baby kicks vigorously against the still-enlarging abdomen, on which striations, or stretch marks, usually appear. Skin color on the abdomen and face may darken slightly, but not permanently. A few drops of fluid—colostrum, a precursor of mother's milk—may begin to flow from the breasts. Weight gain continues.

9th Month. The abdomen no longer enlarges. The fetal movements are felt less often, less vigorously. This is nothing to worry about. The enlarged uterus may cause pressure symptoms on other abdominal organs and on the veins, giving symptoms of temporarily enlarged veins in the legs. The need for frequent urination is common. However, the expectant mother is often filled with unusual energy at this time. She cleans house, buys clothes, gets ready for the baby.

About 2 weeks before childbirth, the infant's head may begin to sink into the pelvic cavity and the uterus correspondingly descends with it. This is the "lightening." The woman usually feels more comfortable.

At last, somewhere around 280 days after conception, labor begins and the baby is born.

The Date of Birth. When will the baby be born? In round numbers, 280 days, 40 weeks, or 9 months after the day of conception. But there is no way of foretelling this *exactly*, because no one yet knows what sets off the trigger mechanism of normal labor. Unless the labor is artificially induced or Caesarean section done, the exact date of birth cannot be assured. A common method of predicting birth date (Naegle's rule) is to add 7 days to the date of the first day of the last menstruation and then count back 3 months. Only 1 in 10 babies is born on this calculated calendar date. But 75% are born within 2 weeks of this time.

Prenatal Care

Pregnancy is a natural, normal physiological process. The hazards of pregnancy are today comparatively few, and the discomforts are more often determined by the woman's own psychological attitude toward her particular pregnancy than by anything else.

Some women are depressed by their pregnancies, especially if they have had any trouble before or have borne many children. Other women find their health improved during pregnancy (relief from arthritis or migraine, for example, often occurs).

Nulliparas (women who have not been pregnant nor had a child before) are likely to be

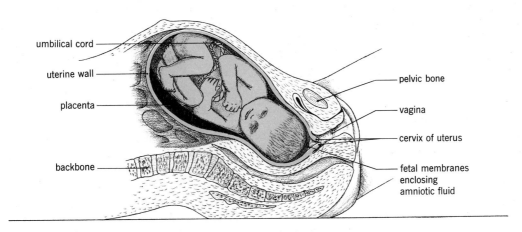

NORMAL SPONTANEOUS DELIVERY I. At term, as the first stage of labor begins. This illustration shows the position of the fetus in the uterus at the beginning of labor. The cervix has not begun to dilate (open up).

overenthusiastic, overmeticulous, and overfearful. Such anxiety in the presence of what is, after all, a profoundly important experience is natural and to be anticipated.

From the standpoint of the patient, prenatal care looks deceptively simple. From the doctor's standpoint it often requires consummate skill to keep the patient and her human freight out of trouble.

Personal hygiene during pregnancy is the same as good health care at any other time, magnified by the responsibility for the life and health of two (or more) lives instead of one.

A patient receiving adequate prenatal care from a private physician or a clinic is expected to:

1. See the doctor regularly—once a month during the early months of pregnancy, twice a month or oftener in the later stages.

2. Bring urine samples when requested.

3. Do what her doctor tells her and not listen to old wives' tales, the misinformation peddled by well-meaning friends, sensational magazine articles, or half-baked books.

4. Report promptly to the doctor any unusual signs or symptoms of disease or any sudden changes in her condition.

Repeated urinalyses are performed because the kidneys are under special strain in pregnancy; the waste products from the fetal circulation are passed back into the mother's blood stream by way of the placenta, and these wastes are removed from the maternal blood by the kidneys.

Childbirth

Pregnancy normally terminates in labor, that is to say, in the spontaneous delivery of a healthy, well-developed, full-term infant.

Labor. *Labor* is well named. The uterine and other muscles work hard. The mother sweats, sometimes losing several pints of fluid. A normal fatigue usually follows labor. Women accustomed to hard physical labor every day may be less affected by childbirth.

Labor is normally divided into three stages. The *first* stage extends from the beginning of labor pains to the time of full dilation (opening) of the mouth or neck of the womb. It is the longest stage, lasting perhaps 10 to 16 hours with the first baby. The *second* stage extends from the time of the dilation of the cervix until the actual birth of the baby. It may take anywhere up to 2 hours. The *third* stage extends from the birth of the baby to the expulsion of the afterbirth (placenta). It may be completed in 2 or 3, but usually 5 to 10 minutes.

The length of labor varies in different women and in the same women in different pregnancies. Rarely it may be over in less time than it takes

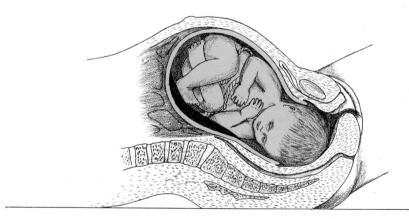

NORMAL SPONTANEOUS DELIVERY II. At the end of the first and the beginning of the second stage of labor. The rupture of the membranes ("bag of waters") usually occurs at the end of the first stage of labor. The cervix of the uterus is now completely dilated.

for a taxicab to get to a hospital. On the average, a woman bearing her first child will be in labor for about 18 hours; if she has already had a child, about 12 hours.

Labor pains usually begin in the small of the back and progress to the abdomen. True labor pains are always associated with contractions of the uterus. Between pains (contractions) there is usually no discomfort. The first contractions may occur every quarter or half hour and last a quarter to half a minute. The pains gradually begin to last longer, to become more frequent and intense, and to come at more regular intervals. As soon as they become *regular* it is time to call a doctor and, on his advice, to be off to the hospital. *False* labor pains often occur, frequently about a month before the baby is born. The diagnosis here is a problem for the doctor. False labor pains are usually irregular.

Delivery. Most women are admitted to the hospital while still in the first stage of labor. The woman is immediately put to bed and prepared by nurses for an aseptic delivery. Pubic hair is shaved, an enema usually given. Members of the hospital house-staff of physicians may look in and perhaps examine the patient. Her pains are timed by an attendant. If necessary, one or more drugs may be injected to help relieve pain or discomfort.

When examination reveals that the cervix is fully dilated—it has a temporary diameter of about 4 inches—the mother-soon-to-be is taken into the delivery room, usually on a wheel table, and placed on the delivery table. It has elevated leg rests, or stirrups, on two corners.

The woman lies on her back, her feet elevated by the leg rests. Her body is draped with sheets.

About this time the bag of waters breaks, and amniotic fluid pours out of the vagina. This sometimes happens early in the first stage of labor, causing a so-called *dry labor.* In other cases, the doctor has to puncture a thick amniotic membrane.

The rhythmic contractions of the uterus continue, exerting a powerful force squeezing the child out into the world. The contractions or pains cannot be voluntarily controlled by the mother. She can, however, "bear down" by using abdominal muscles to help along the contractions. Or she can relax and let the uterus work.

At length, in about 95 out of 100 cases, the top of the baby's head appears at the vaginal orifice. It recedes somewhat as the contraction that brought it down subsides. With each new contraction, the baby's head comes out farther and farther—and finally does not recede between pains.

At this point the doctor grasps the child under the chin. He turns the head gently to one side and then the other as he releases the shoulder.

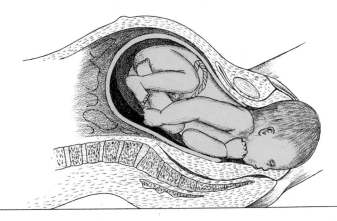

NORMAL SPONTANEOUS DELIVERY III. The second stage of labor, when the child is actually born. The infant's head is impelled into the birth canal (vagina), now greatly enlarged, by the force of uterine contractions. The top of the infant's head appears here at the vaginal orifice.

The rest of the child can be easily lifted out of the birth canal. The infant is still attached to his mother by the umbilical cord.

While waiting for the third stage of labor to be concluded (delivery of the afterbirth), the doctor immediately swabs out the baby's mouth and waits for the first cry. Most infants cry lustily as soon as they are born (a few, even, just before). If regular breathing is not quickly established, the doctor may hold the baby upside down, give him a few gentle slaps on the buttocks, or if necessary, apply a tiny oxygen mask. Breathing air is the first of the many new experiences that await the baby. Rapid changes occur in his lungs and heart while he is getting used to it.

After a final surge of blood from the placenta, the umbilical cord is tied off, about 3 inches above the navel, and cut. The cord stump is covered with a sterile dressing and placed over the abdomen. Infection must be avoided.

Drops of silver nitrate or other acceptable antiseptic (e.g., penicillin) are immediately put into the baby's eyes to protect against possible blindness from gonorrheal infection. The baby is cleaned off as much as necessary, wrapped in a blanket, weighed, footprinted, encircled with an identification bracelet (so that babies can't possibly get mixed up), and placed in a warm crib.

When the afterbirth is expelled, the physician examines it to be sure that it is all out. Imme-diately after the child has been expelled, the uterus begins to contract. In so doing it squeezes off the blood vessels that were broken when the placenta was torn off. To speed this process and prevent needless bleeding, the doctor may give drugs (ergot and pituitrin), which are called *oxytocics*. Only $\frac{1}{4}$ to $\frac{1}{2}$ pint of blood is usually lost. If more, it can be promptly replaced by transfusion.

Following delivery the new mother usually sleeps. Doctors now make every effort to get the mother back on her feet as soon as possible after childbirth—anywhere from the first day on. A few days' to a week's convalescence in the hospital is usually enough—if there are no complications. Many women are anxious to leave earlier. The maternity ward is usually the gayest one in the hospital. A gradually increasing schedule of activity and social life is desirable. Visitors with colds or other communicable infections should not be welcomed. It takes about six weeks for the mother's body to return to the size and shape it had before pregnancy.

Complications of Childbirth. These do occur, but most of them are prevented by adequate prenatal care. Approximately 95% of all babies present themselves to the world head first and go through the normal spontaneous delivery just described. In about 4% the buttocks show first (breech presentation). In the other 1% a shoulder, leg or arm may first present. All these presenta-

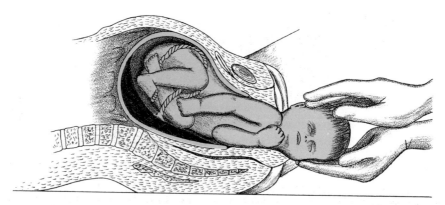

NORMAL SPONTANEOUS DELIVERY IV. The moment of birth, the end of the second stage of labor. The physician gently grasps the head of the infant and prepares to help the rest of his body into the world.

tions can be handled by appropriate obstetric maneuvers ("turning the baby"), delivery by the breech, or by Caesarean section.

"Painless Childbirth." *Painless childbirth* has been a goal of obstetrics since the middle of the nineteenth century, shortly after the discovery of ether as a surgical anesthetic. In 1853 Queen Victoria accepted obstetric anesthesia during the birth of her seventh child—and women everywhere have since demanded painless childbirth. The Queen got intermittent doses of chloroform, just enough at each labor pang to ease the pain but not enough to make her unconscious.

A great variety of anesthetic agents are now available for obstetric anesthesia and analgesia (painkilling without loss of consciousness). Used with discretion they have relatively little effect on the baby. Present-day *"twilight sleep"* is produced by a mixture of an analgesic (painkilling) drug, such as Demerol, with an amnesic drug, like scopolamine, that temporarily wipes out memory. Other methods are nerve-blocking injections of local anesthetics in the pelvic region, for example, caudal anesthesia, in which injections are made at the tail end of the spinal cord.

Education for childbirth is another direction of effort to reduce labor pains. These are the techniques that have been given the name *"natural childbirth."* Their aim is to reduce false fears about childbirth and thus greatly diminish the pains associated with it. In many cases, it may help to reduce pains, but it rarely eliminates them. Hypnotism has also been tried in a few selected cases of childbirth.

Needless fear of childbirth has been bred into many young women by their families and associates—and blithely accepted by their husbands. A classic cartoon shows a young husband and his wife, who is ready for delivery, entering the admitting office of a hospital. The caption reads, "Honey, are you sure you want to go through with this?" Some women (and men) fear childbirth because they heard their mothers and other female relatives complain of it. Others fear childbirth because it is associated with what Guttmacher calls "the larger, terrifying fear of sex." Childbirth is no picnic, but abnormal, neurotic fear undoubtedly tightens up the muscles employed in childbirth and makes it seem more difficult.

Abortion. A high percentage of pregnancies—perhaps one-third—terminate in abortion, a word of ugly connotation. When applied to induced, criminal abortions ("illegal operations"), this connotation is correct. However, it should be noted that there are also therapeutic abortions and spontaneous abortions. Scientifically, abortion may be defined as the "detachment or expulsion of the previable ovum, embryo, or fetus."

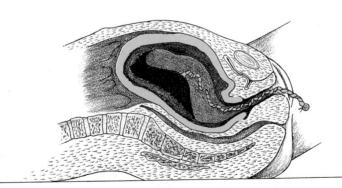

NORMAL SPONTANEOUS DELIVERY V. The third stage of labor. The child has already been born and the umbilical cord cut and tied. In the third stage of labor the placenta, loosened from the uterine wall, is expelled from the uterus along with the remains of the fetal membranes. Note that there is already a thickening of the uterine walls as the uterus begins to shrink and return to its normal, nonpregnant size and shape.

A therapeutic abortion is generally defined as one undertaken, on appropriate medical indications, "to save the life and health of the mother." If performed in a licensed hospital, two licensed, competent physicians must sign an affirmation and diagnosis.

The terms "spontaneous abortion" and "miscarriage" are synonyms. They describe the involuntary, undesired expulsion and loss of the embryo or fetus and hence the termination of pregnancy through the first seven months (28 weeks) of pregnancy. If this event occurs after the seventh month, it is called premature birth. When an infant is born dead, it is termed a stillbirth.

Miscarriages, or spontaneous abortions, usually occur during the first three months of pregnancy. The causes are imperfectly known and difficult to attribute to specific cases. More than half are owing to some abnormality in the formation or imbedding of the egg. It can be said, however, that falls, jars, violent blows, and other forms of physical trauma must be classed as secondary or precipitating rather than primary causes of miscarriage. Spontaneous abortion is a medical problem; induced abortion a social problem, and an ancient one.

It is the consensus of opinion in the United States today that a criminal, induced abortion is the worst way out of an "unwanted pregnancy." And yet the latest Kinsey figures show that among American wives 17% of pregnancies end in induced abortion.

Sterility. Approximately 1 in 10 to 15 marriages in the United States appears to be sterile; that is, the married couple desire children, have marriage relationships over a period of a year or more, but the wife does not conceive. Much medical research has been directed at this problem of sterility. For a third to a half of the couples who would formerly have been doomed to involuntary childlessness, proper medical treatment now makes conception, pregnancy, and the birth of a healthy child possible.

The causes of sterility, infertility, or barrenness, as it is called, are various. In almost half the cases the husband is at least partially at fault. In very many instances sterility is *relative* rather than absolute. Either mate might be able to have a child with a different partner, or after suitable treatment, or after a lapse of time. Occasionally, a long-childless couple finally manage to adopt a baby and shortly thereafter have a baby of their own.

SUMMARY

In Summary: In life before birth every human being recapitulates the evolutionary history of the human race. Starting as a one-celled creature, the single fertilized egg cell or zygote, he proceeds through stages and phases of multicellular life. For example, in the second month of intra-uterine life, he can be described as a "human tadpole"; he briefly develops and gets rid of a tail. At an astonishing rate of growth, however, the embryo and then the fetus develop anatomical structures and physiological functions that can be scientifically explained only as the outcome of the organic evolution of the human race. In the specialized cells and tissues and in the integrated body systems of the newborn infant resides repeated evidence that, from any point of view, the human being is "fearfully and wonderfully made."

In the process of childbirth, labor, and delivery the mother goes through a process and experience which links her with all other mothers. The usual outcome of pregnancy is a normal, spontaneous delivery.

SUMMARY REVIEW QUESTIONS

1. What is the difference between Victorian and modern attitudes toward pregnancy and childbirth? How do you account for them?
2. How would you describe in some detail the process of life before birth?
3. What temporary anatomical structures—embryo excluded—develop in the uterus during pregnancy? What is the function of each one and what happens to it at childbirth?
4. How is a diagnosis of pregnancy made? Be explicit.
5. How does the "timetable of pregnancy" correlate with the intra-uterine life of the infant-to-be?
6. From the standpoint of either (*a*) a prospective father or (*b*) an expectant mother, what do you consider to be the essentials of "adequate prenatal care?"
7. Beginning with the first suspicion of "labor pains," what are the subsequent stages or steps of normal spontaneous delivery of a newborn child?
8. How do you distinguish between (1) spontaneous, (2) induced, (3) therapeutic, and (4) criminal abortion?
9. Are the following statements sense or nonsense? Why? *The process of childbirth is and forever will be a mystery. . . . Childbirth is exclusively a woman's business. . . . Sterility is incurable. . . . A healthy human embryo weighs at least one pound within one month after conception. . . . The very best man in the world/ Must take his child on faith alone;/ The very worst woman in the world/ Knows her child's her own.*
10. What do the following terms mean to you: zygote, embryo, fetus, premature infant, relative sterility, ossification, "natural childbirth," the "quickening," "rabbit test," miscarriage.

Worth Consulting: *The Story of Human Birth* by Alan Guttmacher, M.D. *Childbirth without Fear* by Grantly Dick Read, M.D. *Biography of the Unborn* by Margaret Shea Gilbert. *Expectant Motherhood* by Nicholas Eastman, M.D. For more complete references, see Appendix E.

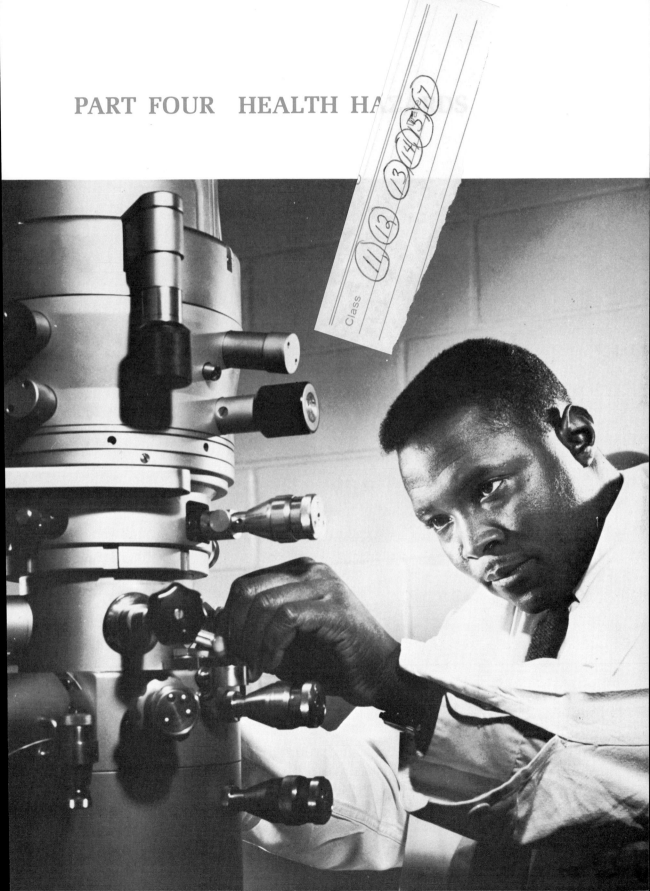

This cancer researcher utilizing an electron microscope exemplifies another step in the long march to control disease. (Photograph courtesy of Chas. Pfizer & Co., Inc.)

16

THE BIG KILLERS:

HEART DISEASE AND CANCER

IF YOU ARE NOT KILLED MEANWHILE BY ACCI-
dent, the chances are 2 out of 3 that you
will die either of heart disease or cancer—the two
degenerative diseases that are now far and away
the big killers of Americans. The older you grow
the more likely you are to die of one or the other.

Principal Causes of Death

In 1900 the five principal causes of death in
the United States were, in order: (1) tuberculosis,
(2) pneumonia, (3) diarrhea and inflammation
of intestines, (4) heart disease, and (5) diseases
of infancy and malformations.

Today the list of the big killers runs: (1) heart
and circulatory diseases, (2) cancer, (3) stroke, (4)
accidents, and (5) certain diseases and conditions
of early infancy.

The causes of death differ at different ages in
life. Accidents, however, top the list from childhood through age 45.

The leading causes of infant mortality (under
1 year of age) now rank as (1) premature birth,
(2) postnatal asphyxia and atelectasis, (3) congenital malformations, (4) other diseases of early
infancy, and (5) pneumonia and influenza.

Among preschool children (ages 2 through 4)
the five chief killers are, in order: accidents, cancer, congenital malformations, pneumonia, gastritis and enteritis.

Elementary and junior-high-school students
(ages 5 through 14) succumb, in order, to: acci-

dents, cancer, congenital malformations, and
pneumonia.

In the senior-high-school and college-age
bracket (ages 15 through 24) the picture changes
to: accidents, cancer, suicide, heart disease, and
murder.

Young adults and parents (ages 25 to 44) die
chiefly, in order, from: accidents, heart disease,
cancer, suicide, and stroke.

The middle-aged (ages 45 to 64) are fatally
stricken with, in order: heart disease, cancer,
stroke, accidents, and suicide.

The aged (65 and over) are killed by, in order:
heart disease, cancer, stroke, hardening of the
arteries, and accidents.

Heart Disease

In the United States heart disease is now responsible for close to 700,000 deaths a year,
approximately 40% of all deaths. Related diseases
of the circulatory system kill 250,000 more people. In total these conditions are the primary
cause of more than one out of every two deaths
in the United States.

We must consider diseases of the heart, blood
vessels, and kidneys together since they operate
that way. Disease or damage in any one of these
three sets of organs is sooner or later reflected in
the other two. We speak therefore of the *cardiovascularenal* system: "cardio" for heart, "vascular"
for blood vessels, and "renal" for kidneys. When

we talk about heart disease, we are really talking about cardiovascular diseases.

Over 90% of all cardiovascularenal deaths are associated with hardening of the arteries— (arteriosclerosis and atherosclerosis) and high blood pressure (hypertension). Blood-vessel damage in the brain—commonly called "stroke"— accounts for about 200,000 deaths a year in the United States.

At any given time somewhere between 10 and 11 million people in the United States are walking around with cardiovascularenal disease. (Only about 5% of the victims are confined to bed.) If you add to the count varicose veins, minor vascular ailments, and unobserved "little strokes," you can calculate that well over 10% of the American population is afflicted with cardiovascularenal ailments.

Discounting the Statistical Picture. Yet, the average person faces no greater risk of dying of heart disease than his grandfather did in 1900. The increase in cardiovascular deaths reflects the success of medicine and public health in preventing earlier deaths from infectious diseases. It also reflects the increased life span of the American population. Approximately two-thirds of cardiovascularenal deaths occur after the age of 65. The death rate from cardiovascular disease has remained constant for the last twenty years.

The hardworking circulatory system is usually the first to wear out as life forces diminish. When we announce that cardiovascularenal diseases account for 55% of the total mortality in the United States, we must also remember that the final total is 100%. Man is mortal. If the Angel of Death were not now using this big cardiovascularenal scythe, he could equally well use others, and more painful ones, as he has in the past. Indeed it has been stated that a high percentage of deaths from stroke is an index of a generally healthy community.

The real problem in cardiovascularenal diseases is the effective treatment and management of patients who come down with these conditions in the prime of life, or earlier. Here great advances have been and still are being made.

It was not so long ago that cardiovascular syphilis accounted for 25% of all heart disease. Today it is considerably less than 1%. Rheumatic heart disease is also on the wane, thanks largely to improved antibiotics, used effectively and widely as a preventive measure. Rheumatic fever control programs, now in operation in many states, afford an excellent example of the wedding of personal and community health.

Research Developments. The dramatic highlights of recent research progress in cardiovascularenal diseases lie in the fields of heart surgery, the discovery and development of new drugs, and in a better practical understanding of the treatment of the *complications* of high blood pressure and hardening of the arteries. The causes of these vascular conditions, however, still remain obscure and unproved.

Entirely new and life-saving types of heart surgery are now being routinely developed. These have been made possible by new pumping machines, "artificial hearts," that keep up the blood circulation of the body during an operation on the heart, and by techniques for actually stopping the heart. The surgeon can now work with a heart that lies still instead of wiggling and jumping out of his hands.

A triumph in heart surgery came in 1968. Surgeons then succeeded in transplanting a "healthy" heart from one person, just deceased, to another person whose heart was so barely competent that early death could be predicted. Many patients did not live too long after the operation, for they were "bad risk" patients to begin with. However, Dr. Christian Barnard of the Union of South Africa succeeded in transplanting a human heart into a 69-year-old dentist, Philip Blaiberg, who lived for many months after the operation.

Just a few years ago there were no drugs that could safely and effectively reduce blood pressure. Now there are scores—including reserpine and other rauwolfia derivatives.

The complications of hardening arteries can also now be better managed with newly developed drugs. Among them are anticoagulants, drugs which help prevent the formation of blood clots; other drugs which forestall or suppress abnormal heart rhythms, the fatal flutter that sometimes follows heart attacks; and drugs which dilate the arteries of the heart, so that new pathways of circulation can be opened.

High Blood Pressure. Blood pressure represents the force of the blood beating back against the walls of the blood vessels. High blood pressure (hypertension) means added pressure on these walls. This makes the heart pump harder, eventually weakening it, and it increases the risk that blood vessels will break. In hypertension the systolic blood pressure may creep over the 200 (millimeters of mercury) mark. This might not be too serious if the blood vessels and the rest of the cardiovascularenal system could take it. Some people's can, but most cannot. Something has to give—commonly an artery in the heart or brain.

If you do have a tendency toward high blood pressure, there is a good chance that you inherited it. This will be especially true if you are short and stocky in build, plump, and "just can't sit still." The average life expectancy of an individual who suffers from high blood pressure is around 20 years from the onset of the disease. However, in any given case, the outcome of the raised blood pressure will depend on three factors: (1) how high the pressure goes, which is the least important of the three factors; (2) how long it stays up—the number of months or years is an important but not the decisive factor; and (3) how well the blood vessels can take it—this is the crux of the matter. Here too heredity counts. You may inherit blood vessels that can take the higher pressure and not break.

Frequent nosebleeds or, in women, excessive menstrual flow (menorrhagia) sometimes indicate that blood vessels cannot take high pressure very well. Other common, but not necessarily definitive, symptoms of high blood pressure include: headaches, fatigue, dizziness, lightheadedness, vertigo (you seem to be spinning around or the world is spinning around you, and a blackout sometimes follows), and a tendency to easy and blotchy blushing, often accompanied by rumbling of the bowels.

Hardening and Fattening of the Arteries. If death from heart or blood-vessel disease has to be pinned on to a specific cause, the right one is usually hardening of the arteries (arteriosclerosis) or fattening of the same (atherosclerosis). It will be remembered that each artery or arteriole has three coats or layers: an inner lining, thin and smooth as mucous membrane and called the intima; a middle layer, the media; and an outer layer, the adventitia. These living tissues get their nourishment from tiny capillaries and from the blood plasma they are carrying. The middle and outer layers of the arteries and arterioles are subject to hardening—getting arteriosclerotic. Sometimes they get as hard as pipestems.

Something else happens to the inner lining. It fattens. In more exact terms it suffers from *atherosclerosis*. It loses its smoothness; it becomes thickened, roughened and studded with little projections, which are primarily fat (lipid) particles.

The accumulation of these fat particles on the inner lining of the arteries has several unfortunate consequences. In the first place it narrows the bore or diameter of a vessel, clogging it up like a deposit of lime or rust inside a water pipe. This decreases the amount of blood that the vessel can carry and therefore increases the pressure necessary to force it through. Second, these extraneous fat particles stuck in the arterial walls invite the formation of blood clots.

Blood tends to clot far more easily when in contact with rough or scarred surfaces. If a clot stays where it forms on the inside of a blood vessel, it is called a *thrombus*. If it breaks away, it becomes an *embolus*. Both thrombi and emboli can clog blood vessels.

The fatty material that tends to stick in the inner walls of the arteries is primarily the chemical substance known as cholesterol, although fatty substances, notably triglycerides, are also involved. One important explanation of the mechanism by which atherosclerosis occurs begins with the obvious fact that fats (or lipids) cannot be dissolved in water. These fats can only be brought into water solution, and thus managed by the blood stream (plasma) and other body tissues when they are combined with proteins; thus they become "lipoproteins."

These are relatively large molecules and unstable in the sense that the bond between the fat and the protein is not always a strong one. These larger molecules may tend to get stuck in certain artery walls; furthermore, after they are stuck, the protein tends to get washed away by the blood plasma, while the fat particles of the molecule remain in the artery wall—and make trouble.

With the facts at hand, it is probably fair to consider atherosclerosis itself a metabolic disease, or at least a metabolic defect in the body's handling of certain fats (lipids) and lipoproteins. It should be noted that atherosclerosis is rare in women before the menopause. This may be attributed to the large quantities of female sex hormone in their bodies. Indeed, it has been shown that the administration of female sex hormone to *men* will inhibit atherosclerosis; but this process has a feminizing effect and reduces libido—to which the men object.

The relationship of female sex hormones to the inhibition of atherosclerosis and the importance of the relationship of atherosclerosis to cardiovascular disease and deaths explains why heart disease kills one and a half times as many men as women. Between the ages of 45 and 65 nearly three times as many men as women die of heart disease.

Types of Heart Disease

There are at least 20 kinds of *organic* heart disease that actually affect the heart muscle, the valves of the heart, or its inner or outer linings. There are also a number of functional disorders of the heart in which its function or action is altered. Heart trouble may be primary, or secondary to other diseases. The most common and serious forms of organic heart disease are those affecting the coronary arteries, which supply blood to the heart.

A *heart attack* is usually a case of *coronary thrombosis,* described below. *Heart failure* may be a late consequence of this or other conditions. This group of heart troubles is predominantly, but not exclusively, associated with the middle and later years of life.

Infections present the second large class of causes of organic heart disease. *Rheumatic fever,* or rheumatic heart disease, associated with certain streptococcal ("strep") infections, heads the list. Syphilis, diphtheria, tuberculosis, typhoid fever, and other infections can also injure the heart. Fortunately, these diseases can usually be treated (or prevented) before they cause heart damage.

Congenital heart defects, which develop before birth and are usually discovered shortly thereafter, account for about 2% of all heart defects. "Blue babies" have a congenital defect that permits the bluer venous blood to mix with arterial blood. Surgical operation for the correction of this condition is now commonplace.

Functional murmurs of the heart, sometimes heard through the physician's stethoscope, have little, if any, significance and should not be taken as a focus of worry. Some people also suffer from an irritable heart; they become acutely conscious of premature or extra beats of the heart. Generally speaking, this condition is not serious in the absence of organic lesions.

Other functional disorders of the heart include disturbances of psychic or emotional origin. In these cases the patient fears and believes that he has heart disease when he does not. He nevertheless develops symptoms associated with it, such as palpitation, shortness of breath, extreme fatigue, and dizzy spells. This condition has many names; for example, in World War I it was labeled "soldier's heart."

Because heart disease can be so specifically classified and so much more accurately diagnosed today, more specific and effective treatment is possible for each kind of heart disease. Not so many years ago coronary thrombosis was often diagnosed as acute indigestion.

Heart Attack. Every minute of the year somebody in the United States has a heart attack. Heart attack is the popular term for what physicians call *coronary thrombosis* (also coronary occlusion, coronary closure, and myocardial infarction). Heart attacks can be suddenly fatal, but the great majority—an estimated 85%—are not. The patient recovers under proper treatment and goes on to live many useful years. A heart attack is not a sentence to permanent invalidism.

The *average* life expectancy following a heart attack is better than 10 years. The younger the victim, the greater the future life expectancy. At least one-third of all heart-attack victims will be able to return to their full schedule of previous work and activity. Another third will have to take life easier than they did before. Still another thir [w] ha e t(tak it r ıcl ·as' r. C ıly about _____ invalid.
_____ onditions
_____ years. For
_____ (intima)
_____ hickened
_____ as *athero-*
_____ h supply
_____ changes.
_____ e flow of
_____ provides
_____ form on
_____ a throm-
_____ the blood
_____ ttack oc-

_____ ıly closed
_____ , in most
_____ ocked ar-
_____ s is called
_____ recovery.
_____ attack is
_____ onary ar-
_____ common
_____ "Women
_____ men de-
_____ arteries."
_____ nufacture
_____)ods that

_____ special diets cannot be depended on to prevent atherosclerosis or heart attack.

Most heart attacks occur while a patient is at rest in bed or working quietly. Vigorous exercise by a person unaccustomed to it may perhaps precipitate the final blood clotting in the coronary artery, but even if he had not exercised strenuously, the chances are the clot would soon have appeared. Hence it is foolish to indict any single event as the cause of a heart attack.

If you ever happen to be present when a heart attack occurs, call a doctor at once. Help the patient take the position that is most comfortable for him. This will probably be halfway between lying down and sitting up. He usually cannot breathe comfortable if he lies flat. Loosen tight clothing, such as collar and belt. See that the patient does not become chilled. Do *not* attempt to lift or carry the victim or give him anything to drink unless a doctor tells you to.

Heart Failure. When the heart is unable to pump blood efficiently to all parts of the body, the condition is described as *heart failure.* It may accompany or be the result of coronary-artery disease or other types of heart disease. Though serious, the condition is not necessarily rapidly fatal; many patients live 10 to 20 years or longer after congestive heart failure is first noted.

The cardinal symptom of heart failure is shortness of breath or difficult breathing (dyspnea). Another common and often early sign of congestive heart failure is swelling of the ankles, although this does not always betoken heart disease. When it is related to heart failure, however, it occurs because the heart is not pumping efficiently enough to get fluids out of the spaces between and within the body cells.

The treatment of the failing heart comprises efforts to reduce its work load, improve its action, and get rid of excess body fluids. Digitalis and diuretic drugs are commonly used. Furthermore, the patient must truly learn to live within his physical means, his cardiac reserve.

Rheumatic Heart Disease. Although by no means yet eliminated, rheumatic fever and its sequel, rheumatic heart disease, no longer pose the threat to life and health they recently did. Scarcely 1 in every 40 cardiovascularenal deaths can now be charged against either acute or chronic rheumatic fever.

Rheumatic fever is a serious disease because the valves of the heart can be damaged and scarred during the acute phase. Scarred valves produce heart murmurs, but they are not necessarily significant. The first attack of the disease usually occurs between the ages of 6 and 8, but it may sometimes be delayed to adolescence or early adulthood. The exact cause of the disease remains unknown, but it is now certain that attacks are associated with streptococcal infections—usually "strep throat." This fact gives an effective means both for treating and preventing the disease. With proper treatment at least two-thirds of the children attacked by rheumatic heart disease recover with little, if any, limitation on their future work and play.

The first step in the prevention of rheumatic heart disease is the prompt treatment of all "strep" infections. The second step is the regular use, often over long periods of time, of small, protective doses of sulfa drugs or antibiotics whenever the threat of strep infections is around. Injections of slow-acting, long-lasting penicillin appear to be particularly useful in preventing reinfection.

Blood-Vessel Surgery. One of the promising new lines of attack on the "villains" of the cardiovascular picture, the blood vessels, is to be found in the development of new surgical techniques (micro-surgery in some cases) to correct defects, evident or developing, in these "lifelines" of the human body. It was once thought that surgery for the relief of vascular disease would be practically impossible, owing to the smallness of the operative field and the narrow margin for error in operating on even the larger blood vessels. There are more than 60,000 miles of blood vessels in the average human body. They range in size from the aorta—which has about the diameter of an ordinary garden hose where it issues from the heart—to tiniest capillaries of so small a bore that only a single blood cell can pass through at a time.

Much of the progress in the new blood-vessel surgery has come from the development of seamless, flexible tubing (vascular prostheses) to replace damaged blood vessels. Greater ability to visualize the blood vessels by X-ray has also aided the operating surgeons. Blood-vessel surgery has already been successfully performed in

dealing with aneurysms (balloon-like pouches or sacs that puff up at weak points along the walls of the arterial blood-vessel system), in removing plugs from some arteries, in correcting defects of the aorta with which some infants are born, and in removing blood clots that have formed inside veins. Especially promising is surgery on blood vessels outside the brain because this gives new hope for the treatment of *stroke*.

Protecting Your Heart. *The symptoms of heart disease* have a unique characteristic: in general, the more serious the condition, the more remote from the heart are the symptoms. Periodic medical examinations—including electrocardiograms—offer one line of defense against heart troubles. Prompt attention to the twenty danger signals (see page 12) is a second approach. Early treatment of infections and other disease conditions that may eventuate in heart disease offers further protection against it.

Several years ago the question of whether fats (especially hard or saturated fats) should be included in the diet of those who wanted to escape heart diseases was a very live issue. The excitement has somewhat simmered down as it has become apparent that you cannot keep cholesterol out of the bloodstream simply by not ingesting it. The body is quite capable of manufacturing its own cholesterol. In September 1962, the Surgeon General of the U.S. Public Health Service observed that it would probably take a generation to prove whether any diet can reduce deaths due to heart or blood-vessel disease. In October 1962, the American Medical Association issued a press release, as follows:

Dieters who believe they can cut down their blood cholesterol without medical supervision are in for a rude awakening. It can't be done. It could even be dangerous to try. . . . Willy-nilly substitution of a few food items without over-all control of the diet accomplishes little if anything in reducing cholesterol.

Success in reducing blood cholesterol by dietary regulation so far has been achieved only in strictly controlled experimental groups, and use of this method remains largely experimental. The carefully calculated diets used in medical research to lower cholesterol are not yet of practical importance to the general public. The current concern about diet . . . should be directed away from hopeless pursuits to a worthwhile goal that can be attained by most individuals—maintaining normal weight. Overweight is the villain.

The simple rules of hygiene also help in avoiding heart disease. Be moderate in food intake and the use of tobacco and alcohol. Keep your weight within normal limits. Get reasonable amounts of rest and exercise in the rhythm of daily living. Avoid nervous tension so far as possible—and don't worry about getting heart disease.

The advice given in the famous "Regimen of Salerno," a twelfth-century Latin poem here rendered in sixteenth-century English, still applies:

Use three physicians still: first, Doctor Diet,
Next Doctor Merryman and then Doctor Quiet.

Stroke

Stroke is the term generally applied to apoplectic stroke, or apoplexy—the sudden breaking or clogging of a blood vessel in the brain. The effect of this vascular accident is either discouraging brain damage or sudden (and usually quite painless) death. People who are found dead in bed are frequently victims of stroke. Stroke generally occurs late in life and, like other cardiovascularenal damage or fatality, is associated with hardening of the arteries and high blood pressure.

Stroke appears as a sudden loss of consciousness (coma) followed by paralysis, generally of the side of the body opposite the side of the brain affected (hemiplegia). Face, arm, or leg may be paralyzed. A few victims of stroke die immediately; others linger on for a few weeks, if the lesions are extensive. But many recover more or less completely and live for years. The great Louis Pasteur did some of his best work after he had suffered a stroke.

Dr. Walter Alvarez has called attention to the frequency of "little strokes," which often go unrecognized for what they really are: brain damage. The victims of little strokes do not fall unconscious, but they lose their former mental sharpness. This is sometimes mistaken for or called senile dementia or "softening of the brain."

It is estimated that there are almost 2 million victims of stroke alive in the United States. The problem with most of these people, partially paralyzed hemiplegics, is to rehabilitate them so that they can still get much out of life.

Cancer

While cancer is a frightening word, the facts about it, as we shall see, are less fearful than the image of the disease.

Cancer begins insidiously and kills slowly—sometimes painfully, often expensively, and over half the time *needlessly*. It is the second great killer of Americans. Yet death from cancer is not inevitable. To a greater degree than with many other diseases it can be said that cancer is curable.

For example, if you had been present in the U.S. Senate Chamber in Washington, D.C., on April 1, 1958, you would have witnessed the first "Cured Cancer Congress" ever assembled. Men, women, and children gathered there were living testimony of many different types of cancer that can now be cured if caught in time. They represented 800,000 other living Americans who had already been saved from untimely death from cancer. (A "cured" cancer case is one in which the patient survives for at least five years without evidence of the recurrence of the disease.)

There is a blacker side to the cancer picture, but the occasion of the first "Cured Cancer Congress," sponsored by the American Cancer Society, dramatically illustrated that among all the major personal and community health problems cancer is susceptible of the earliest and most substantial improvement. Why?

Cancer Is Curable. Cancer untreated, or treated too late, is almost universally fatal. However, cancer treated in time and properly—by surgery and radiation—can be cured in at least one out of every two cases and usually in a much higher percentage. Here is the tragic and yet hopeful cancer story told in percentages:

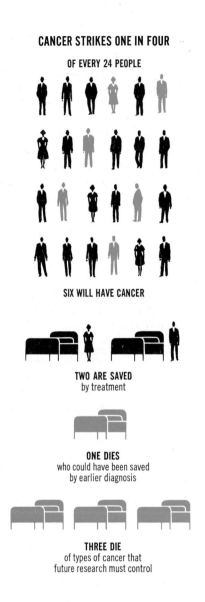

CANCER STRIKES ONE IN FOUR

OF EVERY 24 PEOPLE

SIX WILL HAVE CANCER

TWO ARE SAVED
by treatment

ONE DIES
who could have been saved
by earlier diagnosis

THREE DIE
of types of cancer that
future research must control

Cancer of the breast and uterus, which account for most cancers in women, can be cured in 80% of the patients afflicted. But only 45% of the breast cancers and of the uterine cancers, are being cured now.

The same sad story in percentages applies equally to the other common sites of cancer in the male and female bodies. Skin cancer—the most obvious and accessible form of cancer—can be cured in 95% of all cases, but the present percentage of cure is only 90%. Rectal cancer can

be cured in 70% of the cases, but only 35% are cured. When cancer of the mouth, evident both to dentist and physician, is a small lesion confined to the oral cavity, a 65% cure rate is possible; the present cure rate is only 35%. Lung cancer patients present the sorriest picture of all; 35% could be cured; only 5% are cured. The basic reason for the difference between what is and what could be lies in delay on the part of the patients in seeking early medical diagnosis and treatment.

What Is Cancer? Cancer is usually described as a degenerative disease. Its incidence, like that of heart disease, increases sharply with age. While cancer does occur at earlier ages, and even in children, the vast majority of cases occur after age 45. Most college students, therefore, first become personally aware of the cancer tragedy when it strikes their aging parents, relatives, and family friends. It is sometimes one of the bitterest of tragedies of youth to have to stand by helplessly for months while a beloved parent or relative, cancer-struck, expensively hospitalized, and beyond hope of cure by surgery or radiation, wastes away.

Cancer is not really one disease; it is a whole class of diseases with one characteristic in common: irregular cell growth. Cancer is primarily a disease of cells rather than of body parts or systems.

Microscopically, a great many different varieties of cancer can be identified. Cancer is therefore a *group* of diseases characterized by abnormal, uncontrolled, "lawless" growth of body cells. Plants and animals are also subject to cancerous growths.

Cells are the fundamental units of all living matter. In the normal process of growth and repair, cells grow and take their places in the economy of the body according to what may be called the "rules of nature." Cell growth and development is an extremely complicated process whose central secrets have not yet been fathomed.

Sometimes, for reasons still unknown, a cell or group of cells breaks the ordinary rules of nature. They behave in a disorderly way; they grow wildly. There is no place for them in the normal structure and function of the body. Like weeds in a garden, they crowd out normal, useful cells and steal their food supply. When enough of these wild cells cluster together, they can sometimes be felt as a lump. Unless the growth of these abnormal cancer cells can be checked by some means (usually outside intervention), they oust so many normal cells that eventually the body can no longer function and the victim dies. For example, when cancer cells invade the stomach, they crowd out the specialized stomach cells necessary for digesting food. Hence the patient eventually starves to death.

Cancer cells can start in any part of the body, but some sites are more favored. Unfortunately these cells rarely remain where they originate. Clusters or clumps of cancer cells break off and travel in the blood stream to other parts of the body—from the breast to the armpits, for example. This spread of cancer cells is called *metastasis*.

Cancer cells are definitely different from ordinary cells, and these differences can be observed in tiny sections of tissue removed from the body by surgical techniques (biopsy) and examined under a microscope. Identifying cancer cells is an important part of the job of the pathologist.

Not all new growths are *malignant,* as cancerous growths are described. Many, if not most, new growths are *benign*. They do not spread wildly; they can be safely removed. Since benign tumors are so common, the presence of a lump should not awake wild, unrealistic fear. It should simply send you promptly to a physician. *Tumor* is another word for new growth or swelling.

Where Does Cancer Usually Strike? Nearly one-third of the cases begin in the alimentary canal, most commonly the stomach. The genitourinary system appears to be the next most vulnerable site (mainly the uterus in women and the prostate gland in men); about one-fifth of the cases begin in these sites. The breast is the third most common area, accounting for about 10% of the cases. Next come the blood-forming organs, where leukemia originates. The rest of the cases occur in the respiratory system, mainly the lung; in the urinary system, most frequently the bladder; in the brain and spinal cord; and on the skin. There are significant differences between men and women in the most important sites of cancer attack. For example, fatal cancer of the breast is 90 times more frequent in women; fatal respiratory (lung) cancer is 6 times more frequent in men, although the rate for women is rising.

What Causes Cancer? Nobody yet knows. However, many contributing and predisposing factors have been sorted out. One of the best known is prolonged irritation by chemical, physical, or thermal (heat) exposures. It has been abundantly demonstrated that coal tars are carcinogenic (cancer-invoking) agents. However, there are many other potential carcinogens in the environment, including solar rays, X-rays, and radioactive substances. For example, prolonged exposure to sun and wind seems to predispose to skin cancer. Certainly skin cancer is more common among outdoor workers, like ranchers and sailors, than among housewives.

Research has wiped out many cancer superstitions, giving assurance that there are many things that *don't* cause cancer. Dismiss the notions that cancer is caused by any specific kind of food or beverage, by blows or violence, by bacteria, or by such far-fetched circumstances as kissing, cooking in aluminum pots, or contact with animals.

Cancer is definitely not a germ (bacterial) disease; it is neither contagious nor communicable. You cannot "catch" cancer from cancer patients.

Many lines of research into possible causes are now under way. In essence they must deal with the factors that cause cells to grow and break down (cell metabolism). Among the factors being investigated are the chemical composition of cells, cell nutrition, the effects of viruses, hormones, and enzymes on the cells, environmental stresses, and the problem of heredity.

Cancer research is now a gigantic, multi-million-dollar annual undertaking. In 1959, for example, the federal government alone appropriated over $75 million for this purpose. But no specific "breakthrough" into discovery of the multiple causes of cancer then seemed imminent. Important progress, however, has been made in the development of cytologic techniques (examination of cells removed from the body) for the earlier diagnosis of cancer.

Is Cancer Inherited? This is an extremely complex question. With inbred strains of mice, elaborate patterns of the hereditary influences in cancer have been worked out. However, it cannot be assumed arbitrarily that what applies to inbred mice necessarily applies to man. There are no such pure, inbred strains of the human species. It is possible that a tendency to develop cancer can be inherited by human beings. However, it does not now appear that heredity is the critical or most important factor in human cancer. Dr. Clarence Cook Little, an outstanding authority in cancer research, has summed up the situation: "The role which heredity plays is so complex, so well concealed, and so difficult of evaluation that it is both unnecessary and unwise for individuals to consider it a personal problem."

Cancer Treatment. Cancer is treated by two basic and approved methods: (1) surgery and (2) radiation, which includes the use of X-ray, radium, and radioactive isotopes. Other methods of treatment are constantly being tested by research teams, and many become the subject of popular reports. However, legitimate scientific experiment should be distinguished from the false claims of cancer quacks, who advertise and promise cures.

Surgery, X-ray, radium, and radioisotopes are used alone or in any combination, depending on the particular case. The aim of surgery is to remove all cancer cells. Modern surgery, including extensive preoperative preparation and postoperative care, has made it possible to invade deeper and deeper recesses of the body to cut out cancerous tissue. Lung surgery affords a remarkable example.

Radiation treatment depends on the fact that many types of cancer cells are more radiosensitive than normal cells; they are destroyed while nearby normal cells are not severely injured. However, great caution is required in administering radiation treatment, and normal cells are shielded so far as possible from the rays. A radio-active isotope, cobalt 60, is now frequently used in place of radium or X-rays for radiation treatment.

Cancer Research

Chemotherapy in Cancer. For many years researchers have followed thousands of leads in the search for a drug that will affect the course of cancer once it attacks the human body. Notable progress was recorded in 1961 in the search for a drug.

The drug methotrexate was found to be effective in arresting some 50% of the cases of a highly malignant tumor, choriocarinoma, which originates in the pregnant uterus. In one series of 63 women with choriocarinoma, 30 of them lost all traces of their disease and on the last check-up had been well for periods up to five years.

This particular form of cancer is itself exceedingly rare, and its cure means little in the overall cancer picture. However, the effectiveness of methotrexate represents a forward step in the search for chemical agents that will block cancer.

Other drugs have helped reduce virulence of breast cancer and have helped prevent further spread of breast cancer after surgery.

New Remedies and Old. An ancient cancer remedy, for example, was found in 1962 to contain a chemical that slows the growth of tumors in mice.

The tumor-inhibiting chemical, called aristolochic acid, was isolated from a plant grown in Madras, India, known as *Aristolochia indica*. Species of this plant in the Mediterranean area were supposedly used as cancer remedies by the ancient Greeks and Romans.

The acid is unrelated to any drug presently used against cancer, and if further tests are successful a whole family of similar compounds will by synthesized and tested, according to Professor S. Morris Kupchan of the University of Wisconsin, who conducted this investigation.

The National Cancer Institute of the U.S. Public Health Service's National Institutes of Health at Bethesda, Maryland has reported progress in the chemotherapy (chemical treatment) of cancer. Its report, "Progress Against Cancer—1961," called special attention to definite (though limited) success in the treatment of advanced breast cancer. The report stated:

One of the standard agents for the treatment of advanced breast cancer (in women) is the male sex hormone called testosterone propionate. About 25 to 30% of patients who receive this drug experience objective responses to it—that is, the spread of their disease is halted temporarily, the size of the tumor itself is reduced, and the need for painkilling drugs is minimized.

However, this potent male hormone produces masculinizing effects that are often so distressing to the female patient that the treatment has to be abandoned. A new compound has been developed which has virtually the same anticancer action as the other but is much less masculinizing. This new agent is now available on (physician's) prescription and is coming into progressively wider use.

Virus Research. The possibility that some if not all forms of cancer in man might be caused by viruses, and that these viruses might be rendered and harmless by drugs, became one of the most intriguing prospects before cancer investigators in the mid-1960's. If research in this area proves successful and lives up to its early promise, it opens up the possibility of definite and effective control, through prevention or treatment, of whole categories of malignant disease, such as leukemia, which are now either invariably fatal or poorly responsive to any other treatments so far devised.

"Progress Against Cancer—1961" pointed out: "We are moving into virus-cancer research with the human problem in mind because of the mounting, undisputed scientific evidence that many cancers in animals are caused by viruses. . . . The investigation of viruses in relation to human cancer must be based on what is learned about viruses and cancer in animals. . . . There is a possibility that a vaccine against virus-caused animal cancer may emerge from large-scale laboratory operations. This would be of great importance in the event that even one form of human cancer should prove to be caused by a virus."

Progress in research against cancer continues on an international scale. There is an International Union Against Cancer, a world-wide organization on this vital subject.

In all this research, however, one must not forget the unfortunate cancer patient—still the victim of the disease. Many patients who suffer from the disease become so depressed at the very presence of this potential killer that they lose all heart to live. Their deaths, according to some clinicians, may be attributed as much to loss of morale as to the cancer process. For these people in particular the new research in cancer therapy offers a priceless thread of hope.

"Time Is of the Essence." This standard legal phrase might well be applied to the entire problem of cancer control. Delay on the part of the patient in seeking a medical check-up for "minor" symptoms is the greatest single factor in the causation of early, untimely deaths from cancer. Untimely? Cancer is the leading cause of death in women between the ages of 25 and 55.

Why the delay? Ignorance, fear, superstition, and false modesty are the principal reasons. Too many people are still ignorant of the present high curability of cancer, and fear that a visit to a doctor's office will mean hearing a "death sentence" pronounced in terms of a diagnosis of cancer.

Personal Protection against Cancer. You cannot escape the undesirable growth of cancer cells in your body, but you have many ways of escaping damage or death from them. Make sure that, if cancer strikes, you discover it early and get treatment promptly. Cancer can be diagnosed only by a physician. Your problem is simply to make sure that you get to the doctor in time for him to make an early diagnosis.

Monthly self-examination of the breasts is also to be recommended to women over 35. These are the findings that should send her promptly to the doctor: painless lump in either breast, best felt with fingers held flat and pressed against the breast; change in shape of either breast; one breast higher than the other; nipple retracted or discharging; skin dimpled or pulled in; glands in the armpit enlarged.

An intelligent person should be equipped with a high "index of suspicion" against early cancer. This does not mean, however, a constant fear of cancer (cancerophobia, as it is sometimes called). He should be aware of the twenty danger signals of disease, which include those that may betoken cancer. The list begins on page 12.

The American Cancer Society has provided a list of seven danger signals of cancer. These are not signs by which a layman can make a diagnosis of cancer. Their purpose is to get the person in whom one or more signals are noted to a physician for investigation and diagnosis.

The danger signals:[1]

1. Unusual bleeding or discharge.

2. A lump or thickening in the breast or elsewhere.

3. A sore that does not heal.

4. Persistent change in bowel or bladder habits.

5. Persistent hoarseness or cough.

6. Persistent indigestion or difficulty in swallowing.

7. Change in a wart or mole.

If any of these danger signals last for two weeks or more, you should be sure to see your doctor for diagnosis—or reassurance.

Some Cancer Comments (by Site). *Breast Cancer.* Leading cause of cancer deaths in women. Danger signal is lump or thickening in the breast which can be detected in annual check-up or as the result of monthly breast self-examination.

Colon and Rectum Cancer. Considered detectable and highly curable when digital and proctoscopic examinations are included in routine check-ups, which should be at least annually. Danger signal is change in bowel habits or rectal bleeding.

Kidney and Bladder Cancer. Almost always preceded by urinary difficulty or bleeding, for which reasons you should see a doctor. Annual check-up with urinalysis is a safeguard against this condition.

Lung Cancer. Now the leading cause of cancer

death among men—cigarette smoking is charged with being the chief cause. Get protection by annual check-up, with chest X-ray, and by giving up or never starting smoking. Danger signal is a persistent cough or lingering respiratory ailment.

Mouth, Larynx, and Pharynx Cancer. Many more lives should be saved because the mouth is easily accessible to visual examination by physicians and dentists. An annual check-up, including examination of the larynx, is a safeguard. Danger signals include a sore that does not heal, difficulty in swallowing, and hoarseness.

Prostate Cancer. Occurs mainly in men over 60. It can be detected by palpation and urinalysis at annual check-up. Danger signal is urinary difficulty.

Skin Cancer. Readily detected by observation and diagnosed by simple biopsy. Annual check-up recommended. Overexposure of skin to sun should be avoided. Danger signals include a sore that does not heal or change in a wart or mole.

Stomach Cancer. There has been a 40% decline in deaths from stomach cancer in the last 20 years—for reasons yet unknown. The condition can be detected in an annual check-up. Indigestion is the prime danger signal.

Uterine Cancer. Mortality of uterine cancer has also declined 40% in the last 20 years. The chances of reducing it to a negligible cause of death are enhanced by widespread use of the "pap" (Papanicolau) smear for its early detection. Safeguard against uterine cancer is annual check-up, including pelvic examination and "pap" smear.

Leukemia. Leukemia is cancer of blood-forming tissues; it is characterized by abnormal production of immature white blood cells. Acute leukemia mainly strikes children, in whom it can be treated by drugs that may extend life from a few months to a few years. Chronic leukemias usually occur after age 25 and progress more slowly.

Lymphomas. These diseases arise in the lymph system and include Hodgkin's disease and lymphosarcoma. Some patients with lymphatic can-

[1] From *Cancer Facts and Figures,* New York: American Cancer Society, 1962, p. 3.

cers can lead normal lives for many years. If drugs or vaccines to cure or prevent cancer are found, the cancer experts believe that they will first be successful in treating leukemia and lymphomas.

Pain is not a signal of early cancer; when it occurs, the condition may be well along. If the seven danger signals are heeded and a physician promptly consulted, chances of untimely death from cancer are greatly reduced.

The college student who has learned the true facts about cancer and heart disease has a lifelong responsibility as a citizen for spreading this information to others. The educated must be the educators.

As with the figures for heart disease, the doleful statistics on cancer incidence and deaths in the United States can be read two ways. True enough, over half a million new cases of cancer are reported annually in the United States, and over a quarter of a million deaths from cancer occur. But cancer is principally a degenerative disease and a disease of old age. Increase in cancer deaths is a price American society pays for having eliminated many other causes of disease and thus having lengthened average life span from around 47 years in 1900 to around 70 years at the present time.

A National Program for Conquest of Heart Disease, Cancer, and Stroke. The federal government has taken important, recent steps toward the "conquest of heart disease, cancer, and stroke." A President's [Lyndon B. Johnson's] commission on heart disease, cancer, and stroke was appointed in March 1964, and rendered a first report in December 1964. Its primary recommendation was the establishment of a national network of Regional Heart Disease, Cancer, and Stroke Centers for clinical investigation, teaching, and patient care in universities, hospitals, research institutes, and other institutions across the country. Specifically the commission recommended that over a 5 year period there be established 25 centers for heart disease, 20 for cancer, and 15 for stroke. By 1970 a total of 55 Regional Medical Programs for the treatment of these conditions were in operation.

In addition, the commission recommended the establishment of another national network of Diagnostic and Treatment Stations in communities across the nation to bring the highest medical skills in heart disease, cancer, and stroke within the reach of every citizen. Specifically, the commission asked for 150 such stations to be established over a period of five years for heart disease, 200 for cancer, and 100 for stroke.

Altogether the commission made 33 recommendations for steps necessary in its opinion to make a successful, nationwide thrust at heart disease, cancer, and stroke. Among them were the establishment of a national stroke program unit, of a national cervical cancer detection program, of statewide programs for heart disease control and of biomedical research institutes. The commission further recommended expanded education and training of health manpower, such as training of health technicians and specialists in health communication; and additional facilities and resources, such as more medical libraries and a national medical audiovisual center.

To put all these recommendations into effect over a five-year period would cost billions of dollars. But this would be a small outlay in comparison with the annual losses from these three diseases, which now account for more than 70% of the annual death toll in the United States. Dr. Michael E. DeBakey, chairman of the President's Commission, stated that the heavy losses which these three diseases inflict on our economy are close to $40 billion a year in lost productivity and lost taxes due to premature disability and death.[2]

Implementation of all the Commission's recommendations would undoubtedly increase the average length of life of American citizens. It might even change the order of the principal causes of death in the United States. But it would not eliminate the three conditions against which it is directed. Man is mortal. If he doesn't die

---

[2] *National Program to Conquer Heart Disease, Cancer and Stroke: A Report to the President by the President's Commission on Heart Disease, Cancer and Stroke.* Washington, D.C.: U.S. Government Printing Office (December 1964).

of heart disease, cancer, or stroke, he will have to die of other causes.

Smoking

Tobacco smoking has had its proponents and opponents ever since it was first introduced—from America to Europe. One of its first opponents was King James I of England, who in 1615 issued a "Counterblaste against Tobacco," in which he called it a "filthy habit . . . dangerous to the lungs."

In spite of the terms of criticism, tobacco smoking was until recently something that you could take or leave without undue worry that smoking presented any obvious risk to life or health. The situation is no longer so clear-cut. Physicians and other scientists have already demonstrated the hazards in smoking, especially cigarette smoking, although some controversy over this subject continues. Cigarette packs must now be labeled "hazardous to health." Over 100,000 physicians have given up smoking in recent years.

On the basis of its own and other statistical studies, the American Cancer Society is convinced of the risk of cigarette smoking as a cause of lung cancer. Already in 1962 the Society issued the following statement:

Another cancer risk you can avoid is excessive cigarette smoking. Research findings have convinced most scientists and the American Cancer Society that cigarette smoking is a cause of lung cancer. . . . Facts show that the more cigarettes smoked, the greater the risk of lung cancer. Ingrained personal habits are hard to change and you alone can decide whether to smoke or not to smoke.

Smoking and Health: U.S. Public Health Service Report

Cigarette smoking is a health hazard of sufficient importance in the United States to warrant appropriate remedial action. So concluded and reported an advisory committee to the Surgeon General of the U.S. Public Health Service in January, 1964. The statement was part of a 387-page, detailed report and study, published under the title *Smoking and Health*. To get an official view about tobacco smoking in the United States, it will be worthwhile to quote directly and indirectly from this extensive report,[3] as follows:

Nearly 70 million people in the United States consume tobacco regularly, principally in the form of cigarettes. While per capita consumption of other forms of tobacco has gone down, cigarette consumption has increased and stood at 3986 per person in 1961. It is estimated that roughly two-thirds of the men and one-third of the women over 18 smoke.

In order to judge whether smoking and other uses of tobacco are injurious to health or related to specific diseases, the Surgeon General's committee evaluated three main kinds of scientific evidence: (1) animal experiments, (2) clinical and autopsy studies, and (3) population studies. In the course of the animal experiments seven cancer-producing (carcinogenic) compounds were noted in the tobacco smoke and tars. The clinical and autopsy study on thousands of patients showed that many kinds of damage to body functions and to organs, cells, and tissues occur more frequently and severely in smokers. The population (epidemological) studies were both retrospective, looking back on what had happened to smokers, and prospective, getting smoking histories—or non-smoking histories—and then comparing what happened in the future.

The retrospective studies revealed several things; namely, that proportionately more cigarette smokers are found among lung cancer patients than among control populations without cancer; and that specific symptoms and signs—chronic cough, sputum production, breathlessness, chest illness, and decreased lung function—consistently show more often in cigarette smokers than in non-smokers.

[3] *Smoking and Health;* report of the Advisory Committee to the Surgeon General of the Public Health Service, U.S. Department of Health, Education, and Welfare, Public Health Service, Public Health Service Publication 1103. [For sale by the Superintendent of Documents, U.S. Government Printing Office, Washington, D.C. Price $1.25.]

The seven prospective studies examined by the Surgeon General's Committee included 1,123,000 men who provided usable histories of smoking habits and other data. A total of 37,391 men died during subsequent months or years of the studies. Tabulations in these studies were set up to permit ready comparison of the mortality experience of smokers and non-smokers. By these figures, the mortality rate for male cigarette smokers compared with non-smokers for all causes of death taken together is 1.68, representing a total death rate nearly 70% higher than for non-smokers. An excess mortality (over what would have been expected) was also noted sharply in a number of specific disease conditions among the smokers. For example, the mortality ratio of cigarette smokers to non-smokers was particularly high for such conditions as cancer of the lung (10.8), bronchitis and emphysema (6.1), cancer of the larynx (5.4), other circulatory diseases (2.6), and coronary artery disease (1.7).

The Surgeon General's Committee recognized that no simple cause-and-effect relationship is likely to exist between a complex product like tobacco smoke and a specific disease entity in the variable human organism. It also recognized that often the coexistence of several factors is required for the occurrence of a disease. Nevertheless, the Committee found these things:

¶ Cigarette smoking is associated with a 70% increase in the age-specific death rates of males. The total number of excess deaths cannot be accurately estimated.

¶ Cigarette smoking is causally related to lung cancer in men; the magnitude of the effect of cigarette smoking far outweighs all other factors. The data for women, though less extensive, point in the same direction. The risk of developing lung cancer increases with duration of smoking and the number of cigarettes smoked per day; it diminishes by discontinuing smoking. In comparison with non-smokers, average male smokers of cigarettes have approximately a nine- to tenfold risk of developing lung cancer and heavy smokers at least a twentyfold risk.

¶ Cigarette smoking is the most important of

the causes of chronic bronchitis in the United States, and it increases the risk of dying from chronic bronchitis and emphysema.

¶ Cigarette smoking is associated with a reduction in ventilation function. Among males, cigarette smokers have a greater prevalence of breathlessness than non-smokers.

¶ Cough, sputum production, or the two combined are consistently more frequent among cigarette smokers than among non-smokers.

¶ Male cigarette smokers have a higher death rate from coronary artery disease than non-smoking males, but it is not clear that the association has causal significance.

¶ Women who smoke cigarettes during pregnancy tend to have babies of lower birth weight. [But] it is not known whether this decrease in birth weight has any influence on the biological fitness of the newborn.

¶ No clear-cut "smoker's personality" has emerged from the studies.

¶ Overwhelming evidence points to the conclusion that smoking—its beginning, habituation, and occasional discontinuation—is to a large extent psychologically and socially determined. This does not rule out physiological factors especially in respect to habituation, nor the existence of predisposing constitutional or hereditary factors.

Physiological Effects of Smoking. Smoke, a product of combustion, is a mixture of gases, various vaporized chemicals, and millions of minute particles of ash and other solids. These are drawn into the nose, throat, and lungs during smoking. The smoke includes some vaporized nicotine, a toxic substance found in tobacco, although much of it is destroyed by heat. . . . A smoker gets more nicotine and tar if he smokes a short butt.

Pathologists have found that smoking affects both the respiratory system and the circulatory system. For example, it has been found to thicken the lining membranes of air passages and to obstruct them with secretions.

To smoke or not to smoke is a matter of individual choice. Most authorities would agree that never smoking was preferable; and further, that

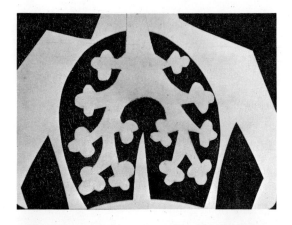

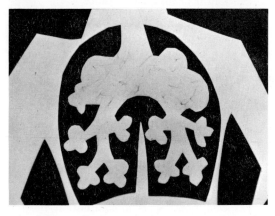

THE INJURY that cigarette smoking does to the tiny air sacs of the lungs is illustrated here. The top drawing represents normal lungs; in the bottom drawing, continuous smoking has caused the air sacs to balloon outward. Eventually their walls break down, resulting in difficulty in breathing and frequently in emphysema, a serious disabling disease. (Illustration courtesy of American Cancer Society)

moderation was a must. The American Medical Association has stated: "If you haven't started the habit, you should carefully consider all the facts concerning your future health before doing so."

Further Opinions on Smoking. In June 1964, the House of Delegates of the American Medical Association adopted a reference committee report which said that the American Medical Association "is on record and does recognize a significant relationship between cigarette smoking and the incidence of lung cancer and certain other diseases and that cigarette smoking is a serious

health hazard." The report went on to urge that the AMA should develop programs to disseminate educational material on the hazards of smoking "to all age groups through all available means of communication."

The American Heart Association has also given some pertinent answers to questions about the relationship between cigarette smoking and the circulatory system.

Are there more heart attacks among smokers than non-smokers? The heart attack rate [is] three times as high as in nonsmokers, pipe and cigar smokers, and former cigarette smokers.

Are there more deaths from heart attacks among smokers? The average increase is 70%. It can be estimated that about 60,000 men (40 to 69 years of age) die prematurely in the United States each year from heart attacks associated with smoking.

Does cigarette smoking cause heart disease? It has not been proved that cigarette smoking is a direct *cause* of heart disease. However, studies strongly suggest that it contributes to or speeds up the development of coronary artery disease which leads to heart attacks.

How does smoking affect the circulatory system? In most people who have been tested, smoking makes the heart beat faster, raises the blood pressure, and narrows the blood vessels of the skin, especially in the fingers and toes.

Social and Psychological Effects. Many social and psychological factors related to tobacco smoking have been noted. For example, many young people begin smoking in imitation of older people, sometimes those just a few years older. Smoking may offer many psychological satisfactions. For example, it may satisfy the infantile desire to have something in the mouth; the infant sucks his thumb if nothing better is available. In some cases lighting up a cigarette may be a means of relaxation; in others, it may represent an act of self-expression. To still others the cigarette represents a kind of "reward" that the smoker can offer himself whenever he wishes.

Tobacco smoking begins early in American youth. By the time they reach their senior year in high school, 40 to 55% of all children are found to have done some smoking. By the time they leave high school one in every four boys (25%) and one in every 8 girls (12.5%) are smokers. The boys are the heavier smokers. An equal if not greater number of young people take up smoking in their college years. It may be recalled that about 65% of American men and 35% of American women do smoke.

Present Status. Tobacco manufacturers are trying to reduce the hazards of smoking by modifying tobacco, cutting down its nicotine content, and filtering out the tars. They have also initiated research to isolate harmful substances so that those who smoke may continue to smoke safely. The results to date have not been too encouraging.

So long as millions of Americans continue to smoke, it cannot be assumed that the last word on the tobacco controversy has been said. Millions of dollars are being granted annually by the U.S. Public Health Service, the American Medical Association, and others for further study of tobacco and smoking. One hope is that this research will come up with a truly "safe cigarette." The filtertips currently used on cigarettes are not considered to be an adequate safeguard.

The United States government has put itself in an awkward position in the tobacco controversy. One branch of the government (U.S. Public Health Service) condemns cigarettes while another branch (Department of Agriculture) supports the price of tobacco, and still a third (Bureau of Internal Revenue) collects large amounts in taxes from the sale of tobacco.

A National Clearinghouse for Smoking and Health has been established in the U.S. Public Health Service. It serves an important educational and coordinating function. It was one among many organizations concerned with a World Conference on Smoking & Health, sponsored by the National Interagency Council on Smoking and Health, and held in New York in September, 1967. The Summary of the Proceedings of this conference is a mine of useful information on the proved relationship of smoking and diseases of the heart and lungs.

On the basis of statistical evidence now available, it can be categorically stated, "Don't smoke." Tempered by current practice and professional experience, this categorical statement might be modified thus: "Don't start smoking. Don't smoke excessively. Don't inhale."

SUMMARY

In this chapter we have come face to face with the principal killers of Americans at different ages; notoriously, heart disease (more exactly, cardiovascular disease) of many kinds, cancer at many sites, and stroke striking the brain. We have noted the crucial disease-producing role of the blood vessels, which may harden, inducing *arterio*sclerosis, or fatten, yielding *athero*-sclerosis. We have presented the many hopeful as well as the discouraging facts about diseases of the heart and blood vessels.

We have discussed the nature of cancer ("cells gone wild"), its many types and sites in the human body, its curability by early treatment (surgery, radiation, and possibly some day drugs), and the seven danger signals which, if respected, can lead to early diagnosis of cancer.

Finally, we have presented the current evidence on, and largely against, tobacco (especially cigarette) smoking. Tobacco is considered a crucial factor in the causation of lung cancer and cardiovascular disease—but nearly 70 million Americans still smoke.

SUMMARY REVIEW QUESTIONS

1. What are the principal causes of death in the United States today? What were they in 1900? Why the difference? What are the principal causes of death in the college age bracket?

2. What reasons, if any, are there for believing that the present statistical picture of heart disease and associated conditions is not so frightening as it might appear if taken at face value?

3. Why is heart disease more properly described as cardiovascularenal disease? What relationship does it have to high blood pressure, hardening of the arteries, and kidney disease?

4. What is a heart attack? What is its *immediate* cause? What are the possible outcomes of a heart attack? What is heart failure? What is rheumatic heart disease? How, if at all, can it be prevented?

5. What is the difference between arteriosclerosis and atherosclerosis? In what way may these conditions be responsible for various forms of cardiovascular disease? To what extent is a fat-free diet a protection against such diseases?

6. What is a stroke? What are the usual outcomes of this event? In what areas does new hope for stroke victims lie? What grounds are there for saying that a high death rate from stroke is an index of a generally healthy community?

7. What is cancer? How does it actually kill and cripple? How does it spread? Is it inherited? How is it treated? What are the new hopes for cancer treatment?

8. What is your attitude toward cancer? Have the facts you now have about it changed your attitude from what it used to be? If so, in what way? If not, why not? Do you think your attitude is different from your parents' attitude? If so, why; if not, why not?

9. What are the seven danger signals of cancer? What should you do when any of these warning signals flash?

10. What are some (name at least six) of the most common sites of cancer in the human body? What specific protective measures, if any, can be taken to minimize the risk of cancer occurring or progressing at each of these sites?

11. What are the arguments for and against tobacco smoking? What arguments against smoking impress you most strongly? How would you defend your personal decision to smoke?

12. In light of the fact that nearly 70 million people in the United States smoke—principally cigarettes—what practical and workable measures would you suggest for decreasing, if not elimminating, the smoking habit?

13. Do you think the present statistical picture of "big killers" of Americans is likely to change during your lifetime? Why or why not?

14. Are the following statements sense or nonsense? Why? *Cancer is curable. . . . Women deposit their fat under the skin while men deposit it in their coronary arteries. . . . A heart attack is a sentence of death or permanent invalidism. . . . Eating food cooked in aluminum pots and pans is the cause of cancer. . . . A man is as old as his arteries. . . . The satisfactions of smoking are worth the risks.*

15. What do the following terms mean to you: cholesterol, lipoproteins, hypertension, vascular accident, aneurysm, malignant, benign tumor, metastasis, chemotherapy, "Counterblaste against Tobacco"?

Worth Studying Further: *You and Your Heart* by H. M. Marvin, M.D., and others. *Common Sense Coronary Care and Prevention* by Peter Steincrohn, M.D. *The Truth About Cancer* by Charles S. Cameron, M.D. *Cancer* by R. J. C. Harris. *Smoking and Health:* Report of the Advisory Committee to the Surgeon General of the U.S. Public Health Service. *Tobacco and Health* by G. James and T. Rosenthal For more complete references, see Appendix E.

The Physician and the Cigarette

Robert H. Browning, M.D.

It's an intriguing group of very human psychological and physiological reactions which has made cigarette smoking such a pervading practice in the United States. The impulse of young people to start smoking has been assiduously cultivated over many years by massive advertising, for which close to $300,000,000 per year is now being expended. Evolving from a practice which was morally condemned forty to fifty years ago, cigarette smoking has acquired social respectability and desirability. Generally speaking, social pressures, and not love of cigarette smoke, produce the new recruits among smokers.

People continue to smoke because they are "hooked." Most of them can't quit, even when they want to. This is a manufacturer's dream: to start a habit among millions of people, because of social pressures, and to have it continued for a lifetime because of habituation or addiction.

The ancient custom of tobacco smoking has been suspected of injuring health for a long time. Only in the last several decades, however, have researchers been able to document the ravages of this lethal habit. Now the evidence is so overwhelming that no informed person can logically deny the association between cigarette smoking and a number of disabling and fatal diseases.[1] A recent survey showed that more than 95 per cent of U.S. physicians accept the evidence which incriminates cigarettes.

The literature includes the results of a great many carefully performed research studies, which provide more than adequate scientific proof of the association of cigarette smoking with morbidity and mortality from a number of diseases. While physicians and informed laymen recognize the danger, many of them do not realize the magnitude of the health problems involved in cigarette smoking. Many are not acquainted with the political and economic power of the tobacco industry.

The statistics shown in "The Toll of Cigarette Smoking" (Table 1) and "People-Cigarettes-Dollars" (Table 2) represent recent United States estimates by qualified observers in official and voluntary organizations concerned with the nation's health.

One cannot measure the toll of cigarette smoking in terms of "excess deaths" alone. From a study of a population sample of 42,000 households by the National Center for Health Statistics during the year ending June 1965, it was found that cigarette smokers in a recent one-year period suffered some 11,000,000 more chronic illnesses than would have been expected if the entire U.S. population were non-smokers. A partial breakdown is shown in Table 1.[2,3]

The statistics in these tables may be incomprehensible, but no one would call them insignificant. They represent the greatest man-made epidemic of disease in human history. They pose a mighty problem for the present and future health of our people. Most deaths in the U.S. are not preventable in the light of our present knowledge. The

SOURCE. Robert H. Browning, M.D. is Professor of Medicine at the Ohio State University in Columbus, Ohio. This paper is adapted from one presented at the 156th Annual Scientific Assembly of the Rhode Island Medical Society, at Providence. It includes small revisions of the original article printed in the Rhode Island Medical Journal (50: 753–756) of November 1967. The version reprinted here appeared (with permission of the Rhode Island Medical Journal) in *The Journal of School Health*, 38: 5 (May 1968).

TABLE 1. THE TOLL OF CIGARETTE SMOKING[2,3]

Premature Deaths associated with cigarette smoking—300,000 annually
      —Coronary heart disease   —50%
      —Cancer of lung   —14% Rough
      —Cancer (other)   —14% estimates
      —Emphysema, bronchitis and other—22%
Longevity—as compared to non-smokers—reduced by:
  4 years—all cigarette smokers
  7 years—2 packs per day smokers
Disease Incidence—per year, among cigarette smokers
    280,000—"Extra" cases of heart disease
  1,000,000—"Extra" cases of chronic bronchitis and/or emphysema
  1,800,000—"Extra" cases of sinusitis
Days of Disability—per year, among cigarette smokers
 77,000,000—Excess man days lost from work
          —19% of the national total
 88,000,000—Excess sick or disabled days spent in bed
          —10% of the national total
306,000,000—Excess days of restricted activity
          —13% of the national total

"excess" deaths experienced by cigarette smokers *are preventable:* in smokers, by the simple but often difficult decision *not to smoke;* and in the case of non-smokers, by the decision *not* to start. Here, then, is the greatest opportunity we have in Preventive Medicine: the chance to prevent massive disability on the part of millions of smokers, and to prevent thousands of deaths each week—300,000 per year. We hear a great deal about "slaughter on the highways." Smoking kills six times as many people!

Our problem is a dual one.

TABLE 2. PEOPLE—CIGARETTES—DOLLARS[2]

Present Cigarette Smokers in U.S.	69,000,000
Ex-smokers in U.S.	19,000,000
New Smokers Recruited per year	1,500,000
Quit Smoking—	
"cigarette dropouts" per year	1,000,000 adults
Farm Families Growing Tobacco	650,000 (1963)
Cigarettes Sold	541,000,000,000 (1966)
—74 million packs/day	
—17,154 cigarettes/second	
Cigarettes—retail value	$8,200,000,000 (1966)
Taxes—federal, state, local	$3,700,000,000 (1966)
Advertising expenditure	$ 300,000,000 per yr.
Anti-cigarette Program of the U.S. Public	
Health Service	$ 2,000,000 (1967)
Fires caused by matches and smoking	163,900 (1965)
—deaths in these fires	1,800 (est.)
—property loss from these fires	$ 80,400,000

First and, in our opinion, the more important is how to prevent the recruiting of *new* smokers, now estimated at 4,000 or more a day, or 1,500,000 a year. In the minds of many of our young people, smoking has become the symbol of the "he-man" or the sophisticated woman. It is part of being "grownup"—a status that is illogically yearned for by the younger generation. In a home where there are smoking parents, it appears to be part of the normal pattern of life.

Smoking cigarettes is not only socially acceptable, but almost compulsory, in many of the school and other living situations of our young people. Add to these social pressures the influence of almost $300 million spent yearly in advertising, which tells us endlessly—with love and nature added—that one can hardly enjoy life and be a success at it if he doesn't smoke cigarettes!

With the *established* smoker, the scene is different. Glamour and social pressures have long since ceased to play a part. He is "hooked" by a dependence on the physiologic effect of nicotine, and in most cases the still stronger demands of a habit pattern which is in control during his waking hours. Cigarettes have become a crutch—something to use pleasureably in a social situation or to provide a little break in the course of work or play, but more commonly just to satisfy the habit pattern and the nicotine dependence.

In a recent survey, 85 percent of a large group of smokers stated they were dissatisfied with their smoking. How many of these, fortified with facts about their dangerous habit and encouraged by their physicians, would be able to quit cigarettes? We don't know!

The whole thing is quite complicated. To some people smoking is more important than life itself—for instance, prisoners of war who were starving, but traded their food for cigarettes. To others quitting may not be difficult, once the hazards are understood.

One of the facets of the smoking problem is the long delay in the development of smoker's diseases. If coronary heart disease or emphysema or cancer of the lung were to appear 6 or 12 months after beginning of smoking, instead of 20 or 30 years later, the recruiting of new smokers would be impossible.

Filter cigarettes, which comprise about two thirds of the total output, give smokers the illusion that they are buying protection although recent analyses[4] show that filter brands of some manufacturers have more tobacco tars and nicotine in their main stream smoke than the non-filter cigarettes produced by the same companies. The most that can be truthfully claimed for filters is that some of them do partially remove some of the harmful ingredients. It can be assumed that the future will bring filters of improved capacity, perhaps greatly improved. But the "new and better" filters, will give no assurance that *all* harmful ingredients have been removed. This will have to wait until the desired reduction in morbidity and mortality from smokers' diseases have been demonstrated by long years of use. It remains to be seen whether smokers will buy and smoke cigarettes whose flavor has been changed by a new filter. It is contradictory to expect the tobacco smoke "taste" to remain the same when major components are filtered out.

The Smoker As a Patient

Smoking clinics, attended by smokers who *want* to quit, are successful in the long run in only 10–20 per cent of subjects, usually those with short smoking histories and low cigarette consumption.

Each smoker comprises a distinctive and individual problem. The response to his physician in regard to cigarette smoking will depend on a number of factors, not all of which can be controlled by the physician. A few of these are: 1) The patient's temperament and psychological makeup; 2) The duration and daily consumption of cigarettes —the more cigarettes consumed in the patient's lifetime, the greater the problem of quitting; 3) His attitude toward his doctor; 4) His knowledge of the dangers of smoking; and 5) The physician's skill in dealing with the individual patient in accord with the factors above.

What are our tools, then: *Education? Personal example? Fear? Appeal to pride? Authority?* Certainly, *education* is our first and best technique. Example is important—"Do as I say, not as I do" is hardly to be recommended. The *scare* technique, or *appeal to pride* may work with some smokers. *Authoritarian* attitudes are commonly ineffective and may actually produce a reverse response.

"Education", as mentioned

above, includes not just a dry recital of statistics on the morbidity and mortality of smokers' diseases. The promoters of cigarette smoking tend to stay away from facts in their advertising. Their ads, often sexually oriented, promote cigarettes on the basis of social status, sophistication, manliness. To combat this approach, one must be prepared to point out the essential irrationality and stupidity of cigarette smoking; to say in various ways, it is neither "smart" nor intelligent to smoke.[5]

Organizing For Action

As part of the growing campaign to reduce and control cigarette smoking (alas, it can't be wiped out), a number of actions have been taken:

The National Interagency Council on Smoking and Health[6] was formed in July 1964. It is composed of 16 voluntary and official agencies which, while carrying on individual activities, have banded together to aid and coordinate the campaign against cigarettes. These agencies are: American Association for Health, Physical Education and Recreation; American Association of School Administrators; American Cancer Society, Inc.; American College Health Association; American Dental Association; American Heart Association; American Pharmaceutical Association; American Public Health Association; American School Health Association; Association of State and Territorial Health Officers; Department of Classroom Teachers of the NEA; National Congress of Parents and Teachers; National Tuberculosis Association; U.S. Children's Bureau; U.S. Office of Education; and U.S. Public Health Service.

Forty State Interagency Councils have been organized and are affiliated with the National. The same sort of cooperative action is being developed in cities and counties. These are areas where the individual physician, as well as his medical society, should participate.

The United States Public Health Service has formed the National Clearinghouse for Smoking and Health,[7] a Federal agency to collect and provide tobacco information on a national basis. In organized medicine about 40 State Medical Societies have passed resolutions of support to the anti-cigarette campaign and have joined State Interagency Councils on Smoking and Health.

National and State Parent-Teachers Associations are making an organized effort to promote pupil education on this subject. There is increasing individual and group education on smoking especially in schools.

The Federal Communications Commission has ordered radio and television stations to present information about the dangers of cigarette smoking as a counter to cigarette advertising. There have been Congressional efforts to stop cigarette advertising by legal action—so far unsuccessful due to regional political factors.

What Are the Prospects?

The campaign against cigarette smoking is building up all over the country. The penalties in human illness and death are so great that this campaign will not fail. The energy and resources of many agencies and individuals are required now. In the end, the consuming public will learn the basic facts about cigarette smoking and will react accordingly.

Far from being discouraged, we should feel only impatient at slow progress. We may not be able to measure the effectiveness of our personal efforts to educate our patients and our communities about smoking. We may be disheartened at times because of our inability to make converts. But every effort we make will contribute to the sum total of public understanding and will hasten the day when cigarette smoking will generally be considered unintelligent and socially unacceptable. *Only then* will we have removed the glamour and social pressure. Only *then* will we acquire the social and political power to stop cigarette advertising and radically reduce the recruitment of new smokers.

REFERENCES

1. Smoking and Health—Report of the Advisory Committee to the Surgeon General of the Public Health Service, 1964; Public Health Service Publication No. 1103.
2. The statistics given in Tables 1 and 2 originate from a number of sources including National Clearing-House for Smoking and Health (see Reference #7); The Tobacco Institute, 1735 K. Street,

N.W., Washington, D.C.; Smoking and Health—Report of the Advisory Committee to the Surgeon General of the Public Health Service; various comprehensive statistical studies, especially those of the Epidemiology and Statistics Division of the American Cancer Society, Dr. E. Cuyler Hammond, Vice President; research reports of several investigators.

3. National Clearinghouse for Smoking and Health, Public Health Service Publication No. 1662.

4. Moore, George E., Roswell Park Memorial Institute, Buffalo, New York, March 1967 report issued by American Cancer Society.

5. Modern Concepts of Cardiovascular Disease, American Heart Association, Vol. XXXIII, No. 10, October 1964.

6. P.O. Box 3654, Central Station, Arlington, Virginia 22203.

7. 4040 North Fairfax Drive, Arlington, Virginia 22203.

17

PROTECTING AGAINST
COMMUNICABLE DISEASE
AND OTHER HEALTH HAZARDS

THE CONQUEST OF COMMUNICABLE DISEASE achieved in the last quarter of the nineteenth century and the first half of the twentieth was one of the greatest achievements of human mind and effort. The number of individual lives saved by this quiet victory far exceeds those lost in the wars of the same period.

Scores of heroes and thousands of devoted microbe hunters and disease fighters were involved in the winning of the Great War against communicable disease. Probably the most significant of them all was the French chemist, Louis Pasteur, who demonstrated in the 1860's that microbes or "germs," visible only under a microscope, were actually the cause of the most serious diseases then plaguing mankind. The application of his germ theory of disease has resulted in the fact that the major degenerative diseases have now, in the Western world, replaced communicable, infectious, and childhood diseases as the big killers.

Worldwide victory over communicable diseases is far from complete. Malaria and tuberculosis are still number 1 and number 2 killers throughout the world. Even in scientifically advanced countries of the world, such as the United States, some typical communicable diseases like venereal infections and the common cold—which we shall shortly discuss in detail—remain significant but manageable problems.

In this chapter we shall also consider the practical lines of protection available to you against the hazards of communicable and other diseases. Making proper use of available medical service is one important line of protection. So we shall also discuss the matter of selecting a physician and using his services to greatest advantage.

Pasteur: The Turning Point. The great turning point in the history of mankind's ability to control communicable disease came between 1865 and 1870, and it is associated with the greatest name in French science, Louis Pasteur. A modest, patient, intuitive genius, Pasteur was actually trained as a chemist and employed by the French government as an industrial trouble shooter. When the wine in Orleans was turning to vinegar, they sent for Pasteur. He showed the vinters how to keep their wine from spoiling by heating it to 55°C. This process has since been called pasteurization; its effect is to kill off and slow up the multiplication of microbes that infest both wine and milk.

When silkworms in Alais were dying of *pébrine,* they sent for Pasteur. Here, between 1865 and 1870, when he found that the silkworms were suffering from two diseases, not one, he evolved the idea that unique kinds of microorganisms caused different, specific diseases. This is the essence of the germ theory of disease.

It is hard for us today to recapture both the

incredulity and the delight with which the general public grasped the idea that "little animals," invisible except through a microscope, were the cause of disease. Pasteur went on to equally great triumphs: for example, the demonstration in 1885 that the human body could be immunized against such a disease as rabies (hydrophobia) transmitted to humans from the bite of a rabid animal. Pasteur is certainly the founder of the modern science of bacteriology. Before Pasteur the attempts to control communicable diseases were few and were only rarely successful. Inability to control malaria, for instance, helped undermine the "Golden Age" of ancient Greece between 500 and 300 B.C. The lawgivers among the Biblical Hebrews, promulgated a few sanitary ideas which did help to control disease, notably isolation of diseased persons and rules of cleanliness which required that human excrement be buried. Roman

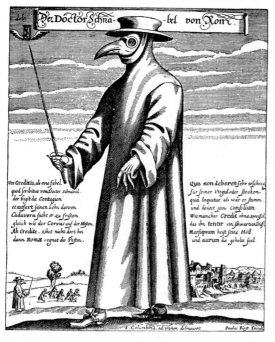

THIS SEVENTEENTH CENTURY GERMAN ENGRAVING shows the "protection cloth" of a plague physician. Theories of communicable disease at that time ascribed epidemics to visitations of divine wrath, miasmal and night airs, or a "conjunction of planets over the Indian Ocean." (Bettman Archive)

baths and sewers undoubtedly reduced filth-borne diseases, but they had no effect on insect-carried malaria.

In the Middle Ages leprosy was controlled by the cruel expedient of banishing lepers from human society. Quarantine, the forty-day detention of incoming ships and travelers, adopted by various Mediterranean ports during the late fourteenth century to escape the introduction of Black Death (bubonic plague), was scientific as far as it went. But it did not effectively keep out the rats whose fleas spread the plague from rat to rat and from rat to man. The theory of communicable diseases was then hopelessly inadequate. It ascribed epidemics variously to visitations of divine wrath, to miasmal and night airs, or to a "conjunction of planets over the Indian Ocean."

Men Ahead of Their Time: The Pioneer Epidemiologists. There were, as always, a few men ahead of their time in their explanations of and their recommendations for the control of communicable disease. Among them were Girolamo Fracastoro, Richard Mead, John Snow, Ignaz Semmelweis, Oliver Wendell Holmes, and Lemuel Shattuck. Fracastoro is best known as the author of the suave Latin poem, "Syphilis sive Morbus Gallicus," published in 1530, which fastened that name on the venereal disease thus known. Syphilis, literally translated "hog-lover," was the name of a mythical shepherd boy in the West Indies, whence the disease was supposed to have originated.

However, Fracastoro did much more to justify his title of the "father of epidemiology." A mild-mannered student at the famous medical school of Padua, he saw more clearly than anyone for the next three centuries that epidemics in communities are the result of infections in individuals. He outlined a theory of "seeds" ("seminaria") of contagion, concerning which he wrote: "These seeds are the carriers of contagion, and that they are the first origin of the disease there can be no doubt. . . . It may be considered that the force of the disease lies in these seeds since they have the power to propagate and reproduce their own kind."

Fracastoro also recognized three modes of infection: (1) by contact with the sick; (2) by contact with their garments, droppings, and exhalations, for which he invented the word *fomites;* and (3) at a distance by dissemination of the original "seeds" (germs) of the disease.

Dr. Richard Mead was a London physician and patron of the arts. In "A Short Discourse Concerning Pestilential Contagion," published in 1720, he suggested that the overseers of the poor should do less police work but "should take care by all manner of provision and encouragement, to make them more cleanly and sweet."

Dr. John Snow, also a London physician, appeared as a modest stranger before the vestrymen of St. James's parish in London (in September, 1854) and suggested that if they wanted to stop the epidemic of cholera that was raging about them, they had only to order the removal of the handle of the Broad Street pump. The vestrymen were incredulous; but, having no other solution for the epidemic, they agreed to remove the pump handle. This immediately stopped the distribution of drinking water containing cholera vibrio in the neighborhood and promptly stayed the epidemic.

Snow conclusively proved that cholera was a water-borne disease, and he inferred that there were others similarly transmitted. His epidemiological maps of the city of London were strong arguments for safe metropolitan water supplies.

Semmelweis and Holmes were instrumental in reducing the incidence of deadly childbed fever in the early nineteenth century. Since their time, childbirth has become increasingly safe.

The Long Fight to Control Disease

Until Pasteur's time, and even during his life, introducing scientific measures for the control of disease was always an uphill struggle. Florence Nightingale, for example, in the late nineteenth century had to fight her way in the British War Office before she was able to introduce sensible sanitary measures and bedside nursing for soldiers wounded in the Crimean War.

Earlier there had also been considerable public opposition to the introduction of vaccination against smallpox, although Jenner's work was undoubtedly the greatest milestone before Pasteur on the road to modern preventive medicine. Jenner originally noted that many dairymaids were immune to smallpox in an age when lack of pock marks on the face was a characteristic so uncommon that criminal identification could be made by it. He noted that the dairymaids' immunity was due to previous attack of the mild disease called cowpox. On May 14, 1796, he began his historically critical experiment. In his famous "Inquiry into the Causes and Effects of the Variolae Vaccine (Cowpox)," Jenner wrote:

I selected a healthy boy, about eight years old, for the purpose of inoculating for cowpox. The matter was taken from a sore on the hand of a dairymaid, who was infected by her master's cows, and it was inserted into the arm of the boy be means of two superficial incisions.

Thereafter many attempts were made to give the boy genuine smallpox by the method of inoculation commonly in vogue. He couldn't get it or "take it," as the saying went; the cowpox had made him immune.

Inoculation against smallpox had been introduced in England nearly three-quarters of a century earlier by the fashionable influence of Lady Mary Wortley Montagu, who had discovered it in Turkey, where she had gone as wife of the British Ambassador. Her "Letters from the East" (1718) talked about "smallpox parties."

When she returned to England in 1722 she persuaded the then Prince and Princess of Wales to have their two children inoculated too. Inoculation thus became fashionable and acceptable; it paved the way for Jenner's safer vaccination. Inoculation represented safety to the individual but danger to the community, since the infection was genuinely smallpox, though of a mild strain, and might easily have gotten out of hand.

It should be noted that all the conquests over epidemic disease before Pasteur were sporadic, practical, empiric, and pragmatic. They worked, but no one really knew why.

Microscopy: Forerunner of Bacteriology. It

was scientific research, development, and instrumentation in a field apparently far removed from clinical medicine that made proof of the germ theory of disease possible. This was the science of optics, which produced crude microscopes in the seventeenth century and achromatic microscopes in the nineteenth. If Pasteur was the father of the science of bacteriology, Leeuwenhoek was its grandfather, and Robert Hooke, curator of experiments for London's Royal Society and author of *Micrographia* (1665), its great uncle.

Anton van Leeuwenhoek, born in 1632, was once a petty shopkeeper and town official in Delft, Holland. For his own amusement he ground lenses and constructed some of the earliest microscopes. Through them he was the first human being ever to observe the teeming world of microorganisms. He reported his findings in rambling letters to London's Royal Society and willed them twenty-six of his jealously guarded microscopes.

"In the year 1675," he wrote, "I discovered very small living creatures in rain water, which had stood but a few days in a new earthen pot glazed blue within. . . . Those little animals appeared to me ten thousand times less than those . . . called water fleas or water lice, which may be perceived in the water with the naked eye." In addition to bacteria Leeuwenhoek was the first to see blood capillaries—in a tadpole's tail—and human spermatozoa. The sciences of microscopy and bacteriology have moved forward hand in hand.

A Half-Century of Excitement in Bacteriology. Following Pasteur there was a mad scientific scramble to discover and identify microorganisms causing specific diseases. We can mention only some of the men who led this exciting search, which has since turned up practically all the kinds of microorganisms associated with the production of disease. The first great name is that of Robert Koch, a German physician, who in 1876 isolated the bacillus of anthrax, a disease that attacks both men and animals.

Koch also developed culture media (gelatin and later agar) on which colonies of bacteria could be cultured and grown for further study.

He also pioneered the staining of bacteria so that they could be seen more plainly under constantly improved microscopes. He developed postulates for proving the specific infectiousness of various types of bacteria. His great moment came on a March evening in 1882 when he was able to announce to a hushed meeting of scientists in Berlin: "I have succeeded in discovering the real cause of tuberculosis. It is a parasite, the tubercle bacillus."

Eight years later Koch made another dramatic announcement—that he had discovered a "cure" for tuberculosis in tuberculin, an extract of the tubercle bacillus. He was tragically wrong; tuberculin did not cure tuberculosis, though it later proved useful in testing for the disease.

Nevertheless, hope for the control of communicable disease continued to reside in the discovery of the specific bacterial agent of each one. Thus for almost half a century there continued great scientific and sometimes public excitement as the invading microorganism of each important disease was ticked off the list of the unknown. Some of the highlights of the roll call are shown in the table on page 353.

The excitement of bacteriologic discoveries gradually died down. The etiologic agents of the major plagues of mankind were one by one discovered. But then the realization came that in order to control a disease more than its bacteriologic agent had to be known. Furthermore, it came to be recognized that in many of the increasingly devastating diseases—notably cancer and the most prevalent forms of heart disease and mental illness—no causative microorganism could be demonstrated.

The species, types, and strains of microorganisms, it further turned out, were more complex than the early investigators dreamed. In addition, not all the microorganisms of disease could actually be seen under optical microscopes, improved as they were.

The Russian investigator Iwanowski made a far more important observation than he originally realized in 1892 when he reported a "filterable virus" as a disease-producing agent. A filterable virus is a living organism so small that it

Brief Chronology of Discovery of Disease-Producing Microorganisms, 1865–1910

An asterik (*) means that these matters are further elaborated in the text.

1865*

Pasteur recommends heat treatment (pasteurization) to prevent wine spoilage.

1871*

Pasteur concludes work on silkworms, confirming his tentative "germ theory" of disease.

1876*

Koch demonstrates that anthrax bacillus causes the disease *anthrax*.

1879

Hansen and Neisser identify the organism associated with *leprosy* (Hansen's bacillus).
Neisser discovers the agent of *gonorrhea*, the gonococcus, and the disease is promptly named after him and politely called a Neisserian infection.

1880

Pasteur and Sternberg discover the pneumococcus, causing *pneumonia*.
Koch and Eberth find the bacillus causing *typhoid fever*.
Laveran discovers the plasmodium whose presence in the blood causes *malaria*.

1882*

Koch discovers the tubercle bacillus, as noted; and with Ogston discovers the streptococcus, common agent of such infections as *childbed fever, strep throat,* and then so-called *blood poisoning*.

1883

Koch discovers the organism of Asiatic *cholera*.
Klebs sees the *diptheria* bacillus, which Loeffler soon obtains in pure culture.

1884

Nicolaier discovers the bacillus of *tetanus* (lockjaw).

1887*

Bruce describes the causative agent of the disease named after him, brucellosis. It was originally called Malta fever, from the island of Malta, where Bruce found it, but is now generally known as *undulant fever*.

1892*

Iwanowski demonstrates a "filterable virus."

1894*

Kitasato and Yersin discover the *plague* bacillus, whose ancestors in the days of the Black Death had decimated Europe.

1905*

Schaudin and Hoffman describe the wriggly, spiral agent of *syphilis—treponema pallidum—*which they see finally in a dark-field microscope.

1910

Bordet and Gengou discover the agent of *whooping-cough, Bacillus Pertussis.*

can pass through the pores of an unglazed porcelain filter, which catches larger microorganisms. In the brief chronology on the next page a number of important communicable diseases are *not mentioned*. It was later demonstrated that these diseases were caused by viruses, for example smallpox, chickenpox, mumps, measles, rabies, yellow fever, poliomyelitis, and the common cold.

Present-Day Microbiology

The science of bacteriology has grown so complex that it has been forced to change its name to describe its present scope and functions. *Microbiology* includes both bacteriology and virology, and it verges into the field of antibiotics. This is in consonance with the idea that prevention and treatment of disease are not completely separated processes. By curing disease in one individual, its host, you can thus prevent it from being transmitted to another individual in the chain reaction that creates an epidemic.

Prevention by cure was the line of attack taken by Paul Ehrlich when he sought his "magic bullet." Chemotherapy and antibiotic therapy depend for their development not only on the science of chemistry but also on the knowledge of the life cycles of microorganisms provided by modern microbiology.

Two important generalizations about modern microbiology must be made: First, it deals with all types of microorganisms, not only those which are disease-producing (pathogenic) and which, in comparison to the total, are few in number. Secondly, its range extends not only to microorganisms which infest man but also to those which invade plants, animals, and other microorganisms.

Many microorganisms are helpful not harmful to man—for example, soil bacteria and the *Lactobacillus acidophilus* which makes buttermilk. Some microorganisms, including some of those that commonly inhabit the lower gastrointestinal tract of man, are almost essential to him. It is not only man who suffers from pathogenic bacteria; the plant and animal kingdoms are often even more seriously ravaged. Many diseases of plants have a virus origin.

The science of microbiology obviously depends upon instruments by means of which microbes can be visualized; but even those too small to be easily seen can be studied by their effects. The most important new tool of the microbiologist is the electron microscope. We speak glibly of microorganisms, but except to the specialist it is difficult to convey how really tiny they all are.

Microorganisms are measured, in so far as they can be, in microns and millimicrons. A micron is 1/1000 of a millimeter, or 1/25,000 of an inch; and a millimicron is 1/1000 of a micron. The polio virus, one of the smallest, measures 10 millimicrons in length. About 6000 polio virus particles could therefore be lined up on the point of a pin, which is about 1/20 of a millimeter in diameter. The largest of the "true viruses" is that of cowpox (vaccinia). Microorganisms of the same type may vary tremendously in size and shape.

Under circumstances favorable to them, microorganisms multiply rapidly; they often begin to reproduce when they are less than half an hour old. The common method of bacterial reproduction is by simple cell division, called fission; one cell divides into two, the two into four, and so on. Some microorganisms, for example the tetanus bacillus, go through a reproductive cycle by forming spores, which are more resistant to destruction than the complete cell.

The life requirements of the microorganism include proper nourishment, proper temperature, either the presence *or absence* of oxygen or air, moisture, and absence of direct sunlight and of chemical and biological antagonists. In general pathogenic microorganisms can be called unwelcome parasites on the cells of their hosts; many require very special conditions for existence and growth.

The attack on pathogenic microorganisms, therefore, sums up to the often technically difficult problem of interfering with their life requirements. Antibiotics, for example, interfere with their metabolism and nourishment. Heat sterilization makes unlivable temperature conditions for them. Chemical antagonists, like sulfa drugs taken internally or chlorine in drinking water, either kill them outright (bactericides) or stop their growth and reproduction (bacteriostatics).

The principles here are quite simple, but elaborate techniques and methods are often required to carry them out for the practical control of communicable disease.

Microorganisms

There are approximately one hundred different communicable diseases that are now recognized—under far more than a hundred names. We have all had contact with and undoubtedly suffered from one or more. The cold and the common diseases of childhood—for example, chickenpox, measles, and mumps—are among their number. But mankind has now escaped the dreadful sense of pestilence and despair that the very names of many communicable diseases once conjured up—the Black Death, the white plague, the choking sickness (diphtheria).

Communicable diseases are invariably caused by pathogenic (disease-producing) microorganisms, commonly called "germs," infecting and multiplying in a susceptible host. Comparatively few of all the known microorganisms, however, are pathogenic for man, animal, or plants.

Even for the specialist, classification of microorganisms is difficult and often confusing. The student need not try. At least sixty different systems of classification have been proposed.

Many of the names attached to microbial organisms are patronymics, (proper names) in Latinized form, of the individuals who first described the microorganisms. Thus the class of organisms known as *rickettsia* are named after Howard Taylor Ricketts (1871–1910), an American pathologist who first identified them and who died investigating them.

The following loose classification of disease-producing microorganisms, tabulated roughly in ascending order of size, may prove helpful in understanding them. See also illustrations on pages 356 and 357.

Disease-Producing Microorganisms, Arranged in Order of Increasing Size. *Virus.* The smallest; shaped like rods or crystals; present in such diseases as smallpox, yellow fever, polio, common cold.

Rickettsia. Barely visible under highest-power optical microscopes; present in such diseases as typhus fever, Q fever.

Bacteria. Visible in characteristic shapes and groups under the microscope as follows:

a. Rod- or pencil-shaped; the most numerous kind; including organisms present in such diseases as typhoid fever, tuberculosis, leprosy.

b. Spherical shape, but sometimes concave or flattened, appearing: (1) in chains or single file, such as the streptococcus associated with "strep" infections; (2) in pairs or double file, such as the gonococcus present in gonorrhea and the encapsulated pneumococcus present in pneumonia; (3) in clusters, like grapes, notably the staphylococcus often present in boils.

c. Spiral shaped, including the corkscrew-shaped spirochete of syphilis and the comma-shaped vibrio of cholera.

Fungi. Plant-like organisms, including yeasts and molds, larger than bacteria and present in such fungus infections as athlete's foot (epidermophytosis).

Protozoa. Ranging in size from that of bacteria to several centimeters; single-celled, primitive animals and parasites; most importantly the malarial parasites.

Worms (metazoa). Many-celled animals usually visible with the naked eye and hence not strictly microorganisms; including flatworms (tapeworms) and roundworms like the hookworm and the trichina causing trichinosis in hogs and men.

Diseases in Transit

For an infection to travel from a source or reservoir to an uninfected human being, disease-producing microorganisms must have both a means of conveyance or transmission and a portal of entry into the human body. For several important diseases, the mode of transmission is still unknown or at least undecided. The portals of entry of infection are obviously few: the body orifices and the skin. Infection can be introduced through the mouth by ingestion of contaminated food or liquid. It can be transmitted to the mouth, nose, or other orifices by unclean, unwashed hands. Infectious agents can also be inhaled through the nose. Some infective agents can pass through the unbroken skin barrier. Others enter through breaks in the skin (wounds and cuts).

In the final analysis infection can be con- veyed only by contact with the infecting orga- nism, but this contact may be either *direct* or *indirect*.

Direct contact means actually touching or being touched by the infecting person or natu-

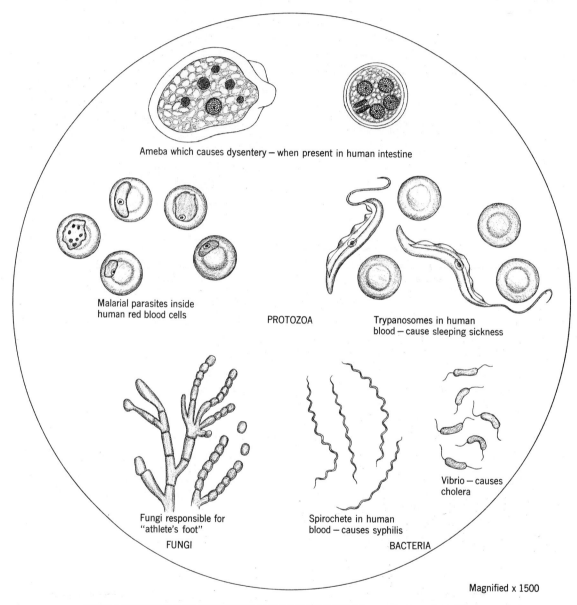

Ameba which causes dysentery — when present in human intestine

Malarial parasites inside
human red blood cells

PROTOZOA

Trypanosomes in human
blood — cause sleeping sickness

Fungi responsible for
"athlete's foot"

FUNGI

Spirochete in human
blood — causes syphilis

BACTERIA

Vibrio — causes
cholera

Magnified x 1500

SOME LARGER DISEASE-PRODUCING MICROORGANISMS. The smallest speck visible to the human eye is about 1/250th of an inch long. If such a speck were enlarged 1500 times, it would be the size of the circle used as the background of this illustration. At that magnification (× 1500) the microorganisms responsible for amebic dysentery, malaria, sleeping sickness, "athlete's foot," syphilis, and cholera look about as they are shown above.

ral source of infection. This includes hand-to-body and hand-to-mouth contact, sexual intercourse, kissing, and inhalation of the air containing droplets of infective material within a range of three feet or less.

Indirect contact takes place by means of contaminated surface articles, or matter, or vehicles of infection, including floors, food, clothing, and utensils; by air convection, usually only for a few feet, the particles remaining infective usually

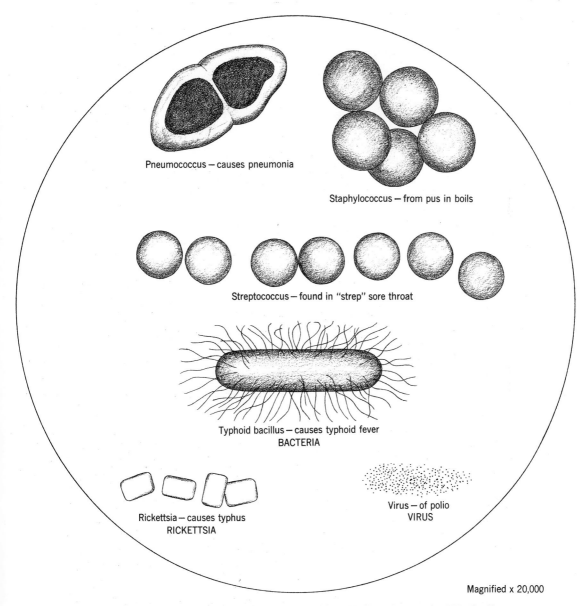

Pneumococcus – causes pneumonia

Staphylococcus – from pus in boils

Streptococcus – found in "strep" sore throat

Typhoid bacillus – causes typhoid fever
BACTERIA

Rickettsia – causes typhus
RICKETTSIA

Virus – of polio
VIRUS

Magnified x 20,000

SOME SMALLER DISEASE-PRODUCING MICROORGANISMS. If one of the red blood cells shown in the illustration on the facing page was enlarged to 20,000 times natural size, it would be about the size of the circle used as the background for this illustration. At that magnification (× 20,000) certain bacteria (pneumococcus, streptococcus, staphylococcus, typhoid bacillus), rickettsial bodies, and the very small polio virus appear about as they are shown above.

for only a short period of time; and by insect or animal vectors.

Venereal Disease

Venereal diseases are so designated because they are usually the outcome of venery, a word whose origin goes back to Venus, the Roman goddess of love. The five commonly recognized venereal diseases are syphilis, gonorrhea, chancroid, lymphogranuloma venereum, and granuloma inguinale. The last two mentioned are comparatively rare and chiefly tropical diseases.

The principal venereal diseases are syphilis and gonorrhea, two quite different infections but occasionally acquired at the same time. Untreated syphilis is a long-range, sometimes fatal disease. Untreated gonorrhea is a shorter, sometimes crippling disease. Chancroid describes a soft chancre or ulcer on the genital organs.

When a "hush-hush" attitude toward venereal disease pervaded society, the venereal diseases altogether were politely called "social diseases." Then it was both conscientiously believed and vindictively taught that venereal diseases were "the wages of sin." With all that is known about them today they might more properly be described as "the wages of ignorance." Intelligent community health organization, better treatment (antibiotics), and public education have all helped to change community attitudes toward venereal disease.

The extreme fear in which these dieases have been held was undoubtedly more justified in earlier generations than in our own. Like other communicable diseases, their etiologic agents were then shrouded in mystery, and there was no effective treatment for them.

Unquestionably, moral and social issues such as promiscuity, prostitution, and personal sex conduct are associated with the spread of venereal disease. However, since we have previously dealt with these problems (Chapters 11 and 12), we shall limit our discussion here to venereal diseases as communicable diseases that fall into the province of the physician and the public health officer and his staff. With the introduction

in the 1940's of penicillin and other antibiotics for the treatment of venereal diseases, the incidence of these diseases fell sharply. However, in the mid-fifties the incidence of the venereal disease began to rise again.

Syphillis. The antiquity and origins of syphilis are still disputed by scholars. According to some it originated in the Western Hemisphere and was imported from America to Europe by the sailors of Columbus. At any rate the disease first came to serious public attention in France and Italy shortly after the discovery of America. It followed the Armies of Charles VIII at Naples in 1495— and it has been following armies ever since.

Syphilis has been called by many names: historically, the French pox, the English pox; scientifically and politely, lues (for which the adjective is luetic); vulgarly, "bad blood," "the dog," and other names. In the late 1800's Sir William Osler gave it the nickname of "the great imitator," for in its final stages syphilis can produce signs and symptoms which mimic almost every known disease.

The specific causative agent of syphilis is the corkscrew-shaped microorganism called *Treponema pallidum,* formerly *Spirochaeta pallida.* It is capable of invading all tissues of the human body and does not, as some believe, stay only in the blood stream. It is an eager parasite on a human host, but outside the human body it is relatively delicate and fragile. Dried up, it dies. Exposed for any length of time to temperatures as high as those of an extremely hot bath, it perishes.

The source of infection in syphilis is always another infected human being. The sphirochete travels to its new victim in discharges from his or her obvious or concealed lesions on the skin or mucous membranes. Spirochetes can also be discharged in semen and in blood. Direct contact with infected persons is the chief means of transmission of syphilis.

How Syphilis Is Spread. In well over 90% of all cases this direct contact is by sexual intercourse. It is occasionally contracted by professional workers in the course of their duties— through dental, surgical, or technical accidents.

Indirect contacts are responsible for the trans-

COMMON MEANS OF TRANSMISSION OF SOME COMMUNICABLE DISEASES

1. By respiratory discharges ("droplet" infections and/or contact).

   Common cold
   Pneumonia and influenza
   Tuberculosis
   Septic sore throat and scarlet fever

   So-called childhood diseases:
   Mumps
   Measles
   German measles (rubella)
   Diptheria
   Whooping-cough (pertussis)
   Chickenpox

2. By discharges from the intestinal tract (and therefore often by contaminated soil or water).

   Cholera
   Typhoid fever
   Paratyphoid fever

   Hookworm diseases
   Dysentery (amebic and bacillary)
   Schistosomiasis (snails carry it)

3. By contaminated food or milk.

   Food infections (e.g., salmonellosis)
   Botulism
   Cholera
   Typhoid fever
   Trichinosis

   Undulant fever
   Tuberculosis
   Streptococcal infections (eg., septic sore throat and scarlet fever)
   Intestinal worms

4. By association with animals.

   Actinomycosis ("lumpy jaw")
   Anthrax
   Undulant fever (e.g., cow)

   Plague (e.g., rat)
   Tularemia (e.g., rabbit)

5. By insects (usually by insect bite).

   Malaria (mosquito)
   Yellow fever (mosquito)
   Typhus (louse)
   Plague (rat-flea)

   Filariasis (mosquito)
   African sleeping sickness (tsetse fly)
   Sandfly fever (sandfly)
   Dengue (mosquito)

6. By sexual intercourse, usually; or intimate contact.

   Syphilis
   Gonorrhea

   Chancroid (soft chancre)
   Lymphogranuloma venereum

Note: These are not to be considered the exclusive means of transmission of each disease.

---

mission of syphilis only in the rarest of instances. Articles freshly soiled with discharges or blood containing the spirochete might transmit the disease if the second person touched them within just a few minutes after they left the infected individual and they were still moist. Towels, toilet articles and articles held in the mouth, such as pipe stems or some musical instruments, are,

practically speaking, about the only objects on which a viable spirochete might be conveyed.

The fear of contracting syphilis "innocently" by touching doorknobs or coming in contact with bathtubs, eating utensils, or toilet seats is *unwarranted*.

The only other way of getting syphilis is congenitally—through the placenta during intra-uterine life from an infected mother. However, the protection of the unborn infant by treating the mother is very effective. Even if treatment is begin as late as the fourth or fifth month of pregnancy, the chances of preventing congenital syphilis in the child are 90% or better.

The individual who has syphilis is not always capable of transmitting it. The disease is communicable during its primary and secondary stages. Infrequently the skin lesions of secondary syphilis later reappear, within a year usually, and these too may be infectious. Technically these lesions are designated as mucocutaneous relapses. The most important period of communicability is during the first few months or year or two of infection. Yet inadequately treated patients *may* transmit the infection through sexual intercourse for a period up to approximately five years.

Like many other communicable diseases, syphilis is carried along through a chain of infected individuals. A single infected prostitute might give the disease to 100 men. There is no such thing as a "safe" prostitute or call girl even though they receive periodic medical inspections.

The Stages of Syphilis. If untreated, syphilis runs a long course and goes through the following stages: primary, secondary, latent, and tertiary.

Primary Stage. This is marked by a sore at the site where the spirochetes entered the body. It is usually found on the sex organs, but occasionally in the mouth. This sore, called a chancre (pronounced shanker), is generally hard and painless. It may look like a small pimple or ulcer, ranging from pinhead size to an inch or more. It is often concealed and may pass unnoticed.

The chancre appears anywhere from 10 days to about 3 months after exposure, but on the average in about 3 weeks. By this time the spirochetes have spread through the body, but there are no general symptoms of disease. Treatment of syphilis should begin promptly whenever a chancre is discovered, for this is the best time to drive out the spirochetes. The disease is highly communicable while the chancre is present.

Secondary Stage. Even without treatment, the chancre disappears in about 3 to 6 weeks. The secondary stage of syphilis begins as the chancre is disappearing; at this time the spirochetes diffuse themselves throughout the body, and can be found in the circulating blood. The secondary stage lasts for a variable period of time, usually a few months but sometimes for several years. The disease is still readily curable in the secondary stage.

Latent Stage. The signs and symptoms of secondary syphilis gradually pass away although no treatment be given. This disease then lapses into a latent or quiescent stage, which usually lasts from 5 to 20 years but may range from 2 to 50 years. There are no symptoms in the latent stage, but the spirochetes are still present in the body and can be discovered by serologic ("blood") tests.

Tertiary (third) Stage. In this final stage of syphilis, the untreated disease often comes to a hideous flower and imitates many other diseases. It may attack the brain and spinal cord (neurosyphilis), the heart and blood vessels (particularly the aorta), the bones, and the skin.

The effects of late syphilis on the nervous system go under such names as paresis, general paralysis of the insane, dementia paralytica, locomotor ataxia and tabes dorsalis. Late syphilis can be treated—but not so effectively as the earlier stages of the disease.

Diagnosis and Treatment. The diagnosis of syphilis requires laboratory confirmation. In the primary stage it is confirmed by examining fluids from the chancre under a dark-field microscope and actually seeing the pale, wriggly spirochetes. In the subsequent stages the diagnosis is made by serologic tests, (*blood tests*). Spinal fluid is also used. The best-known of these laboratory tests for syphilis is the Wassermann test, but there are a great many others also named after the laboratory men who developed them—for example, the Kahn, Kline, Kolmer, Hinton, and Eagle tests. A four-plus Wassermann signifies a completely positive reaction on the test.

Syphilis at all stages is now effectively treated and usually cured with penicillin and other antibiotics. The treatment period is *short,* and the injections can be given easily and painlessly in any doctor's office. A series of four or five injections of penicillin in the course of a week can change a positive Wassermann to a negative Wassermann in that time. Relapses are few, although reinfection can occur.

Gonorrhea. Gonorrhea is both the most common and the most readily curable venereal disease. Its incidence is about five times higher than syphilis. It is an acute, communicable disease, specifically caused by infection with the gonococcus microbe (*Neisseria gonorrheae*). Untreated gonorrhea may have a chronic, serious, and crippling aftermath, resulting in sterility, arthritis, or blindness.

The only source of gonorrheal infection is discharges from lesions of the mucous membranes or lymph nodes of persons currently afflicted. Hence the disease is almost always transmitted by sexual contact or direct personal contact with the discharges. In rare instances articles freshly soiled with discharges—wash cloths, towels, and other bathroom accessories—may transmit the disease. Little girls under 6 are especially susceptible to vaginal infection with such discharges, and epidemics of vulvovaginitis sometimes occur in girls' schools. These are the principal instances in which gonorrhea is innocently acquired.

Symptoms. The symptoms of gonorrhea appear from 1 day to 2 or 3 weeks (usually 3 to 5 days) after exposure. In the male the symptoms of the early and acute disease include pain—stinging or burning—when urinating, some slight swelling and discomfort in the urinary region, and the discharge of a few drops of pus from the tip of the penis. These symptoms grow worse as the infection of the mucous membranes of the urinary system and adjacent organs progresses.

In women the early symptoms are likely to be less acute. In addition to pain on urination (which is less acute because the female urinary tract is shorter than the male), the early symptoms may include a yellowish vaginal discharge and a painful swelling or abscess of the glands (Bartholin's glands) at the mouth of the vulva.

Even without treatment, the acute, painful symptoms of gonorrhea gradually fade away. But there is no absolutely positive way of knowing that the gonococcus has completely disappeared from the body. Chronic or recurrent inflammation with discharge is a common occurrence in untreated gonorrhea even after the initial, acute stage has passed. So long as the gonococcus persists, the infected individual can transmit the disease.

The mucous membranes of the eye are particularly susceptible to gonorrheal infection. Newborn babies were once frequently infected during the process of birth. "Babies' sore eyes"—gonorrheal ophthalmia—was once a common cause of blindness. This condition has been practically eliminated by laws requiring silver nitrate or other equally effective gonococcus-killing drugs to be instilled in infants' eyes immediately after birth.

Treatment. Present-day treatment of gonorrhea is swift and sure. Cure rates approaching almost 100% have been reported. Any doctor can give the treatment. Most cases can be cleared up in a day or two by a single injection of delayed-action penicillin or administration by mouth of some other antibiotic drugs.

Control of Venereal Disease. Syphilis case rates in the United States and other parts of the world fell precipitously to new low levels when penicillin and other antibiotics highly effective in the treatment of venereal diseases were first introduced in the 1940's. The effectiveness of these drugs has not diminished, but their consistent application apparently has. For a variety of reasons the rate of reported syphilis has been increasing in the United States since 1957.

About 60,000 *new* cases of syphilis are now reported yearly; and there are about 2 million cases still needing treatment. There are about 1 million *new* cases of gonorrhea in the United States every year. Very few of them—perhaps 10%—are reported by private physicians to public health authorities.

The control of venereal disease has many ramifications—moral, legal, social, educational, medical, and personal. Guided by knowledge and by moral and common sense any alert individual can guarantee himself freedom from contracting venereal disease or suffering its consequences.

This is more than can be promised for almost any other class or type of disease. The rules for freedom from venereal disease, or perhaps more properly the precautions against them, can be summed up simply as follows:

Precautions Against Venereal Disease. Avoid exposure to venereal diseases and to the circumstances inviting them, especially alcoholic indulgence.

If exposed, take prompt prophylactic measures.

Watch out for the danger signals of infection—the chancre of syphilis, the pain and pus of gonorrhea.

Seek treatment promptly from a reliable physician.

Continue treatment until pronounced cured.

Have a blood test taken as part of a medical examination.

Prophylaxis may be mechanical (the rubber sheath), chemical (ointments and solutions for application to the genitals), or chemotherapeutic (antibiotics). As one of several methods of control of syphilis and gonorrhea the American Public Health Association's official *Control of Communicable Diseases in Man* recommends: "teaching methods of personal prophylaxis applicable before, during, and after exposure."

Theoretically—if every person with venereal disease was immediately put under adequate treatment—it would be possible to eliminate these diseases entirely. In Sweden, where the police power of the state has been invoked for this purpose, this goal is nearly attained.

In the United States, public health authorities have not thought it wise to press for such drastic power. Legal action is confined to setting up free clinic programs, repressing commercial prostitution, forbidding sale of liquor to minors, requiring premarital and prenatal blood tests (which some authorities believe are no longer worth the cost and effort), and regulating the conduct of taverns.

Unfortunately, with respect to many other communicable diseases, such as the cold, there are no laws which can possibly wipe them out.

The Cold

A most eloquent description of the cold was given by Charles Dickens thus: "I am at this moment deaf in the ears, hoarse in the throat, red in the nose, green in the gills, damp in the eyes, twitchy in the joints, and fractious in temper from a most intolerant and oppressive cold."

The symptoms of the cold represent attempts of invaded tissues of the eyes, ears, nose, and throat to get ride of the invaders. The stuffy nose is suffused with extra blood; its air passages are partly shut off with extra mucus released to wash out the invaders. Sneezing and coughing are attempts to dislodge irritations in the respiratory tract.

A dry, scratchy, irritated feeling in the nose or the back of the throat is usually the first sign that a cold is coming. From this point it may be a half day to three days before the cold really blooms. A slight elevation of temperature, chilly sensations, and a general feeling of fatigue frequently mark the first day or two of a cold.

The cold is a communicable and infectious disease. Indeed, it is the most common of such, and it has been estimated that its incidence outnumbers other diseases by about 25 to 1. The infecting agent of the cold is a virus—or a number of them. Research is beginning to identify certain groups of viruses with the onset of the cold, but there is no agreement yet on these findings. Secondary infection with bacteria is often superimposed on tissues softened up by the viruses. This usually prolongs the cold for two to three weeks and is responsible for the thick, yellow nasal discharge.

Catching Colds. Susceptibility to the cold is practically universal. Only inhabitants of small, isolated communities seem to escape—and even they don't when an infected individual enters the community. Few people are completely free from colds. In the United States almost everyone has at least one cold a year; about half the population has at least two; and 25% have three or more colds.

Basically you catch a cold from someone who has a cold. But colds may also be indirectly transmitted by handkerchiefs, eating utensils, and other articles. The virus picked up from the throat can be conveyed on the hands. This is one of the strong arguments for hand washing as a disease-preventive measure.

Colds are most communicable in the early stages, usually the first day. By the third or fourth day, it is unlikely that the virus will be transferred. It is almost certain that it will not be after the first week.

Many factors beyond the presence of the virus are involved in catching a cold. Physical environment and resistance of the host are concerned. Overfatigue, malnutrition, and other illness may have weakened the body's powers to resist the virus and bacterial invasion.

Weather plays a part. Frequent moving from dry, warm interiors to cold, wet outdoor weather and vice versa (the normal living process for most sedentary workers) seems to help the process of catching cold. Cold weather itself does not seem to induce colds, as recent experience of explorers in Antarctica confirms.

Treating Colds. A cold should be treated with respect. If any of the following "danger signals" appear—chills and fever, rapidly rising temperature, difficult breathing, or pain in the chest or side—medical attention should be promptly obtained. These symptoms may betoken the onset of pneumonia.

There are no specific remedies against the viruses of the cold, although most secondary bacterial invaders can be controlled with modern sulfa drugs and antibiotics.

The sovereign remedy for the cold is rest in bed during the early stages, which enables the body to mobilize its resources to throw off the infection. Unfortunately, too many people refuse this remedy; indeed they take the opposite course of fighting the cold, sometimes with disastrous results.

An old adage had it that the duration of a cold was 2 weeks if treated, or a fortnight if untreated. Actually, most people recover in 5 to 10 days. If a cold hangs on for more than 2 weeks, treatment for secondary invaders is probably indicated.

Preventing Colds. There is no guarantee that common colds can be prevented, but the following suggestions are common sense.

Keep away from people who have colds, especially those who cough, sneeze, or talk in your face.

Mind the weather. Dress properly for it. Keep your feet dry.

Avoid overheated rooms, sitting in drafts, and becoming needlessly chilled.

Get adequate rest and sleep. Do not become overfatigued. Maintain adequate nutrition with a well-balanced diet.

Aspirin may make you more comfortable and bring down fever. Use of disposable paper tissues instead of cloth handkerchiefs may prevent reinfection.

Most time-honored treatments are worthless. Little help can be expected from forcing (or restricting) fluids or fruit juices, or from cathartics, antiseptic gargles, hot or cold compresses, mustard plasters, exercise ("sweating out a cold"), or inhaled vapors.

Put little faith in highly touted and advertised methods of cold prevention. Scientific evidence has discredited most of the fads that have periodically swept the country. You will not prevent colds by overdosing yourself with vitamins, exposing yourself to ultraviolet light, hardening yourself by taking cold baths or sleeping in cold rooms, ingesting antihistamine drugs or other medications, or getting "cold shots."

Virus Diseases

The cold is the prototype of acute respiratory diseases caused by or associated with viruses. But there are many others, as well as many virus diseases which have their principal lodgement in other parts of the body—in the skin, for example, as in smallpox, and in the gastro-intestinal tract and the nervous system, as in polio. Table 1 describes respiratory viruses associated with major manifestations in other systems of the body, and Table 2 lists a number of respiratory viruses associated with acute respiratory manifestations— that is to say, these viruses lodge and show their effects principally in the lungs and nasopharynx.

Viruses lodging in the respiratory tract are the principal cause of acute illness in the United States. The National Health Survey estimates that approximately a billion respiratory illnesses occur in the United States every year—and the overwhelming majority of them are virus infections.

Great progress has been made in recent years in identifying the viruses—such as the adenoviruses and the viruses responsible for psittacosis (which originally described just "parrot fever" but has been extended in meaning to cover many forms of respiratory virus illnesses transmitted by birds). Such identifications lead to the hope that vaccines to prevent or ameliorate these virus diseases may soon become practical.

New Vaccines and Pharmaceuticals Against Communicable Diseases. A live-virus polio vaccine, perfected by Dr. Albert B. Sabin, was licensed against two of the three types of polio during 1961. The Sabin vaccine against Types I, II, and III polio is now being manufactured.

Polio vaccine has remained a source of some controversy. One school of thought holds that only the live-virus vaccine can finally eliminate polio as a threat. On the other side are those who maintain that the killed-virus vaccine, perfected by Dr. Jonas Salk in 1954–1955, can do the job equally well.

A measles vaccine developed by Dr. John Enders and associates was successfully tested during 1961. Other types of vaccine since developed now offer the definite possibility that within a few years measles can be eliminated from the United States as a threat to children. Other types of vaccine against some other viral diseases, mumps and rubella, were introduced in the 1960's.

TABLE 1. RESPIRATORY VIRUSES ASSOCIATED WITH MAJOR MANIFESTATIONS IN OTHER SYSTEMS*

Virus	Clinical Manifestations
Herpes simplex	Fever blisters; encephalitis
Varicella	Chicken pox; herpes zoster
Variola	Smallpox
Rubeola	Measles
Myxovirus mumps	Parotitis; orchitis; meningitis
Enteroviruses	Undifferentiated febrile illness
Poliovirus	Meningitis; paralysis
A	Meningitis; rash
Coxsackie	
B	Meningitis; myocarditis; pleurodynia
ECHO	Meningitis; rash; diarrhea
Salivary gland	Cytomegalic inclusion disease

TABLE 2. RESPIRATORY VIRUSES ASSOCIATED WITH ACUTE RESPIRATORY MANIFESTATIONS*

Group	Subgroups or Types
Myocoplasma	Eaton agent
Psittacosis-LGV	Psittacosis
Myxovirus	Influenza A, B, C
	Parainfluenza 1, 2, 3, 4
Adenovirus	Types 1–7 and 14
Unclassified	Respiratory syncytial (CCA)
	Coxsackie A
	Coxsackie A21 (Coe)
	ECHO 7
	ECHO 11 (U virus)—?
Enterovirus	ECHO 20 (JV-1)
	ECHO 28 (JH-2060)
	Salisbury strains
	HGP, FEB
	?Total No. types
Reovirus	Types 1, 2, 3
Infectious nasal secretions	At least 5 types

*Tables from William S. Jordan, Jr., M.D., "Acute Respiratory Diseases of Viral Etiology 1. Ecology of Virus Diseases, 1961," *American Journal of Public Health*, **52**: 6, 897–945 (June 1962). Reprinted with permission of the *American Journal of Public Health*. Copyright 1962 by American Public Health Association, Inc. (1790 Broadway, New York 19, N.Y.).

Viral Hepatitis: A New Threat Among Communicable Virus Diseases. Medicine's battle against the viruses has not been all triumph even in this "golden age" of virology. The human virus disease hepatitis has been on the increase for many years. In the mid-sixties over 1000 cases a week were being reported to the U.S. Public Health Service, and it ranked third, behind measles and streptococcal infections, in such reports. Hepatitis was first recongnized as a major public health problem in the United States in 1951. Within ten years the disease reached an all-time high, with 73,000 cases reported in 1961.

Hepatitis is usually spread from person to person. Some cases have been transmitted by the uses of contaminated syringe needles, surgical instruments, and blood products. However, some outbreaks have been traced to contaminated food or water.

The disease is particularly serious in adults. It sometimes requires weeks or months of bed rest and can result in permanent liver damage. Because a yellow tinge in the skin is a common symptom, it is often called "yellow jaundice." Not all patients develop jaundice, however, and because symptoms are varied and vague, the disease is often difficult to diagnose.

Immunity

One attack of the cold does not prevent another from occurring at a later date. Nor, incidentally, does the human body invoke any defenses aginst reinfection with venereal disease. Fortunately for the survival of the human race, however, there do eixst some natural lines of protection against many communicable and other diseases. These go under the general heading of *immunity,* although they are also described as *resistance* to disease and *tolerance* of noxious agents.

It is impossible to explain yet why or exactly how immunity, resistance, and tolerance occur or develop. A teacher with active tuberculosis stands daily before a class of 30 children—3 become infected; 27 do not. Why? During a poliomyelitis epidemic, practically everyone in

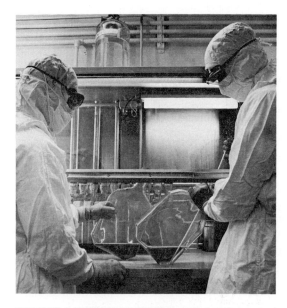

TO MAKE A MEASLES VACCINE, pure strains of virus must be grown in large quantities, and this can be done only in living cells. Monkey kidney cells are grown and multiplied to serve as hosts for the virus. Flasks of tissue cultures are inoculated with live measles virus and incubated. After the incubation period, technicians harvest the virus-laden fluid, which will then be filtered to remove the kidney tissue. The virus is inactivated with formalin and precipitated to make the finished vaccine. (Photograph courtesy of Chas. Pfizer & Co., Inc.)

the community is infected with polio virus. But the polio virus "crashes" the blood-brain barrier and causes paralysis in only 1 in 200 or more residents. Why? Most of the common childhood diseases induce a relatively life-long immunity against reinfection. Why? Some people get poison ivy if they barely brush against a leaf. Others can wade in it with impunity. Why? The answer to all the "Why's" in this paragraph is that nobody yet really knows.

Immunity is a strong word which might imply complete resistance to any attack of a specific disease of pathogenic microorganism. Practically speaking, immunity is relative. Under some circumstances even a very high degree of immunity may be broken down.

The opposite of immunity is *susceptibility* to disease. A person is susceptible in the degree that he is not immune; never 100% either way. The ability of combinations of multiple factors to overcome the body's resistance to disease depends upon the interaction between the host, the agents of disease, and the internal and external environments of both.

Natural and Acquired Immunity. We speak of several kinds of immunity: (*a*) natural and acquired immunity, (*b*) active and passive immunity. *Natural immunity* is an inborn trait which renders a species, a race, or an individual highly resistant to certain infections or stresses. For example, human beings are naturally immune to hog cholera. The newborn baby enjoys a high degree of acquired immunity from antibodies given to him through the blood stream of his mother. These immunities in general apply only to the diseases to which the mother herself was immune and, except for natural immunity, rarely last beyond a period of a few months to a year.

A less pleasant way of acquiring immunity (*natural acquired immunity*) is to suffer an attack of or exposure to a disease involving specific microorganisms. This situation is more or less true of the common diseases of childhood, especially those caused by viruses, but there is no guarantee that a given individual cannot contract the same disease twice.

Finally, immunity can be acquired by deliberate immunization (*artificially acquired immunity*). This requires inoculation or injections—so-called shots. The first practical success in this direction was smallpox vaccination, introduced in England by Edmund Jenner in 1798. The list of diseases for which artificial immunization is considered practical is still short. It includes—routinely for infants—smallpox, polio, diphtheria, tetanus (lockjaw), whooping cough, and measles; and—for adults or children where the risk warrants—cholera, plague, typhus, typhoid and paratyphoid fever, influenza, yellow fever, "German measles" (rubella), and rabies (for anyone bitten by an animal known or strongly suspected to have rabies). Mumps vaccine has recently been added to the list.

Active versus Passive Immunity. In every case of *active immunity* the body cells and tissues of the host *themselves react* to produce a specific immunity to the infective agent (antigen) to which they

were exposed. Active immunity is acquired slowly but lasts a relatively long time—from months to years. Once exposed to the infecting agent in some form, the body cells appear to acquire experience which permits them to fight off later invasions of the same or closely related agents. This "experience" usually means the ability to produce specific antibodies to fight the disease.

In passive immunity the body cells and the tissues take no part themselves in producing the immunity. The individual receives the protection by substances injected into his body, such as gamma globulin or convalescent serum derived from human beings or antitoxins from animal sources.

Passive immunity is generally used in treatment of an acute infection, such as the administration of diphtheria antitoxin or tetanus antitoxin in the actual presence of the disease. Passive immunity generally lasts only a short time—from hours to months, because the body rejects foreign substances.

Control Measures in Communicable Disease

While official public health agencies have many functions, as we shall soon see, the original and continuing basis of their support derives from their position in the control of communicable disease—largely through environmental sanitation.

Modern measures for the control of communicable disease may be summed up under four general headings:

Preventive measures are applicable to individuals generally and to groups when a disease appears in sporadic, epidemic, or endemic fashion. They can and usually should be applied whether or not the disease appears as an active threat at the time. Such measures include vaccination against smallpox, chlorination of water supplies, pasteurization of milk, control of rodents and insects (arthropods), animal control (e.g., the dog pound), and immunization.

Control of the infected individual, his contacts and environment is a measure designed to prevent infectious matter present in the person and environment of the infected individual from being conveyed to other persons, insects, or animals in such a way as to spread disease. This may require isolation of an individual, quarantine of his premises, immediate and terminal disinfection of his excretions and belongings, passive immunization, or even enforced treatment backed by police power.

However, these methods are employed selectively; none applies to all diseases. Investigation of the source of the infection is almost always in order; this is often of special importance in the venereal diseases and tuberculosis. The person or persons with whom an infected individual has been in contact should be kept under surveillance throughout the assumed period of incubation of the disease under investigation.

Epidemic measures are emergency procedures designed to limit the spread of communicable disease which, on the basis of continuing reports of incidence, appears to be developing widely and perhaps rapidly in a community. Such epidemic measures are unnecessary and unjustified when the disease is sporadic, occasional, or comparatively rare. For example, a widespread epidemic of typhus fever might be cut short by compulsory delousing of an entire population, but such a drastic measure would not be acceptable when there were only a few cases. Then it would be enough to apply inseticides with residual effect simply to the effects of people known to have been in contact with infected persons.

International measures include controls of population movements, commerce, and transportation of immigrants and travelers across national boundary lines. Such controls may be agreed upon through international conventions or conferences. They are means of affording protection for the uninfected inhabitants of one or more nations against known and notified risks of infection from another nation where a particular disease may be present in endemic or epidemic form. Also part of the picture of international measures are precautions concerning vaccination and immunization, quarantine, surveillance of travelers, and animal control (e.g., hoof-and-

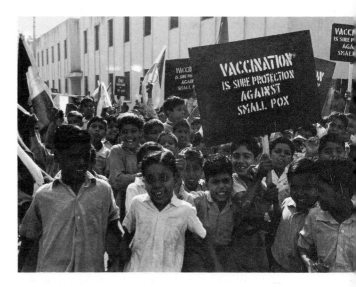

VACCINATION against smallpox is gaining acceptance all around the world as the fervor of these schoolboys in India illustrates. (Photograph courtesy of World Health Organization)

mouth disease quarantine regulations). The World Health Organization provides a central office for the international reporting and notification of endemic, epidemic, or pandemic disease.

Travel Precautions. American travelers abroad must be prepared for the fact that many foreign countries, especially less developed ones, do not maintain the same high sanitary standards as these well-plumbed United States. In particular, water supplies are often contaminated with microorganisms to which the natives have apparently developed a tolerance but which bring the foreign traveler down with troublesome and sometimes dangerous intestinal ailments (various forms of dysentery).

There are some locales in the world where water cannot be safely drunk unless it is boiled or chlorinated in the sight of the drinker. Even bottled water is not safe. The temptation to refill fancy bottles with the local water supply cannot always be resisted. In these countries light wines are often the common beverage.

In the countries where "night soil" (human feces) is used for fertilizer the eating of "fresh" vegetables may also have dire effects. Travelers have reported situations where even lettuce had to be boiled before it was safely edible!

The foreign traveler should take two other important precautions: (1) be immunized against diseases often endemic in the area to which he is traveling (if immunizations are available, see page 366) and (2) carry along an adequate quantity of medications and first-aid supplies.

Environmental Sanitation

Environmental sanitation is today primarily a job for experts and professionals—sanitary engineers, public-health staffs, food and drink processors, architects, and plumbers. The average citizen in a metropolitan community has little to do with environmental sanitation except to keep his garbage can covered and refrain from spitting on the sidewalk. Even in rural areas the householder does not have much more to do than to keep his premises clean, to have his private water supply tested and inspected, and to be sure that his privy is insect- and vermin-proof and located at least 100 feet away from his well-water supply without risk of seepage.

The professional workers in the fields of environmental sanitation face huge and continuing tasks. They are concerned, for example, with public water works and the best methods of purifying public water supplies. This can be done by impounding, which includes exposure to sunlight, by filtration, by aeration, or by chlorination and treatment with other chemicals.

They are also concerned with water-pollution control in running streams, with problems of air pollution ("smog"), with sewage treatment, with garbage and refuse collection, with the disposal of radioactive wastes, with insect and rodent control, and with milk and food sanitation. They must further look into matters which concern the health-safety of the public at home and at work; on the streets, in schools, in offices, and in industrial plants; traveling by auto, train, or plane; bedding down in tourist camps, tourist courts, or motels; or swimming in public swimming pools.

The specific exercise of these manifold func-

tions is divided up by law among local (city or county) and state health departments and the U.S. Public Health Service, an agency of the federal government. The divisions are historical rather than logical. See Chapters 20 to 23 for more detailed information on these subjects.

Self-Protection Against Health Hazards

At risk from so many communicable and other diseases, how then can you protect yourself against these health hazards?

¶ You can take advantage of the immunizations available against some specific diseases, as we have just noted.

¶ You can be alert to the common danger signals of disease and see a doctor when they flash. (See pages 12 and 13.)

¶ You can seek and accept the best available medical advice in time and on time. Conversely, you can stay away from the folly of self-medication.

¶ You can avoid so far as possible the *causes* of disease and accident. For instance, you can consciously avoid exposure to venereal disease. With a mature philosophy of life you may even avoid some of the anxieties that are *precipitating* factors in many diseases. Again, by understanding the normal reactions of the body, you may correct some of the *predisposing causes* of disease, for example, the neglect of a common cold or needless fatigue which could predispose to pneumonia.

¶ You can escape and *postpone the effects* of disease. With proper medical guidance and the use of insulin or tolbutamide, as prescribed, you need not die prematurely of diabetes.

¶ You can support those *community and public health activities* which do for individual citizens and their families what they cannot possibly do for themselves, for example, protect community water and milk supplies against contamination. You can take leadership in voluntary health agency activities. You can support your local health department.

Selecting a Physician

It is sad that far too many people neglect and disregard the opportunities open to them for their own health protection.

Many people, for example, hesitate to call on or visit a physician at times when they could most profit by his services. One common rationalization for this is, "Why should I spend the money?" Actually, the fear of the physician has deeper roots. The ill person may fear "bad news." He may not want to be told that he is really sick. He may secretly rebel against giving up so much of his independence as to obey the doctor's orders. As a result of childhood associations, and for other reasons, physicians often stand in the role of parent substitutes to their patients. Unresolved hate, fear, and aggression directed against parents may therefore be unconsciously transferred to the physician, and powerful resentments against him and his treatments built up.

When should you see a doctor? The answer to the question would be elementary if it were not so often disregarded. Obviously, you should call a doctor when you are sick, and as early in the course of illness as possible. It is very hard, however, for some people to admit they *are* sick even when they *feel* sick—eat poorly, sleep poorly, run a temperature, and the like.

Medicine is an art tempered by science, and there are still mysteries in the healing process. However, needless ignorance about the ethics and mechanics of the practice of medicine often separates patients from physicians and impairs the vital doctor-patient relationship. Medical ethics are based on the Hippocratic oath, which puts the welfare of the patient first.

Medical treatment has advanced more in the last 100 years than in the previous 2000, but all methods of treatment still fall under five major headings: (1) surgery, (2) drugs, (3) physical medicine, (4) psychotherapy, and (5) regimen. We turn now to consider the actual selection of a physician.

The physician who is good for you is one in whom you personally have implicit faith and confidence. Most of the physicians in the United States are in private practice, either alone or in a group or clinic. All you have to do to see a doctor is go to his office or summon him by telephone to your home if you are too sick to visit him. Physicians *expect* calls from patients whom they have never seen before, and they are accustomed to emergencies.

Five out of six colleges and universities in the country have some kind of college (or student) health service—an emergency service at the very least. If you do not already know how or where to reach it in your own institution, you can easily find out by calling the central administrative offices or the central switchboard of the college and asking to be connected with the college health service, the college medical office, or the college physician.

Whenever you need a doctor in a genuine emergency, pick up the telephone and ask for the Physicians' Emergency Service or, that failing, the city (or county) hospital, the city (or county) health department, or the police department. In many places emergency ambulance service is dispatched through the police department.

Ideally, of course, a person should select his physician before an emergency arises, but it must be admitted that this is not common practice. Comparatively few people give their doctors a chance to keep them well.

Sources of Recommendations. The most common practice in selecting a physician is to ask friends or associates to recommend one. Often you don't even have to ask! However, if you hesitate to ask your friends, you can call or write the local county medical society, which will give you a list of names and addresses of three or more general practitioners of medicine whose offices are reasonably near to your residence. Sometimes the county medical society will release its entire roster for your perusal. Names and addresses of nearby physicians will also be supplied to you in most instances by the superintendent of a hospital or by a local health department.

Almost all the physicians whose names are given you will be general practitioners. Do not ask for the names of specialists. See the general practitioner first. He will refer you to any specialists your condition requires.

"Shopping around" for medical specialists on your own initiative is likely to be both a frustrating and expensive practice. Your general practitioner's first choice will generally be better than your first guess. If you don't like the first specialist to whom he refers you, he can always recommend another.

Factual data about any physician—M.D.—in the United States can be obtained from the American Medical Association, 535 North Dearborn Street, Chicago, Illinois. It is usually more convenient, however, to consult the latest massive volume of this association's *Directory of Physicians,* available in many libraries. Beyond these simple facts, the only positive way in which you can select and evaluate a physician is through your personal contact and experience with him.

The Periodic Medical Examination. Periodic medical examinations or "check-ups," on every birthday or on certain "threshold" birthdays, for example, have long been recommended. The logic of the idea, however, has not yet in America been able to overcome general public inertia toward it. Its value is attested on many sides. Leading insurance companies provide periodic health examinations for some (or all) of their policyholders. The armed forces insist on such examinations repeatedly. In many industries, notably the transportation industry, they are commonly performed. Airline pilots and railroad engineers, for example, cannot afford to have physical or mental impairments which may endanger the lives of passengers.

Yet, in spite of all the arguments in its favor, it must be admitted that the periodic medical examination has not "caught on." There are psychological and economic arguments against it. Most disappointing is the fact that the people most in need of periodic health examinations are the ones who most often resist having them, and not because of cost. People just don't want to "know the worst," as they wrongly put it.

SUMMARY

In Summary. The control of communicable disease since the middle of the nineteenth century is one of mankind's greatest success stories, though it is still an unfinished story. Worldwide victory over communicable disease, notably malaria and tuberculosis, is still far from complete.

In this chapter we have briefly told the story of the sciences of bacteriology and microbiology after Louis Pasteur, in the 1860's, had established the "germ theory of disease." We have pictured and described some of the common disease-producing microorganisms (microbes, germs) and indicated the common means of transmission of a number of communicable diseases. By way of examples of the nature of infectious diseases, we have discussed in considerable detail two of the venereal diseases, syphilis and gonorrhea, usually transmitted by sexual contact; and the common cold, an almost universal virus disease, transmitted by respiratory discharges ("droplet" infection).

We have noted the important role of immunity and immunization in protecting against communicable diseases, and we have noted the many other control measures necessary to complete the task—for example, environmental sanitation. Finally, we have outlined the numerous methods available for *self*-protection against health hazards, not the least of which are intelligent selection of a personal physician and periodic medical check-ups.

Since the ills to which human flesh is heir are so many and so varied, no individual, acting alone, can hope to protect himself or herself entirely from them. We all need the community health organizations delineated in Chapter 19.

SUMMARY REVIEW QUESTIONS

1. What is communicable disease? How is it caused? How is it spread? Among the 100 known communicable diseases of man, name six for which you can state (a) the specific microorganism that causes it and (b) its common mode of transmission.

2. What measures for the control of venereal disease do you *personally* advocate? What measures—briefly—do you think you would emphasize if you were: A police chief? A public health officer? A physician? A clergyman? A parent of teenage boys or girls? An army officer? A high-school principal? The proprietor of a public dancehall?

3. What are the early and evident signs of syphilis? How is the disease spread? What are the stages of the disease?

4. How does gonorrhea differ from syphilis? What are the presenting symptoms of gonorrhea? In what way, if any, is the treatment of the two diseases different?

5. What methods of preventing or treating a common cold would you now personally employ or recommend to a friend? What other virus diseases besides the common cold are responsible for acute respiratory distress? Name at least three and their causative agents.

6. What is immunity? How would you distinguish between (a) natural and acquired immunity and (b) active and passive immunity?

7. In what six general ways can you protect yourself against the hazards of disease? Which way, if any, seems most important to you? In what four general ways do public health authorities safeguard you against communicable disease?

8. How would you go about selecting a personal physician for yourself? What do you expect of your doctor? Do you have a doctor now? If not, why not? If so, how did you choose him?

9. What was the turning point in man's long uphill fight to control communicable, infectious disease? What specifically were some of the great discoveries made in this direction after the turning point had been reached (name at least five)?

10. Can you identify the following men and indicate the principal contributions of each one toward the control of communicable disease: Girolamo Fracastoro, Anton van Leeuwenhoek, Edward Jenner, Oliver Wendall Holmes, Louis Pasteur, John Snow, Robert Koch, Paul Ehrlich, Howard Taylor Ricketts, Jonas Salk?

11. Are the following statements sense or nonsense? Why? *All microorganisms are germs.* . . . . *Gonorrhea is no worse than a bad cold.* . . . . *It's easy to tell whether a person has a venereal disease.* . . . . *The periodic health examination is the best way of guaranteeing continued good health.* . . . . *"The devil was sick. The devil a monk would be./The devil got well. The devil a monk was he."*

12. What do the following terms mean to you: rickettsia, microbiology, the germ theory of disease, "indirect transmission" (of diseases), chancre, four-plus Wassermann, "babies' sore eyes," predisposing cause of disease, viral hepatitis, periodic medical examination?

Worth Looking Into: *The Control of Communicable Disease in Man,* an official report of the American Public Health Association. *The Conquest of Epidemic Disease* by C. E. A. Winslow. *The Family Medical Encyclopedia* by Justus J. Schifferes. *Communicable Disease Control* by Gaylord W. Anderson, M.D., and others. *Snow on Cholera* by John Snow, M.D. *Rats, Lice and History* by Hans Zinsser, M.D. For more complete references, see Appendix E.

18

ACCIDENT PREVENTION—SAFETY

I N THE THREE SECONDS IT WILL TAKE YOU TO read this sentence, somewhere in the United States somebody has been seriously hurt in an accident. In the five minutes that it will take you to read this page and part of the next, someone has been killed in an accident. More Americans have been killed in traffic accidents than in all the nation's wars.

The accident picture in this country is so grim that we tend to repress knowledge of it. We often react by saying that the topic of accidents is boring—until we ourselves are somehow caught. Then, often too late, we want to know what caused the accident and how it could have been prevented. Not wanting to talk about accidents is quite a common reaction.

We should not want to live constantly with the threat of death by violence hanging over our heads. Reasonable safety-mindedness is fine; rational steps to avoid accidents can then be taken. But overanxiety or constant fear about being involved in an accident is a symptom of mental disturbance and sometimes mental illness.

In this chapter we shall deal with the highlights of the broad subject of accident prevention and safety education. The emphasis will be on the prevention of motor-vehicle accidents, since they are the greatest single hazard to young men and women. There are, of course, many points of view from which the subject of accident prevention can be considered; the traffic policeman has one point of view, the safety engineer another, the accident statistician a third, and so on.

However, since all statistical records reveal that the "human element" is the great unpredictable factor in accidents, or, in more obvious terms, that the cause of accidents is people, we shall direct our discussion largely to the kind of people who are most liable to have accidents and to the psychological, *unconscious* drives and circumstances most likely to bring them on. Far too many accidents, we shall see, only *appear* as accidents. They were *purposeful* attempts at self-injury or self-destruction. These accidents can be prevented only by attention to the mental health of the individual *before* he would otherwise be involved in them.

Even today there is still a good bit of superstition about the causes and prevention of accidents. Many people still carry charms, such as a rabbit's foot, or wear amulets to ward off accidents. Even more carry in their minds a vague belief in some magic formula that will save them from harm, from accident, from violence.

When an accident happens to them, they may attribute it to "gremlins"—invisible imps of disaster first "noticed" by British aviators during World War II. This explanation is not so foolish as it looks at first glance; it is an externalization of the fact that the fundamental causes of accidents are *people*, often ourselves. Since we are unwilling to admit this horrible, guilt-producing thought to ourselves or others, we conveniently project the blame for accidents on the gremlins.

We speak glibly of the "causes" of accidents. Our safety engineers have gone a long way in identifying the *scenes* of accidents, the places and the situations in which they are most likely to occur. Much can be done with this information to prevent future accidents; for example, the accident record on a particular street intersection may make it imperative to install stop lights. But neither the engineers nor the accident statisticians can tell us why a particular accident has happened or is going to happen.

The reason is this. Accidents have causes; but the causes are often so personal, so obscure, so complex, so unrelated to the scene of the accident that we cannot see or find an explanation until after the tragedy has occurred

Accident Proneness

Accidents can happen to anybody, but the fact is that some people are more liable to accidents than others. They can sometimes be identified by their accident records and, with greater difficulty, by their personality patterns. It is easier to label a person "accident prone" than to prove it. Nevertheless, where careful records are kept, as in some industries, it soon becomes evident that the greatest number of accidents cluster around a comparatively few people who are called—rightly or wrongly—accident prone.

It appears that the person who has already had an accident is most likely to have another; further, the person who has lots of little accidents appears to be going to meet a big one. Uncorrected defects of sense organs, poor vision, and partial deafness, for instance, account for some cases of accident proneness. But modern psychiatry offers a deeper explanation.

Some psychiatrists believe that most truly accident-prone persons unconsciously wish to have accidents happen to them, for the accident victim at least gets sympathy. Having an accident resolves intolerable conflicts in his unconsious mind, just as drinking does for the alcoholic. A repeated pattern of accidents, not just an occasional accident, can be considered a poor and damaging pattern of life adjustment that accident-prone people are internally driven to find and accept. This escape into accidents is possible because having an accident is still socially acceptable.

Every accident-prone individual has his own specific personality structure and unconscious

motivations, but psychoanalytic study has revealed some of the broad emotional characteristics of the type, thus:

He was often brought up in a strict home. He deeply resented parental authority and often flouted it. He carries this resentment of authority into early adult life; he hates bosses, policemen, and all other symbols of authority. Seeking his own pleasure, he is a law unto himself. Many people admire him for daring, bravado, and the air of excitement he creates. But he himself rarely feels strong emotional attachments to other people. His school and work records are likely to be spotty; he tries to escape responsibility and the association with authority that it entails.

As an adult, he usually responds to stimuli with action rather than thought. But he is more likely to respond quickly and impulsively to his own inner needs and feelings than to the realistic facts and situations that confront him. He looks to accidents as solutions of his emotional torments because the accidents may bring him love and sympathy—and sometimes money—without requiring the assumption of responsibility or exertion on his part.

The broad-stroke picture of this personality type fits the description of social misfits other than the accident-prone individual. Dr. H. Flanders Dunbar, an authority on psychosomatic medicine, says: "When this personality pattern is set beside those of other groups in the population, it turns out to match very precisely that of the juvenile delinquent and the adult criminal. The behavior characteristics of the persistent breaker of laws is virtually identical with that of the persistent breaker of bones—right up to the point where the one commits a crime and the other has an accident."[1]

What Accident Statistics Tell Us

Every year in the United States somewhere between 9 million and 10 million people are accidentally injured and somewhere between

[1]H. Flanders Dunbar, *Mind and Body: Psychosomatic Medicine*, (New York: Random House, 1947).

90,000 and 100,000 are killed by accident. Around 350,000 people are permanently disabled to some extent by accidents every year. For many years the accident death rate in the United States remained almost constant (at about 72 deaths per 100,000 population). It is an amazing fact that, when organized safety efforts or other conditions push the death rate from accidents down at one point of the compass, it appears to rise up at other points. For example, during World War II, when auto driving was restricted, the motor-vehicle accident death rate declined. At the same time, since war production and military training were being pushed, the industrial accident death rate increased, the military training accident death rate (especially airplane accidents) increased, and the over-all accident death rates during the war years were just about the same as before. The postwar trend was substantially downward. The accidental death rate fell to a low of 50 (per 100,000 population) in 1961.

Yet it is fair to assume that, without organized safety efforts and continuing safety education, America's accident record would be even more shocking than it is. After diseases of the heart, blood vessels, and kidneys (the cardiovascular-renal diseases), and cancer, accidents are the fourth principal cause of death in the United States. *In school and college years, from five to twenty-five, they are the first cause of death.*

We often think of accidents in terms of catas-trophes, because these are the events that make newspaper headlines. A catastrophe, statistically speaking, is an accident in which five or more lives are lost. However, a careful record of national catastrophes reveals that less than 2% of all accidental deaths occur in them.

Another key fact is that only about 10% of the catastrophes are due to the uncontrollable forces of nature—floods, hurricanes, tornadoes, and the like. Your chances of being struck fatally by lightning during any year, for example, are only about two in a million—even less if you are a city-dwelling woman. Ninety percent of the head-line catastrophes are the result of some kind of human failure or neglect, engendering confla-grations, explosions, railroad wrecks, airplane crashes, mine accidents, building cave-ins, ma-rine accidents, and the like.

But, wherever you turn in the accident picture, the failure in the human factor stares you in the face. For example, in traffic accidents, defects in the vehicle are reported in less than 10% of the cases. That is why it has been often stated, with-out serious challenge, that 90% of all accidents are preventable. Yet fatal and crippling accidents continue to occur daily. Over the years, un-heralded, unspectacular, foolish accidents out-strip catastrophes fiftyfold; and as a cause of death they outrun the sum of war deaths, mur-der, suicide, and legal executions combined by a ratio of at least 4 to 1.

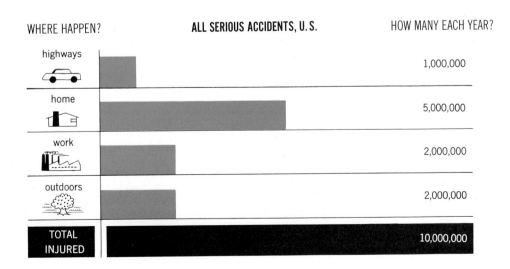

WHERE HAPPEN?	ALL SERIOUS ACCIDENTS, U.S.	HOW MANY EACH YEAR?
highways		1,000,000
home		5,000,000
work		2,000,000
outdoors		2,000,000
TOTAL INJURED		10,000,000

A Philosophy of Accidents. We often speak of the accident problem in purely numerical terms, forgetting both the human and philosophical concept behind the word "accident." Material on the psychology of accidents has been included in this chapter, but a Frenchman, Professor Jean L' Hirondel, of Caen, speaking at the 1962 International Conference on Health and Health Education put the accident problem in its proper philosophical perspective in the following terms: (Translation from the French original by this author.)

Accidents are only one aspect of the human drama and the constant struggle of man against the universe [about him].

Three kinds of perils menace us:

1. Those arising from ourselves and especially from the imperfections of our bodies;

2. Perils presented by other human beings;

3. Finally, the attack [or agression] of the elements of nature outside man [on man], where such elements can be schematically identified, namely:

—the attacks of microbes and viruses; these are the infectious diseases; and

—the aggression [or violence] of physical agents; these precisely are accidents.

Even with such "classifications," so to speak, it is often difficult to give a precise definition or description of an "accident." [For example:]

A hunting "accident" may be accident, suicide, or murder depending upon the motivation of the protagonist [the man who fired the gun].

Snakebite [with the injection of venom] is termed an accident. The toxins [spread through the body] by microbes are said to cause a disease.

Frostbite [or freezing to death] is called an accident, but injury to the lungs [pneumopathology] due to cold is classified as an illness.

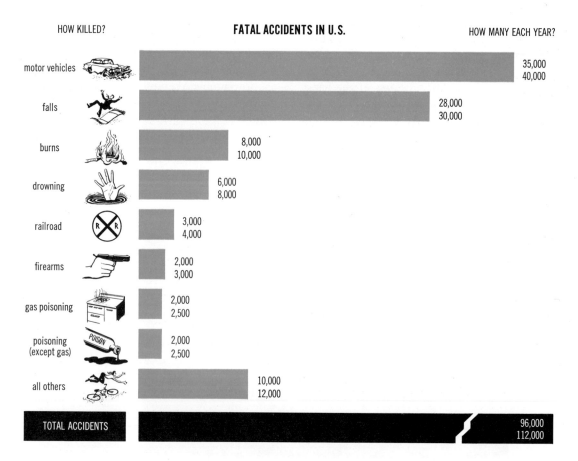

HOW KILLED?

FATAL ACCIDENTS IN U.S.

HOW MANY EACH YEAR?

motor vehicles	35,000 / 40,000
falls	28,000 / 30,000
burns	8,000 / 10,000
drowning	6,000 / 8,000
railroad	3,000 / 4,000
firearms	2,000 / 3,000
gas poisoning	2,000 / 2,500
poisoning (except gas)	2,000 / 2,500
all others	10,000 / 12,000
TOTAL ACCIDENTS	96,000 / 112,000

Where		How many each year
highways		35,000 / 40,000
home		30,000 / 35,000
work		15,000 / 18,000
outdoors		16,000 / 19,000
TOTAL KILLED		96,000 / 112,000

With this philosophy, Professor Hirondel concludes that accidents are a check on the development of mankind by the forces that both surround (threaten) and motivate him. He quotes the Biblical injunction of the Lord to Adam: "People the earth and subdue it."

The International Conference dealt in practical as well as philosophical concepts of accident prevention. "The National Child Cycling Proficiency Scheme in the United Kingdom," submitted on behalf of the Royal Society for the Prevention of Accidents, advised that if you teach 10-, 11-, and 12-year-olds how to ride bicycles safely, you will save them from millions of motor vehicle accidents when they are allowed to drive cars eight to ten years later.

Prevention of Motor Vehicle Accidents

There are enough automobiles in the United States so that every man, woman, and child could be riding simultaneously. Yet in 1895 there were just four gasoline motorcars in the country—a Ford, a Haynes, a Duryea, and an imported Benz. People were shocked that these cars could travel at a speed of 11 miles an hour; automobiles have since been clocked at a speed of over 600 miles per hour.

With more than 83 million powerful cars on the streets and roads, and probably 100 to 125 million drivers, it is a traffic problem of first magnitude to keep them out of each other's fenders. The modern automobile is a powerful instrument; but the driver is its brain. Without a driver, a motorcar is useless. But with a careless, thoughtless, inexperienced driver, it can become an instrument of death and a tool of destruction.

Practically all college men and a high percentage of college women know how to drive, or think they do. Actually there are great differences in skills and attitudes. Many are excellent drivers all the time and enjoy respect for their ability. Still more are fair to good drivers, with occasional lapses into trouble. A few are poor and dangerous drivers, partly responsible for the high fatal accident involvement rates recorded in drivers under 25 years of age. Sample studies indicate that the safest drivers are the 35 to 50 age group. Younger drivers, between 16 and 25, are involved in fatal accidents much more often.

What does it take to be a good driver—one whose invitations to ride with him are more welcomed than feared? First and foremost, a proper *attitude* toward driving, its risks, responsibilities, and opportunities. After that, mental and physical fitness, knowledge, judgment, skills, and habits based on good instruction and intelligent experience.

What Makes a Good Driver? *Knowledge.* An important part of the knowledge that makes a good driver is that of the physical and physio-

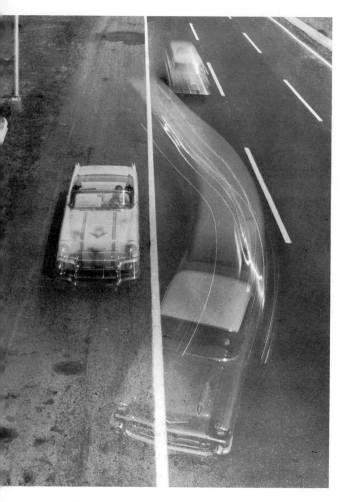

TRAFFIC ACCIDENTS are caused by people, who are frequently driven into them by unconscious motivations—such as regression, an infantile disregard for personal safety or the rights of others. Motor vehicle accidents are the principal cause of death in the college-age population.

logical laws or principles that govern the motion of the car and the driver behind the wheel. The most fundamental traffic laws are the laws of nature: gravity, friction, force of impact, and centrifugal force.

The entire control of a moving automobile depends on the grip which four small areas of tire surface have on the roadway at any given moment. These four points of contact are no bigger than the palm of the hand which grips the steering wheel. The coefficient of friction be-

tween tires and roadway is itself dependent on many factors, including the condition of the tires, the condition of the brakes and brake pressure, and the kind and condition of the road surface, which is often further dependent on weather conditions. A good driver knows and respects all these conditions. He is also aware of the centrifugal force that operates on curves; this force inexorably tends to push the moving car off the road, just as a rock whirled on a string tends to break the string.

Most important, the good driver is aware of the tremendous amount of kinetic energy developed by a moving automobile and the real difficulty of changing its motion—specifically, stopping the car. Modern engineering genius has made it seem deceptively simple to stop an automobile. Only when the car collides with something or someone else before stopping is the poor driver jolted into a realization of what a powerful force he was directing.

The kinetic energy packed into the moving automobile is a function of the weight of the car and the speed at which it is being driven. Speed too high for driving conditions is usually the killing factor in motor-vehicle accidents; it is associated with fatal accidents more than twice as often as any other observed factors. The relationship of speed to death in auto accidents has been worked out by A. N. Kerr, a California mechanical engineer, in terms of *danger units*. At a speed of 25 miles per hour an automobile has developed 1 danger unit of kinetic energy. This amount of energy also represents just about the "shock limit" of a human being, the equivalent of a fall from a second-story window.

At 25 miles per hour an automobile can be stopped within an average street's width, and if it turned over upon hitting an obstacle, it would roll over only once. As speed is increased, danger units increase, but the danger increases faster than the speed. In fact, the danger units are proportional to the square of the speed. Thus, at 35 miles the car packs 2 danger units; at 50 miles, 4 danger units; at 75 miles, 9 danger units. The human body was never engineered to take such shocks.

Just as there are danger units packed in the momentum of a moving automobile, we can likewise speak of a danger zone always projected in front of it. This danger zone can be easily pictured by imagining the hood of the car stretched out ahead of it for literally hundreds of feet. The good driver is always aware of this danger zone and knows the various factors that determine its length. Both physical and physiological factors are involved. The danger zone is the distance ahead within which the car can be brought to a complete stop.

The actual stopping distance is the sum of the braking distance *plus* the reaction-time distance. The braking distance depends upon pure physical laws already mentioned, the factors affecting the coefficient of friction. The braking distance is the distance the car will travel after the brakes are applied. At 10 miles per hour, on a hard-surfaced road with brakes in "good" condition, it is 7.5 feet; at 25 miles, 46.9 feet; at 60 miles, 270 feet.

But, before you even begin to push your foot down on the brake pedal, the foot must respond

DANGER ZONE AHEAD OF A MOVING AUTOMOBILE*

Stopping distance calculated at the following speeds:

Miles per hour	Distance in feet before car stops
10	18.5
20	52.0
25	74.4
30	100.5
35	130.4
40	164.0
50	242.5
60	336.0

Stopping distance is sum of (1) braking distance, calculated for brakes that just meet the requirements of the Uniform Vehicle Code (44.5 percent efficient); and (2) braking-reaction-time distance, calculated at an average of three-fourths of a second.

*This table is an abridgement from Table I, "Stopping Distances," in *The Driver,* first volume in the Sportsmanlike Driving Series published by the American Automobile Association, Washington, D.C., 1946, p. 30.

to a signal from your brain. This takes time; the nerve impulse must travel from the original stimulus on eye or ear to the brain and from the brain to the leg and foot muscles. The length of time required for this action is called the braking reaction time. It varies in different individuals, and in the same individual at different times. It can be measured with a fair degree of accuracy by various testing devices. Under ordinary driving conditions the average braking reaction time is about $\frac{3}{4}$ second. A car traveling 25 miles per hour will have moved ahead about 27 feet in that split second.

However, even young people with comparatively fast reaction times on ordinary tests slow down under many conditions, notably fatigue; drinking of alcoholic beverages; inattention owing to daydreaming, conversation, or listening to an auto radio; eye strain; low visibility; and indecision possibly reflecting emotional strains. The good driver knows all this and guards against most of these hazards.

If he is drowsy or tired while driving, he pulls off the road and takes a nap. If he drinks, he doesn't drive. If he finds himself distracted by "back-seat driving" or other conversation, he refuses to go on until it stops. If he is required to wear glasses while driving, he always wears them. He constantly takes visibility conditions into account; he slows down at intersections; he does not pass cars on hills; he doesn't overdrive his lights, that is, he doesn't drive at night or in a fog at a speed which makes the inescapable danger zone ahead of him greater than the distance he can see ahead.

Daydreaming and indecision are more difficult factors to control. About the only possible advice that can be given here is not to drive on days that you find yourself acting absent-minded or feeling "jittery." Physical condition is a factor in safe driving; sometimes a toothache may be at the root of an auto accident.

Sound Driving Practices and Habits. The good driver is habitually aware of adverse driving conditions and their effect on shortening the danger zone ahead of his car. He compensates for these adversities by driving more slowly. For example, he knows that, when he is wide awake and alert and his car and tires in tiptop shape, he can safely drive at 50 miles per hour on a hard, smooth, dry, level, straight road in clear daylight. He further recognizes that changes in any combination of these conditions will require proportionate reduction in speed. Thus, when feeling fatigued and driving at night with fogged-up headlights on a wet pavement with a 5% down grade and then suddenly subjected to the glare of oncoming headlights which cut his visibility to only 100 feet, the good driver habitually reduces his speed to about 15 miles an hour.

Three "C's" can be used to describe the habits of the good driver: Courtesy, Commonsense, and Caution. Courtesy on the highway undoubtedly prevents many accidents; some authorities believe that, if it were commonly practiced, highway accidents could be cut in half.

Rude, discourteous, unsportsmanlike violation of driving rules is associated with a high percentage of accidents. In one reported series of accidents, for example, the drivers involved were guilty of the following violations of sportsmanlike driving rules: demanding the right of way (11%), exceeding speed limit or safe speed (8%), driving on the wrong side of the roadway (6%), disregarding warning signs and signals (4%), passing improperly (3%), turning improperly (3%), driving while under the influence of alcohol (3%), following too closely (2%), failing to signal or giving improper signal (2%), parking or starting improperly (2%). To sum up, in 56% of these traffic accidents, the offending drivers did not observe courtesy, caution, or common sense. Afoot, where it is more annoying than dangerous, no one is permitted to use the sidewalks as rudely and bumptiously as many drivers use the highway.

The character of the good, safe driver can be summed up in his observance of these six habits:

¶ Through experience under instruction, he has developed mechanical and technical skill in controlling his car.

¶ He knows what to expect of his car under both favorable and adverse driving conditions.

¶ He avoids taking foolish chances; he *never* overdrives the danger zone projecting ahead of his car.

¶ He has a courteous and sportsmanlike regard for the rights of all other users of the public highway, including pedestrians, bicyclists and motorcyclists, and other motorists.

¶ He signals his intentions to all persons who may be affected by the course of the car of which he is the brain; he does not expect other people to be mind readers.

¶ He is alert for the mistakes of other people, and he does what he can to compensate for them; he does not demand the right of way to his own or anyone else's hurt.

The Unconscious Causes of Auto Accidents

Attitudes. The good driver, as we have described him, always knows what he is doing when he is at the wheel of his car. His safe driving habits are "automatic" reactions or responses to stimuli without interference or misdirection by unconscious motivations of which he himself is not aware. Under conditions of emotional stress, an ordinarily good driver may become temporarily a poor and dangerous driver. The big pool of poor drivers, however, and the still-wider stream of "accident-prone" persons, is made up of individuals who do not really know what they are doing because they are unaware of or will not accept the deep unconscious motivations, the dangerously overworked mental mechanisms, that control their attitudes and their conduct.

To understand the attitudes which make some people exceptionally bad risks as auto drivers, it must be frankly recognized that in modern American society the automobile is regarded as more than a cheap and convenient means of transportation and its value is measured in terms other than either the weight of metal in it or even its cost in dollars.

The automobile is used as a symbol of many factors in the life of the American individual. The kind of car a man drives is often taken as a measure of his status or prestige in the community, although this is by no means universally so. Equally true, the right of a young man to drive the family car is a token of the independence he has achieved and a measure of the degree of maturity and responsibility which his family thinks he has attained.

The more basic fact is that almost every single mental mechanism of which the human mind is capable can be expressed in feeling and action related to driving or owning an automobile. The car becomes not only an extension of the ego; it also symbolizes other family relationships, and it substitutes for both love and hate objects. Many people become poor, dangerous, accident-prone drivers because they use the role of driving as an outlet for subconscious reactions whose origins have nothing to do with the realistic act of transporting themselves from one place to another.

We will not repeat the list of the mental mechanisms here (see pages 41–45). We shall simply give a few examples of how they relate to bad driving and auto accidents:

Repression. A poor driver may really hate driving because, for example, he may be trying to repress memory of an auto accident of which he was once a cause, a victim, or a witness.

Identification. A poor driver may identify the act of driving a car with a family member, usually a father, toward whom he still has unresolved aggressions. He may subconsciously want to hurt his father by getting into an accident and hurting his car.

Extroversion. Some people "drive like mad" in a hopeless attempt to escape inner conflicts. Reckless driving is an excellent example of unreflective action.

Fantasy. Daydreams of attaining an unassailable height of power often incorporate fantasies of driving or riding in a long, sleek automobile with limitless speed and power. The car rides easily over all obstacles and opposition, and there is no one powerful enough to bid the driver to stop. Confusing fantasy with fact, the driver steps on the accelerator and sometimes speeds to his death.

Rationalization. The poor driver invariably rationalizes the factors that led him into an accident. He was driving too fast, he asserts, not because he started for an appointment too late but because "he absolutely promised to be on time."

Regression. Almost every type of regressive, childish behavior can occur in that driver whose infantile ego reasserts itself in hogging the road, insisting on the right of way, double parking, speeding—all with an infant's complete disregard for the rights and presence of other people. This can be a fatal form of emotional infantilism.

Projection. The poor driver projects the blame for his accidents onto everything and everyone except himself. His accidents are *always* "the other fellow's fault," or they were caused by bad roads, poor visibility, faulty brakes, or any other driving condition for which the driver himself failed to make proper allowance.

Isolation. The driver who segregates and isolates his thinking and feeling into logic-tight compartments is often the most dangerous and hopeless of the lot of poor drivers. He honestly cannot see that his demoniac conduct behind the wheel is completely at odds with his polite and often mild-mannered conduct in other situations. So he continues to charge pedestrians, speed up when another car tries to pass him, and take chances in passing other cars.

Symbolization. The false "sense of power" that this poor driver gets when he steps on the gas symbolizes the feeling of importance he would like to have but has failed to achieve in other areas of living. For him especially the car symbolizes the ego, and he shows off by reckless driving.

Substitution (or Displacement). In this class of poor drivers we sometimes find the introverted, over-obedient child who was afraid to talk back to his parents, the henpecked husband, and the Mr. Milquetoast who doesn't dare speak up to his boss. He displaces his hidden feelings of resentment against them by madcap driving and a cavalier disregard for the rights of others. He weaves carelessly in and out of traffic lanes; he shows other cars his dust. After all, they can't talk back.

Inferiority Feelings. Many a poor driver handles his car with an attitude of superiority that represents overcompensation of the wrong kind for feelings of inferiority and inadequacy. Driving makes him feel like the proverbial "Mister Big," and he shows it in many ways. He won't move over when other cars want to pass him; if they finally do succeed in passing, he immediately speeds up to overtake them and "get even."

Highway Safety A Mental Health Problem. Accident records incontrovertibly show that it is the drivers with poor attitudes who have the most accidents. Highway safety thus becomes in great part a problem of mental health. The poor and dangerous driver, unfortunately, does not usually recognize himself as such. His unconscious reactions and motivations toward the automobile are part of his total personality pattern.

From a personal standpoint, you can make yourself a better driver by understanding your personality pattern in all respects and thus becoming a more mature individual. From the standpoint of the public safety, however, since the poor driver is a menace to others as well as himself, the problem must be approached differently. Only a few, bad-risk drivers are weeded out by checking their repeated accident records and refusing them further driving privileges or a driver's license.

Theoretically, it might be possible to test all drivers for mental and emotional difficulties before they were allowed to get on the road and cause accidents; but this task of plumbing the unconscious minds of probably 115 million automobile drivers is far beyond the practical resources of public safety officials. Only the crudest beginnings have been made, and then only in a few states, by refusing licenses to people with frank mental illnesses and mental deficiencies.

An Engineering Problem. It is clearly recognized that highway safety is also an engineering problem. This takes into consideration the design and construction of motor vehicles themselves and the design and upkeep of the streets and highways on which they ride. Important, relatively recent engineering contributions to automobile safety are the seat belt and harness. Prop-

erly installed and used regularly, they can cut death and accident injury tolls. The National Safety Council estimates that if everyone used seat belts and/or harnesses regularly, at least 5000 lives a year could be saved and the number of serious injuries could be reduced by one third.

Are automobiles today designed with the maximum concern for the safety of their drivers and passengers? It is often claimed that they are not. Such an attack was made in 1966 in the book, *Unsafe at Any Speed,* by Ralph Nader, a young Washington attorney. Some of the safety factors that he recommended have since been incorporated in the design of new automobiles.

Cost of Accidents. The immediate and accumulating costs (e.g., loss of earnings) of motor vehicle and other accidents run into billions of dollars a year. The National Safety Council regularly calculates the money costs of all types of accidents involving deaths and injuries in the United States. The estimated cost for the year 1963 was $16.5 billion. This figure includes wage losses, medical fees, and hospital expenses, insurance costs, property damage and destruction (e.g., fire), and production losses. About half the total costs were charged against motor vehicle accidents; about a third against work accidents. In 1963 the total number of disabling accidental injuries reported was over 10 million; the number of deaths 101,000.

Young men between the ages of 16 and 25 are most likely to be involved in auto accidents. They, or their parents, pay for this hazard in the form of much higher insurance rates. An insurance company[2] has averaged out the projected accident record, and costs of these accidents, 50 years ahead, for a young man who starts driving at age 16. By the time he is 23 he will probably have had 4 accidents, 1 involving injury; by 40 he will have had 9 accidents, 3 with injuries; at 66, a total of 13 accidents, with 4 injuries, costing altogether about $6500. Assuming that the young man at 23 takes a 23-year-old bride, who also

[2]Kemper Insurance Company, quoted in editorial in *Safety Education,* A National Safety Council Publication (January 1964), p. 22.

has been driving since she was 16, and that they have three children, plus grandchildren, the lifetime grand total at age 66 for this *one* man and his family will be 38 accidents, 12 involving injuries, at a cost of about $19,000.

Motorcycle Accidents. An increasing number of motor vehicle accidents can be assigned to motorcycles and their smaller versions, the motorscooter and motorized bicycle. In 1967 it was estimated that unless the upward trend of motorcycle registrations and fatal motorcycle accidents abated, somewhere between 4000 and 5000 motorcycle deaths could be expected annually in the 1970's. (About 1 in 7 of these would be with the lighter vehicles, which are rapidly increasing in number.)

The U.S. Bureau of Public Roads estimates that there will be a total of at least 5 million motorcycles registered and on the roads in 1970. This would bring about a ratio of one motorcycle to every 40 people. In Europe, where motorcycles have long been more popular, the ratios in seven countries run from 1 in 9 persons to 1 in 29.

The hazards of motorcycling are made evident by observing the statistics on motorcycle accident fatalities. The number of passengers and drivers killed per 100,000 motorcycles registered was $2\frac{1}{2}$ times the corresponding rate for all other types of motor vehicles. The National Safety Council estimates that the accidental death rate for motorcyclists ranges between 20 and 40 per 100 million vehicle miles, compared with 5.6 for drivers, passengers, and pedestrians in all motor vehicles.

Experience is of prime importance for safe handling of motorcycles, motorscooters, and motorized bicycles. In one British study it was shown that drivers under age 21 with less than 6 months experience had higher accident rates than those with more than 6 months experience. A Minnesota hospital study of motorcycle accident injuries found that 1 in 5 of the injured persons had been riding a motorcycle for only the first or second time! About $\frac{3}{4}$ of them were on borrowed or rented vehicles.

In a typical motorcycle accident the driver is usually thrown forward so that his head sustains the impact with another vehicle, object, or pavement. Injury to the head occurs in 50% or more motorcycle accidents. Accordingly, motorcycle riders are now wearing more protective headgear (crash helmets), and efforts are now being made to require special drivers' tests and licenses for the motorcycle operators. The highest rates for motorcycle accident deaths occur in the college ages between 15 and 24. About 10% of these are females.

A Word About Pedestrians. Though the poor driver is the central figure in all auto accident records, it should be noted that pedestrians are also sometimes at fault. From 9000 to 12,000 pedestrians of all ages are killed in traffic accidents every year. Some jaywalk to death. There is alcohol on the breath of about 1 in every 5 adult pedestrians killed in traffic accidents. Two out of every three pedestrians killed are either violating traffic laws or acting in a patently unsafe manner. The following simple rules for pedestrians, if obeyed, will save lives:

Cross streets only at crosswalks. Three out of five urban pedestrian deaths occur between intersections.

Watch those first few steps into the street.
Obey stop signs.

Make sure you're clear *before* you attempt to cross a street or road. Learn to judge the speed of approaching automobiles, and don't try to beat them on foot.

Walk on the *left* side of country roads where there are no sidewalks. You will be in a better position to see cars approaching on your own side of the road.

At night on country roads wear or carry some light-colored object so that your visibility in an oncoming driver's eyes will be increased.

Other Kinds of Accidents

Not all fatal accidents occur on the highway. They also take place at work, at play, and, most frequently, at home.

Home Accidents. Over half of the fatal accidents that take place at home strike people over 65, and one-fifth of them happen to children under 5. The highest accident rates are recorded for two-year-old boys. Among the causes of home accidents we must therefore put physical frailty or handicap and poor judgment high on the list, although psychological mechanisms are also at work. Falls are the principal type of fatal home accident. Every home should be repeatedly checked for accident hazards; for example, poor lighting, unsafe electrical fixtures, stairways without railings, slippery floors, scatter rugs that slip underfoot, untidy housekeeping that leaves bundles and objects lying around on floors and staircases.

The kitchen is the most dangerous room in the house, according to accidental-injury records. All types of home accidents occur there: falls, burns, scalds, explosions, internal poisoning, gas poisoning, and suffocation. After the kitchen the chief danger spots around the house, roughly in order of accident frequency, are: outside stairs, inside stairs, living room, porch, bedroom, basement, dining room, bathroom, and hallways. Comparatively few fatal accidents, except for carbon monoxide poisoning, occur in the garage. But the outside yard, statistically speaking, is just as dangerous as the kitchen. The essence of accident prevention in the home is good housekeeping coupled with common sense.

Industrial and Occupational Accidents. More thought is probably given to the prevention of accidents in industry and at work than in any other area. Safety engineering has done a tremendous job in cutting down the risks of injury even in hazardous employments, such as mining and quarrying. The human factor, however, remains the uncontrollable element. Poor housekeeping in the shop and horseplay around machinery are important causes of industrial accidents. So also are improper use of machinery or other equipment and failure to use protective devices. It is significant that proportionately more people are killed working on farms, where they are more or less their own bosses, than working in factories. Because accidents cost money, organized safety work in industry has gone to great pains to identify accident-prone individuals before they hurt themselves or others.

When industrial safety measures were first introduced, it was feared that safety measures, such as wearing goggles, would slow production and cut efficiency. It has turned out, however, that the safe way of doing a job is also the most efficient way.

College Accidents. Lest college students think that problems of environmental health, safety, and occupational health are far removed from their immediate sphere of interest, they may be surprised to learn that only a small percentage of the nation's colleges and universities operate environmental health and safety programs— whose purpose is the conservation of the human and physical resources of the college population. Few colleges even believe such a problem exists. As an example of tragic failure to face up to such problems it is worthwhile to describe a scene from the campus of a midwestern university [*Student Medicine*, **10**:4, 504 (April 1962)]:

Two students who were enrolled in a chemistry course took some chemicals from the laboratory which could be used to make smoke in their dormitory. The chemicals, mixed in the lab and placed in a small sealed jar, exploded when the jar was bumped. The student who bumped the jar was permanently blinded in both eyes. . . .

Outdoor Accidents. Sports accidents kill hundreds of men and boys over fifteen every year. Most of the deaths are accounted for by the so-called "milder sports": swimming, fishing, and hunting. Very few deaths, numerically speaking, result from rough or vigorous sports like football, boxing, wrestling, baseball, and auto racing. This is partly the good result of more adequate supervision of vigorous sports. Responsible coaches and athletic directors take it as their primary jobs to instruct team candidates in skills that will keep them from getting hurt. The first thing a football player must learn, for example, is how to fall properly. Unsupervised recreation is more likely to invite accidents.

Drownings make up the largest category of fatal outdoor accidents. These could be substantially reduced in number if poor swimmers and non-swimmers obeyed water safety rules and stayed out of deep water. Good swimmers most frequently drown when they attempt feats beyond their powers. The same psychology, applies here as in motorcycle accidents, where the expert riders are more likely than the novice riders to try stunts leading to fatal accidents. Experience sometimes induces overconfidence and carelessness.

Organizing for Safety

Consistent and organized safety efforts have over the years reduced the toll of accidents that might otherwise have been rung up. The water safety programs of the American Red Cross is an example. Reduction in Fourth of July fireworks accidents as a result of legal restrictions on the sale of fireworks is another example. Public safety departments, including traffic policemen and fire inspectors, are constantly at work to reduce accident and fire hazards.

Many national organizations cooperate in safety promotion and accident prevention efforts; among them may be listed the National Safety Council, the American Automobile Association, the American Red Cross, the National Board of Fire Underwriters, the National Committee for Traffic Safety, and the International Association of Chiefs of Police—Safety Division. They emphasize in varying degrees what safety workers call the "three E's" essential to the public safety: *E*ngineering, *E*nforcement, and *E*ducation. But in the final analysis it is up to the individual who wants to beat the law of averages concerning the occurrence of accidents to educate himself to be above average in alertness, safety-mindedness, and self-possessed maturity.

Emergency Medical Identification

One positive step that the safety-minded individual can now take, if he requires it, is to provide himself with adequate emergency medical identification. Probably 40 million people in the United States have physical conditions or disabilities serious enough to warrant wearing or carrying emergency medical identification.

Emergency medical identification is provided

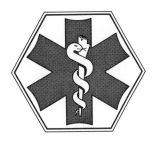

STANDARD (American Medical Association) symbol for emergency medical identification devices.

by medallions, bracelets, lockets, purse and wallet cards, and other signal devices warning of physical conditions, such as diabetes or penicillin sensitivity, afflicting the particular individual. Then, if he is ever found unconscious, the police officer or attending physician will immediately know what to do—or often, very importantly, what *not* to do—for him. Epileptics and diabetics are sometimes mistaken for drunks; the emergency identification device immediately sets the record straight.

Following pioneering efforts by such organizations as the Medic-Alert Foundation, the American Medical Association in 1963 adopted a standard symbol for emergency medical identification. It is a hexagon enclosing a six-pointed "star of life" on which is emblazoned the staff of Aesculapius, symbol of medicine (see illustration). The American Medical Association (Emergency Identification, 535 N. Dearborn St., Chicago, Ill.) will upon request supply a list of manufacturers and vendors of emergency signal devices.

Who needs emergency medical identification? Essentially people with "hidden" medical problems who might fail, without it, to receive proper first-aid and emergency treatment. Your physician is the one to determine finally whether you should wear or carry emergency medical identification. The records of the Medic-Alert Foundation, compiled since 1956, show that there are over 200 specific conditions in which emergency identification is extremely important, if not imperative. These conditions include: *diseases,* such as diabetes, epilepsy, hemophilia, myasthenia gravis, multiple sclerosis, glaucoma, and amnesia; *allergies* to penicillin, horse serum (in tetanus antitoxin), insect bites, and a long list of common drugs; *medications* being currently taken, such as antabuse, cortisone, and digitalis; *previous surgery,* such as the laryngectomy which creates the "neck breather"; and various *miscellaneous conditions,* for instance, contact lenses, deafmutism, practices like skin and scuba diving which may cause "the bends." For individuals in all these major categories, emergency medical identification may be life-saving.

SUMMARY

In summary, in the United States accidents are the principal cause of death between ages 1 and 45! This fact alone makes safety education and safety engineering mandatory. The principal cause of accidents is people—not gremlins, unsafe equipment, or natural catastrophes. Accident-prone individuals, who can be identified, are more likely to have accidents than other people; but no one is immune.

More *serious* accidents occur in the home (especially to children and old people), but more *fatal* accidents occur on the highways. Excessive speed is the factor most commonly associated with motor vehicle fatalities. Good driving habits, including courtesy, caution, and common sense, are the primary bulwark against auto accidents.

Yet it must be recognized that there are many unconscious or subconscious causes of automobile, home, work, and outdoor accidents. He who would escape, or at least minimize, the risks, disabilities, and costs of accidents must learn not to take needless chances.

SUMMARY REVIEW QUESTIONS

1. What are the primary causes of accidents? How and where, therefore, should efforts to promote safety begin?
2. What are the characteristics of the "accident-prone" individual? With what other types of characters can this individual be compared? Why?
3. What accident statistics quoted in this chapter registered most vividly on your mind? Quote them.
4. What are the characteristics of a good automobile driver? What makes a poor driver?
5. What are some of the unconscious causes of automobile accidents? In what ways, if any, are these unconscious causes related to the symbolic roles which the automobile plays in American life?
6. What are some simple safety rules for pedestrians? (Give at least five.)
7. Why is "poor housekeeping" such an important cause of accidents at home and at work? How does "good housekeeping" serve to prevent accidents?
8. What are the "most dangerous" rooms in a house or home? What is the relative order of frequency of accidents in all the different rooms of a house (most frequent site of accident first)? Why should the list run in approximately the order you have given?
9. What can be done to prevent various types of sports and outdoor accidents? Whose responsibility is it?
10. With reference to safety and accident prevention, what are the "three E's"? The "three C's"?
11. Are the following statements sense or nonsense? Why? *Safety first. . . . Accidents are necessary. . . . The safest place is home. . . . If you drink, don't drive; if you drive, don't drink. . . .*

Accidents are an insignificant cause of death and injury among college students. . . . A good driver can afford to take chances on the road.

12. What do the following terms mean to you: gremlins, safety engineering, catastrophe, stopping distance, danger unit, shock limit (of a human being), RoSPA, jaywalk, scatter rugs, reaction time?

Worth Looking Into: *Accident Facts,* published annually by the National Safety Council. *Sports Illustrated Book of Safe Driving* by the Editors of *Sports Illustrated. First Aid Textbook* by the American National Red Cross. *Life Saving and Water Safety* by the American National Red Cross. For more complete references, see Appendix E. *See also Appendix B, on First Aid.*

Drinking and Driving: New Approaches

A. R. Roalman

Can I have a few drinks and drive safely? ☐ What does a blood alcohol level of 0.10 (or 0.04 or 0.15) percent mean in terms of the number of martinis or bottles of beer I might drink? ☐ Is there some simple procedure I can use to check my blood alcohol level to make sure I'm safe when I slide behind the wheel of my car? ☐ Am I more likely to be arrested and charged with drunken driving than I was five years ago? ☐ What is likely to happen to me if I am arrested and charged with drunken driving?

These are a few of the questions brought up by an unusual research project—questions almost any driver might ask himself. Some of the answers might surprise you.

For example: Yes, you are more likely to be arrested and charged with driving while intoxicated today than you were five years ago. But before we examine the reasons why, and take a look at answers to the other questions above, let's consider the public confusion that exists regarding drinking and driving. Talk to any two drivers at random and you might get comments like these:

"If you drive, don't drink."

"I can drive better after I've had a few drinks. I'm more relaxed."

Much of this confusion is justified. Here's why:

—The subject of drinking drivers is, basically, a complex one, and rarely have there been attempts to clarify it for a broad-scale public reading.

—A great deal of emotion tends to emerge any time drinking and driving is discussed. Probably 93 million Americans drink alcohol, according to Seldon D. Bacon, head of the Rutgers Center for Alcohol Studies. Most people past 16—about 100 million—drive. Criticize the drinking driver and you find large numbers of people thinking that you are trying to take from them one of two popular pastimes—drinking and driving. Many people remember prohibition and think that anyone who discusses a curtailment of drinking while driving is, at heart, a prohibitionist. Neither assumption should be made about this article.

—Broad scale public pronouncements about the drinking driver have smacked of prohibitionism, tended to oversimplify the problem and, facts now document, were based on

erroneous information. For years the most common statement from safety organizations was "if you drink, don't drive." Now, fortified with new research, they are subtly, but substantially, modifying that stand. No longer are they relying on such slogans. Armed with new knowledge, they are spending more time explaining some of the nuances of the drinking and driving problem.

—Rock-hard information about the drinking driver has only begun to emerge in motivating quantity during the past decade. This new information has helped effect substantial changes in official attitudes about drinking and driving compared with what they were 10 or 20 years ago.

For example, the National Safety Council, after studying scientific reports, has changed its position on the matter. The 1946 edition of *Accident Facts,* the Council's annual compilation of accident information, said: "According to state reports, nearly 18 percent of all drivers involved in fatal accidents had been drinking." (Note that it did not say that alcohol was a factor in 18 percent of the accidents; it merely said that 18

SOURCE. A. R. Roalman is a writer on health subjects. This article, slightly condensed, is from the March 1968 issue of *Today's Health,* published by the American Medical Association.

percent of the drivers had been drinking.)

In the 1966 edition of the same publication, the Council said: "Alcohol—a leading factor in fatal accidents. Drinking may be a factor in as many as half of the fatal motor vehicle accidents."

Probably the most dramatic emergence of new information occurred in New York state. There, as recently as 1957, official publications were stating that alcohol was a factor in one or two percent of all fatal motor vehicle accidents.

To see how change took place in New York and to get a good perspective on the drinking and driving problem, let's go back a few years and look over the shoulder of a man—Dr. William Haddon, Jr.—who was the director, from 1957 to 1961, of the Driver Research Center supported by the New York State Department of Health and the state's Bureau of Motor Vehicles. Part of Doctor Haddon's job was to get hard facts on which decisions about driver controls might be made.

Doctor Haddon, like any good researcher, started his study by asking a lot of questions. He went out on the highways and began asking policemen what they thought caused highway accidents.

Drinking, they said. There was little variation in the first answer they gave.

"But official records show that only one or two percent of all fatalities involve drinking drivers," said Doctor Haddon.

In a recent interview, he told how highway partolmen scoffed when he said that. A common reply he got from policemen,

when he countered with the official statistics, was: "I don't care what the statistics show; I know how many drunks I pull out of wrecks."

This inconsistency bothered Doctor Haddon and led him to conduct a study that, in medical and professional safety circles, is considered one of the landmarks of new and recent knowledge about drinking and driving.

Doctor Haddon, who now is director of the National Highway Safety Bureau and one of the top safety voices in the world, began searching for scrupulously scientific evidence. He decided that the way to get hard facts to answer some of the disturbing questions he had about drinking and driving was to get blood samples of drivers in single-car fatal accidents.

He chose not to rely on official reports, which too often did not include scientifically valid information about the intoxication level of drivers involved in crashes. (Police at an accident scene have several duties—help the injured, prevent more crashes, and get obvious information about the people involved in the accident—and they seldom are able to conduct scientifically solid tests to determine whether or not a motorist is legally intoxicated.)

Doctor Haddon found, in New York's Westchester County, a medical examiner who had been obtaining and testing blood samples of drivers killed in single-car fatal accidents for eight years. When Doctor Haddon found the Westchester information, he recognized it for what it was: an irrefutable collection of hard facts about drinking and driving. He ar-

ranged to have the information analyzed. What he found from the analysis was to start a national modification in thinking about drinking and driving.

What did the Westchester study, first published in *The Journal of the American Medical Association* in 1959, show?

1. Forty-nine percent of the dead drivers had blood alcohol levels of 0.15 percent or more. (Subsequent tests by other researchers have shown that most people are incapable of operating an automobile safely after their blood alcohol has reached 0.04 percent, and there isn't anyone likely to be able to drive safely after his blood-alcohol level has reached 0.08 percent.)

2. Twenty percent of the drivers had blood alcohol levels of from 0.05 to 0.14 percent.

3. Only 27 percent had no alcohol at the time of the tests.

While the study did not end all arguments about drinking and driving, it did substantiate that the drinking driver is a far greater problem than most people had thought.

Other, more recent, investigations confirm Doctor Haddon's findings.

One study by the U.S. Air Force found that, while only 5.3 percent of drivers *not* involved in accidents—a "control" group selected at random along the highways—had had two drinks or more, almost 65 percent of people involved in wrecks had had two drinks or more. Ninety percent of these drinking drivers had had at least three drinks, and an astonishing 60 percent at least six.

Also worth noting is that pedestrians involved in road or street accidents tend to have comparably high blood alcohol levels.

To return to arrests for drunken driving, let's see what has happened in the last five years. Police now have new laws to help them convict the drunken driver. Today, 44 states have laws that clearly specify at what blood alcohol level a driver is presumed to be under the influence of intoxicating liquor. The other six states also use chemical tests capable of determining the blood alcohol levels, and their courts accept results of such tests as evidence in all driving-while-intoxicated cases.

But more significant is the fact that a substantial body of law, developed during the past five years, has changed the attitude of the police toward formal charges of driving while intoxicated. While police might have been wary of making arrests for drunk-driving five years ago, now they have a much stronger body of legal authority for obtaining convictions. Five years ago, after arriving on the scene of an accident and finding a driver who appeared to be intoxicated, the police officer might have had no recourse except to say that the driver appeared drunk or to ask the driver to submit to a chemical test of his breath, blood, or urine. If—without the results of a valid chemical test—he merely said in court that the motorist had been drinking, it was difficult for the prosecuting attorney to obtain a conviction. There were many loopholes through which a defense attorney could obtain release of his client if no chemical test was involved.

Five years ago, in most states,

even if the arresting officer asked the suspected drunk to take a chemical test, the driver generally could refuse without fear of punishment. He could draw himself up, talk about his constitutional right against self-incrimination, and reject the request.

This situation is changing rapidly. Twenty-four states now have "implied consent" laws which say, in effect, that, if you drive in that state, you either submit to a chemical test if you are suspected of being drunk while driving, or you lose your privilege to operate a motor vehicle. Eight of those 24 states passed the implied-consent laws during the past two years. . . .

The reason for this change in attitude about the implied-consent law is partially the result of a 1966 Supreme Court decision relating to the administration of chemical tests for intoxication.

—You should know that, once you have more than 0.04 percent alcohol in your blood, you are mechanically not as able to drive safely as you are when you do not have any alcohol in your system.

—You should know what the legal limits for intoxication are in your state. Most states specify that, if you have more than 0.15 percent alcohol in your blood, you, legally, are intoxicated. Seven states (Florida, Illinois, Minnesota, North Carolina, North Dakota, Rhode Island, and Vermont) have set the legal limits at 0.10. One state—Utah—has said you are legally intoxicated if you are found to have more than 0.08 percent alcohol in your blood. The federal government, in June 1967, asked

all states to set 0.10 percent as the legal limit. (The American Medical Association has set 0.10 percent as a point of intoxication, but recognizes that drivers may be impaired at points as low as 0.05 percent.)

In any case, you should know what the legal limit is in your state and stay below it, so you can avoid serious legal consequences in case you are stopped on the highway. (You do not have to be involved in an accident to be arrested and convicted of driving while intoxicated. Mere operation of a motor vehicle while legally intoxicated is ground for punishments that vary from extended loss of your license to heavy fines or imprisonment.) . . . .

Generally, the body will eliminate alcohol at a constant rate of one-third to one-half of an ounce of alcohol (about an ounce of whiskey, vodka, gin, or other common alcoholic beverages) per hour. Theoretically it is possible for most people to sip half an ounce of alcohol an hour for 24 hours straight and not be intoxicated.

But the AMA Committee on Medical Aspects of Automotive Safety doesn't think much of this idea, or even of drinking four or five drinks and then waiting for the effects to wear off. Dr. H. A. Fenner, Jr., of Hobbs, New Mexico, the Committee chairman, says that "it is true that you eliminate about one drink an hour. But if you take even three or four drinks in a short period, your judgement might become impaired to the point where you will not wait the required length of time before driving."

The important things are that

you be familiar with your personal tolerances, that you avoid going beyond them when you are planning to drive, and that for the benefit of your friends, you apply the broad rules described here.

As for knowing your tolerances, listen to this advice from the AMA: "Studies reveal that test subjects, after consumption of alcohol, almost unanimously believe that their performance is unimpaired or even better than usual, whereas objective testing demonstrates that performance is impaired."

Especially remember that only time can return an intoxicated brain to normal, so parties where alcoholic beverages are served should end with a period of an hour or so when guests are eating, talking, or drinking coffee rather than drinking alcohol. The odds are always against the drinking driver.

19

HEALTH FRAUDS

W E HAVE DELIBERATELY RESERVED MATE- rial on medical misinformation and health rackets to such a late point in this text because it should serve as a kind of summary and review of everything that has gone before. To be an intelligent health-fraud-and-nonsense detec- tive, you must first have a solid background of legitimate, scientific health and medical infor- mation. It is difficult today to escape exposure to unreliable, misleading, and even dangerous health and medical misinformation. But you should now be able to begin to detect the differ- ence, and join the fight against quacks and non- sense.

Identifying Medical Misinformation

The rest of this chapter is devoted to the ex- position of certain perennial health rackets, frauds, fads, and hoaxes. They can be described as expensive and often dangerous nonsense which needlessly increase medical costs. There are some guidelines for detecting these health rackets.

Incredible amounts of health and medical in- formation—and misinformation—find their way into print in newspapers, magazines, brochures, pamphlets, leaflets, and books, are broadcast in television and radio programs, or pass by word of mouth. People are hungry for this kind of information. A survey on science news, conducted in 1958 for the National Association of Science Writers and New York University, revealed that 42% of the men and women interviewed wanted more medical news. Women, whose medical bills are higher, wanted even more than men. The survey also indicated that people get most of their medical news from newspapers (64%) and television (41%).

For the most part this is reliable news. Yet on many occasions an experiment is reported as a cure, a hope stretched into a promise, a research lead twisted into a clinical result, or a sensational headline made out of a routine finding. The fallacies in this type of medical misinformation are difficult to detect.

The best, but not an infallible, test for the accuracy of medical news is to look to its *source* rather than the medium in which it is published. If the news emanates from a convention of a recognized medical or voluntary health organi- zation, or scientific society, from the official publication of such an organization, from a uni- versity, or from a well-known hospital, and if it is written or bylined by an established science writer or reporter, the story is probably reliable and worth credence. If the information is released by an insurance company or a well-recognized pharmaceutical company, its credibility is also high. However, the statements of self-styled "doctors"—not M.D.'s—fly-by-night companies with pills, powders, or other remedies, systems, or devices to sell directly to the public should be viewed with judicious suspicion.

The most reliable single source of information on medical subjects is still your own physician. He better than anyone else can tell you whether some newly reported remedy is really appropriate for you. Many of them are not. Often they are dressed up with meaningless statistics—the better to fool you.

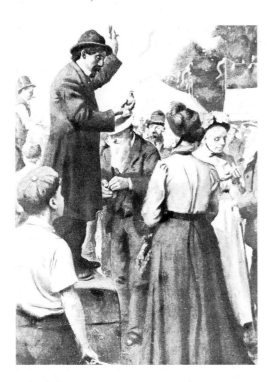

Fighting Health Frauds and Rackets

Although no area of human suffering is exempt, the areas in which the health racketeers most blithely ply their trade are food and nutrition fads, weight-reducing schemes, cosmetic quackery, dental nonsense, mental-health cults, cancer hoaxes, and drug panaceas for the "relief" of minor, annoying, or non-existent chronic illnesses. They don't dare legally to say "cure." But, ah, to "be regular"! To escape the "misery" of colds, piles, and rheumatism!

Among the types of products often dangerously and ridiculously "puffed" are stomach tablets, "tonics" with and without alcohol, liver pills, breath sweeteners, eyewashes, cough medicines, cold "preventives," and laxatives. As for so-called "testimonial advertising," the kind that reads, "I took a bottle of your medicine and now feel like a million dollars," the Bureau of Investigation of the American Medical Association has collected numerous examples of such testimonials that appeared in the same issue, and sometimes on the same page of a newspaper, as the obituary notice of the testimonial giver. It should be made clear, however, that advertising abuses of public confidence are limited to a small minority of the drug industry and that the majority has made strong efforts to tone down the offenders.

Probably the most tragic of health frauds and hoaxes are alleged cancer cures. These seem to attract devoted followers who defend them to the death. Yet in 1956 the Federal Food and Drug Administration was forced to issue an official public warning against one cancer hoax as worthless and "dangerous to those who rely on it instead of obtaining competent medical treatment." Many so-called "cured" cancer patients treated by quacks never had cancer in the first place.

One of the most amusing of the modern hoaxes, expensive but not dangerous, is the "royal-jelly" cosmetic nonsense. "Royal jelly" is the substance that queen bees feed on; it is a well-investigated mixture of common proteins and vitamin B complex. Some astute merchandisers have discovered that if you put 20 cents' worth of royal jelly in an ounce (10 cents' worth) of cold cream, you can sell the combination for $10 an ounce as a skin beautifier. The secretary of the American Medical Association's Committee on Cosmetics has stated several times that the committee has *no* evidence that royal jelly "in any way affects the cosmetic appearance of the skin."

Lines of Protection against Fraud. The situation today is not so blatant or scandalous as it was a few decades ago. In 1938, partly as a result of a series of deaths from an inadequately tested "elixir of sulfanilamide," Congress passed long-overdue laws strengthening the original pure food and drug laws of 1906 and giving the Federal Trade Commission (FTC) increased jurisdiction over advertising claims of foods, drugs, and cosmetics. Since then the drug and pharmaceutical industries have for the most part cleaned house.

As more powerful and effective drugs are introduced into medical practice, increased precautions in testing them for both direct effects and side effects are called for. Realistically this is a joint responsibility of the pharmaceutical manufacturers, the medical profession, and the governmental agencies that license the use of new drugs. More stringent criteria for testing drugs are constantly being developed, but there have been some tragic examples in the use of drugs whose possible side-effects were not sufficiently explored in advance. One relatively recent example was the tranquilizer, thalidomide, the use of which by pregnant women in the early stages of pregnancy resulted in deformed babies. It should be emphasized that drugs prescribed by physicians are (with the rarest exceptions, as noted above) safe under the conditions of prescribed use. The patient who far more frequently gets into trouble is the one who prescribes drugs for himself.

No unsafe drug can now be legally marketed in the United States, though many foreign countries do not enjoy such protection. The enforcement of the pure food and drug laws is in the hands of the Federal Food and Drug Administration, which cooperates with the American Medical Association and leading universities in establishing standards for drug safety.

The flagrant type of drug and cosmetic scandals which were sensationally exposed in the United States in the 1930's, in such books as *100 Million Guinea Pigs,* have for the most part disappeared. Still, subtle abuses of public confidence continue to arise. In 1951 the *Journal of the American Medical Association* still felt called upon to castigate some advertising of home remedies in the following words—which have not lost their cogency when applied to some of the publication and television advertising still with us today.

Undoubtedly the untruths are not as blatant as a few decades ago [in the heyday of proprietary medicine advertising], but clever writing and careful display more than compensate for the limitations on deliberate fabrication. . . . The advertising copywriters probably are well aware that comparatively few people read fine print when large bold-face words are near by to distract their attention.

Superlatives appear to be the order of the day. . . . By clever wording, promises are suggested which leave the reader believing that his health and other problems can now be solved without risk of failure. . . . It is time to clean up advertising.[1]

As far back as 1957, the chief inspector of the U.S. Post Office Department was moved to declare: "Medical frauds are today more lucrative than any other criminal activity." He cited weight-reducing schemes as the most profitable racket. A subcommittee of the U.S. House of Representatives found that in the city of Washington, D.C., alone the public was "wasting about a million dollars annually on useless and sometimes dangerous reducing drugs, pills, candies, and gums." The door-to-door vitamin subscription racket is also a juicy plum for its promoters.

A spokesman for the American Dental Association's Council on Dental Therapeutics addressed another House subcommittee in 1958. He described false toothpaste advertising as "reckless" and "vicious" and gave a host of specific examples. He named one dentifrice advertising campaign as "outright deception," called another "not only misleading and deceptive but also harmful to the public," and said of a third, "If [this toothpaste] is claimed to have twice the decay-germ-killing power [of others], then [its] advertisements may be considered twice as misleading."

The FDA is Getting Tougher. Its hand strengthened considerably by extensive (and admittedly sometimes controversial) U.S. Congressional subcommittee hearings (the Kefauver committee) in 1960 and 1961, and by new enforcement laws passed in 1962, the Federal Food and Drug Administration (FDA) moved forward more sternly than ever before in the mid-sixties to enforce laws against quackery and stamp out fraudulent and racketeering practices. It began to name names and take successful court action against notorious quacks and charlatans, their

---

[1] *JAMA* (editorial), March 31, 1951.

publications, "drugs," "health foods," and fake devices.

In 1962, for example, the FDA undertook a nationwide seizure campaign against a fake diagnostic machine, of which some 5000 had reputedly been sold at a price of $875 each in preceding years. This machine was supposed to diagnose a long list of serious medical conditions; all it actually did was to measure the amount of perspiration on the skin of the unlucky patient hitched up to its electrodes.

In 1962, also, the deputy director of Bureau of Enforcement of the FDA could say with confidence:

The quacks are being challenged on many fronts by a growing number of individuals and organizations. Public health officials no longer fear the quacks and are speaking out against them at the risk of time-consuming and costly damage suits. . . . We in the Food and Drug Administration are not only talking about the quacks but we are being specific and naming names. . . . The time is gone:

. . . when a self-styled nutritionist can use the air to spread his false teachings and promote nutritional products, without being challenged;

. . . when a health food propagandist can use the printing press to flood the country with nutritional nonsense, without being challenged;

. . . when a health writer can use the daily press to spread false medical theories that are used to promote the sale of sea water for the treatment of serious diseases, without being challenged;

. . . when doorstep diagnosticians like the thousands of salesmen of health foods can use the privacy of the home to sell their wares for the treatment of every known and unknown disease condition, without being challenged;

. . . when the publications of physicians containing unorthodox and unproven theories can be used in commercial promotions of foods or drugs, without being challenged;

. . . when charlatans can sell worthless articles for the treatment of cancer and arthritis, without being challenged;

. . . when promoters can launch nationwide promotions of unproven articles for the treatment of any disease condition, without being challenged;

. . . when our food manufacturers and drug manufacturers can promote their products by meaningless, confusing, and false nutritional and therapeutic claims, without being challenged.

Yes, we have challenged all these and many more to prove their theories in the Federal courts where they move from the sunny land of the copy writer to the cold, objective atmosphere of scientific fact.

The FDA's Role. The Federal Food and Drug Administration (FDA, an agency of the Department of Health, Education, and Welfare) has a large and varied task. Its main job is to enforce the Federal Food, Drug, and Cosmetic Act. To this end it makes sure that foods are safe, pure, wholesome, and made under sanitary conditions. It checks all drugs and therapeutic devices to be sure that they are safe for their intended purposes. It checks cosmetics to be sure that they are safe and prepared from appropriate ingredients. Finally, it scans the labels of all these products to be certain that they are honestly and informatively labeled and packaged.

To give a good hint on how the FDA carries out its manifold responsibilities for purity, quality, and labeling of foods, drugs and cosmetics, we have listed a few of the many specific things the FDA does:

1. Makes periodic inspections of food, drug, device, and cosmetics establishments and tests samples from interstate shipments of these products.

2. Assists industry in voluntary compliance with the law and in setting up controls to prevent violations.

3. Requires manufacturers to prove the safety and effectiveness of "new" drugs before they are put on sale to the public.

4. Tests every batch (except for exemptions) of antibiotic drugs and insulin for safety and effectiveness before they are sold. The manufacturers pay for such tests.

5. Enforces the law against illegal sales of prescription drugs.

6. Sets up standards of identity, quality, and fill of a container for food products in line with the congressional mandate "to promote honesty and fair dealing in the interest of consumers."

7. Passes on the safety of food additives, and checks to see that safety rules are followed.

8. Sets safe limits on the amount of pesticide residues that may remain on food crops, and checks shipments to see that these limits are observed.

9. Passes on the safety of colors for use in foods, drugs, or cosmetics, and tests and certifies each batch manufactured.

10. Checks imports of foods, drugs, devices, and cosmetics to make sure they comply with the laws of the United States.

In addition to its Washington, D.C., headquarters, the FDA has 18 district offices, where it can perform scientific analyses and investigations of the multifold products it is required to check. The FDA has about 800 scientifically trained inspectors in the field. Its cost to taxpayers (for 1962–1963) was estimated at 15 cents a person, representing a total appropriation from Congress of $28,280,000. Products covered by laws enforced by the FDA have a sales value of more than $117 billion! They are disbursed in probably 100,000 factories and warehouses and about 700,000 retail establishments.

During the sixties, in an average year, 60,000 establishment inspections were made, and 75,000 samples of products made in the United States were collected for analysis. An additional 15,000 samples were collected from shipments offered for importation into the country. It can be seen that this adds up to coverage of only a fraction of the foods and drugs bought by the American public. Enforcement of the food and drug laws must therefore be intelligently selective.

Though they have been notably rewritten and modernized on several occasions since—notably in 1938—the first federal "pure food and drug laws" actually date back to 1906. Dr. Harvey W. Wiley led the crusade for the new law and later undertook its enforcement. It is hard for us to realize the shocking conditions under which food was being commercially manufactured at the turn of the century and the bland, useless "cure-all" promises of that day's patent medicines.

State law enforcement officials are also getting tougher on the health racketeers. The New York State Attorney General, for instance, has taken legal steps to bar many shady fund-raising schemes in the name of health from plying their profitable promotional charlatanry. In at least one case the Attorney General demonstrated to the satisfaction of the courts that shady promoters were pocketing 90% of the funds raised for an apparently worthy, but secretly racketeered, health cause.

"Patent Medicines." Half of the drugs sold over the counter in the nation's nearly 60,000 drugstores can be purchased without a doctor's prescription. Sales of these drugs reach a volume of over $1 billion a year. Some of these drugs are heavily advertised; others are not. None of these products is likely to be directly harmful, except insofar as they delay treatment of the causes rather than the symptoms of a specific disease.

It is still common to speak of these non-prescription drugs as "patent medicines." Few of them are actually patented, because that requires a public registration of the exact content, proportion, and mode of manufacture of the drug. So-called secret-formula drugs are properly described as *proprietary drugs*. Their chief value is in their advertised brand name. Any competent pharmacological chemist can break their "secret" formulas.

There are no secret, undiscovered remedies for disease available for sale in drugstores or by mail. No matter how heavily and fancily advertised, they contain some old-fashioned drug long known to medicine or some new drug in such tiny doses as to be impotent. You can find this out by reading the fine print on the label. The real "miracle drugs" are not for sale without a prescription. Nor are they heavily advertised to the public.

The most widely sold "over-the-counter" medication remains aspirin, cheap in ordinary tablet form but often inflated in price when combined with other questionably useful ingredients and sold under a trade name. Aspirin production in the United States reached an all-time high in 1963, when nearly 30 million pounds were manufactured. The public paid a record $350 million for straight aspirin tablets and mixed ingredient products that year. Something like 16 *billion* aspirin tablets were consumed!

Practically all non-prescription analgesics ("painkillers") contain aspirin as their only, or chief, active ingredient. The London *Lancet* counted and published a list of 322 of these mixed-ingredient pain relievers, each sold under its own brand name!

The sums paid for aspirin *alone* in its various guises equalled 10% of the total sum ($3.5 billion) paid by the American public in 1963 for *all* prescription drugs, including the so-called wonder drugs.

The source of effect in some non-prescription remedies is alcohol. Many of the so-called "women's tonics," at one time very popular in "dry" states, had a comparatively high proportion of alcohol and represented a socially acceptable way for a professed teetotaler to take a drink.

An occasional dispenser of unreliable medical information is the "counter-prescribing druggist." Ethical pharmacists, it must be remembered, eschew and condemn this practice, but there remain a few clerks who are flattered to answer the question, "Hey, doc, what can you give me for a cold?" The person who expects to get reliable medical information for the price of a bottle of medicine is gambling dangerously with his health.

"Kind" friends and relatives, because they enjoy our personal trust, are often as dangerous health advisers as the few unscrupulous advertisers. Avoid them like poison, for that is what their suggestions frequently amount to.

The purchasers of quack products are not always aware that they are being victimized. Just one company had 75,000 agents using pseudo-scientific vitamin literature to sell its products! After proving that it contained false claims, the FDA destroyed 50 tons of this literature in the Chicago area alone. The quacks have no hesitation about claiming that their products are good for diseases and conditions that no legitimate remedies can cure—for example, cancer, multiple sclerosis, muscular dystrophy, Parkinson's

disease, cataracts, cirrhosis, baldness, and sterility. To cure one of these conditions, the luckless victim is often given nothing more than a bottle of seawater—at a price of $3.75 or higher. The peddler argues that taking a little seawater a day is providing the body with a "chemical smorgasbord" and that its "rich" supply of minerals has a "vaccinative" effect against so-called deficiency diseases!

The American public apparently has a high degree of gullibility when it comes to reaching for useless, valueless health products. At the National Congress on Medical Quackery, jointly sponsored by the FDA and the AMA in Washington, D.C., in December 1963, it was conservatively estimated that the public wastes at least $1 billion a year on falsely promoted, worthless or dangerous products or methods of treating disease. Over half this was considered to be wasted on falsely promoted vitamin products and health foods. The FDA has records of protein products that contain little or no protein; cholesterol capsules that do not prevent cardiovascular disease; high potency vitamins which are *im*potent. On the regulatory front the FDA brings scores of legal actions. But an active educational and informational program is more rewarding.

Folly of Self-Medication. *He who has himself for a physician has a fool for a patient.* Except by physicians, who never treat themselves and rarely minister even to their own families, this ancient and appropriate warning is still lavishly disregarded.

Why do so many people continue to fall chronic victims to false or at least exaggerated hopes and claims that some particular remedy is "good for whatever ails them"? The remedy may be a heavily advertised specialty sold in drugstores, a "natural" food not commonly found in the American dietary, or even a nauseous herb concoction cooked on the kitchen stove according to a recipe that "grandmother brought from the old country."

The answer lies in the mental mechanisms. The victims first project all their troubles on "poor health," and secondly identify and idealize their salvation with their faith in a particular remedy.

They feel better, they say, if they take the medicine—or the exercises, or the mechanical treatment, or whatever other nonsense is offered them. The astonishing part is that they often feel better! But only for a short while.

This fact has long been recognized in the practice of medicine by the occasional prescription of *placebos,* sugar pills or bitter medicines that have no real effect on body functions. Vitamins sometimes serve as self-prescribed placebos.

Quacks, Cults, and Fads. Many of the same psychological factors which drive individuals to the danger and folly of self-medication also push them into the arms of irregular healing cults and outright quacks. And the same unhappy results often obtain. The strength and persistence of healing cults and quacks throughout the centuries lie in several facts:

At least eight out of ten cases of illness are self-limited. The patient will recover regardless of what is done or not done for him. Recovery follows treatment; therefore treatment caused recovery. That is what the quacks and cults persuade their patients, who gratefully swallow their utterly fallacious reasoning.

There is still an element of mystery—facts beyond present knowledge—in how recovery from disease is brought about by the healing force of nature (*vis mediatrix naturae*). The quack and cult exploit this mystery. They practice magic in modern dress and make irrational appeal to superstition and fear of demonic powers, sometimes recounted in a pseudoscientific vocabulary.

In the United States, at least, the general standard of living is high enough so that many people can afford to patronize irregular healers at good fees. These charlatans prey upon human ignorance. Often they "cure" diseases that never existed in the first place, such as "lost manhood." One stigma of the healing cult is its belief in a single "cause" or a single "treatment" for all varieties of disease.

It is, of course, illegal to practice medicine in the United States without a state license to do so. To this extent, certainly, the public is protected from irregular, untrained, self-styled doctors. But weird healing cults tend to spring up from time to time without claiming to practice medicine. They sometimes put forth extremely fancy names and set up elaborate establishments and machinery to draw business to themselves. They advertise. Perhaps the most protective single piece of advice that can be given to the person who wants to stay out of the hands of quacks and charlatans is to avoid any practitioner who publicly advertises his ability to heal or cure.

The truth is that there is nothing that a charlatan (or group of them) can do for a patient that a doctor of medicine—M.D.—cannot do better and more safely. Certainly the M.D. is far better trained in the rational diagnosis of disease, and there is less chance of a serious underlying source of pathology being missed while idle manipulations go on to relieve surface symptoms.

Some distinction, perhaps, should be made between fads and cults. A fad becomes a cult when its founder sets up a school to teach others how to practice a system of healing which the founder is already purveying directly to the public. Food faddists are legion, each with his own special brand of diet. Bulgarian buttermilk or yogurt is an old standby. The food faddists rarely, however, set up schools but instead make their money through books, lectures, and direct sale or endorsement of foods. Safflower seed, its oil, and other derivatives, are among the newer nutritional "gimmicks."

Very few licensed physicians have ever fallen into out-and-out quackery; the very unusualness of this situation has made such rare falls from grace both newsworthy and historical. When controversy over a medical treatment gets into the newspapers, there is usually some politician or editor trying to make a case or a story out of a dangerous fallacy.

Don't waste too much sympathy on the "persecuted" innovator who uses newspaper publicity and the courts to advertise products and methods whose worth he has been unable to prove to his professional colleagues through professional channels always open. Fakes and quacks thrive on the publicity arising out of lawsuits.

We cannot predict under what fancy names

or titles or claims the fads and cults of the future will be established. We can only predict that they will occur. Quackery is a classical example of history repeating itself.

We also venture to predict that the ads of the fads of the future, like those of the present, will be heavily interlarded with false phrases like "Science says" and "Doctors prove" and that they will wave meaningless statistics under their readers' noses.

How to Lie with Statistics

In his highly entertaining but thoroughly sound little book, *How to Lie with Statistics,* Darrell Huff has pointed out a number of statistical tricks which, he says, the crooks already know and honest men must learn in self-defense. He calls attention to biased samples, meaningless averages, purposeful omissions ("the little figures that are not there"), apples-and-peaches comparisons, illogical correlations ("semi-attached figures"), the *post hoc, propter hoc* fallacy (this happened after that; therefore this caused that), the cut-off ("gee whiz") graph, the deceptive map, and the two-dimensional picture to express three-dimensional facts.

If you want to analyze a statistical statement, says Huff, ask questions: Who says so? How does he know? What's missing? Did somebody change the subject? Does it all make sense? He cites, among scores of amusing examples an "amazing new dentrifice" headline ("23% FEWER CAVITIES") based on just *six* experimental cases, a "proof" that railroad travel is "dangerous" (the "proof" omitted to say that 95% of the fatalities were among hobos riding the rods), and a nonsense demonstration that milk causes cancer (more people drink milk, more people get cancer; therefore, milk causes cancer).

Huff points out that many a statistic is "false on its face." "It gets by," he says, "only because the magic numbers bring about a suspension of common sense." A *New Yorker* cartoon amusingly makes the same point. A tough tycoon is shown saying to his yesman, "All right, then, get another *independent* laboratory report." The moral is plain: buyer, voter, patient, BEWARE!

Sources of Reliable Information. Your own knowledge, intelligence, and common sense must be your first and best line of protection against health frauds and rackets. If you are unsure of your ground, however, and skeptical about some of the things you hear and see, you can obtain reliable, accurate, unbiased information from the following sources:

1. Your own physician.
2. Officers of your local county medical society, or your public health officer.
3. Your local Better Business Bureau.
4. The American Medical Association, 535 North Dearborn Street, Chicago, Illinois.
5. The Federal Food and Drug Administration, Washington 25, D.C.
6. The Federal Trade Commission, Washington 25, D.C.
7. Local chapters or national headquarters of voluntary health agencies or professional societies (e.g., National Foundation, American Dental Association) on questions which fall within their particular sphere.

Health frauds and rackets, quacks and charlatans provide an alarmingly interesting chapter in the long history of human gullibility. You may expect to meet again in modern dress the fakery associated with such ancient princes of quackery as Valentine Greatrakes, Elisha Perkins (and his magnetic tractors), Mesmer (parlor hypnotist), Cagliostro, and Sylvester Graham (who gave his name to graham crackers).

SUMMARY

One foolish way to increase your health and medical expenses needlessly is to patronize the perennial health quacks, cults, fakes, fads, and frauds. Probably half of these are in the field of nutrition. Unnecessary vitamins are shamelessly peddled; bottles of seawater are sold as cure-alls!

The Federal Food and Drug Administration (FDA) and other agencies offer you some protection against these rackets. In the final analysis, however, it is your own understanding of the scientific facts about health and medicine—information we have sought to present in this book—that will guard you against the pseudoscientific lies and statistics with which present-day frauds are usually embellished.

In the next chapter we shall go still more deeply into the general topic of environmental health, of which the subject of consumer health is an integral part.

SUMMARY REVIEW QUESTIONS

1. What are the best tests for the accuracy and reliability of medical news? Where does this news usually appear? Why is medical news so popular?
2. What are some of the perennial health rackets to which the American public is exposed? (Give at least six examples.) Why do these rackets persist?
3. What legal protection against health frauds and rackets does the American public now have? How did this come about? What other protection is possible? What is the role of the FDA?
4. How would you distinguish between health rackets and (*a*) health cults, (*b*) health fads, and (*c*) health quacks? How, if at all, would you defend any one of these as being "more innocent" than the others?
5. How can you lie with statistics? (Give at least six examples.)
6. Are the following statements sense or nonsense? Why? . . . *He who has himself for a physician has a fool for a patient. . . . Seawater is a good remedy for many minor illnesses. . . . Vitamins every day keep the doctor away. . . . You can prove anything with statistics.*
7. What do the following terms mean to you: consumer health, socialized medicine, shaman, Federal Trade Commission (FTC), quackery, patent medicine, yogurt, *post hoc, propter hoc?*

Worth Looking Into: *How To Lie With Statistics* by Darrell Huff. *Devils, Drugs, and Doctors* by Howard W. Haggard, M.D. *The Medicine Show* by the Editors of Consumer Reports. *Folk and Modern Medicine* by Don James. For more complete references, see Appendix E.

SEE SPECIAL EXERCISE ON THREE FOLLOWING PAGES

WHICH OF THE FOLLOWING NEWS STORIES AND ADVERTISEMENTS DO YOU BELIEVE? ▶

Which do you disbelieve? Which are you in doubt about?
Why? When you have *finished* this exercise, see page 482.

WHICH OF THE FOLLOWING
NEWS STORIES AND ADS
DO YOU BELIEVE?

DOCTORS CARRY DISEASE

The practical point to be illustrated is the following: the disease known as puerperal fever is so far contagious as to be frequently carried from patient to patient by physicians and nurses.

This long catalogue of melancholy histories assumes a still darker aspect when we remember how kindly nature deals with the parturient female, when she is not immersed in the virulent atmosphere of an impure lying-in hospital, or poisoned in her chamber by the unsuspected breath of contagion.

OCEAN GIVES UP SECRET

Resembles Outer Space, Jap Admiral Says

NEW LONDON, SEPT. 8—Conditions at the bottom of the sea resemble outer space more closely than anything else on earth, the voyages of polar (atomic) submarines have revealed. A report given today at the Navy's New London Submarine Base uncovered this startling fact. The report was given by Rear Admiral Foni Gey of the Japanese Naval Airforce Medical Corps. The admiral is both a flier and a diver. "What I have seen at the bottom of the ocean is the same thing I have seen at the top of the sky," he said.

The admiral's report was part of a classified symposium on the medical problems of confinement in a space sealed completely against the outside atmosphere. Approximately 200 leading authorities on environmental medicine, from North and South America, Europe and Japan, were invited to attend the conference, which opened today.

The Navy's public-relations officer at the conference, Captain U. S. Ess, would make no comment on what the Japanese admiral said he saw. "I said, nothing," he shouted when a reporter put the question to him for a second time.

*be beautiful
with*

BEE BEAUTIFUL
brand of royal jelly

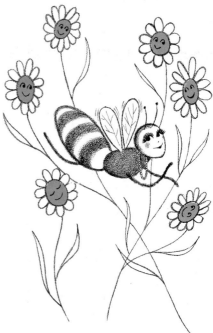

Be a honey.
Try BEE BEAUTIFUL TODAY.
Don't listen to to the buzz-buzz of the skeptics.
Make up your own mind!

Science has proved that ROYAL JELLY,
the secret food of the queen bee,
is the quickest, easiest way to a skin that
any man (even a drone) would love to touch.
It stands to reason, doesn't it?
The queen bee outlives her sisters
forty times over! Explain that!!

But you really don't have to bother
to explain anything when you have
that skin loveliness that only
BEE BEAUTIFUL can give.

So be beautiful . . . . with

BEE BEAUTIFUL

On sale at all drug and department stores
$10 for #1 beauty-bound package (1 oz.)

NEW TRIUMPH FOR MEDICINE?

Soviet Reports Alleged Cancer Cure

MOSCOW, APR. 1 (QRS)—Soviet scientists have discovered a cure for cancer, sources close to the Kremlin revealed unofficially last night. No official comment could be obtained from the Ministry of Health. The superintendent of a Moscow hospital, where proof of the alleged cancer cure is rumored to have been established, denied that a former high government official, sent to Siberia in a recent purge, was now a patient in the hospital.

Confidential sources, whose names cannot be revealed, disclosed that the exiled government official had brought the cancer cure back from Siberia. He was dying of the disease, the story goes, when a Siberian peasant woman offered to cure him. She gave him a brew of unknown ingredients and he recovered within a month.

"I know that the Western World will not believe this new triumph of Soviet medicine," the informant declared, "because it comes from behind the Iron Curtain. But what is so different from the fact that the English doctor William Wuthering discovered digitalis, the sovereign remedy for heart disease, in a brew of herbs he bought from an old woman?"

CONTROLLED SLEEP FOUND EFFECTIVE IN PEPTIC ULCER

WASHINGTON, D. C.—The success of a carefully controlled regimen of sleep therapy, in which 120 patients with peptic ulcers slept an average of 14 hours per day for 14 days, was reported in a paper presented to the World Congress of Gastroenterology here by Dr. Jan Roguski of Warsaw.

Dr. Roguski said that the crater disappeared in 16 out of 24 patients with gastric ulcer and in 36 out of 96 patients with duodenal ulcer after similar treatment.

Significant increase in weight and improvement of appetite were noted in nearly all patients, said Dr. Roguski, who called the results "satisfactory, considering the short duration of therapy."

The therapy was conducted in especially adapted clinical wards. Sleep was induced by 0.1 Gm. phenobarbital three times daily in the first two days, with the dosage gradually diminished to 0.1 Gm. once a day by the second week. The drug was replaced by a placebo thereafter without apparently affecting depth or continuity of sleep.

Dr. Roguski said that the study was conducted over a four-year period. The 14 days of sleep therapy were preceded by a hospital stay of three to seven days for physical examination and selection of the patients best suited for the study.

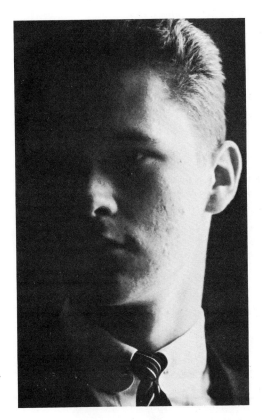

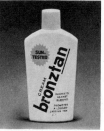
404   Health Hazards

20

COMMUNITY HEALTH ORGANIZATION
AND CONSUMER COSTS

No man is an *Iland*, intire of itselfe; every man is a peece of the *Continent*, a part of the *maine;* if a *Clod* bee washed away by the *Sea, Europe* is the lesse, as well as if a *Promontorie* were, as well as if a *Mannor* of thy *friends* or of *thine owne* were; any mans *death* diminishes *me*, because I am involved in *Mankinde;* And therefore never send to know for whom the *bell* tolls; It tolls for *thee.*
                                    John Donne, seventeenth century

THERE IS NO ESCAPE FROM PERSONAL RE- sponsibility for personal health. But no man lives alone. For fullest protection from the normal health hazards to life, we must join with our fellow men in support of community health organizations. Indeed, it is through these orga- nizations—operating largely behind the scenes of everyday life—that the life-saving, health-build- ing benefits of modern science are delivered to us.

From a more exact understanding of commu- nity health organization, it is useful to distinguish between "public health" and "community health." *Public health* traditionally stands for health authority, for health laws derived from the essential police power of the state, and for tax support of its activities. *Community health* is a broader concept, implying voluntary cooperation of all elements of the community, including public health departments, the medical profes- sion, and the general public, in finding and meeting its health needs.

Community Health

Community health proceeds on the assump- tion that citizens will willingly devote their time and contribute their funds voluntarily toward the support of community health measures. Leader- ship in the community health movement has been taken by voluntary health agencies, by in- surance companies, by social and welfare agen- cies, by civic organizations, and more recently by community health councils.

Probably the most successful single effort at voluntary cooperation in the utilization of com- munity health resources throughout the United States was the development of the Blue Cross group hospitalization plans, begun in the early 1930's.

The concepts of public health, in the early nineteenth century, were embodied in the picture of the sanitary policeman. He was armed with the authority to enforce compliance to public health statutes. The health inspector is still with us. But public health authorities, together with voluntary health agencies, all learned in the course of the twentieth century that you cannot club a man into mental health, quarantine him against heart disease, or officially warn him against most of the important hazards to life and health that man in modern society faces.

The modern concept of community health is best exemplified in the community health coun- cil. It can be described as a group of people in a community anxious to learn the real health needs of that community and to find ways of meeting them. It is a representative, democratic body, drawn from all segments of the commu- nity—the healing arts and professions, public

HEALTH PROFESSIONS:

Physicians (in active practice) 325,500
    M.D.'s 314,000
    Osteopaths (D.O.) 11,500

Dentists (in active practice) 100,000

Pharmacists (in active practice) 125,000
    86% in local drugstores

2. **Nurses** (and related services) 1,960,000
    RN's (Registered Nurses) 725,000
    Practical nurses 352,000
    Nursing aides, orderlies, and attendants 880,000
    Home health aides 14,000

Administrators of health services 50,000

Basic science in health field 57,000
    Researchers other than physicians, dentists, or veterinarians

Biomedical engineering 11,000

Clinical laboratory services 110,000
    Laboratory directors (M.D.'s and Ph.D.'s) 4500
    Clinical (medical) laboratory technologists 43,500
    Clinical laboratory technicians or aids 63,000

Dental hygienist 17,500

Dental assistants 100,000

Dental laboratory technicians 28,000

Dietitians, nutritionists, technicians, and food supervisors 37,000

Environmental control 39,000
    Environmental engineers 10,000
    Industrial hygienists 2,300
    Other environmental specialists (e.g., pollution control) 9,700
    Sanitarians and sanitarian technicians 17,000

Food and drug protective services 23,000

Health and vital statistics 2,500

Health educators 22,000
    Public health educators 2,000
    School health educators and coordinators 20,000

UNITED STATES, 1970

Health information and communication	5,000
Medical librarians	3,500
Medical library assistants	5,500
Medical record librarians	14,000
Medical record technicians	27,000
Midwives	3,000
Orthotists and prosthetists (Making and fitting artificial limbs and braces)	3,500
Occupational therapists and aides	13,000
Physical therapists and aides	22,000
Podiatrists (chiropodists)	8,500
Psychologists (clinical, counseling, etc.)	10,000
Radiologic (X-ray) technologists and technicians	110,000
Secretaries, office assistants	275,000
Social workers (clinical) and assistants	23,500
Rehabilitation services (includes corrective, educational, manual arts, recreational, and music therapists)	10,000
Speech pathology and audiology	18,000
Veterinarians (in active practice)	25,500

Vision care (excluding 9,000 ophthalmologists already counted under M.D.'s and D.O.'s)

Optometrists (O.D.)	17,000	
Opticians and optical technicians)	25,000	
Orthoptists (give eye-exercises)	500	

Vocational rehabilitation counselors	9,000
Inhalation therapy technicians (administer oxygen)	8,000
EKG (electrocardiograph) technicians record heart waves	7,000
EEG (electroencephalograph) technicians record "brain waves"	2,500
Surgical aides (operating room assistants)	21,000

HEALTH RESOURCES: UNITED STATES, 1970

Hospitals and other in-patient health facilities		31,000
Short-stay hospitals (general hospitals)	6,500	
Short-stay hospitals (specialty hospitals)	300	
Long-stay hospitals		
General hospitals	200	
Psychiatric hospitals	475	
Geriatric and chronic hospitals	300	
Tuberculosis hospitals	125	
Other (chronic disease, rehabilitation, obstetric, etc.)	175	
Nursing care and related homes	20,000	
Other inpatient health facilities		
Institutions for the mentally retarded	1500	
Other (for deaf or blind, for unwed mothers, for dependent children, etc.)	3300	
Public waterworks, serving well over 150 million people		17,000
Drugstores, through which the American public buys $4 billion worth of health goods annually-produced by drug, pharmaceutical and allied industries		52,000
Food stores, providing essential elements of a nutritionally adequate diet to American public		50,000
Health departments, local, county, and state		1,800
Local chapters of voluntary health associations		20,000
Community health councils, coordinating health care patterns in a community		750
Institutions of higher learning, colleges and universities, including *89 medical schools,* and other graduate schools, which supply most of the advanced and specialized professional training for the health professions		2,200
Nurse's training schools, operated in connection with hospitals		1,100

health agencies, voluntary health agencies, business, industry, labor, schools, churches, consumer groups, and all other civic organizations that recognize their stake in the health of the community. About 750 community health councils are now operating in the United States.

Community Health Resources

When community health problems are identified, community health resources must be mobilized to meet them. What are the community health resources?

Fundamentally, they are the community itself, whether neighborhood, college, or nation. It has often been said that the wealth of a nation is the health of its people, through whom its total productivity is achieved. In a community of any size competent professional workers are needed to organize and deliver all manner of health services.

But the healing arts and professions do not

create the health of a community. They simply channel its resources. Through its professionals, the community not only employs its own wealth in the interest of its own health, but it is also able to draw upon an international fund of scientific knowledge, inherited from earlier generations the world over.

Community health resources are both tangible and intangible. To get you well, if you are sick, and to keep you well, if you are now in good health, the United States has a corps of at least 3½ million professionally and technically trained individuals directly serving the health needs of other people and deriving their own livings from this service.

There are many interesting health careers beyond the practice of medicine. College students who have not yet settled on their own future vocations are well advised to investigate them. (See "Health Career Opportunities".)

The accompanying table (page 406) categorizes the more than 3½ million people serving in the healing arts and professions in the United States. From them you may receive specific kinds of health service, health counsel, and health education. The figures given are estimates for the beginning of the decade of the 1970's.

More than thirty so-called "paramedical" specialties are now recognized. These are made up of the individuals who help physicians toward the complete diagnosis, treatment, and rehabilitation of their patients. Almost a million persons are now employed on a full-time basis in American hospitals. The lower echelons, such as maintenance men and laundresses, are not classified as professional.

Another vital set of intangible health resources is the wealth of scientific knowledge and training stored in the members of the healing arts and professions. This implies a whole network of educational resources that can eventually turn out trained technicians and highly educated specialists from whom new advances in health science can be expected. Colleges and universities supply most of the brains, libraries, space, and facilities for medical and scientific research on which medical progress rests.

Tangible Resources. The tangible health resources of a community, in people and in buildings, equipment and supplies, are comparatively easy to count, yet exceedingly difficult to evaluate in terms of dollars. Beyond the level of the institutions and organizations that provide immediate health services and direct health education, we can estimate only crudely the health resources of any community. For whatever such estimates are worth, and they give at best mere orders of magnitude, we may approximate the direct health resources of the United States in the decade of the 1960's, exclusive of personnel and the wealth of scientific knowledge, approximately as shown in the table on page 408.

America's 8000 registered hospitals represent the largest fixed capital investment among its numerous direct health resources. This is estimated at over $25 billion. A well-run modern hospital is a masterpiece of organization of health services for the benefit of the patient. The status of the hospital today is the reflection of the triumphs of twentieth-century medicine and surgery.

Beyond the health resources already enumerated, we must include such community resources as parks, playgrounds, and recreations centers; churches of all faiths that minister to the spiritual, social, mental, and sometimes directly to the physical health of their parishioners; and good homes, which undoubtedly top the list of health resources.

Health Career Opportunities

While the fully trained physician—doctor of medicine, M.D.—remains the key player (and usually the quarterback) on the health team, it can be clearly seen that the non-physician members of the team now outnumber the doctors by 7 or 8 to 1. College students who may be interested in pursuing health careers in any number of interesting specialties (as suggested in the table *Health Professions: United States, 1960's*) may write to the National Health Council, 1740 Broadway, New York, N.Y. for booklets, pamphlets, and brochures fully describing the opportunities and requirements for entry into these health professions.

Health Careers Guidebook, published by the National Health Council, outlines in considerable detail more than 150 health career opportunities at various levels of professional and semi-professional skills. The following alphabetical listing of areas in which training and careers in health services may be sought is derived from this publication. The purpose of this listing is to *suggest* where opportunities lie; not every possible job is mentioned, nor are the many present-day medical specialties (e.g., orthopedic surgeon, radiologist, etc.) described.

Administration of health services offers such careers as hospital administrator, administrative assistant, business manager (many types), voluntary health agency executive or field representative, and public health administrator (at many levels).

Basic sciences related to health provide numerous career opportunities, especially in the areas of laboratory research. Among the specialties here are biophysics and biochemistry, bacteriology, virology, physiology, and toxicology.

Chiropody (or podiatry), dealing with care of the feet, is another area of opportunity.

Dentistry and its allied services, including the dental assistant, dental hygienist, and dental laboratory technician, afford increasing career openings.

Dietetics and nutritional services provide many opportunities for qualified dietitians, nutritionists, food technologists, food service supervisors, and other food service workers.

Environmental health services, growing in importance, offer many jobs to sanitary engineers and sanitarians.

Food and drug inspectors and analysts are constantly needed in government jobs.

Health education offers excellent prospects both for the public health and school health educator.

Information and communication services in the health fields provide many opportunities for writers (e.g., science writers), editors (e.g., medical editors), medical illustrators, and photographers.

Health statistics require the services of statisticians, biometricians, actuaries, and (on a lower level) statistical clerks. The rapid growth of *health insurance* has multiplied all kinds of employment related to this field.

Medical librarians are in growing demand, as are medical record librarians and technicians.

Medical secretaries and medical assistants usually have a wide choice of jobs in physicians' offices, clinics, and hospitals.

Medical technology, a field which is becoming increasingly specialized, offers many opportunities to the trained medical technologist. It is especially suited to women who wish to work part time.

Nursing and related services provide the bulk of health occupations—around one and one-half million jobs. The nursing team includes not only the professional, graduate, registered nurse (R.N.), who has many choices for specialization and place of work, but also practical nurses, nursing aides, orderlies, and attendants.

Occupational health services offer a wide range of employment in industry to safety engineers, industrial hygienists, and industrial nurses.

Occupational therapists, who direct "curing by doing" in creative, recreational, and educational activities, enjoy great opportunities for speeding ill and convalescent patients on the road to recovery.

Optometry provides useful, well-paid professional careers. The optician also provides essential services and may eventually go in business for himself. Orthoptic technicians supervise eye exercises.

Orthopedic and prosthetic appliance work, providing artificial limbs and fitting braces, is the increasingly professional task of the orthotist and prosthetist.

Osteopathy is a profession allied to medicine but with some differences in theory and practice.

Pharmacy—the science of drugs—offers many career opportunities in retail, hospital, and manufacturing pharmacy (the pharmaceutical industry).

Physical therapy is a rapidly growing profession. The physical therapist is a key member of the health team which undertakes the *rehabilitation* of the crippled and disabled.

Psychology is a profession which is increasingly dealing with problems of mental health. Many opportunities are open to the clinical psychologist, counseling psychologist, social psychologist, and psychometrist (who specializes in testing).

Social work includes two specialties which are important health careers: medical social work and psychiatric social work.

Speech and hearing therapists practice a gratifying profession which helps thousands of children and adults to overcome speech defects, frequently associated with hearing difficulties. The speech pathologist concentrates on speech rehabilitation, the audiologist on hearing conservation.

Veterinary medicine, though dealing primarily with

the health of animals, plays an important role in disease prevention among humans beings.

Vocational rehabilitation counseling, undertaken by skilled and trained counselors, offers still another place on the rehabilitation team.

X-ray equipment operation calls for increasingly well-trained X-ray technicians, who actually take the X-ray pictures (roentgenographs) which the physician interprets.

Health Teaching in Schools

Both the elementary and secondary school teachers have responsibility for the teaching of their pupils in the areas of health.[1] They must acquire knowledge of this area, and techniques. A teacher should develop an understanding of how children grow and develop, for their continuous health and guidance and the adaptations that must be made in teaching them are illuminated by this knowledge. A teacher should be able to identify significant health problems which exist among school-age children and should be able to take some steps to help them alleviate these problems. Obviously the teacher's own health status, attitudes, and knowledge will forward the cause of good health among her own pupils.

Teachers should also be aware of health services which their communities and schools provide. For example, the teacher should understand the purposes and appreciate the value of the various health-screening procedures to which children are admitted. The teacher may also have to perform a role in preparing children for various health appraisal experiences, such as health examinations, tuberculin tests, and vision

and hearing tests. The teacher must understand the functions of other members of the school health staff; in particular, the school nurse. The teacher should be informed about school policies relating to emergency care and know his or her responsibilities in carrying out this program. The teacher should also be well informed of the school's policy related to excusing pupils from school for medical, dental, or other health reasons.

The teacher must be able to take some responsibility for the physical, emotional, and intellectual health of the school environment. She must know how to maintain a classroom environment which is conducive to comfort and efficiency within the limits of school equipment. In emergencies she must be able to conduct exit and security drills. She must recognize the normal health and safety hazards to the children on the way to school and in the vicinity of the classroom. She must encourage sanitary practices in school lunch programs. She must be aware of potential hazards and must urge protective practices in providing school water supply and sewage disposal.

The teacher must be aware of the opportunity of forwarding health knowledge whenever it arises in a special situation or as part of a program that naturally integrates health instruction with such other areas as science, social studies, and art education. The teacher must learn how to motivate health teaching so that desirable changes in health habits and behavior take place.

The secondary school teacher does not have as much or direct responsibility for health education as the primary and elementary school teacher. Nevertheless the secondary school teacher must understand the total growth and development pattern of her students; must accept where necessary responsibilities for their health protection, including appraisal and counseling; must help them assume increasing responsibility for their own health; must meet emergencies created by illness or accident; must help maintain a healthful school environment and schedule; and must incorporate some specified areas of health education within their course content.

[1] "Teaching Classroom Teachers to Teach Health," by H. Frederick Kilander, (deceased) Dean, Graduate School, Wagner College, Staten Island, New York. This article was taken from the *Proceeding of the Fifth Pre-Convention Session on School Health,* sponsored by the American Medical Association and the American School Health Association, Atlantic City, N. J., (June 16, 1963). Published by the Department of Community Health and Health Education, Division of Environmental Medicine and Medical Service, American Medical Association (535 N. Dearborn St., Chicago, Ill).

The elementary or secondary school teacher may be called upon to teach in one or more of some ten or a dozen areas of health and safety. The areas in which the teacher should have preparation in content may be summed up as follows: personal health, community health, safety education, first aid, nutrition, mental health, family living, alcohol and narcotics education, and home nursing. If the prospective teacher is not able to cover all these subjects in a busy undergraduate curriculum, it is recommended that he or she fill in the gaps with inservice training after beginning teaching.

There are a limited number of teachers who take majors in health education. However it is recommended that minors in health education be taken by students majoring in physical education, biology, or general science, since it is the teachers from these departments in the high school and junior high school who are often detailed to teach health courses.

Public Health Departments

A local public health department or unit serves six basic and essential functions and may, with funds and leadership, take on many more. The horizons of public health are broadening. The six essential functions are:

1. *Collecting, tabulating, and analyzing vital and public health statistics*
2. *Providing for the control of communicable diseases.*
3. *Providing for the control of environmental sanitation—and policing it.*
4. *Maintaining a public health laboratory.* All varieties of biological, chemical, and physical tests are now provided by such laboratories. Typical are blood tests for syphilis, examination of adulterated foods suspected of causing an outbreak of food poisoning, bacterial counts on milk products, and, more rarely, tissue examinations for early detection of cancer or blood typing of expectant parents. The first public health laboratory in the United States was established in New York City in 1894. The public health laboratory is primarily at the service of the physicians in

a community who send specimens for laboratory examination.

5. *Maintaining services for maternal and child hygiene.* So-called Well Baby Clinics were among the first efforts in this direction. This field now embraces public concern for the health of mothers and for the health of children from birth through all the years of required school attendance. School health services fall into this category, as do prenatal clinics, marriage-counseling centers, and all other activities centering about human reproduction and an "improved human product."

6. *Enlarging the horizons of public health education.* Every function of a health department has educational implications; people learn something about health through every contact with it. However, as the techniques of education have gradually reduced the importance of the police work of a public health department, special methods of public health education have been required. For example, establishing schools for food handlers does a better job in providing sanitary eating facilities in a community than simply arresting and fining proprietors of substandard eating establishments. The techniques of health education include newspaper, magazine, radio, and television publicity—keeping the public accurately informed of health conditions and needs within a community—pamphlets, posters, exhibits, meetings, special classes, and the like.

In addition to these six vital functions some local health departments also concern themselves, especially educationally, with major disease problems such as cancer, mental illness, heart disease, and diabetes. In this area the health department cooperates with other agencies, usually voluntary health agencies, and serves as one of the many health resources of the community.

How to Identify Community Health Problems. The identification of community health problems—the diagnosis of what ails a body politic, if you will—is no easier than diagnosing the personal ailments or health hazards that add up to total community health problems. In both cases, as we have pointed out, various degrees of health and disease may exist side by side.

Some of the techniques of identifying community health problems, however, are in many ways quite different from the usual tools of medical diagnosis. The community techniques have of necessity relied heavily on statistical methods and have therefore been subject to the serious limitations of this method.

Nevertheless valid statistical tools must be employed to make honest appraisals of a community's health status and its current or impending health problems. Community health surveys usually turn up problems, needs, or situations that demand community action. Communities are sometimes shocked into making health surveys. A suicide on a college campus, for example, may lead to the discovery of the inadequacy of its mental health and personal counseling resources.

Vital Statistics (Biostatistics)

Vital statistics are basically public records of a number of vital facts in the life cycles of individual members of a community, including records of birth, marriage, death, and cases of certain illnesses. The records are based on direct reports of physicians, midwives, and others to a duly appointed *registrar* of vital statistics in a local community. The final statistics can never be more informative than the original reports. The registrar's job is both to validate the accuracy of the original reports and to tally up the figures: for instance, the number of births per month, the number of deaths per year. This is simply human bookkeeping.

Church and parish records of christenings and burials were the roots from which the modern, complicated science of vital statistics grew. The scientific interpretation of vital statistical records dates back only to the seventeenth century and points to England. In 1662, in London, Captain John Graunt and Sir William Peatty published a thin little book entitled, *Natural and Political Observations on the Bills of Mortality.*

Most startlingly, they observed that 36% of the children born in London in the seventeenth century died before the age of six. They also noted a fact, which has yet to be fully explained, that the ratio of births of boys to births of girls was 106 to 100.

Great improvements in the methods of keeping and tabulating vital statistics were made in the nineteenth century, particularly in the Scandinavian countries and in England. Massachusetts was the first state in the United States to begin keeping reliable vital statistics, about the middle of the nineteenth century. A *U. S. Registration Area for Deaths* was formulated by the Bureau of the Census in 1900; at first it included only the New England states, New York, New Jersey, and Indiana. By 1933 it included all states. A *Birth Registration Area*, inaugurated somewhat later, now also includes all states.

The final task of tabulating and analyzing the data originally collected by local registrars and transmitted through state departments of public health to the federal government falls upon the National Office of Vital Statistics.

Cause of death must be certified by a physician. He signs a death certificate, without which a legal burial cannot proceed. The causes of death are now listed under some 200 major headings (called rubrics) according to the International Statistical Classification of Diseases, Injuries, and Causes of Death. The availability of accurate, national vital statistics has been of major importance in defining America's health problems.

Rates Are Ratios. Vital statistics are collected and tabulated in numbers, but they are usually reported in terms of *rates*. A rate is essentially a mathematical ratio. Confusions sometimes arise between the numbers and the rates: between, for example, the total number of births in a community during a year and the birth rate of the same community. Rates are usually figured on the basis of population and expressed in proportions of round whole numbers: 1000, 10,000, 100,000, and 1,000,000. These round numbers are called the base of the rate and must be stated or unmistakably understood in every expression of the statistics. Crude death rates, for example, are commonly stated as *X deaths per 1000 population*. The mathematics of this formula is simply expressed as follows:

Crude death rate =

$$\frac{\text{Total number of deaths} \times 1000}{\text{Total number of population}}$$

In 1962, about 1,757,000 United States residents out of an estimated population of about 170,000,000 died. The United States crude death rate for that year could therefore be calculated as 9.5 deaths per 1000 population.

The use of rates instead of whole numbers makes possible valid statistical comparisons between different places, different groups, and different times. Thus the death rate from tuberculosis in New York City, with a population of over 8 million people, can be compared with the same rate in Manhattan, Kansas, with a population of about 17,000. Again, New York's death rate in 1900 can be compared with its death rate in 1970 even though the population of the city has grown. In making any kinds of comparisons, great caution must be taken that the same kinds of rates, and the same bases of the rates, are being used.

Corrected and Adjusted Rates. Whereas *crude* death rates are usually figured on a basis of 1000 population, *specific* death rates, that is, death rates accountable to a specific disease—say tuberculosis—are reckoned on a base of 100,000 population. For usefulness and accuracy both crude and specific death rates usually have to be *corrected* for the actual residence of the deceased and *adjusted* for the age and sex composition of the population.

For example, unadjusted, uncorrected, specific death rates for tuberculosis appeared for many decades to be higher in the states of Arizona and New Mexico than anywhere else in the United States. These rates had to be *corrected* for residences of the deceased before they could be properly interpreted. Many of those who died came from out of the state because they already were afflicted with advanced tuberculosis, and died in New Mexico and Arizona; but the native residents of New Mexico and Arizona were not more

susceptible to tuberculosis than people elsewhere.

Adjusted rates require calculations of the age, sex, and color composition of populations that are being compared. Thus, for example, specific death rates in a population composed of the members of the United States Army cannot be properly compared with specific death rates in the general population. The absurdity of such comparison would be even more evident if we attempted to compare birth rates. We have elaborated this point of adjusted and corrected rates so that students may never in the future be deluded either by peaches-and-pears comparisons or by deliberately "doctored" rates.

Rates in any statistical comparison must have a sensible base.

Thus, *maternal mortality rates* usually represent the number of maternal deaths *per 1000 live births*.

Infant mortality rates express the number of deaths of infants *under 1 year of age per 1000 live births in the same period.*

But the figures can trick the unwary. In some places maternal mortalities are figured on total numbers of births (including stillbirths) and infant mortalities include infants up to 2 years of age.

Crude birth rates are expressed in total number of *live births per 1000 population.*

Statistical information is often presented in the form of graphic charts, diagrams, and maps. These should be scanned for accuracy even more closely than published tables, for they are more subject to distortion and error.

Precautions in Using Statistics. The following precautions should be taken in using and interpreting vital statistics:

1. Examine the source of the statistics. Thus, for example, material actually published by the National Office of Vital Statistics can be taken as reliable, but juggled figures simply "based" on its publications should be viewed more critically.

2. Check the bases of the rates on which the figures are given. Unless they are on the same base, or can be put on the same base of population, they cannot be compared.

3. Estimate the accuracy of the original raw

data or information from which the statistics were tabulated. Thus, for example, statistics about the incidence of gonorrhea are extremely inaccurate because this disease is very incompletely reported by physicians.

4. Do not accept statistical evidence based on a small number of cases.

5. Do not reason falsely on statistical premises. Statistical correlations are often accidental and coincidental; they may sometimes *suggest* a cause-and-effect relationship, but they absolutely never prove it.

The case against delusion by statistics was put most vigorously by one of America's greatest vital statisticians, demographers, and biometricians, the late Raymond Pearl of Johns Hopkins. In a simple example he pointed out that he could calculate extensively on the probability of the color the next born baby in the city of Baltimore. However, if he had possession of one crucial, causative fact—the color of its mother—he could give a correct answer without any statistical calculations at all. He said:

The statistical knowledge on which a statistical prediction is made is essentially the most sterile kind of knowledge that one can possible have *so far as concerns the individual event*. It merely gives one the betting odds for or against the occurrence, and absolutely nothing more. Now a wager, however large, in the scientific sense neither discovers, expounds, nor is a criterion of the truth. Bets, in other words, are not evidence—though the statistician sometimes seems to forget this.

The statistical method is a descriptive method only and has the limitations as a weapon of research which that fact implies. . . . The theory of probability grew up about the gaming table, not in the laboratory.

The chief usefulness of the statistical method, Pearl states, is in furnishing "shorthand descriptions of groups" and in offering one kind of test of the probable reliability of conclusions.

Vital statistics remain valuable pointers in identifying community health problems; but unless they are properly used and understood they can be fashioned into booby traps for the unwary and the innocent. At the head of every table of vital statistics there should probably be printed the legend: "Shake well. Use with caution.

Functions of Local Health Departments

The Philadelphia Story. The organization and functions of a local health department can perhaps best be illustrated by a case history of one such department. We have chosen to describe briefly the Philadelphia Department of Public Health, since this up-to-date health department received a national award (the Crumbine award) in 1961 as an outstanding local health unit. The student should recognize that not all local health units have—or even require—the same extensive organization that Philadelphia, a large metropolitan area, has achieved. This description will, however, give you an accurate picture of the kinds of problems any local public health department might be called upon to face and handle.

One of the first jobs of a health department, as noted, is to keep the vital statistics for the community—an accurate record of births, deaths (and causes of death), incidence of illness, and other bio-statistical facts. These facts are often graphed or plotted on maps to show exactly where the problems lie. The four maps of Philadelphia (by wards) on pages 416 and 417 show how precisely the Philadelphia Department of Public Health has spotted four major areas of public health concern in its community: air pollution, infant mortality, syphilis, and tuberculosis. The Philadelphia department has, for example, an air pollution control board, based on an Air Pollution Control Ordinance adopted in 1948. (Such a board would be a superfluity in the health departments of small farm communities.)

The key unit in the Philadelphia health department is its division of community health services, which deals with, among other things, venereal diseases, tuberculosis, polio, chronic and other diseases, mental health, dental health, community nursing service, mosquito and rodent control, radiation hazards, health centers, and cancer detection (called its "save-a-life" campaign). In Philadelphia the important office of medical examiner, replacing the coroner, is under the health department. The medical examiner's office does studies and reports on causes of death (especially when criminal causes are suspected), but it also operates a poison information center, supervises the city cemetery, engages in research, and processes data. The Philadelphia Department of Public Health has a large general hospital, the Philadelphia General Hospital, under its jurisdiction. Through the hospital the depart-

ment maintains affiliation with local medical schools and centers, supports research in medicine and public health, assists in the training of nurses, and provides an "alert" plan to cope with any civilian disasters that the city might suffer.

Noise Abatement—Health Codes. The Philadelphia health department also operates an annual campaign of noise abatement, for which it has several times been honored, with the advisory help of a Mayo's Committee for Noise Abatement. This is primarily a big city problem. It is doubtful whether a junior high school in a mid-

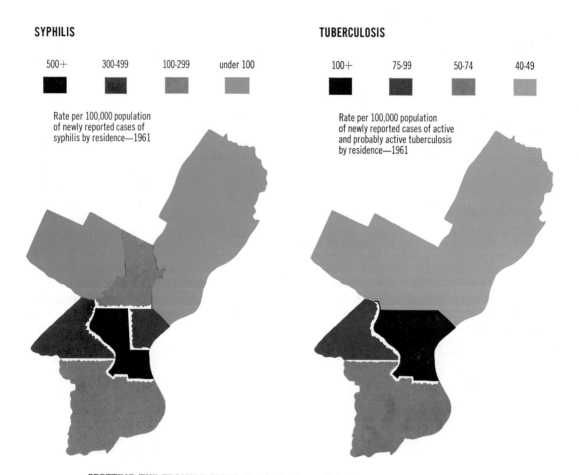

SYPHILIS

500+   300-499   100-299   under 100

Rate per 100,000 population
of newly reported cases of
syphilis by residence—1961

TUBERCULOSIS

100+   75-99   50-74   40-49

Rate per 100,000 population
of newly reported cases of active
and probably active tuberculosis
by residence—1961

SPOTTING THE TROUBLE SPOTS. By plotting in ward divisions on the map of the city of Philadelphia, the relative rates (or incidence) of air pollution, infant mortality, syphilis, and tuberculosis, the statisticians of the Philadelphia Department of Public Health are able to spot where these important areas of public health concern are concentrated. Special attention to the control of these conditions can then be directed to the trouble spot areas pinpointed or outlined on the maps.

western town would put up signs spelling "Quiet" in a number of foreign languages—as one Philadelphia junior high school did as its contribution to the city's noise abatement campaign. The largest category of complaints against unnecessary noise in Philadelphia is industrial noise, followed by animal noise (such as barking dogs), and vehicular noise.

The major responsibility of the Philadelphia Board of Health, now a part of the health department, is the maintenance of a Health Code, a codified body of laws and regulations (based finally on the police power of the health commissioner) which are developed and enforced to protect the public health. The following list of new regulations passed by the Philadelphia Board of Health since 1955 will give you an insight into the kinds of matters which the public health department is concerned with:

Operation and Maintenance of Apparatus Used for Shoe-Fitting Fluoroscopy.
Eating, Drinking, and Catering Establishments.
Slaughter, Handling, Inspection, and Preparation of Meat and Meat Products.

INFANT MORTALITY

40+	30-39	25-29	under 25
⬛	⬛	⬛	⬛

Rate per 100,000 live births by residence—1961

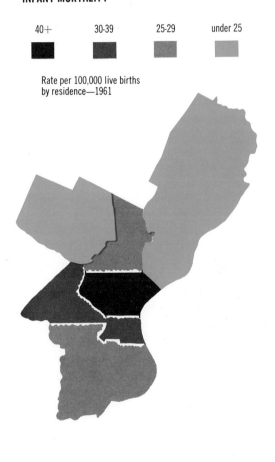

AIR POLLUTION

	Heavy	Med. heavy	Med. light	Light
	⬛	⬛	⬛	⬛
WINTER	75	55	35	25
SPRING	60	40	25	15
SUMMER	50	35	20	10
FALL	65	45	30	20

Average seasonal values of "settled dust" (tons per sq. mile per month)

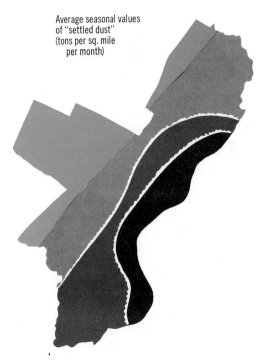

Bacteriological Quality and Disinfection of Water in Swimming Places.

Operation and Conduct of Barber and Beauty Shops, and Schools and Colleges for the Training of Barbers and Beauty Culture Operators.

Conduct, Operation, and Maintenance of Rendering Plants.

Food Establishments with Permanent Location.

Private Dumps and Landfills.

Food Stores.

Milk, Milk Products, and Frozen Desserts.

Food Processing and Food Manufacturing Establishments.

Repair and Reconstruction of Alleys, Driveways, and Retaining Walls to Correct Public Health Nuisances.

Isolation for Tuberculosis in its Communicable Stage.

Milk Derivatives.

Control of Rabies in Animals Subject to Rabies.

Sale of Foods and Beverages through Vending Machines.

Control of Communicable and Non-communicable Diseases and Conditions.

How many of these health-protecting subjects have you ever thought about? Of most local health departments it can fairly be said: They work while you sleep.

State Health Departments. State public health departments are organized on the same general basis as local health departments. Their services are usually advisory to the local units, but their subdivisions and facilities may be greater than those of the local departments. The Michigan Department of Public Health, for example, has divisions of (1) local health administration, (2) laboratories, (3) disease-control records and statistics, (4) tuberculosis and venereal disease control, (5) engineering, (6) industrial health, (7) administrative services and (8) local health services designed to strengthen and promote the state's approximately 50 full-time local health departments and 40 health districts. The local health services section is further subdivided into sections concerned with (1) maternal and child health, (2) nutrition, (3) public health nursing, (4) dentistry, (5) cancer and adult health services, and (6) recruitment and training of public health personnel.

The functions of state health departments vary greatly beyond those originally conceived to be primary public health functions. State legislatures are constantly adding additional responsibilities. In Nebraska, for example, the state health department has the task of examining, licensing, and inspecting twelve vocations in the business and professional fields whose practice within the state requires a license: namely, medicine, dentistry, osteopathy, pharmacy, optometry, veterinary medicine, chiropody, chiropractic, barbering, cosmetology, embalming, and funeral directing. The Nebraska health department also has the job of licensing and inspecting all boxing and wrestling matches in the state.

U.S. Public Health Service

The U.S. Public Health Service has a long and honorable history. It began in 1798 as the Marine Hospital Service, authorized by Congress to provide hospital care for sick or disabled seamen at various ports. It still operates about 65 hospitals, and other establishments (including a leprosarium at Carville, Louisiana); and the principal beneficiaries of its *direct* medical services are still the seamen of the U.S. Merchant Marine. However, since 1912, when the name of Public Health Service was first given to it, its size and scope have steadily expanded as Congress has given it a hodgepodge of specific responsibilities aimed at the maintenance and improvement of the nation's health. To carry out its manifold and diverse tasks, Congress now appropriates over $2 billion a year for the Public Health Service.

In practice the Public Health Service is principally a consultative, research, and fund-granting agency, which gives very little direct medical service. In 1953 the Public Health Service became a constituent of the new Federal Department of Health, Education, and Welfare—along with the Food and Drug Administration and other agencies.

The present organization of the U.S. Public Health Service reflects the wide variety of specific health problems with which it deals. It has been reorganized (since 1967) into five operating bureaus and three other major components; notably (1) the office of the Surgeon General of the U.S. Public Health Service, (2) the National Library of Medicine (with over 1 million volumes), and (3) the National Center for Health Statistics.

The five operating bureaus and their separate divisions are listed below:

I. *Bureau of Health Manpower* includes: (1) Community Health Services, (2) Hospital and Medical Facilities, (3) Nursing; and (4) Dental Health. This Bureau is concerned with all activities and grants related to meeting the needs of health manpower on a national scale. This leads the Bureau into educational research, utilization of professional and *auxiliary* manpower (for example, physician's aides), and the endowment of traineeships, student loans, and training facility grants.

II. *Bureau of Health Services* includes the following divisions: (1) Chronic Disease, (2) Community Health Services, (3) Hospital and Medical Facilities, (4) Medical Care Administration, (5) Hospitals, (6) Health Mobilization, (7) Indian Health, and (8) Medical Care—for designated groups. In addition to care for American Indians and merchant seamen, the Public Health Service also gives direct medical care to the ship and shore establishments of the U.S. Coast Guard and the Maritime Administration, Alaskan Indians and Eskimos, members of the Peace Corps, and federal prisoners.

III. *Bureau of Disease Prevention and Environmental Control* includes the following divisions and offices: (1) Communicable Disease Center (in Atlanta, Georgia), (2) Accident Prevention, (3) Chronic Diseases, (4) Arctic Health Research Center (in Anchorage, Alaska), (5) Environmental Engineering and Food Protection, (6) Pesticides, (7) Solid Wastes, (8) Air Pollution, (9) Occupational Health, (10) Radiological Health, and (11) Foreign Quarantine. All domestic and foreign quarantine regulations are the responsiblity of this Bureau. Also vested in it are activities related to prevention, detection, and control of

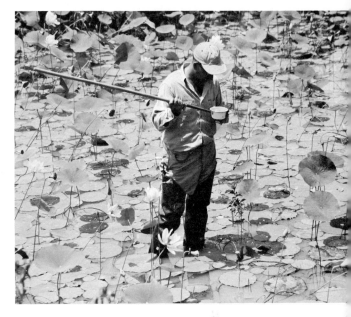

A TECHNICIAN dipping for mosquito larvae. This is one of the many activities of the U.S. Public Health Service. (Photograph courtesy of National Institutes of Health)

chronic and communicable disease and accident hazards.

IV. *National Insitutes of Health* (NIH) includes the following divisions: (1) Allergic and Infectious Disease, (2) Arthritis and Metabolic Disease, (3) Cancer, (4) Child Health and Development, (5) Dental Research, (6) General Medical Sciences, (7) Heart, and (8) Neurological Diseases and Blindness. NIH also operates a large Clinical Center—a 500 bed research hospital with extensive laboratory facilities—at Bethesda, Maryland, and the National Environmental Health Sciences Center, as well as the following divisions: (a) Biologic Standards, which licenses the manufacture of biological products, such as insulin and penicillin (b) Research Grants; (c) Research Facilities; and (d) Research Services. Through its thousands of grants, costing millions of dollars, for research and training, NIH supports research in hundreds of medical schools, universities, and teaching hospitals.

V. *National Institute of Mental Health* is involved in the large-scale problems of mental health—especially the prevention and treatment of men-

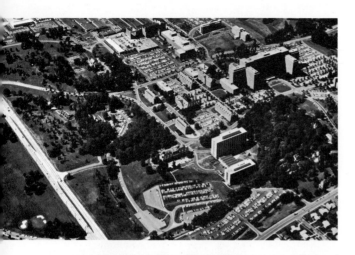

NATIONAL INSTITUTES OF HEALTH. A 300-acre cluster of buildings at Bethesda, Maryland, which serves the U.S. Public Health Services as its main research center. (Photograph courtesy of National Institutes of Health)

tal illness and the rehabilitation of the mentally ill. It provides funds for further programs on mental health at state and local levels. It operates an Alcoholism Center and has under its control two large neuropsychiatric hospitals, one at Lexington, Kentucky, and one at Fort Worth, Texas (both of which had formerly been devoted exclusively to the 'treatment of drug addiction).

The Public Health Service has between 35,000 and 40,000 employees. About 5,000 of these are officers of the Commissioned Corps, who, like officers of the Armed Services, are commissioned by the President of the United States. The largest share of Public Health Services staff is located in and around the National Institutes of Health at Bethesda, Maryland. The permanent field stations of the Public Health Service include 9 regional offices, 65 hospitals, 25 clinics, 51 major foreign quarantine stations, 42 Indian Health Centers, three large specialized research centers, and a number of smaller laboratories concerned with specific problems of environmental health.

It represents the United States in international health matters, particularly in conjunction with the World Health Organization.

The Veterans Administration. It has long been American policy that war veterans be cared for.

Indeed, the Pilgrims in 1636 enacted in their court: "If any man shallbee sent forth as a soldier and shall return maimed hee shalbee majntained competently by the Collonie during his life."

Except for the armed services, the vast bulk of direct medical services provided by the federal government for its citizens is through the Veterans Administration, which operates the largest hospital system in the country and one of the largest in the world (166 hospitals with 108,000 beds). More than half of the hospitals are associated with schools of medicine.

The Veterans Administration has a large medical staff: approximately 5000 full-time physicians, 3500 residents and interns. In addition it has 2000 part-time physicians and 10,000 private practice physicians who serve as consultants. Furthermore 40,000–50,000 physicians treat veterans with service-connected disabilities.

More than half of the cases are psychiatric and a good many others are persons over 65 with chronic conditions. It should be noted that there are 26 million living veterans who, with their families, comprise about one half of the population in the United States.

Voluntary Health Agencies

Voluntary health agencies are non-profit organizations in which the medical profession and the public have formally joined together for the solution of specific health problems.[2] Some are the outgrowth of specialized medical societies—for example, the American Cancer Society, the American Heart Association, and the American Diabetes Association. Others owe their origin to the grit and determination of interested laymen—especially the National Foundation [for Infantile Paralysis], the National Association for Mental Health, and the American Social Hygiene Association. The oldest agency is the National Tuberculosis Association; the largest and richest is the American National Red Cross, which is both

[2] See Appendix A for description of diseases with which some of these agencies are concerned.

a voluntary agency and a semi-governmental organization.

Origins of Voluntary Agencies. The forerunners of the present-day voluntary health agencies were the temperance societies and welfare organizations which flourished in the nineteenth century. The temperance societies, for example, forced state legislatures to pass laws requiring schools to teach the "evils of drink." From this unpromising beginning, however, the broader concept of school health education arose. It received impetus also from the original concept of "progressive" education and from reactions to draft and selective service examinations of young men, an appalling number of whom were found physically unfit for military service.

The first voluntary agencies that concentrated their interests around specific health problems came into being around 1900. In the 1890's a "modest society" was formed in Philadelphia to give people the best available information about the "cure" of tuberculosis, then the Number 1 killer of Americans. With leadership from the distinguished physician Dr. Edward Trudeau, this little group mushroomed into the first of the important *national* voluntary health agencies. Its original name was the National Association for the Study and Prevention of Tuberculosis, and Dr. Trudeau was its first president. Somewhat later is was called the National Tuberculosis Association. Now, as tuberculosis has declined, it has become the National Tuberculosis and Respiratory Disease Association.

One of the great community discoveries of the National Tuberculosis Association was that many people would give small, but in the aggregate substantial, sums of money as gifts for the control of disease. The familiar Christmas-seal-sale idea was originated by a Danish postal clerk, Einar Holboell, and introduced into the United States in 1907 by Jacob Riis.

Some of the voluntary health agencies aptly fit Emerson's description that an "institution is the lengthened shadow of a man." The present National Association for Mental Health is a case in point. It goes back to one man, Clifford Beers, who, in 1900, attempted to commit suicide by jumping out of a fourth-story window. He lived—but he spent the next three years committed to various mental hospitals. His experiences were horrible.

Then he did a most daring thing—he wrote a book about them. The title of this frank book was *A Mind That Found Itself.* The book stimulated respectable and conscientious help when, in 1908, in Connecticut he founded a "Society for Mental Hygiene." The purpose of this organization was "to work for the conservation of mental health; to help prevent nervous and mental disorders and mental defects; to help raise the standards of care of those suffering from any of these disorders." This platform is still as valid as the day it was written.

The American Social Health Association, organized to combat venereal disease, owed its origin in part to the shock suffered by a Harvard president, Charles Eliot, when he saw the destruction a fulminating venereal infection had caused in a promising young graduate.

The National Foundation [for Infantile Paralysis] was founded by and owed its success to the interest of President Franklin D. Roosevelt, himself a victim of the disease. The "President's Birthday Balls" and the "March of Dimes" for polio, beginning about 1938, demonstrated that there was still more money voluntarily forthcoming for the support of voluntary health agencies than had been dreamed possible.

After that many new agencies were started and old ones expanded. The National Multiple Sclerosis Society, for example, originated in a two-line classified advertisement in the *New York Times.* The relative of a victim of the disease advertised that she would like to contact any other patients suffering from this particular malady. Unexpected hundreds responded to this appeal to their common interest, and a formal organization grew out of this early correspondence.

Present Status of Voluntary Health Agencies. By their very nature voluntary health organizations tend to be established in the areas of un-

Special Exercise—A Pictoquiz*

WHICH OF THESE HEALTH-AGENCY SYMBOLS DO YOU RECOGNIZE?

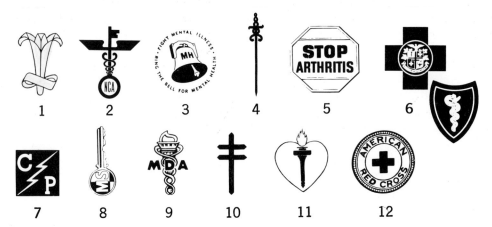

1   2   3   4   5   6

7   8   9   10   11   12

*Answers on page 434

solved health problems, and for diseases whose causes are unknown and whose treatment is uncertain. These are largely the chronic diseases, such as heart disease, cancer, arthritis, and hayfever, and in particular the unsolved neurological disorders. That is why we have the National Multiple Sclerosis Society, the United Cerebral Palsy Associations, the Muscular Dystrophy Associations of America, Inc., the Parkinson's Disease Foundation, the National Association for Retarded Children and many others. An Acute Appendicitis Foundation would be ridiculous.

There are now approximately 75 recognized, national voluntary health associations in the United States, of which about a quarter are members of the National Health Council. New ones, however, are constantly being organized. There are approximately 20,000 local chapters of the leading voluntary health agencies. It is estimated that somewhere between 5 and 10 million people a year volunteer their services to these agencies, chiefly but not exclusively for their educational fund-raising campaigns. Thanks to these voluntary workers, the agencies' administrative expenses are generally quite low, and most of the money collected goes back into service and education in the communities from which it was collected.

The programs of voluntary health organizations change with the times—particularly as the disease problems for which they were founded fade in importance. Thus, after it had successfully promoted the development of the Salk vaccine, which—together with the Sabine vaccine—have largely eliminated paralytic polio, the National Foundation for Infantile Paralysis was forced to decide whether to disband or expand. It decided on the latter course and announced in July 1958 that under the shortened name of the National Foundation, and without abandoning polio patients, henceforth it would devote its March of Dimes funds and professional know-how to the unsolved problems of virus diseases in general and birth defects.

As the tuberculosis problem waned, the National Tuberculosis Association devoted more and more attention to the problem of health education in general. With the temporary decline in venereal disease, following introduction of antibiotic drugs, the American Social Health Association undertook a more positive program of education for marriage and family living.

Role of Voluntary Health Agencies. The role of the voluntary health agencies in the development and utilization of America's health resources is unique—unduplicated in any other country. Most people tend to think of them primarily as fund-raising organizations. The acrimonious debates that go on among the agencies and in the press as to whether fund-raising should be "separate" or "united" helps to create this "dollar-image" of voluntary health agencies. More importantly, however, the voluntary health agencies are educational organizations. They are *catalysts* of all other health resources, stirring, prompting, and cajoling them into action to help solve specific health problems. They are pioneers in search of new solutions.

The test of a successful voluntary health agency is not how it raises its money—nor how much money it raises—but rather how wisely it spends its funds in the direction of education—public and professional—research, and service to patients.

Fund raising and education are complementary functions. Contributions to voluntary health agencies represent expressions of interest in the work of the organizations and the problems they are seeking to solve. This could not be so widely, personally, or directly expressed in any other way. The average man or woman cannot personally go into a research laboratory and hope to discover the multiple causes of cure of crippling, chronic, killing diseases. But he can express his personal interest and contribute to the support and morale of the scientists capable of doing the job through his gifts to specific voluntary health agencies.

Contrary to popular opinion, the voluntary health agencies are neither "big business" nor major financial contributors to medical research and service. All the health agencies together (exclusive of the Red Cross) collect around $275 million a year. Furthermore, the agencies contribute far less than 10% of the sums now expended on medical research.

But their role in unlocking huge sums for medical research and service is priceless. The agencies may not be rich, but they are influential. Nearly two-thirds of the $1.5 billion now spent annually on medical research in the United States comes from the federal government. It is expended principally through the U.S. Public Health Service, the Department of Defense, and the Atomic Energy Commission, and is appropriated by Congress. Congressional appropriations are made in response to demonstrated public interest in a specific disease (or other) area. This is where the voluntary health agencies perform their great educational service. They demonstrate public interest *confirmed* in voluntary money contributions by millions of individual citizens.

Thus, for example, in 1955–1956, the federal government was willing to appropriate about ten times as much money for the distribution of polio vaccine as the National Foundation for Infantile Paralysis gave away.

Criticisms of Voluntary Health Agencies. In their very success—which is based on a combination of fear and social consciousness, vanity, and a sense of civic duty—the voluntary health agencies have made new problems for themselves. Programs sometimes overlap and duplicate. An attack on one disease partially discredits the modern medical concept of treating the patient, not the disease. A disproportionate amount of human energy goes into the sheer mechanics of "fund raising," which often amounts to an exchange of dollars among friends. More seriously the clamor for attention in the press and through other media of publicity by separate organizations with the same general goal—health—tends to diffuse the appeal of any one. In some places the public has not only begun to complain about a "pernicious multiplicity of drives" but, even worse, to be indifferent to all of them. Nevertheless, whole-hearted and single-minded concentration on specific diseases or groups of diseases, with public cooperation, has achieved results much more rapidly than any impersonal, diffuse approach might accomplish.

Are the Health Resources of the United States Adequate? The listing of community health resources in this chapter should give you perspective on the numerous agancies for health protection and improvement available to you in the United States. Almost without exception these agencies have grown rapidly in number, wealth, and services in the first half of the twentieth century, and the trend is still up. In terms of total health resources it is probably safe to say that the residents of this country are better off than the inhabitants of any other. (Only one country, Israel, has more physicians per capita.)

Are United States health resources adequate to meet all the health needs of the nation? It is certain that they are not yet adequately proportioned to all sections of the country and all classes of the population. Nonwhite Americans certainly receive a smaller share than whites. Geographical inequities and maldistribution arc common. Much reamins to be done in providing fuller health resources for the nation. The limit is psychological: How much is the American public eventually willing to pay, either in fees, gifts, or taxes, for the great but intangible value called "health"?

A particular gap in the health resources of the United States in the 1960's was the lack of adequate facilities for long-term care and treatment of patients with chronic illnesses. While more long-term-care facilities (e.g., nursing homes) are essential, another essential step is the modernizing of obsolete hospitals (particularly in big cities) and integrating them with systems of "progressive medical care"—in which patients are gradually moved from more-expensive-to-operate to less expensive facilities as their physical condition improves. The chief of the Hill-Burton Hospital Construction program of the U.S. Public Health Service (provided by an act of Congress under which local funds for building hospitals and similar institutions are matched by federal funds according to certain financial formulas) estimated in 1962 that a program of modernization or replacement of America's older hospitals would cost about $4 *billion.* Yet the chronic illness still prevalent in the United States is far costlier than this.

Chronic Illness

The increase in our aged and aging population has meant an increase in the prevalence of chronic, or long-term, illness in the United States. Chronic illness is not, however, a problem solely of old age. Approximately half the chronically ill in the United States are under the age of 45.

Many chronic diseases have an acute phase, followed by an aftermath of chronic illness or disability, for example, paralytic polio and heart attack. Other chronic illnesses begin insidiously and progress slowly but inexorably, for example, cancer. Many of the other conditions already discussed in this text either do or can have longstanding effects—notably mental illness, heart failure, rheumatic fever, stroke, and syphilis. These conditions can and often are classified as chronic illness, although this is a somewhat vague term. How a disease is treated or managed will often determine whether or not it is or becomes chronic. This is one of many reasons why good medical care is so essential and why quack or self-medication is such great folly.

When we speak of chronic illness, we are saying in effect that health itself is a relative matter. Many people with chronic illness may function better than others who are presumably in good health. Thus, the epileptic under competent treatment is as good a workman as his colleague; the deaf woman with a hearing aid can get along as well as her sisters; the hayfever sufferer can usually escape most of his discomfort in an air-conditioned room.

Chronic illness, like acute illness, runs the gamut from mild to severe. Some chronically ill patients are definitely disabled, bedridden, or hospitalized, but they comprise only a small fraction of the millions of Americans estimated to suffer from chronic illness. Thus, of the "mentally ill" only 4% are hospitalized; of the heart patients about 5%; of hayfever sufferers and the hard of hearing practically 0%.

The solution to the problem of chronic illness, so far as it can be solved, is good medical care

CHRONIC ILLNESS

Estimated Numbers of People in the United States Who Are More or Less Disabled by Specific Long-Term Ailments (1960's)

Heart and circulatory diseases	25,000,000
Mental illness (in some degree)	20,000,000
Arthritis and rheumatism	17,000,000
Hearing impairments	
(760,000 totally deaf)	15,000,000
Accidental injuries	11,000,000
Kidney disorders	8,000,000
Alcoholism	
(750,000 chronic alcoholics)	6,500,000
Mental retardation	6,000,000
Hayfever and asthma	4,000,000
Diabetes	4,000,000
Orthopedic handicaps	3,200,000
Syphilis	1,900,000
Stroke	1,800,000
Epilepsy	1,500,000
Parkinson's disease	
(shaking palsy)	1,500,000
Sinusitis	1,400,000
Tuberculosis	
(400,000 active cases)	1,200,000
Cancer (under treatment)	700,000
Cerebral palsy	550,000
Chronic throat infections	
(tonsillitis)	500,000
Multiple sclerosis	
(and other demyelinating diseases)	500,000
Peptic ulcer	
(stomach and duodenum)	400,000
Blindness (legally blind)	350,000
Polio (previously crippled)	300,000
Gonorrhea	
(new cases reported annually)	250,000
Muscular dystrophy	200,000

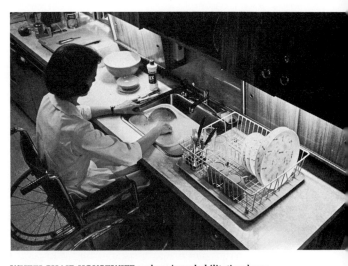

WHEELCHAIR HOUSEWIFE undergoing rehabilitation; learning how to use a specially designed kitchen. (Photograph courtesy of Institute of Physical Medicine and Rehabilitation of New York University—Bellevue Medical Center)

and opportunity for the *total medical care* that may also be called rehabilitation.

Rehabilitation. Rehabilitation can be described as the challenge of helping disabled people make the most of themselves. Practically speaking it poses enormous problems of cost and organization of medical care.

Rehabilitation is one of the most important concepts in modern medical treatment. Although its practice has been spearheaded by techniques of physical medicine, it is not the exclusive property of any single medical specialty, and properly begins with diagnosis.

Good rehabilitation practice usually requires the "team approach" to the disabled patient. It demands the services not only of doctors but also of associate medical personnel—for example, the nurse, the physical therapist, the occupational therapist, the medical social worker.

Though initially costly, rehabilitation of patients with chronic disability has proved to be a most profitable investment. For every dollar a community invests in rehabilitation, at least two dollars are returned by the rehabilitated individual in productive labor henceforth accomplished.

Costs of Medical Care

Few college students have had much experience in paying their own doctor, dentist, drug, hospital, or insurance bills. The years of young adulthood are relatively the "healthiest" of life. Medical expenses are few in this age bracket. Statistically speaking, obstretical costs are the major item. Chronic illnesses, with their repeated drain on the pocketbook, are comparatively rare. Previous medical expenses have usually been met by parents—either through direct payment of bills or regular payments of health, hospital, and accident insurance premiums.

The young married couple or the single person with older parents to assist gradually becomes aware that medical costs are a constant tax on family income.

In the course of your lifetime, you may expect to expend between 4 and 6% of your total income on medical care of *all* kinds. Only about 26% of this sum, however, will go directly for physician's services. The rest will be spent for hospital care, about 31%; drugs and supplies, 16%; dentists, about 10%; health insurance, about 7%; appliances, about 5%; and other costs (including nursing) about 5%.

These medical care bills for the United States as a whole rose to $31.3 billion in 1966, according to figures released by the U.S. Department of Commerce. This sum represents 6.7% of the total personal consumption expenditures that year of $465.9 billion. Other expenses in this category were: food, $93 billion; tobacco and liquors, $22.5 billion; clothing, accessories and jewelry, $48.4 billion; personal care, $8.2 billion; housing, $67.1 billion; personal business and financial, $24.0 billion; transportation, $59.6 billion; recreation, $28.7 billion; other costs (including private education and research, religious and welfare activities, and foreign travel) $16.5 billion.

It is interesting to compare some of these figures; for example, the public's expenses for alcoholic beverages and tobacco ($22.5 billion) was nearly 3 times as much as that paid to physicians ($8.8 billion). The cost which is rising most rapidly is that of hospital care. The hospitals in 1966 collected $9.6 billion—the lion's share of the medical expenses. Increased wages of hospital employees are the big factor.

Here are some figures to note regarding hospital charges: The average charge (1968) was about $58 a day; the average patient stayed an average of 7.8 days, for which on the average, he paid about $450.

For as long as the economic records have been kept in the United States, annual medical-care expenses have absorbed between 4 and 6% of the total national income, whether that figure was at $42 billion, as in 1932, or more than ten times as much, as it was in the 1960's. Whether he pays it directly or indirectly, in insurance premiums, union dues or *taxes,* it is doubtful whether any wage-earning adult over a lifetime can beat the medical-cost percentage. It is the inexorable money price of health, a reflection, if you will, of the inevitability of accidents, ill health, death, and taxes.

Topsy-Turvy Economics. In making comparisons of medical costs with other personal expenditures, it is always necessary to remember that the economics of medical care are topsy-turvy. Peoply buy liquor and tobacco because they want them. What they pay out for medical services represents expenditures for something they did not *want* in the first place and would have infinitely preferred to be able to do without.

Direct payment for medical and health services is probably the most economical in the long run, even though the financial burdens of illness or accident are unpredictable in any given year. One can budget against this unpredictability by purchasing health insurance. The "best deal" on health insurance over a lifetime is almost certainly offered by the non-profit health-insurance plans, of which Blue Cross, for hospital insurance, and Blue Shield, for protection against medical and surgical expenses, are the prototypes.

Differing Cultural and Political Outlooks on Paying for Medical Services. There are distinct cultural, nationalistic, and political tinges to all opinions about the best way to pay for medical services. This is a reflection of the historic tradition that linked the medicine man with the priest in the character of the magic-making *shaman* of the primitive tribe. Systems of native medicine still flourish today in less-developed countries of the globe side by side with the latest "scientific medicine" by Western standards.

The Chinese, for example, have had a custom of paying their doctors to keep them well and depriving the doctor of income when the payor falls sick. (This, incidentally, is a custom reflected in some very modern American sickness and accident insurance policies, which compensate the sick or injured person for loss of income.)

A sophisticated statement on the individual's right to health services at national expense may be credited to the late Aneurin Bevan, the British Labor Party leader, on the occasion of the National Health Service Bill debate in the British parliament. Bevan was the son of a Welsh coal miner and had seen bitter days of unemployment and much misery in the mining towns of his youth. He said, in effect, in the British House of Commons: "We, on this side of the House, are sick of charity; we demand these services as a right, paid for through payroll deductions, contributions by both employer and employed, and through taxes."

Bevan's arguments were repeated in the United States by labor leaders and others arguing for medical care for the aged through payments collected through the Social Security system. Their cry was that only this method of payment "safeguards the dignity and self-respect of the individual" and keeps him off the "charity rolls." How Medicare and Medicaid fare in the U.S. remains to be seen.

The British, however, are not of one mind concerning their present system of medicine. A *British Medical Journal* editorial called it a "pretty ghastly awful system." One Scots physician who fled the British system, Kenneth I. E. Macleod, M.D., F.A.P.H.A., health commissioner of the city of Cincinnati, in 1962 told the city's Academy of Medicine:

The almost unalterable fixity of the bureaucratic methodology [of the British National Health Service], however honorably directed, simply stultifies progress,

for it splutters and chokes when the unusual is presented. . . . It might therefore be profitable for those who would 'nationalize' American medicine after the British model to consider the fact that conditions of service have to be made attractive to encourage men and women to enter medicine, for even in America there is a distinct drift away from medicine, dentistry, and nursing for other fields. . . . The strength of American health care is [its] very diversity of approach. . . . Let us accent the positive, diminish the negative, and work for our patients—and all will be well here in the United States.

Students of this chapter should be aware that except for the brief digressions into foreign opinions just expressed, we are dealing here exclusively with traditions of health care and medical service as they exist in the United States of America. Even our nearest neighbors, Canada and Mexico, have systems different than ours for delivery of health and medical services.

Health Insurance

The term "health insurance" means many different things to different people. It is sometimes called "sickness insurance," or "medical-surgical protection," or "disability benefits," or other names. In general, however, health insurance is the name for any *prepayment* plan by which individuals, families, and larger groups can more comfortably meet the unpredictable costs of illness, accident, and medical care. Health insurance is no guarantee of good health. It is simply a way of paying for, wholly or in part, several kinds of medical services. To the extent that it encourages proper utilization of health resources, it is a boon to personal and community health.

Health insurance has been, and will not doubt again be, the subject of acrimonious political debate. This has been true in every country where it has been introduced—for example, Germany (1870) and England (1945). The fundamental political question is whether the insurance should be *voluntary* or *compulsory*.

Numerous attempts have been made to enact national compulsory sickness insurance in the United States. Until the U.S. Congress passed the Medicare and Medicaid bills in 1965, all bills of this nature were defeated. The proponents say that the health of all the people is the direct concern of the government; therefore tax money should be used to pay for medical care of those who think they can't afford it. The opponents of compulsory sickness insurance have argued that it is "socialized medicine" and that the intervention of government into medical practice would make medical care a "political football," resulting in worse medical care for everyone at a higher cost.

Voluntary Health Insurance. Voluntary health insurance in the United States has shot ahead at a rapid pace since 1932, when the first Blue Cross group hospitalization plans were established.

By 1965 the American public had broader protection than ever before against the risk of medical, surgical, and hospital expenses. The Health Insurance Council reported that as of January 1, 1964 nearly 148 million Americans were protected by some form of voluntary health insurance against hospital or medical expenses. Over 47 million wage earners had insurance or other fomal arrangements protecting them against the loss of income resulting from disability.

In 1969 voluntary health insurance benefits of nearly $10 billion were paid out by Blue Cross and Blue Shield, other medical society plans, independent insuring agencies (such as union welfare plans), and private insurance companies.

There would be no serious problem of meeting medical expenses if every family could be assured that its medical bills would not exceed the normal 4 to 6% of income in any given year. But this is not possible. Illness is still unpredictable. About 7% of American families every year have medical expenses in excess of 20% of their gross income. Higher costs are associated with increasing age. People over 65 consume twice as much hospital care as younger age groups. Women, on the average, have higher medical expenses than men—in a ratio of approximately 8:5.

Voluntary health insurance spreads the risk over a large number of families, thereby reducing the chances that any one will be reduced to penury through catastrophic illness in the family.

Types of Voluntary Health Insurance. Despite the great variety of individual policies, there are basically five types of voluntary health-insurance protection now available, namely:

1. Hospital-expense protection. These policies pay wholly or in part the hospital charges for room, board, miscellaneous, and special services, such as X-ray, laboratory, and drugs. The payment is either in the form of actual *service* (room, board, etc.) rendered to the patient by the hospital, or *cash* indemnity (money) paid to the patient or to the hospital by the insurance company.

2. Surgical-expense protection. Surgical benefits are paid according to a predetermined fee schedule for each type of operation, usually including both preoperative and postoperative care.

3. Regular medical-expense protection. These policies pay for medical expenses other than surgical, including home, office, and hospital calls. Diagnostic examinations, consultations, and periodic health examinations may be included, but usually benefits do not begin until the second or third call on or from the doctor.

4. Major medical-expense protection. This type of policy is designed to protect against unusually large, "catastrophic" medical expenses. It pays 75 to 80% of all medical costs above a "deductible" minimum—from $100 to $500— and up to a high maximum—$2500 to $10,000. The patient or family, called "co-insurers," pays the other 20 to 25% of the medical and hospital bills.

5. Loss-of-income protection. This type of policy is sometimes called sickness-and-accident indemnity or disability insurance. It pays cash benefits, usually weekly, to compensate for loss of income owing to sickness and accident. This money can be used to pay medical costs or living expenses.

These different types of insurance protection are combined in various ways to make different "packages," expressly set down in policies. There are also other types of insurance in force which protect against the economic risks of disease and accident. Among them are workmen's-compensation insurance, which covers occupational injuries and illnesses "arising in and out of the course of employment"; individual and group accident policies, which provide benefits for injuries from accidents; and liability insurance, which covers medical expenses of injured victims of the legally liable party.

Read Policies Carefully! When you buy your own health-insurance policies, deal only with reputable companies and reliable agents, personally known to you. Read the actual policy submitted and compare it for benefits, extent of coverage, cancellation clauses, rates, and the like with similar policies. Choose the one that fits your needs best.

Blue Cross and Blue Shield and other group contracts are usually written through the place of employment. Everyone is bound by a "master policy." Group-insurance premiums are usually lower than individual premiums for the same or equal coverage.

There are no bargains in health insurance. So-called cheap policies are often almost worthless because of the number of exclusions and legal conditions for payment covered in the fine print in their contracts.

It cannot be said that the final pattern of health insurance has been reached in the United States, or anywhere else. Further consideration must be given especially to coverage of older people and those in low-income groups.

Medical Care and Family Income (U.S.)

An interesting view on overall health costs and payments in the United States was provided in May 1964 by the U.S. Public Health Service. In data from the National Health Survey, based on 42,000 household interviews and covering 134,000 persons, the Division of Health Interview Statistics of the U.S. Public Health Service collated and published under the title, "Medical Care, Health Status and Family Income (U.S.)" recent statistics on personal health expenditures, health insurance coverage, the use of dental and

medical services, chronic illness and disability, acute illness and disability days. These facts were also correlated with family income, family size, age, and sex.

It was judged that the figures collected applied to a civilian, non-institutional population of 183 million people during the period July 1962, to June 1963. It was estimated that approximately 12% (23 million) were living in families with incomes of less than $2000. About 18% of the people were in families with incomes from $2000–$3999; 34% were in the $4000–$6999 bracket; and 31% had incomes over $7000. (This income of 5% was not known.)

Health Insurance (Hospitalization). How did they fare for family health insurance (hospital and surgical insurance)? Roughly in correlation with family income, ranging from 34% among those in families of less than $2000 income to nearly 90% in families of $7000 or more family income. Persons of all ages in the lowest income group and older persons in the higher income groups have the least health insurance coverage. In low income families, only 22% of the children have hospital insurance coverage, a figure which for the most part reflects poor coverage in big families.

Interestingly, health insurance protection is related to the educational level of the head of the household as well as to family income, especially in lower income groups. The purchase of health insurance depends on an understanding of the need for insurance and some judgement on how one should allocate his income in dollars to meet various needs. The greatest single factor influencing the rate of health insurance protection is the ability of the family to pay for it. Nevertheless, about 75% of the people in the United States have some form of health insurance, usually basic hospitalization insurance, and frequently protection against surgical expenses.

Practically all segments of the American population are interested in plans to meet the increasing costs of inpatient hospitalization. That this is a large bill is evident from the fact that approximately 23 million short-stay patients (excluding tuberculosis, psychiatric, and other long-term hospitals) are served in the United States every year. The length of a "short-term" hospital stay ranges from about 7.2 to 10.7 days, the lowest income families having the longest stays. Among the hospitalized, insurance pays some part of the bill for about 40% of patients with less than $2000 family income; 60% of patients with $2000–3999 family income; and 80% of patients with higher incomes. Insurance also pays some bills for surgery and delivery. It pays such bills for about 40% of the surgically treated from families with incomes of less than $4000 and for about 75% from families with incomes over $4000.

Medical and Dental Care. It is estimated that there are now in the United States approximately 900 million physician visits (two-thirds at doctors' offices) and 250 million dental visits a year. People in families with incomes under $4000 a year average about 4.6 visits to a doctor a year; those with incomes of $7000 or more average 5.7 visits. Women see doctors more frequently than men. Owing to unequal distribution of medical services throughout the population, however, there are approximately 15% of the people who have not seen a doctor in two years and 18% who have never seen a dentist. Within a year approximately one patient in five receives services of such medical specialists as pediatricians, obstetricians or gynecologists, ophthalmologists, otolaryngologists, psychiatists, dermatologists, or orthopedists.

Chronic Illness and Disability. In evaluating the costs of medical care on the American scene, it is necessary to take a look at the chronic illnesses and disabilities that interfere with normal activity. Heart conditions, arthritis and rheumatism, and orthopedic impairments have the highest prevalence in limiting activity. It is estimated that there are about 81 million people in the United States with one or more chronic illnesses. However, it is judged that only about 23 million are limited in activity because of their 31.5 million chronic conditions. It should be noted that nearly 40% of the chronically disabled suffer from more than one activity-limiting condition. About 7% of the people in the low income

group have some degree of limitation on their mobility, while in the high income group only a little more than 1% are limited in their ability to move around.

A certain number of chronically disabled (about 7 people per 1000 population) are incapacitated to the degree that they require the services, either full time or part time, of a household member, a nurse, or other attendant. In families with incomes under $4000 the rate of persons receiving care at home (10.4 per 1000 population) was about three times higher than the rate (3.7 per 1000 population) for home care among persons in families with incomes of $4000 or higher. It seems that rates of disability days attributable to chronic illness and impairment are highest among persons with the lowest family incomes and decrease consistently with higher amounts of income.

Attitudes Toward Health Insurance. Within the last generation health insurance of all kinds has become increasingly popular. By 1968 there were about 1045 insurance companies, 82 Blue Cross and Blue Shield plans, and 300 independent-type plans offering some sort of health insurance. Approximately 160 million people in the United States now carry some health insurance. the public's willingness to employ an increasing share of its disposable personal income for health insurance is both a gratifying signal of its interest in health and a sensible recognition that health care and protection costs money.

Financing Medical Care. The question of financing medical care is an ancient one. There are "pro" and "con" arguments for every new and old method that has been proposed. The past and traditional way is for the patient to pay the doctor out of his own pocket. But in modern society there is a strong trend—one might almost say a necessity—toward prepayment approach. Among the pro and con methods may be considered Blue Cross and Blue Shield, commerical insurance, co-insurance programs through which deductibles and percentage payments by the patient are arranged, labor union clinic centers, closed panel or capitation plans, contractual arrangements with a hospital or medical school.

The present prevailing attitude is that medical care is a *right* of all citizens and not just a privilege for those who can afford it.

Medicare for the Aged. In 1965 the Congress of the United States passed a law establishing a broad program of health insurance for people 65 and older. This law, popularly known as "Medicare," became effective in July 1966. There are two kinds of insurance available under the Medicare program: (1) hospital insurance which helps pay a large part of hospital bills; and (2) medical insurance which helps pay the bills for physician's services and other specified medical services. The importance of this Medicare program is emphasized by the fact that older people need more medical care and hospitalization than younger people.

All people 65 and over receiving monthly social security (or railroad retirement) checks are *automatically* on the rolls for hospital insurance. Approximately 18½ million United States citizens are now receiving such checks.

This hospital insurance is financed out of special social security taxes paid by people while they work. Matching taxes are paid by employers. Thus the costs of hospital care (and extensions of it—for example, nursing home care) are and will continue to be met for close to 100% of American citizens aged 65 or over.

Medical insurance is *not* automatic. To get it people 65 and older must apply for it with the Social Security Administration in periods of time set forth in the law. The cost of this voluntary health insurance was set at only $3 a month in the original bill but has since been raised. The $3 or more premium is deducted from Social Security checks. The low cost of this health insurance to the recipient is possible because the federal government pays an equal amount toward the costs.

Most of the state and federal insurance payments to older people eligible for hospital or medical insurance have some built-in charges to be paid by the beneficiary, to prevent abuse of the services. Thus, for example, hospitalization is provided for up to 90 days in a "spell of illness." But the patient must pay the first $40 of his care and $10 daily for covered services after 60 days of hospitalization.

In addition to actual hospital care, the hospital insurance program of Medicare provides for outpatient diagnostic services, extended care in a skilled nursing home, and home health services—such as visits by public health nurses or physical therapists, but not physicians.

The medical insurance program pays 80% of the reasonable charges for covered services, except for the first $50 in a calendar year. These services include professional services of physicians and surgeons no matter where rendered; home health visits; and other medical health services—for example, diagnostic tests (X-ray plates and laboratory services), X-ray or radium treatments, surgical dressings, splints, casts, braces, artificial limbs, and so forth. Items *not* covered under Medicare plans include: routine physical checkups, eye glasses, hearing aids, private duty nurses, custodial care, and personal services (such as a telephone or television set in the hospital room).

While the federal government collects and disburses the funds needed to operate Medicare, it has contracted with Blue Cross, Blue Shield, private insurance companies, and independent plans to administer the benefits of the hospital and medical insurance. Many of these organizations offer "complementary coverage" to take care of expenses not covered under Medicare protection.

Medicaid is the term used to describe the system of assisting "medically indigent" persons and families to pay their medical bills. The federal government pays part of their bills but the state governments are also involved. Each state determines what family income level is to be deemed "medically indigent." (These levels differ among the states.) A family or individual is termed "medically indigent" when other bills can be paid, but not the cost of medical care.

Community-Wide Approaches to Health Problems. It is important to note that some communities, bellwethers for others, have made a success of community-wide approaches to local health care problems. An exceptionally fine program of this sort was undertaken in Seattle,

Washington, with the creation in 1961 of a Health Care Commission by the King County Medical Society. Through this commission, the joint efforts of physicians and many civic organizations were brought to bear on the health care needs of the people of Seattle and surrounding King County.

Working relationships were established with civic groups representing labor, management, hospitals, insurance, nurses, pharmacists, dentists, churches, and such other organizations as the Chamber of Commerce, the YMCA, YWCA, and Boy Scouts. The physicians, in discussion with all groups, sought to expose the basic, unmet medical needs of the area and then suggest and undertake some practical solution to the problems.

Prepaid Dental Care Plans. More than a million people in the United States are now covered by some sort of prepaid dental care plan, the U.S. Public Health Service reports. There has been both an increase in the number of plans and the number of people covered in recent years. There are probably 1.5 million people covered for dental care by over 300 different plans. In recent years there has been a tendency for plans to provide a wider range of dental benefits than some of the early ones. One of the largest contracts for dental care was that signed by the California Dental Association Service with Aerojet General Corporation, of Azusa, to provide dental care for its 115,000 employees and dependents. The California Dental Association Service is a non-profit organization sponsored by the dental profession of California. Nation-wide, prepaid dental care plans have been organized, financed, and administered in a number of ways—by labor unions, by employers and by employee groups.

Tax Support Unchanged. In the past generation, dating from 1940, there has been a tremendous, almost eightfold increase in annual expenditures in the United States for health and medical care. This figure leapt from $3.6 billion in 1940 to $31.3 billion in 1966. In spite of this increase in total, the percentage which is derived from tax support has not increased. It has remained steady at about 20% of the total for the past generation. This is to say that the American system of medical care operates 80% as a system of private practice, which is apparently the way the majority of American people want it.

SUMMARY

We have compressed into this single chapter the vast story of community efforts, official (public health departments) and voluntary (voluntary health agencies), to meet the health needs of the American people. We have given considerable attention and a specific example (Philadelphia) of the functioning of local health departments, since it is at this "grassroots" level that public health protection is most genuinely operative. The importance of state and national health departments and agencies—such as the U.S. Public Health Service—should not, however, be discounted.

We have outlined the community health resources of the United States, tangible and intangible. We have also outlined the approximately 30 different health careers open to college students and graduates. The subject of valid vital statistics (biostatistics) has been discussed at considerable length.

Voluntary health agencies are unique parts of the American scene. By their very nature they concern themselves with unsolved health problems and chronic illnesses which disable millions. We cannot hope to rehabilitate every chronically ill person in the country; but with community-wide health efforts embracing the health professions, public health and voluntary health agencies, great progress can be and is being made.

We have looked into the topsy-turvy economics of medical care. We must recognize and accept the fact that about 5% of one's lifetime income must be spent on medical care of all kinds (physicians, hospitals, drugs etc.). The immediate impact but not the final cost of medical care can be softened by health insurance policies (five varieties), wisely purchased. We have noted the advent of Medicare and Medicaid as new types of health insurance, federally financed. We have also pointed out that the higher your income, the more likely you are to have voluntary health insurance.

SUMMARY REVIEW QUESTIONS

1. How do you distinguish between community health and public health? Why, if at all, do you consider this distinction important?
2. What are the present tangible and intangible health resources of the United States? Be specific and list at least ten.
3. What professions, beyond the practice of medicine, contribute to the health of patients? Have you ever considered entering any of these so-called medical auxiliary (or paramedical) professions? If so, why? If not, why not?
4. What precautions should you adopt when using or interpreting vital statistics?
5. In a certain midwestern city, with a population of 150,000, there were in the year 1964 a total of 1500 deaths, of which 15 were from tuberculosis and 90 among infants under 1 year of age. In the same year 4500 live infants were born in the city.
   a. What is the birth rate in this city?
   b. What is the crude death rate?
   c. What is the specific death rate from tuberculosis?
   d. What is the infant mortality rate?
   e. What was the population increase?
   f. On the basis of these figures would you say that in comparison with other metropolitan areas in the United States this city was a comparatively healthy place in which to live? Justify your answer.
6. For what reasons should you be very hesitant about being guided into a belief or course of action on statistical evidence alone?
7. What are the primary functions of a local (city or county) public health department? What other services might it perform? What methods for the control of communicable disease might it employ? How might it be organized?
8. How did the U.S. Public Health Service originate? What in general are its present functions and responsibilities?
9. What is a voluntary health agency? How did they originate in the United States? (Give four specific examples.)
10. Which of the following possible functions of a well-organized voluntary health agency do you consider to be the most important, and why: Research? Professional education? Public education? Fund-raising? Service to patients? Lobbying in Congress? Recruiting volunteers?
11. What are the most common "chronic illnesses" in the United States? What is the relationship of chronic illness to acute illness? To what extent can rehabilitation help to solve the problem of chronic illness?
12. Why is it important that teachers (elementary, secondary, and college) be familiar with the basic concepts of health and health education? What content (or subject matter) does adequate preparation for understanding and teaching health embrace?
13. Are the following statements sense or nonsense? Why? *Give once for all. . . . Stop arthritis. . . . Ring the bell for mental health. . . . A rate is a ratio. . . . Chronic illness is a problem of aging. . . . Public Health is the foundation of prosperity. . . . The doctor is an angel when the patient is sick but a devil when he presents his bill. . . . Health insurance is a racket.*

14. What percentage of your lifetime income can you expect to pay out for health and medical services of all kinds? How does this compare with other expenditures you may be called upon to make? At what ages of life can you expect your *yearly* medical bills to be the largest?

15. What does the term "health insurance" mean to you? What is the purpose of health insurance? What two basic kinds of health insurance are there? Why should health insurance be subject to political controversy?

16. What are the five general types of voluntary health insurance that can be purchased on an individual or group basis? What precautions should you take when individually purchasing health-insurance policies?

17. What percentage of the U.S. population has some form of health insurance? Chiefly what kind? In what ways does the amount of family income influence the amount of coverage of medical and hospital expenses provided through health insurance?

18. Does health insurance decrease the cost of total medical (and hospital) care? If so, how? If not, what justification is there for its increasing popularity?

19. What do the following terms mean to you: Blue Cross, rehabilitation, death certificate, health code, health education, National Institutes of Health, Veterans Hospital, noise abatement, Medicare, Medicaid?

Worth Looking Into: *The Gentle Legions: A Probing Study of the National Voluntary Health Organizations* by Richard Carter. *A Mind That Found Itself* by Clifford Beers. *Medical Biometry and Statistics* by Raymond Pearl. *An Introduction to Public Health* by Harry Mustard, M.D., and Ernest Stebbins, M.D. *A Brief Explanation of "Medicare" Health Insurance for People 65 and Older,* from the U.S. Department of Health, Education and Welfare and the Social Security Administration. Washington, D.C.: U.S. Government Printing Office, 1965. For more complete references, see Appendix E.

Answers to Special Exercise (Pictoquiz), page 422.

1. National Society for Crippled Children (Easter Seal Society). 2. The National Council on Alcoholism, Inc. 3. National Association for Mental Health. 4. American Cancer Society. 5. Arthritis Foundation. 6. Blue Cross and Blue Shield. 7. United Cerebral Palsy Associations. 8. National Multiple Sclerosis Society. 9. Muscular Dystrophy Associations of America. 10. National Tuberculosis and Respiratory Disease Association. 11. American Heart Association. 12. American Red Cross.

The Health Status of the Negro Today and in the Future

Paul B. Cornely, M.D., Dr.P.H., F.A.P.H.A.

Introduction

The first nationwide conference on the health status of the Negro, held on March 13 and 14, 1967, during the Centennial Observance of Howard University, was called for the purpose of having a group of knowledgeable and experienced scholars, researchers, educators, and providers of health services consider the major health problems of this segment of the population, and to suggest guidelines which would be helpful to governmental and voluntary agencies at the local, state, and national levels. Financial support for this conference came from the Public Health Service and the Milbank Fund; about 200 persons from 20 states were in attendance. It should be made clear that this two-day conference was not called for the purpose of finding instant solutions to the many health and welfare problems which beset the Negro.

I have been asked to summarize what occurred at this conference. This is being presented under the following three headings: (a) major health problems of the Negro, (b) possible solutions for selected health problems, and (c) the urgency of the situation.

Health Problems of the Negro in the United States

The major health problems of the Negro were discussed at length at one of the workshops. Although, I shall not go through all of them, nevertheless, it is well to mention three of the many health problems with which the conference struggled so that none of us will entirely forget what is happening to our fellow Americans.

1. *The Widening Gap*—Any objective look at the available data comparing Negro and white mortality and morbidity shows that the gap between the two is getting wider. This is true for most of the important public health indexes used in this country.

2. *Mental Retardation*—The prevalence of inferior intellectual functioning among the Negro community is related by recent studies of Negro school-age children. Eighth grade pupils in Central Harlem were found to have a mean I.Q. of 87.7, while the average I.Q. for New York City eighth graders was 100.1.[1] A normative study of 1,800 Negro elementary school children in five southern states yielded a mean I.Q. of 80.7.[2] According to the most recent classification system accepted by the American Association of Mental Deficiency,[3] which is also used by the U.S. Public Health Service, the average child in the latter study is "borderline retarded." These data do not present any particularly new information; such findings have been reported for over 50 years.[4,5] The

SOURCE: Paul Cornely, M.D., Dr. P. H. is Professor and Head of the Department of Preventive Medicine and Public Health at Howard University College of Medicine, Washington, D.C. He was also elected in 1969 President of the American Public Health Association. This article reports the first nationwide conference on the health status of the American blacks, held on March 13–17, 1967 on the occasion of the Centennial Observance of Howard University (a predominantly Negro university). The presentation here includes the major portions of Dr. Cornely's paper appearing in the *American Journal of Public Health* **58**:4 (April 1968). It is reproduced here with the permission of the American Journal of Public Health.

precursors of and factors associated with mental retardation abound in the Negro community. Mental retardation has been found to be associated with prematurity, complications of pregnancy, low socio-economic status, as well as lower occupational levels, lower educational attainment, and broken homes. Yet, little has been done to alleviate these conditions.

3. *Health Concerns of the Unskilled and Semiskilled Worker*—The unskilled and semiskilled workers have the most serious health problems and receive the least adequate health care. Because of segregation and discrimination, the great majority of Negroes fall into these occupational groups, and their health problems stem mainly from this fact. The health services received by them tend to be obtained from two sources: (1) charity wards and clinics and (2) private care by overworked and harried general practitioners.

Another factor has to do with injury and compensation. Negroes who are largely concentrated in unskilled and heavy labor occupations are often subjected to greater risk of injury and consequent potential loss of health.

Because these workers are largely unskilled, poorly educated, and Negro, even union activity, significant in protecting the workmen's interest in these areas in the past, is largely waning and in some areas has tragically disappeared.

There is a growing tendency in many industries to contest all claims made by injured workmen, particularly where disability results. This kind of activity on the part of industry forces the claimant in many instances to require legal services to establish the merit of his claim or forfeit, through ignorance and inadequate education, the very benefit for which the law originally came into being. The Negro is the greater sufferer.

These three examples are sufficient. The others are indeed known only too well—discriminatory health patterns, shortage of health manpower, organization, delivery and utilization of health services, and so on.

Possible Solutions for Selected Health Problems

Each of the workshops of the Howard University Conference attempted to develop possible solutions and recommendations for many of the health problems which beset the Negro. An effort will be made here to summarize the more salient approaches which came to the fore.

What Can Be Done About the Unfavorable Morbidity and Mortality Patterns of the Negro? The unfavorable morbidity and mortality experiences of the Negro population are not due to any genetic differences, but rather to the socioeconomic and environmental deficiencies, such as poverty, housing, unemployment, non-availability, and/or inaccessibility of health services facilities, discrimination and segregation, and inadequate family structure. Therefore, the major thrust to improve the health of the Negro must be directed at these factors along the following lines:

a. A massive, coordinated, and comprehensive attack on the nation's social, economic, and health problems sponsored by the federal government is critically and urgently needed. A recent press release in Washington reported that Argentina recently sent six Peace Corps volunteers to help in poverty areas in our affluent society. It is possible that after a brief exposure here, these volunteers will ask their country to send surplus beef to feed the starving children in Mississippi.

b. Much of the mental retardation in the Negro community can be alleviated by positive, significant, and lasting improvement in the over-all standard of living. The high incidence of borderline mental retardation among the deprived is acutely susceptible to available remedies. A comprehensive plan of effective action for the Negro community as a whole, and for the functionally retarded individual in particular, is necessary if a notable decline in the incidence of mental retardation in the Negro community is to be observed.

c. Research is urgently needed to determine the many factors which affect the full utilization of health services by the poor, and to find ways and means to develop a health care system which will reach and be accepted by the poor.

d. Negro health professionals should become actively interested in the correction of factors which promote homicide, drug addiction, illegitimacy, and other behavior problems with high incidence among Negro youth. Currently there appears to be considerable apathy among this group.

e. Small regional conferences

financed by the federal government or foundations should be developed to consider some of the health problems of the Negro. These conferences could bring together specialists in the field for a more careful consideration of these problems. Hopefully these would stimulate an increase in research in many neglected areas.

Urgency of the Situation

The salient deliberations and discussions of the Howard University Conference have been summarized above. The Negro revolution and protestations occurring throughout the United States underscore the importance of the health problems of the Negro, and all Americans must be concerned about their urgency. This urgency must be viewed in the light of the following four considerations which repeatedly come into clear focus.

1. Our affluent society is allowing a widening gap to develop between the health of the white and nonwhite population. This adds fuel to the smoldering Negro revolution which explodes intermittently. Those concerned with health care can contribute their skills to the resolution of these conflicts and frictions which are being intensified daily, particularly in our large metropolitan communities.

2. The health of the Negro is both an expression and the result of the social and economic burdens imposed upon him. His health is inseparably connected with poor housing, unemployment, and inadequate educa-tion. But the health problems of the Negro are also the health problems of the poor. There is, therefore, a tremendous justification for setting aside ethnic considerations and making the health of all the poor our major concern. This is the desideratum, but it is impossible to achieve today, or in the immediate future, because of the burdens of a long existent cultural pattern. There is a basic difference between the black and white poor because of discrimination and segregation which continue in our midst. Both the consumer and the providers of health services suffer. This is not a mere physical barrier. More importantly, it is emotional and it alters the attitude and behavior of those who seek health and those who dispense it. The health provider, if he is to serve and aid the black poor, must himself undergo a revolution or conversion in his own thinking. Only in this way will he be able to meet and understand the major changes which are occurring in the attitude of the Negro community. This has tremendous importance to universities and colleges engaged in training members of the health team.

3. Health agencies, whether federal, national, or local, must realize that the health problems of the Negro poor are extremely urgent, and financial support for a nationwide "man in his home" program should equal that of the "man on the moon" project. Unless this is done with dispatch, our communities, particularly the urban centers, will continue to grow into black jungles of unmanageable proportions. The resolution of this is a challenge to the federal government, particularly Congress. This government has not been willing to establish certain social objectives and goals to be accomplished within stated periods of time. Neither has it been willing to face up to the problems of black America because the mentality of the majority of the leaders of this country is still polluted with the miasma of prejudice.

4. The health problems of the Negro poor are many, and have been known for a long time. Yet there is insufficient data, as well as a paucity of studies, designed to answer many of the questions confronting us. How can these problems be attacked if the epidemiology is woefully inadequate? The Public Health Service, the universities, and foundations should address themselves to these problems and stimulate interest in finding answers.

The urgency of the situation is of grave importance to all health workers, and particularly to the leaders of the profession. The American Public Health Association itself has just recently accepted the challenge and the urgency by committing itself to the employment of a staff person who will be concerned with the problems of discrimination and segregation in health matters. But solid achievements in this area cannot take place unless there is the commitment of the almost 20,000 members of this organization, and particularly those of the two Sections (Medical Care and Health Officers). The time has come for the Councils of these two Sections to come together and initiate the procedure whereby they can become an effectively strong unit in order to accomplish three major tasks.

a. Determine and delineate the nature and function of the type of health agency at the local, state, or federal level, which this country needs now and for the future, in order to provide each one of us with the health and medical services which are needed.

b. Define the social objectives and goals which must become part of the political structure of our country.

c. Formulate an approach whereby the APHA can become the effective spokesman for whatever consumer group today or tomorrow is denied the health care which our technology has made possible.

The task is urgent.

REFERENCES

1. Moynihan, D. P. The Negro Family (The Case for National Action). US Department of Labor, Office of Policy Planning and Research, 1965.

2. Kennedy, W. A., et al. A Normative Sample of Intelligence and Achievement of Negro Elementary School Children in the Southeastern United States. Monogr. Soc. Res. Child Development 28, No. 6 (Ser. No. 90), 1963.

3. Heber, R. A. Manual of Terminology and Classification in Mental Retardation (2nd ed.). Am. J. Ment. Deficiency Monogr. Suppl (Apr), 1961.

4. Peterson, J. The Comparative Abilities of White and Negro Children. Comp. Psychol. Monogr. 5:1–141, 1923.

5. Shuey, A. M. The Testing of Negro Intelligence, Lynchburg, Va.: Bell, 1958.

6. Cornely, P. B., and Bigman, S. K. Some Considerations in Changing Health Attitudes. Children 10,1:23–28 (Jan.-Feb.), 1963.

PART FIVE   ENVIRONMENTAL HEALTH

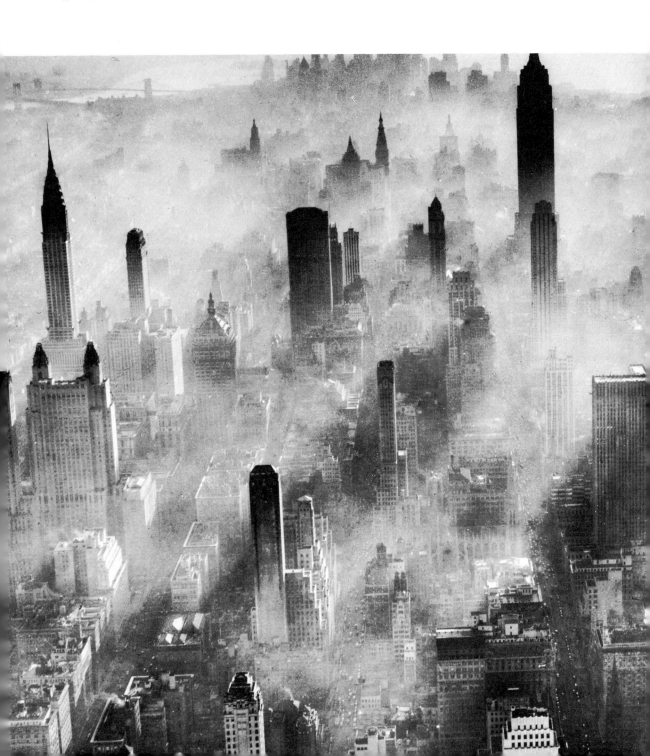

Environmental health problems, differing in kind, arise in all parts of the world. This picture of the effects of air pollution in New York City illustrates a particularly prevalent urban problem. (Photograph by Aero Service Division, Litton Industries)

21

ENVIRONMENTAL HEALTH
AND MEDICINE

MAN, THE THINKING ANIMAL, WHO HAS obtained—almost—complete dominion over the beasts of the field, birds, insects, fish, and other creatures of the deep, nevertheless remains subject to the biological, physical, and social environment that he has created for himself. As human beings have increasingly triumphed over their "natural" enemies of climate, pestilence, and famine, they have created a man-made environment which introduces new hazards to human health.[1]

The accident rate of the human race has probably remained constant since the first cave-man fell out of a tree when he tried to climb it and reach for a succulent fruit. But the present day-by-day instrument of violence and death in

[1]This chapter derives some of its most important concepts from the International Conference on Health and Health Education, held from June 30 to July 7, 1962 in Philadelphia, under the sponsorship of the International Union for Health Education (IUHE) in collaboration with the World Health Organization (WHO) and at the invitation of the American National Council for Health Education of the Public (ANCHEP). The writer attended this conference and had the privilege of serving as a member of the leadership team among the technical study groups devoted to "Health Education of College and University Students." The conference—the largest of its kind ever held—was conducted in three languages, English, French, and Spanish, with simultaneous translations provided. Approximately 1200 delegates from 60 countries arond the world attended the conference. It was obvious that people from the so-called "overdeveloped" nations had much to learn from delegates from the so-called "underdeveloped," or better, "developing," countries.

the most "civilized" countries of the world has in the 20th century become the motor vehicle (see Chapter 18).

We have largely conquered, or are on the way to conquering, epidemic and communicable disease, but in the process of liquidating insect pests, predators, and vectors of disease we now run a risk of upsetting the cycles of nature (the ecology of parts of the globe) to the extent that we may be endangering our eventual food supply.

We wittingly, or unwittingly, pollute the waters we must live by and the air we must breathe. We take into our lungs, air saturated with hydrocarbons from the exhaust of motor vehicles, from the smoke of industrial plants, and from tobacco.

We have developed marvelous new life-saving drugs—the antibiotics, for example—but we often use them unwisely, giving our enemies—microbes like the staphylococcus—a chance to adjust to their antibiotic enemies. The phrase "iatrogenic disease" (disease caused by medical treatment) has come into prominence in recent years. The classic example is blindness owing to retrolental fibroplasia, caused by giving too much oxygen to premature infants whose lives would not be saved without some added oxygen in their early days of life. This, however, is only to repeat in more sophisticated language an ancient saying which probably has a counterpart in all languages and cultures: "The remedy is worse than the disease."

We have a new science of aerospace medicine and a new concept of molecular disease, which promise breakthroughs within a decade or two for conquest over the degenerative and chronic diseases which afflct millions of inhabitants of the globe. But we have not yet licked such down-to-earth problems, whose methods of control are well known, as malaria, tuberculosis, the venereal diseases, and juvenile delinquency.

Further study of man in his biologic, physical, and social environment is certainly indicated— and this is a problem (or set of problems) to which every student of this text may eventually hope to make his own contribution. In presenting this material on environmental health, on which volumes can be and have been written, we must limit ourselves to just a few of the most significant and sometimes man-made hazards to human health, notably accidents; water, food and air pollution; pesticides; radiological health; and world health.

Man's Physical Environment

As Dr. Abel Wolman, speaking at the International Conference on Health and Health Education in Philadelphia in 1962 said: "Within the last ten years, the 'environment' has been rediscovered. [But] man, as an ecological animal, has shown throughout his history a remarkable capacity for adaptation to his external and internal environment. He is, in fact, a result of these persistent and continuing adjustments. The physical environment [however] is only a part of his total constellation. Other impacts are simultaneously at work."

Dr. Wolman has listed as the four main categories which encompass our concept of the physical environment: water, air, earth, and food. He has also pointed out that these categories have been elaborated historically into other subdivisions which at different times in human history have primarily engaged scientific and even political concern. Among these subdivided categories, some of which are current and brand new, others of which represent ancient but still unsolved problems, he lists: water supply and

wastes, food and milk, insect vectors, air, radiation, housing and occupied space, accidents, industry, noise, recreational areas, urbanization, and outer space.

Dr. Wolman has properly cautioned that in reaching for the stars we do not neglect and forget the problems that are underfoot. This too may be considered ancient, though still valid advice, for we have the legend of the ancient Greek philosopher who was so entranced at gazing at the stars that he fell into a well.

Changes in Man's Social Environment

Whatever else historians of the future may say about the twentieth century, they cannot overlook the fact that it is the period of most rapid social change that has been recorded (to date) in human history. The revolutions in communication, transportation, and public health that science and technology have wrought have forever changed the social environment of the globe. And they have affected the juvenile on the streets of New York, London, Moscow, and Paris just as much as they have changed the lives of the native of an emergent Africa.

Dr. Margaret Read, formerly professor of education at the University of London, made the valid suggestion that we keep in mind the three following principles when we look at twentieth-century peoples in their social environment, especially where the emphasis of the century is on areas of rapid social change:

1. The first principle is that the nature of social groups in a society determine the relationships and responsibilities arising from kinship patterns, from patterns of authority depending on knowledge, status, and age, from patterns of making a livelihood based on the environment. [There is an] overriding mutual dependence of individuals upon each other within an accepted pattern of relationships and behavior.
2. The second principle is that [today's] winds of change blow without regard for existing patterns of livelihood and social grouping. Some changes may be directed from above as part of a government program. Others arise from a considered or sponta-

neous desire in a community to alter its way of living. In either case the total social environment is affected in some way or other, and nutrition, child care, homemaking, and personal security are inextricably bound together in the process of change.

3. The third principle is that in all changing cultures, adult human beings can choose between acceptance and rejection, between conformity and nonconformity. This fundamental trait in human behavior appears whether an individual is conforming to traditional practices or to new ones. When a health educator is impatient because, as he says, "people do not readily learn from him," he has to see his program as the community sees it, offering perhaps certain improvements, but demanding a break with traditional custom. Choice in these circumstances involves individuals and communities in a careful and considered weighing up of many related aspects of social living.

Environmental Health: The Range

Environmental health, which possibly derives from the term, "environmental sanitation," represents man's effort to control all those factors in his physical environment which "exercise, or may exercise, a deleterious effect on his physical, mental or social well-being." Taken literally, and as a whole, this is a large order. However, when it is broken down by specific projects, it is well within the realm of official and government agencies. It must also be recognized that much greater progress has been made in some parts of the world than in others.

Environmental sanitation, as we understand the term today, began in England in the mid-nineteenth century when Sir Edwin Chadwick established the first sanitary commission and Dr. Southwood Smith organized a "Health of Towns Association." In the United States the great motivators toward better environmental sanitation were Lemuel Shattuck, Stephen Smith, and, somewhat later, William Thompson Sedgwick. Shattuck was a Boston publisher. His famous "Shattuck Report," as the "Report of the Sanitary Commission of Massachusetts: 1850" has become known, set the stage for a new era of public-health work in the United States. Stephen

Smith was a New Yorker; he called strong attention to the health abominations, such as pigsties next to schools, in the metropolis.

Sedgwick, long a professor at the Massachusetts Institute of Technology, was one of the great apostles of the "sanitary awakening" which swept America in the 1890's. He taught that "the common drinking cup is anathema," which it is, and that "dirt is dangerous," which is not necessarily so true as he believed. The causes of disease, as we have seen, are multiple.

Environmental health today is a matter of broad and complex scope. In one way or another it relates to practically all of man's activities. Major efforts, both by governmental and non-governmental agencies, must be made to attack the environmental health problems resulting from the rapid growth of our highly technological civilization. New problems must continually be studied and more thoroughly understood if measures for their control and ultimate prevention are to be developed. Environmental health is still an open-end topic and in some respects raises more questions than it answers. It is related to many public health and community health services already in operation (e.g., water supply), but it gives a new focus for many of these activities.

A wide range of scientific and operating personnel is necessary to put working programs of environmental health into effect. Biologists, physicians, physical scientists, social scientists, engineers, mathematicians, and members of other scientific disciplines are required for the effort. Among the things they must do is undertake joint research on problems of common interest from many points of view (e.g., air-pollution control); yet they must provide unified mathematical, statistical, data-processing service (together with techniques for information storage and retrieval) and develop new instruments and analytical laboratory procedures for getting a fresh handhold on both old and new problems. This may seem a somewhat abstract approach but it is an essential process for applying the vitalized new concept of environmental health to concrete problems of great diversity.

It would be impossible within the brief scope of these chapters, or of this book as a whole, to cover all the facets of environmental health. We shall therefore present some of the most important and representative areas. Among the topics of environmental health we shall discuss are air pollution, water supply and pollution control, radiological health (protection from radiation), and occupational health. We shall have to pay less attention to problems of milk and food protection and distribution, environmental engineering, and pest control. We can only mention that the field also cultivates analytical methods and instrumentation, mathematical and statistical approaches to environment, and the underlying sciences of pharmacology, toxicology (study of poisons), physiology, and biochemistry.

The field of environmental health already employs the interest and services of many people, although more will be needed. It was estimated that in the United States in the 1960's between 30,000 and 35,000 scientists, engineers, and other professionals were engaged in environmental health activities. These included individuals in the water and sewage fields, in state and local health departments, teaching, research, public works, and in private and consulting practice.

The Historical Pathway.[2] In its narrow sense environmental health is the offspring of public health, which represented, historically, man's effort to protect himself and his community against disease—for centuries primarily against communicable disease. Environmental health broadens the field enormously. It seeks to identify and provide positive protection for healthy individuals against adverse influences that crop up in an expanding society, which is becoming ever more technical and complex.

There have been unprecedented improvements in public health, community health, and environmental health practices and accomplishments in the twentieth century. On a worldwide basis, however, the progress has been spotty. The United States, Great Britain, and Western Europe took giant strides toward health protec-

[2]George Rosen, *A History of Public Health,* (New York: MD Publications, 1958).

tion in the twentieth century. It is fair to say, however, that the so-called underdeveloped nations, at least in an economic and technological sense, are often back in the nineteenth century. They still face problems of preventable diseases which the more fortunate countries learned to cope with 50 to 75 years ago.

The technological advances in the more fortunate countries, however, have brought new problems; for example, automobile accidents. It is another interesting fact that whereas these countries formerly had to deal with water, air, and food contaminated chiefly by *bacteria,* they now have to deal with these elements actually or potentially polluted by *chemicals.* Expanding industrialism brings technical, social, economic, and eventually health problems that must be faced; for example, housing, atmospheric pollution, and use of radioactive materials.

Some Key Questions for the Future

It would be hard to pinpoint exactly the environmental health problems now emerging in the United States and elsewhere. The types of problems can perhaps best be hinted at by asking ourselves some pointed questions. In these questions we give substance to the nature and future of environmental health problems.

How fast will the American and other populations grow during the remainder of the twentieth century?

What special plans must we make for the increasing percentages of older people in our own and other populations?

How can we accommodate ourselves to the ever-expanding complexity of our technology? (How, for example, do we handle the problems and displacements created by automation?)

What will the development of new industries do to our society and environment?

How risky is increasing reliance on nuclear power?

How large and what kind of agricultural efforts must we put forth to feed our populations?

What hazards may arise from the introduction of new chemicals into our food, water, air, clothing, tools, and even toys?

What will be the results of urban sprawl, forming huge metropolitan areas?

What will changes in communication and transportation do to us? (Are we going to have to learn to live with the sonic booms of faster and faster aircraft?)

What will we do with our increased leisure time? What sort of recreation facilities must we plan for?

The health risks, or opportunities, implicit in these questions are obviously greater in some instances than others, but taken altogether the questions suggest the eruption of many diverse problems in environmental health. They will have to be identified and solved—hopefully before they become too acute.

Environmental Health and Medicine. We cannot deny that we live in an era of change—progress if we want to make it so. The twentieth century is not the nineteenth century; nor is the second half of the twentieth century exactly commensurate with the first; to name but one crucial difference—the population explosion. Our outlook on health, its preservation and restoration, and our attitude about the practice of medicine, with as much emphasis on preventive medicine as curative medicine, are being revised as we breast the multiple currents of the present decade.

It has been very wisely said that man's health today depends on his aptitude to meet unexpected challenges in an environment being constantly transformed. From birth, and even before, the human being begins a life struggle to adapt himself to a shifting environment and to an equilibrium which is constantly being threatened. The mass and speed of development of new scientific knowledge, in medical as well as other sciences, have had a strong impact on the present social evolution of man. This advancement has given medicine itself added roles and responsibilities; it must play both an educative and social mission along with and indeed as part of its preventive and healing tasks. This is the essence of environmental medicine. It is practiced not only by physicians but also by public health officers, nurses, educators, technicians, sanitarians, and others. Physicians must treat patients and communities as a whole; and they need the help of everyone else with technical knowledge toward this end.

The twentieth century has boldly set the welfare of the human race as its goal. There are, unfortunately, some stumbling blocks on the path. Today's medical weapons create some new dangers. We cannot expect to wipe out all change and struggle. Education must play an increasing role in helping man to adapt to changing conditions.

In this broad pattern of environmental health and medicine it becomes difficult to formulate a definition of "health." Perhaps as good a definition as we can essay in words is this: Health is a fullness of life, the balanced output, the total harmony in as close accord as possible with the evolving demands of the environment. More briefly, we can say that health is a product of harmony, more or less perfect, between man and his environment: biological, physical, social, and ideological. These are separated here for the sake of analysis; he faces them as a unified whole with many facets. And he must master them—or at least keep them from mastering him.

Physical environment was the first of the environments that man had to master for his survival. This he has managed on an ever-increasing scale. Consider the topography that man has had to conquer: earth, oceans, rivers, mountains, deserts, lakes, swamps. With this geography have come mighty forces of weather to be mastered. Hidden in these physical surroundings were also useful sources of energy, water power, steam, electricity, and nuclear energy, which man finally captured for himself. Now the human race has extended its physical conquests beyond Earth and set out on a conquest of space.

Two historical facts should be noted. Whatever tools, instruments, or artifacts man has created, these technological creations have become an integral part of his environment and pointed to his future. Whatever has increased man's communication and mobility has influenced his appreciation of and loyalty to enlarged areas of physical environment. Thus, sociologically, man has advanced from the tribe, the horde, the village to the modern state, to the international alliance (United Nations), and to outer space.

The *biological environment* of man consists of the animals he has tamed or not, the plants and trees he has cultivated or not, fish, insects (who were recognized as a bother but not as a danger until the nineteenth century), and microbes (including viruses). The ability to master his biological environment, on the one hand to produce food and on the other to minimize disease, has been one of man's new and big steps forward. Of utmost importance was the germ theory of the nineteenth century, which, attached to the twentieth-century recognition that most diseases are the result not of a single cause but of many conditions, has led the way to annihilating a number of disease-producing biological agents. Biologists tell us further that a nuclear catastrophe would upset the biological environment and leave the globe in command of enormously radio-resistant insects, like the cockroach and various bacteria.

The *social environment* of mankind is other people. Mankind now has the largest social environment of its history, and the outcome of this fact is uncertain. The social environment of man has been organized, split up, and sub-divided to provide the political, economic, social, and educational institutions that man manipulates in the conduct of his activities. Since the mental health of living individuals in society must evolve out of and take form from the social institutions of mankind, the social environment of man must remain one of the great banks in which the treasure of human personalities is stored up. The phrase, "a sick society," would describe an unhealthy social environment.

The *ideological environment* is nothing but the set of ideas with which individuals and groups of individuals of varying sizes surround and encase themselves and sometimes worship. A man's ideological world reflects what he believes he represents and stands for in the universe. He may be willing to fight and indeed die for this ideal. It may be the most powerful motivating force to get him to change factors in his physical, biological, and social environment. You can win a man by appealing to his ideals. The advancement of environmental health for the mass of mankind can probably be achieved most effectively by this technique.

The Rediscovery of the Environment

From his earliest history man has been compelled to conform to various environments. However, he also has a record of efforts to tamper with and change elements in his environment, i.e., the men who "captured" fire and invented the earliest tools that made hunting, fishing and killing more efficient. Around 7000 B.C., some primitive men discovered how to sow seeds and domesticate animals and—with this knowledge spread to groups of men all over the world—gradually established the agricultural revolution. Hunters and food-gatherers became farmers and herdsmen, a social revolution occurring with the technical one. We can read in detail about the "industrial revolution," which began in the late eighteenth century and is not over yet. Industry, however, has succeeded agriculture as the chief productive factor in our society; and the relative number of farmers is constantly shrinking. Many—but it cannot be said all—of the problems which mankind faces today stem from the industrial revolution.

We have only to glance about us, at least in the technically advanced countries of the world, to see how grossly and how eagerly man has sought to alter different phases of his present environment. There is no hint that he is going to stop trying to tamper with his environment. We may distinguish, perhaps, between minimal, subsistence economies, where a relatively stable adaptation to the environment is the desiderata, and technologically advanced, industrial economies, where in general whatever is "new" is gauged as "good" and where time for adjustment and adaptation to change is not always sufficiently allowed. On this point there is wisdom in a *Summary Report to the President* of the Committee on Natural Resources of the National Academy of Science, which said:

It is apparent that man must concern himself with a variety of changes in the environment, both those caused by human beings and those reflecting man's responses. Some are good; some may be very harmful. That we often do not have any clear-cut idea of their impact on man, or of man's response, is cause for concern. It would seem unwise to continue to tamper without concurrently striving to determine the real and lasting effects of our actions.

With its new tools (for example, nuclear energy, pesticides) and new ideologies (for instance, communism, "suburban living") the human race in recent decades has begun to bump up against its various environments as it has not done in several centuries. Indeed looking at the immediate past, with its developments in communication, transportation, medicine, and public health (the germ theory of disease), it looked hopefully—but falsely—for a few years as if mankind might become free of dependence on its various environments. This was not to be. The interaction between man and his environments has reached a new and critical stage, which has led to a rediscovery and new awareness of the environment.

We are now facing up to questions and problems that we had left more or less slumbering for many years. This is not to say that there were not always some forward-looking men and groups who recognized and investigated what we now again call environmental health problems; but it is to say that the crucial and rising importance of these problems was not fairly evaluated. Why bother about a few puffs of lingering smoke on the horizon? But how do you relieve a city bathed in "smog"? The fundamental questions about environmental health and medicine are quite simple to ask: What do we know about our environment? What, if anything, are we doing to alter it? How can we adapt to it? If not, how can we adjust it to our own benefit? What laws must we make and live by to manage our environment most successfully? These are simple questions; but the answers are complex, extensive, and usually variant from locality to locality.

The trend toward rediscovery of the importance of the environment in human health and medicine has been emphasized by the number of special conferences and seminars that have been held on this topic and its subtopics, and also by the fact that the U.S. Public Health Service has established an Environmental Control Administration in its Consumer Protection and Environmental Health Service. Legislative proposals, budget increases, and political emphasis have been laid upon environmental health and medicine in recent years. This has been most markedly true in the most heavily industrialized countries but it has also been impressive in less developed regions where an inevitable advance in urbanization has been creating an environmental impact upon health. In whatever country it is located, the large and enlarging city evolves new environmental health problems. Against some of these problems education is the only, and it it is frequently the best, weapon.

Choices in Environmental Health Programs. The choices of environmental health programs to be undertaken in different localities throughout the world vary greatly and depend upon many criteria of need, awareness, and readiness. The dilemma now confronting the environmental health worker or committee is a surfeit of challenges along with a deficit of scientific understanding and underpinning in some highly significant areas of physical environment. In the days when infectious diseases were the principal challenge to the health officer, courses of action could be more clearcut because the nature of the diseases, their modes of transmission, and the techniques for their control were for the most part reasonably well understood.

Today we face a situation, at least in industrialized and urbanized nations, where contamination of land, air, water, and food is frequently easily demonstrable. However, it is much more difficult to show the positively deleterious health results which stem from these more subtle, long-term, and often symbiotic circumstances. It is not enough to know that a possibly hostile physical environment exists. It is more important to be able to evaluate this potentially harmful physical impact so that the wisest measures for its control can be undertaken.

In many areas of the world, with multimillions of inhabitants, infectious diseases that are controllable are still the prime hazards. For these areas environmental sanitation is the easy and obvious choice of environmental health activity. It makes little sense to go pursuing the carcinogenic (cancer-producing) risks of drinking water in a country where half the people do not have bacteriologically safe water in their homes and three-quarters lack anything but the most primitive means of excreta disposal. Sanitation is the first step here. Its techniques are simple, well known, and proved. They are somewhat expensive, but no-where near so costly as the loss of life their absence engenders.

On the easily proved premise that it is often difficult to get people to do what is good for them, Dr. Abel Wolman in 1958 evolved a well-defined set of criteria which might be used for initiating and making choices between suggested environmental health programs in a given community. The program chosen for action in the attack on the environment, he said, should have as many as possible of the following characteristics: (1) It should be a program that can be dramatically "sold" to the community. (2) It gives more than reasonable expectation of easy and prompt execution. (3) It requires minimum expenditure of time and energy for promotion. (4) It brings potentially the greatest public health, comfort, and economic returns. (5) It affects the greatest number of people. (6) It rests to a major extent upon the resources of the people. (7) It requires the minimum education of all the people. (8) It has a strong scientific and technological basis. (9) It requires little or no additional research. (10) It is most timely.

As we review Dr. Wolman's criteria we are reawakened to the vital influence of the social and ideological environment on the physical and biological. In the *practice* of environmental medicine we must make wise choices of programs that work. And yet, because it intersects so many of the advancing frontiers of human life in so many areas of the globe, we cannot expect the same certainties from the practice of environmental medicine that we enjoy from curative medicine (which has its own kinds of uncertainties). We do not have final answers in the broad fields of environmental health and medicine; but we are under obligation to look for these answers and give the ones that have so far been evolved in the various subdivisions of this broad and vital subject.

Pollutions and Contaminations. In one sense we can say that environmental medicine is partly the never-ending struggle against pollutions and contaminations that threaten human health. It is the battle both to prevent them and to eliminate, or at least minimize, them. In this broad and realistic definition environmental medicine touches on and intersects many other established areas of medical practice and scientific research—for example, public health, preventive medicine, industrial medicine, bacteriology, climatology, engineering, and radiant energy (radiology).

The *major* pollutions with which environmental health and medicine now deal are *water* pollution, *air* pollution, *land* pollutuon (bacteriological and chemical), *noise,* and *food* contamination. Some of these pollutions, in some areas of the globe, including the United States, have relatively recently risen or risen to new levels of hazard and significance. We shall deal with the impact of these major—and often new—pollutions in our last two chapters. Here we shall consider other problems that fall into the field of environmental health and medicine: occupational health, environmental engineering, international quarantine.

Occupational Health and Industrial Medicine

The civilian labor force in the United States numbers between 75 and 80 million people, of whom about 4 million are unemployed at any given time. To protect and improve the health of this working population is the role of occupational health and industrial medicine in the United States. Other countries have commensurate responsibilities. It is a task which falls in the province of environmental health and medicine, since the workers spend such a large part of their lives in their working environments. The cooperation of labor, management, and government, and the intercession of both departments of health and departments of labor are necessary to prevent and control occupational diseases, and other health hazards at work, and to promote preventive health services for employees.

Occupation has a significant influence on health, and health has a considerable influence on production. But the value and importance of the everyday practice of occupational health has not yet reached a high state of appreciation. Of the 53 million wage and salary workers in U.S. industry, for example, fewer than 15 million work in establishments with in-plant health services; that is, where a physician and/or nurse is on hand to supply health services. And this is a good record in comparison to most other countries!

The major occupations at which people in the United States now work, as estimated in millions by the U.S. Bureau of Labor Statistics, is about as follows:

Operatives and kindred workers	12,668,000
Clerical and kindred workers	10,564,000
Craftsmen, foremen, and kindred workers	9,283,000
Professional, technical, and kindred workers	7,695,000
Managers, officials, and proprietors (except farm)	7,206,000
Service workers (except private household)	6,978,000
Sales workers	4,344,000
Laborers (except farm and mine)	4,128,000
Farm laborers and foremen	3,082,000
Farmers and farm managers	2,541,000
Private household workers	2,364,000
Total	70,851,000

It is significant to note what a relatively small part of the United States working population is engaged in agriculture—scarcely 5.6 million men and women, or barely 8% of the working population. Again this is in sharp contrast with most of the rest of the world.

The cost in days and dollars of time lost from work as the result of illness and/or accident is appalling. In the United States in 1962, for example, it was calculated that "currently employed" people lost a total of 394 million days from work as the result of illness or accident; and the cost in wages was more than $7 billion! These figures can be put in other ways: On any average working day in 1962 in the United States, 1.3 million working people, or about 2% of all civilian employees, were too sick or disabled to go to work. The number of days lost from work for health reasons in 1962 was more than 20 times as great as the days lost from industrial disputes.

Not all of this time lost can be charged against the industrial environment. Growing problems in health as related to occupation and employment also stem from the changes in the age-composition of the working force. Nevertheless a tremendous amount of investigation of working-environment is still requisite to minimize its hazards. It is not always easy to identify an occupationally related disease; and the mechanisms for reporting and analyzing the incidence and prevalence of such diseases are not yet adequate. Furthermore, rapid technological changes in modern industry are constantly giving rise to new risks and new environmental health problems.

Industry has not shirked its responsibilities. In addition to individual corporate investments in the search for, study of, and elimination of plant hazards, the 4000 + member Industrial Medical Association and the American Industrial Hygiene Association work toward healthier working conditions. Government agencies and departments also play an important role. The Occupational Health and Safety Unit of the U.S. Public Health Service, for example, has established an Occupational Health Information Exchange, a facility that provides for exchange of information on the hazards of industrial products and processes and the methods for their control. This bureau also conducts clinical, environmental, and toxicological studies of factors that might affect the health of workers. It provides technical and consultative services at many levels and generally encourages the development of safe, healthy working conditions.

Occupational Disease—The Historical Conspectus. Medical history, dating back at least to Agricola in the mid-sixteenth century, affords numerous examples of specific, dramatic, and killing occupational diseases that turned out to be caused by one or a small group of environmental factors. In this list we can put such disabling and fatal diseases as lead, mercury, phosphorus, and radium poisoning, tar cancers (e.g. "chimney-sweep's cancer" of the scrotum observed by Sir Percival Pott in the eighteenth century), and silico-tuberculosis. New industrial materials, however, produce new hazards that have to be ferreted out by careful medical and scientific detective work. Except in rare, and really accidental, circumstances, the day of occupational diseases that dramatically kill and maim their victims is probably over. Instead, the working environment may evoke residual diseases and disablements that operate slowly and subtly and may be confused with "normal" processes of aging. The involvement of a given individual may be less, but a great many more people will be involved. Multiple factors, difficult to isolate and demonstrate, will probably each add some burden to the physiology of the exposed worker. Half of today's workers already have some physiological impairment.

With the introduction of labor-saving machinery and automation, heavy physical labor to get the world's work done will decline in importance. This is true even in underdeveloped, largely agricultural areas, where the introduction of even simple farm machinery, long used in technologically advanced countries, saves a tremendous amount of back-breaking physical labor.

On the other hand the psychological stresses on many jobs are increasing and can be expected to continue doing so. As one example, the operators in airport control rooms, plant control rooms, communication centers, and emergency installations are under increasing pressure to handle and interpret masses of incoming information in split-second fashion. Their mental health, which reflects their social environment, is as crucial to their jobs as their physical health. Management will have to become increasingly alert to the evolution of jobs, arising from advancing modern technologies, that would put some men to work under conditions of stress which are beyond the extreme limits of their capacity for adjustment. Jobs must be broken down; men fitted to jobs.

Challenges Ahead in Occupational Health. As with all other fields of environmental health, it is obvious that occupational health is a relatively new endeavor with many challenges ahead. The assignment, difficult to work out in detail, may be simply stated as follows: The future development of occupational health demands (1) a recognition of the environmental factors and potential risks associated with each of the wide variety of human occupations; (2) an appraisal of the favorable and unfavorable factors, and the specific risks, on human health; (3) the working out of means to minimize and eliminate the risks, real or potential, and the unfavorable factors; and (4) the assurance that the available knowledge for promoting and protecting the human factor in industry and agriculture is in fact applied.

Some of the specific challenges that must be met in the future development of occupational health and industrial medicine may be briefly pointed up here:

Evaluation of Trends. Because of the complexity of industrial processes and the changing character of jobs and workers it will be necessary to keep comprehensive and useful records of all trends or developments in industry which might have a health aspect.

Clinical and Epidemiological Studies. A great many "industrial" diseases already recognized still have much to be learned about them. Workers exposed to cotton and other vegetable fibers, to coal dust, to asbestos, to other industrial dusts, to irritant gases, mists, or fumes should be studied—especially to obtain quantitative data of long-term effects of such exposures on the lungs.

Toxicology Studies. There is no *systematic* survey of new materials released to the public—especially by smaller companies. On the other hand many of the larger chemical firms do a considerable amount of study, which should be encouraged. Recent commendable examples are the studies on the toxicology of vanadium, ozone, nitrogen peroxide, fluoride, oil mists, and intermetallic compounds.

Stress Evaluation Studies. More exact measurements, by new methods, must be made of the physiological effort and psychological stress used in work. These processes constitute the basic mechanisms on which the abnormal stresses of the environment operate to produce disease, sometimes by slow but inevitable steps. Effects of heat, climate ("thermal stress"), noise, vibration, and tolerance to chemicals must be investigated.

Monitoring Instruments. There is need for the development of more sensitive monitoring instruments to keep track of various aspects of the physical environment, such as radiant heat, vibration, noise, pressure, and dust counts.

Development of Standards for Working Environment. Determination of the optimal environmental conditions to be recommended for the health, efficient productivity, and possibly "happiness" of the workers is an essential concomitant to the continuing advancement of occupational health programs. Standards mean goals and progress.

Environmental Engineering

Environmental engineering, a relatively new term, may be described as sophisticated sanitary engineering. In a way environmental engineering is the wedding of urban (or metropolitan) planning and "human engineering" to old-fashioned sanitary engineering, whose original responsibilities do not disappear but rather become enlarged. Environmental engineering deals with

problems encountered at each of the four successive levels of public health concern with the environment, enumerated by the American Public Health Association as follows:

1. Insuring the elements of simple survival.
2. Prevention of disease and poisoning.
3. Maintaining an environment suited to man's efficient performance.
4. Preservation of comfort and the enjoyment of living.

Among the challenges which environmental engineering faces are these: more basic knowledge of the effects of *waste* on man, both physical and social effects; more efficient and economic means of water supply, collection, treatment, and distribution; more effective methods of sewage treatment, including onsite disposal; better drainage; more useful and acceptable means for the collection and disposal of garbage and refuse; more healthful housing within the means of those who need it; establishment of health criteria and guidelines for urban renewal, zoning, open space usage, and accident prevention.

The metropolitan factor is the key element in modern environmental engineering. The problems of safeguarding man's life and livelihood, especially in the United States but increasingly so all over the world, stem largely from the fact that modern man wants to live in cities or right next to them, in suburbs. Over 70% of the United States population now lives in urban areas. There are more than 200 Standard Metropolitan Statistical Areas in the United States and the number is increasing annually. Twenty-seven of these metropolitan areas are interstate, including in terms of population the largest such area in the world—the New York City—Northern New Jersey metropolitan area, with an estimated population of 15 million people. Many problems in environmental engineering would be much easier to solve if they were not magnified and complicated by the urban dimensions in which they must be faced.

There are, however, persistent problems in smaller magnitudes. For example: The installation of approximately 300,000 individual sewage

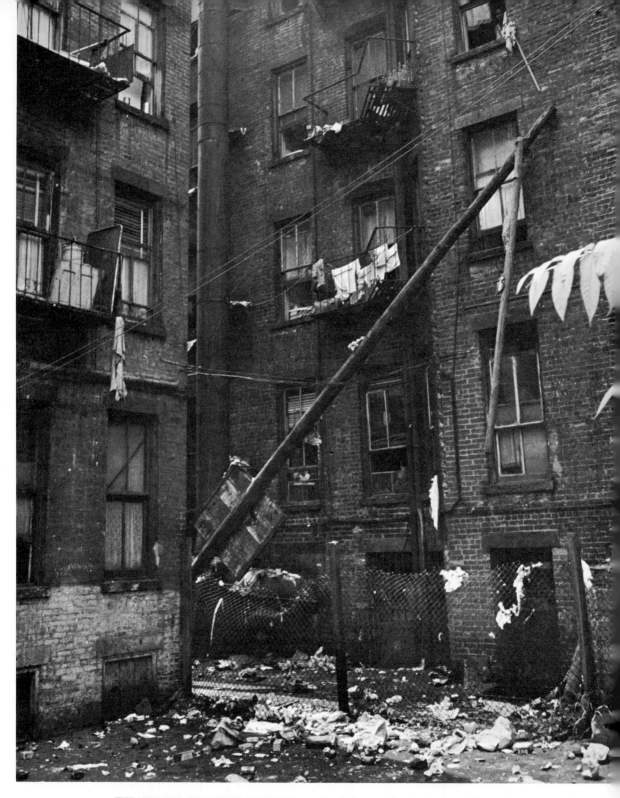

THE NEED FOR HEALTHFUL HOUSING is a major challenge to the community and the environmental engineer. (Photograph by Ken Heyman)

disposal systems every year in suburban and rural areas creates both personal and community health problems. In 90% of the 9000 communities of the United States with populations over 1000, the facilities for refuse disposal are inadequate. To safeguard the health of 1.5 million travelers daily on interstate carriers requires the environmental engineering supervision of the construction, maintenance, and operation of 5000 conveyances and the approval and certification of 4500 sources of water, milk, and food. To be sure that shellfish (produced in 22 states), milk (produced in 40), and certain other foods are free of disease-producing microorganisms and other contaminants when they move in interstate commerce requires an elaborate system of governmental inspection and certification.

The environmental engineer today must be able to handle the problems of environmental health posed by the urbanization and suburbanization of American society. The nature and trend of the population concentration in a given area, the economic and social patterns of these people, their cultural and ethnic traditions, the public and private social institutions with which they live—all these factors enter into the environmental health problems they pose. Consideration of these factors becomes especially important when changes have to be made.

As one example of air pollution, consider Los Angeles. Studies there showed that 69% of the hydrocarbons deposited in the air each day came from automobiles, trucks, and buses. Thus it was obvious that the environmental engineering problem of air pollution is related to commuting habits and patterns, and also to industrial and recreational locations.

New Challenges to Environmental Engineering. Every day brings new challenges to environmental engineering in the area of housing and occupied space, urban and recreational land use, public water supplies from the water-works' intake to the consumer's tap, the accumulation and disposal of solid wastes, the design of safer roads and traffic systems, and many other areas of concern to human safety and welfare. New hazards appear. For example:

Until not so many years ago the principal cleansing agent used in the United States was *soap*. Discharged in waste water, the "used" soap was acted upon by biological agents which changed it into harmless substances that eventually disappeared. Then came detergents. By 1958 people in the United States were using nearly 4 billion pounds of detergents a year. Detergents are discharged to the environment generally by way of drainage to surface or ground waters. The chemicals in them, chiefly the foaming agent which was originally alkyl benzene sulfonate, resist bacteriological and biological decomposition. They passed readily through the usual water and sewage treatment processes. Hence environmental engineers found themselves challenged by the presence of detergents, which had come from great distances, in individual and municipal water supplies.

One approach to this problem has been at the level of "human engineering," persuading and requiring manufacturers of detergents to switch to chemical formulas which decompose more readily under biological action. The members of the Soap and Detergents Association agreed that by January 1, 1966, all alkyl benzene sulfonate would be eliminated from their formulas and products. New "soft" detergents will still not be as decomposable as old-fashioned soap, but they are a great improvement over the hard detergents from a public-health and water-supply point of view.

Other chemical contaminants besides detergents have been occasionally found in public water supplies in recent years. These include such insecticides and pesticides as DDT, aldrin, lindane, dieldrin, diphenyl ether, tetralin, and acetophenone. The new question for environmental engineering that has appeared is whether any of these chemical contaminants are present in water supplies in quantities sufficient to make them potential cancer-producing agents.

The environmental engineer must face these obvious facts: Regardless of political boundaries, air, water, and land resources are fixed. As populations increase, there is less of each for every individual. In some places, especially metropolitan areas, this may create pressures and problems. Increasing populations also mean increasing amounts of waste products (human, agricultural, industrial). Concentrated in and around limited—metropolitan—areas these waste products could eventually choke growth and lead to urban stagnation. The environmental engineer must immediately make plans for the disposal of increasing amounts of waste products.

One of the great practical problems that the environmental engineer faces is to increase the world's supply of potable water. In the final analysis the oceans are the source of virtually all the world's water. They are also a potential source of a great deal larger percentage of the world's food supply than has yet been drawn from them. Chemical processes have been developed for converting fish into odorless, tasteless, nutritious flour; and better methods are being devised for harvesting and converting into human food the billions of microscopic plants and animals—plankton—floating in the seas.

The engineers have gone *directly* to the oceans for increased supplies of fresh water. They have developed large installations to purify seawater. The methods include distillation, freezing and membrane solar distillation. To improve the processes and reduce the costs engineers and chemists are seeking new membrane materials and installing metals, such as titanium and alloys of nickel, which have greater resistance to corrosion. With brackish water the methods used for purification are electrodialysis and solvent extraction. For powering the new desalinization plants, it looks as if nuclear energy will be a practical and economical source of power. The world's (then) largest freeze-desalination plan for the production of "fresh water" was completed at Wrightsville Beach, N.C., in the spring of 1964.

International Quarantine. Quarantine—40-day detention of a vessel suspected of carrying plague—was introduced at Italian seaports in the fourteenth century. This was probably one of the most important concepts and techniques of public and environmental health ever invented. Note that the restriction was put upon a *premise*—the suspected vessel—and not directly upon people. The practice of international (and local) quarantine, with changes based on improved medical knowledge, advances in communication and modes of transportation, and greatly increased numbers of travelers remains part of the environmental health program of every nation. The object of the programs is to prevent the introduction into and the spread throughout the country of quarantinable diseases or any other illnesses that present a significant threat to the public health. The International Sanitary Regulations and the operations of the World Health Organization simplify the everyday practice of international quarantine. It is practiced more diligently and faithfully in some countries than in others. We shall use the figures and practices of the United States as representative of international quarantine.

The increase in international travel, especially in the volume and speed of air transport, has intensified quarantine problems. Medical inspections of arriving aliens continue to increase as a result of more travel for business and pleasure, exchange programs, and immigration, as permitted. There are medical aspects of immigration legislation. The examination *abroad* of alien applicants for visas, who number nearly 200,000 a year, requires the direct services of the U.S. Public Health Service or the supervision of local physicians.

Medical examinations are also required of all the other aliens, something over 3 million a year, who enter the United States. Over 300,000 migratory farm laborers in addition are examined at U.S. Reception Centers near the Mexican border. Where necessary, a smallpox vaccination is given.

The U.S. Foreign Quarantine Service carries out authorized inspection and vaccination programs covering people and certain imports at various points of entry into the country. The object is to prevent the introduction of quarantinable or certain other communicable diseases. Insect and rodent control programs are conducted on ships and airplanes in port areas. A ship sanitation program is also carried out. The headquarters office of the foreign quarantine service collects, analyzes, and disseminates data on worldwide communicable disease prevalence and immunity requirements.

The magnitude of the foreign quarantine service can be seen from these figures for a recent year. Over 400 ports of entry ("points of coverage") were covered. More than 65,000 aircraft inspections were performed and in about one-third of the cases (nearly 20,000) the aircraft were treated for insects. About 33,000 ship inspections were performed. The number of individuals inspected on aircraft was about 2.7 million, on vessels about 2 million, on land via the Mexican border about 1.4 million.

International quarantine as practiced by the United States and other countries is the direct, and largely successful, attempt to keep the diseases prevalent in one environment out of another.

SUMMARY

Environmental health is one of the most significant new fields of scientific endeavor, but it is not yet an exactly defined science. Environmental health and medicine represent man's old and new efforts to control all those factors in his environment which may "exercise a deleterious effect on his physical, mental, or social well-being." Environmental health originated in the much narrower field of environmental sanitation; but today it seeks to attack all the important hazards arising out of man's physical, biological, social (and even ideological) environments.

Specifically, the practitioners of environmental health and medicine today are concerned with the new pollutions of air, water, and food (more fully discussed in the following chapter); the dangers of pesticides and ionizing radiation (delineated in the final chapter); the problems of occupational diseases and industrial medicine, such as the effects of poisons (toxicology) and psychological stresses; the new techniques of an expanded field of environmental engineering, wherein one day the engineer may be called upon to build a new sewage system and the next to design a plant for extracting fresh water from sea water; and the manifold challenges of world health, which demand the operation of efficient international quarantine services. Environmental health may also be taken to include the areas of safety engineering (e.g. highway design) and consumer health (e.g. plans and costs of new hospitals and health facilities).

In the new concept of environmental health, whatever directions it may take, all human activities should be reviewed, revised, and planned on the twin premises that they (1) must not harm and (2) should contribute to human health and welfare.

SUMMARY REVIEW QUESTIONS

1. In what three environments does modern civilized man exist? In which of these three have the greatest changes occured in the twentieth century? What are some of these changes and their underlying causes?
2. What is the range of environmental health as we understand it today? What are some of the most important problems (name at least six) with which environmental health and medicine must presently grapple? What are some of the environmental health problems now emerging with which we shall have to deal more vigorously in the future?

3. How do you interpret the phrase, "the rediscovery of the environment"? What events of the eighteenth and nineteenth century are partially, if not largely, responsible for the twentieth century's environmental health problems?

4. On what basis must public health authorities and many other professionals concerned with environmental health make wise and rational choices of programs to improve environmental health conditions? What factors of location will strongly influence priorities in choices of programs?

5. In what ways may work or occupation injure or endanger health? Can you give some specific examples (at least three) of occupational diseases and tell how they were brought on?

6. What are some of the specific challenges that must be met by safety engineers, industrial physicians, business management, government experts, and others in the future development of the fields of occupational health and industrial medicine? Where is the most attention paid to providing adequate protective measures for workers? The least attention?

7. What are some (name at least four) of the major problems and challenges in the field of environmental engineering? For what purposes have the environmental engineers gone to the oceans?

8. What present-day factors have magnified the problems of international quarantine? What is the purpose of international quarantine? How, briefly, does the United States operate its foreign quarantine service?

9. Are the following statements sense or nonsense? Why? *Dirt is dangerous. . . . The right to work means the right to work safely. . . . The twentieth century has set the welfare of the human race as its goal. . . . It is always easy to get people to do what is good for them. . . . The world's supply of potable water is in danger of running out.*

10. What do the following terms mean to you: urbanization, environmental sanitation, toxicology, topography, monitoring instruments, thermal stress, detergent, the "sanitary awakening," desalinization, "industrial revolution"?

Worth Looking Into: *Man In His Environment,* proceedings of the Fifth International Conference on Health and Health Education, Philadelphia, 1962. *Environmental Health Problems,* report of a committee to the Surgeon General of the United States Public Health Service. *A History of Public Health* by George Rosen, M.D. *The "Shattuck Report,"* report of the Sanitary Commission of Massachusetts, 1850, by Lemuel Shattuck. For more complete references, see Appendix E.

Men like gods . . .?

Environment and Personality

William G. Mather

The relationship of environmental health and human personality is a very poorly defined field in which to browse....

We are aware that certain occupations, for example, have certain physical and mental effects upon the people that pursue them. We may mention the "miner's disease", silicosis, and its effect upon the lung. There is also the miner's attitude toward work—that working and mining are the same, so that a non-mining job is no job at all . . .

We are aware that certain ills have certain types of personality associated with them, almost like diagnostic symptoms: the moody irritability of the diabetic, the worried tenseness of the prossessor of an enlarged prostrate gland, and the detached euphoria of the smoker of marijuana, for examples. That there are environmentally induced, or emphasized, personality effects we know. That they can be neatly identified and classified and assigned specific treatments, we do not know. Our evidence is confused....

Let us begin with our story of the Hay River fishing village and the New Jersey Bar Mitzvah party. [An outbreak of food poisoning in Edison, N.J., traced last year to the Canadian Northwest, with salmonella java the culprit.] Only a group of trained public health workers would have the imagination and the skill to trace that illness to the whitefish, and the whitefish through the channels of trade to the place where the Hay River empties into the Great Slave Lake. So far, it is kept within the family, so to speak.

But this is not an infrequent thing. More and more such incidents are being reported in the daily papers. The Chesapeake Bay was named in a recent dispatch in the New York Times as a possible source of danger to health due to the infection of its fish with germs from man as its in-flowing rivers traverse heavily populated areas. Thus, the fish would become carriers of disease from man to man. Antibodies to such human disease as paratyphoid, pseudo-tuberculosis, bacillary dysentery and other varieties of misery were found in white perch caught in the Bay.

There was Rachel Carson's *Silent Spring,* that shocked the general public to the dangers of careless use of pesticides; and that has been followed by Earl Murphy's *Governing Nature,* which suggests that the Creator could have made a better choice of a gamekeeper for the Garden of Eden. And there is a rather massive volume that has come from a sober seminar of the American Association for the Advancement of Science, *Agriculture and the Quality of Our Environment,* in which thirty-six scientists discuss the deleterious effects of air, water, and soil pollution on plants and animals, including that present day creation of man's genius, radionuclide contamination.

Now, man's environment never was wholly favorable to him, but in earlier days it was visible, close at hand, to be engaged in close range combat. The source of contagion was in the neighborhood, not thousands of miles away among a

SOURCE. Dr. William G. Mather is Research Professor of Sociology in the Department of Sociology and Anthropology at the Pennsylvania State University, at University Park. The article presented here is taken from a talk given before the First Colonial Health Conference of Sanitarians in May 1968. This version appeared in May-June 1968, issue of the *Health Officer's News Digest.*

people unheard of. The danger in the atmosphere was only rain, hail, snow, and possibly strange demons and beasties. For both the illness and the demons man had spells and herbs which we smile at now—but at least they were things to do with his hands, and to give him confidence. False confidence, but confidence just the same.

What environmental disease control efforts do to us today is to scare us. We keep our neighborhood clean and respectable and our kitchen sanitary, and then are laid low by some salmonella java—whatever they are—from some Canuck town a thousand miles from nowhere. We make plans to escape nuclear fall-out by retreating to the peaceful, out-of-the-way coves of our native Ozark Mountains, only to read that it happens to have an unusually heavy dosage of that not-so-gentle rain.

John Doe today feels that he stands naked in a world with no hiding places left. This is not good for man. It makes him feel incompetent, frustrated, lacking in self-respect, the possessor of an inadequate personality. It is not that he knows "he cannot win them all", it has become a question whether he can win any.

Men Like Gods

We have spoken of the fear and the frustration that have come to our society with the discovery of the expansion of our ecosystem, and of the destruction that walks in the noon of our success. There is another effect of the impact of our invironmental problems upon us, and it is almost the opposite of these.

In its lowest form it is the naive assumption that "something will turn up" to save us from our own folly. In its highest form, it is the conviction that we have everything under control, that we are the ultimate among the species of life on our planet, that we have conquered and arrived, have eaten of both the tree of knowledge and the tree of life, and become like Gods . . .

The truth is, a good many of us are not going to handle the problem raised by our advancing knowledge in general and that of environmental health in particular. At the present time our environment is producing many people unable to meet problems and solve them. These people have a tendency to strike out blindly and cover up or run away from responsible problem-solving in the health field.

We could mention that on the average one person from every three homes will at some time need treatment for a disabling mental disorder. We could mention that suicide is the second leading cause of death among college students (accident is the first). We could mention the mixing of alcohol with driving, which seems to be a factor in most automobile accidents involving fatality. We could mention the rising addiction to drugs of various types, now frankly popular as a way of "dropping out" from the troubles of modern life.

But all of these indicate the apparent present inability of our society to produce the kind of personality that can successfully cope with the totality of our environment. In other words, at a time when our problems are great and our knowledge is also great, at a time when we need men like gods, we are producing men like boys.

Environmental health today is far more than restaurant sanitation and garbage disposal. Hay River and Edison, New Jersey, are on the same planet, in the same hemisphere of that planet, on the same continent, and once in man's early days were bedded under the same sheet of glacial ice. The whole earth, in fact, is one great public health district now. Bacteria are contemptuous of national boundaries, and viruses have no racial prejudice. If we bury our heads in the sand on these matters, the rest of our bodies will soon follow them into the grave.

Now, while we have some natural resources remaining; now while we have the knowledge and the skill; now, while there is still a little sand in the hour-glass; now, our species must decide whether it will stand up and live like "man the wise," or mingle its bones in Mother Earth with those "lower" forms of life and be succeeded by some other animal that can adapt to the new environment which we have created, where we have failed.

Benefits of Space Program to Medicine

... **there** is no question about the fact that the space programme is helping medicine become more efficient in providing care for people. Medical research carried out in the course of the space programme has, for example, played a major role in providing computer programmes for recording and retrieving medical data. In 1950, getting medical research data for the simplest clinical survey took hours, if not days. Today, a computer can retrieve the same information in a matter of minutes, and can evaluate the data in several more minutes. Within five years, data will be available indicating the best therapy for most common diseases, thus improving medical care and saving thousands upon thousands of hospital manhours now lost through inefficiency.

One of the greatest bottlenecks in hospital care is laboratory procedures. As knowledge of body chemistry continues to grow, demands on hospital laboratories grow apace. The space programme has already made available automatic techniques for many evaluations of body chemistry, which save time and manpower, and reduce the possibility of human error.

The space programme has even contributed towards easing the nursing shortage. Bio-instrumentation developed in the course of space medical research can automatically record such basic measurements as temperature, respiration, pulse rate, blood pressure, electrocardiogram (ECG) and even electroencephalogram (EEG). It is also interesting to note that space research has been responsible for the development of computer ECG and EEG assessment, a technique far more efficient than the present visual inspection.

Space medical research has also been responsible for a number of important developments in the field of radiation.

One of the most fascinating applications of space research in medicine lies in the use of computer techniques, developed for improving the quality of lunar and planetary photographs, for enhancing the quality of x-ray pictures of patients. Results already achieved through this x-ray enhancement technique have been astonishing.

There are many other examples of such space spin-offs. Hearing aids have been developed which use closed-loop body currents for power, thus eliminating the need for conventional batteries. The "miniscope," a pocket oscilloscope a doctor can carry on his person and use to monitor the heart action of patients who have drowned or been seriously injured in accidents, is already available.

One example of space medical research which could have a significant economic as well as sociological effect in the future deals with human Circadian rhythms, or the so-called "biological clock." The question is whether man can function efficiently during long space flights, in the course of which there would be no night or day and periods for work, rest and sleep would be arbitrarily selected.

The problem was well summarized in an experiment at the Max Planck Institute in Germany, where three men were isolated in underground bunker cells with no clocks and no artificial daily schedules. At the end of 30 days, one of the men was having lunch at the same time another man was eating dinner and the third was sitting down to have his next day's breakfast!

Commercial airlines are aware of the problem and schedule their pilots' flights in accordance with the Circadian cycle.

SOURCE. From *Space Science and Technology: Benefits to Developing Countries*, on the United Nations Conference on the Exploration and Peaceful Uses of Outer Space, held in Vienna, 1968. United Nations, 1968.

There have also been a number of instances in which specific techniques or equipment developed in the course of space research have been used in medicine. Space miniaturization techniques, for example, have been used in transmitters for cardiac sensors; sterilization methods used to prevent planetary contamination have been carried over into surgical rooms; and an air bearing designed for a rocket guidance system has been adapted for use in a ballistocardiograph that floats a man, free from all vibration, while his heart-beat is measured.

Examples of equipment developed in the course of space medical research which are now being used in medicine would include spray-on electrodes, developed for instrumenting pilots and astronauts under vigorous performance conditions, and now used by patients even when they do exercise; a new titanium alloy used in the manufacture of artificial hip and elbow joints which developed out of a need for a more durable material for use in mechanical bearings that must function under space conditions; and the sight switch, actuated only by voluntary movement of the eyes, adapted for use in a motorized wheel chair which can be controlled by a paraplegic, without any body or limb movements.

Somewhat farther in the future, perhaps, but still of considerable interest, is the possibility of using the space environment for therapeutic purposes. Environmental factors such as gravity cannot be controlled in today's bio-medical facilities, and it has not been determined what effect gravity has on various operations and recovery procedures.

The space environment offers an almost ideal opportunity for biological and medical research. The leading environmental characteristic is weightlessness, but space also provides an opportunity for reducing weight below that on the surface of earth and of varying the g-level between zero and one.

Since many human systems are particularly gravity sensitive, physicians have speculated on what the effects of reduced gravity conditions might have on circulatory, skeletal, muscular or metabolic diseases or illnesses. In the case of heart disease, for example, the general opinion is that confinement in a gravity-free or low-gravity environment might prove beneficial. (See page 497.)

22

IMPACT OF THE NEW POLLUTIONS

ONE MEASURE OF THE PROGRESS OF CIVIL-ization might be the progressive removal of hazards from the environment of mankind—physical, biological, psychological, social, and even ideational hazards. We might say, for example, that the ideational hazard of "the divine right of kings" was removed in the eighteenth century, the biological hazard of infectious diseases minimized in the twentieth century.

Historically we can observe an almost fantastic progress in environmental health and medicine from the middle of the nineteenth century to the middle of the twentieth century. It is reflected, among other ways, in the tremendous increases in longevity and life expectancy in the technically and scientifically advanced countries of the globe.

Then, in the middle of the twentieth century, we see a new cloud rising on the horizon. It is a cloud of pollutions; and it is beginning to shadow over some of the bright progress of environmental health and medicine. In many respects it comes as a surprise, an unwelcome surprise. We suddenly find that parts of our environment which we long judged safe and clean and pure are not so. They are polluted, contaminated, distorted. As responsible, intelligent twentieth-century students we cannot run away from the impact of these new pollutions. Indeed we must help to dispel them.

There are three old elements in our environment which now, suddenly, in the mid-twentieth century we discover to be newly polluted and contaminated: air, water, and food. We also come face to face with two major new contami-nants: man-made radioactivity and pesticides. The individual who wants to promote and protect his own personal health and contribute to the improvement of community health must realistically know what hazards he faces in the presence of these five new major risks in his environment: (1) air pollution, (2) water pollution, (3) food contamination, (4) pesticides, and (5) radioactivity. We shall provide a full, up-to-date discussion of these five major topics (and a few more related ones) in this and the next chapter.

The impact of the new pollutions is strong. But it is not necessarily fatal. An intelligent attitude toward these new hazards is to listen and learn where the danger really lies; then to take steps as an individual and a citizen to avoid and help reduce it.

Air Pollution

To sustain his life man needs on the average $4\frac{1}{2}$ pounds of water, 2 to 3 pounds of food, and 30 pounds of air, day in day out. He has some choice of food and drink, but he must breathe whatever air is available to him; and in cities, this may well be partially polluted or unclean. The occurrence over the years of several clear-cut air pollution disasters, with out-breaks of sickness and death associated with air pollution, has indicated that this problem, growing in importance, must be faced.

Possibly the first recorded air pollution disaster occurred in the Meuse Valley of Belgium, in 1930, where many people died. In the United

461

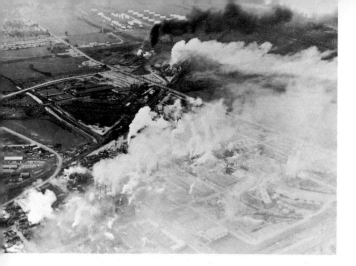

AIR POLLUTION. Smoke from industrial plants and processes is one of the major factors causing smog. (Photograph courtesy of National Air Pollution Administration)

States an air pollution tragedy occurred at Donora, Pennsylvania, in October 1948. Industrial waste so befouled the atmosphere that day was like night; 5000 people fell ill; 17 died. London, England, has reported at least two occasions—December 1952 and December 1962—when it was so blanketed by grime and soot that thousands of "extra deaths" occurred and had to be charged to the occasion.

Far more common than the disasters are the annoyances brought to many cities by their air pollution and smog problems. Los Angeles has suffered from an annoying smog problem for a number of years. One factor in the problem arises from its location, because the mountains east of the coastal plains keep banks of air piled up over the city and county. Under these, man-made pollutants collect from a populous and industrialized city. The Air Pollution Control District of Los Angeles estimates that gasoline-driven vehicles in the county pollute the air daily with 1180 tons of hydrocarbons, 300 tons of nitrogen oxides, and 8950 tons of carbon monoxide. Factories, refineries, and even backyard incinerators contribute to the smoky air pollution.

Speaking at the American Medical Association Congress on Environmental Health in May 1964, S. Smith Griswold, Los Angeles County air pollution control officer, said of the situation there: "We have a basic understanding of what is polluting our atmosphere. . . . Potentially we have the ability to assure an acceptable standard of air quality. . . . Ignorance and apathy are the real limitations upon the control of air pollution. A community endures air pollution because it lacks leadership and the will to act."

Some of the contaminants in fresh air, which is approximately 78% nitrogen and 21% oxygen, can be visualized as soot, dust, and smoke. There are, however, other contaminants that do not make themselves visible or even smellable. Some of these are the combustion products of gasoline; they intermingle in the atmosphere, and in the presence of sunlight they may form unknown aerosols. This complex chemical mixture, sometimes called synthetic or photochemical smog, seems to pose some menace to health.

Meteorological factors sometimes play a role in bringing about air contamination. Generally speaking, the movement of the great masses of air above us is sufficient to replace stagnant air with fresh air. On occasions, however, these currents fail. Masses of air hover motionless for hours and days and accumulate high concentrations of pollutants. Most serious, usually, is a thermal inversion, in which a layer of warm air forms and acts as a lid over the colder air, which is prevented from dissipating its waste products in the usual manner.

Health and Polluted Air. The studies that were made in London and Donora left evidence that acute air pollution is a serious threat to health, particularly to the health of elderly people who have recently suffered from heart or lung ailments. While direct cause-and-effect relationship between contaminated air and disease has not been shown, nevertheless, there is strong evidence that air pollution is associated with a number of respiratory ailments. Among these are non-specific infectious upper respiratory diseases ("the common cold"), chronic bronchitis, chronic constrictive ventilatory disease, pulmonary emphysema, bronchial asthma, and lung cancer.

Much of the cleansing of the larger airway passages of the lungs is done by ciliary action; little hair-like projections (cilia) with a whip-like motion sweep the larger irritants out of the lung. It has been shown experimentally that this important, protective ciliary action can be slowed down by such air contaminants as sulfur dioxide and synthetic smog. Hence when concentrations of irritants build up in the lungs they must be removed by coughing; other symptoms of respiratory difficulty may soon follow.

Another problem in the air pollution field is that of long-term breathing of only "slightly" polluted air. What will happen if this goes on for 10 to 20 years? The general conviction is that long-term, low-level air pollution can contribute to and aggravate certain diseases. The report of the Panel on Health Considerations at the 1962 National Conference on Air Pollution stated:

It would be a mistake to leave this conference with the impression that there is insufficient evidence for action—now. The evidence that air pollution contributes to the pathogenesis of chronic respiratory disease is overwhelming. The classical concept of one agent being responsible for one disease . . . is an investigational convenience.

An Official U.S. Government Study: Summary. In September 1963 a study of air pollution in the United States was published as a staff report to the Committee on Public Works of the United States Senate. The following summary of this report [1] gives a clear picture of why our problem of air pollution is becoming more serious:

The rapid deterioration of the quality of our air has reached the point at which more effective control measures can no longer be postponed. To underline this point, research continues to provide new evidence that air pollution is objectionable, not only for its esthetic and nuisance effects, which we can see and smell, and its economic damages, which are more varied and costly than we had supposed, but also because of its hazards to health and safety.

Pollution is increasing faster than our population increases, because our rising standard of living results

[1] A Study of Pollution—Air, a staff report to the Committee on Public Works, United States Senate (88th Congress, 1st Session). (Washington, D.C.: U.S. Government Printing Office, September 1963).

in greater consumption of energy and goods per person, and our production and transportation activities increase on both accounts.

Technical procedures are available which can prevent the discharge of most contaminants to the air. The application of some of these procedures involves considerable cost. However, failure to use them is now costing the public far more in economic damages, even aside from the nuisances and hazards to health associated with air pollution.

Despite the lack of satisfactory answers to certain specific problems, such as motor vehicle pollution and sulfur oxides from fossil fuels, a significant reduction of pollution from most of our problem sources is now possible through widespread application of proven control principles.

In this country, we have only begun to attack air pollution realistically. The Federal program of research and technical assistance has defined important facets of the problem and provided guidance to States and communities in assessing the nature of their local problem and demonstrating remedial measures.

One-third of the States have established programs to deal with air pollution, but most of these are, so far, quite limited in scope. Local government programs, where they exist, are generally understaffed and without sufficient financial and trained manpower resources to meet their needs properly. Only 34 local programs have annual budgets exceeding $25,000 and 7 of these are in California. . . . In the past decade, despite a 30% increase in urban population, there has been, outside of California, no overall increase in manpower to combat air pollution at the local level.

It has been estimated that in 1961 major air pollution problems existed in 308 urban places. This represents an increase of 84 in a decade. About 7300 places, housing 60% of the population, are confronted with air pollution problems of one kind or another.

The American public looks forward to a growing population, an expanding economy, and an improving state of well-being. Essential to this is clean air. To compensate for past neglect of air quality conservation, a greater effort is required now, by the public, by industry, and by governmental agencies at all levels. The nationwide character of the air pollution problem requires an adequate Federal program to lend assistance, support, and stimulus to State and community programs.

There is a need for the establishment of air quality standards in terms of known and suspected effects on what is necessary for the protection of human health and welfare, agriculture and property.

A number of States do not have air pollution control laws; others have laws which have control authority only, or no control authority, but local option legislation and research and technical assistance authority.

It is quite evident that an aggressive program of research needs to be directed toward providing assistance in developing appropriate State and local air pollution control laws and standards. There is also a need for nationwide enforcement and standards and in addition consideration needs to be given to the international aspect of air pollution.

An International Union of Air Pollution Associations was formed with United States leadership in June, 1964.

The question of air pollution is of greatest concern to residents of large metropolitan and highly industrialized areas, such as the cities of New York, Los Angeles, Philadelphia, and London. With the increasing urbanization of the globe this is becoming a more widespread problem, and its very existence often dictates individual choices of places of residence.

Air pollution occurs wherever industries, cities, and masses of people, moving around in automobiles and otherwise, come together. There are some special cases, such as pollution by volcanic smokes and dusts, as seen in Costa Rica in 1963 and 1964. Air pollution in cities, as we have noted, is usually the result of the emission of a *number* of different gases and particles, notably factory or household smoke and automobile exhausts. It is probable that all metropolitan areas have some limit on their air resources. When and where weather conditions are favorable to dispersal of contaminants, air resources are greater. But even in favored metropolitan areas, acceptable concentration limits of pollutants are sometimes exceeded.

Air pollution affects human life and health and a great many other human interests and activities. We have noted tragic examples in Donora, Pennsylvania, and in London, England. We have also cited increasing evidence that prolonged exposure to even low-level air pollution may aggravate chronic diseases (e.g. bronchitis) which affect large numbers of people. Polluted air also causes enormously costly damage to crops, animals, and buildings.

Some Unresolved Questions About Air Pollution. Hosts of unresolved questions about air pollution remain. To gain perspective on the problem it will be worthwhile to examine a sampling of the observations that have been made and the further lines of research they suggest.

Statistical studies have indicated a higher incidence of lung cancer in urban than in rural areas. The air in cities has been found to contain certain known cancer-producing (carcinogenic) substances, notably benzpyrene. It has therefore been suspected that benzpyrene and related hydrocarbons (aromatic, polycyclic hydrocarbons) in the atmosphere may contribute to the causation of lung cancer. It has been shown that experimental animals exposed both to the virus of influenza and inhalation of ozonized gasoline develop epidermoid cancers in the lung. All this information suggests further investigation; it does not provide definite answers.

Since the respiratory tract is the portal of entry for inhaled substances, diseases of this tract are suspected of being made worse by air pollutants. For example, it has been observed that asthmatic attacks occur more frequently on days when there is smog damage to plants; that patients with emphysema (enlarged air sacs) improve when they breathe filtered air after exposure to several days of smog; and that the condition of patients with chronic, obstructive respiratory disease fluctuates with certain air pollutant levels.

The famous song, "Smoke Gets in Your Eyes," may be taken as common evidence of the effects of atmospheric pollutants on the eyes. Smog is another well-known irritant of the eyes; but exactly which constituents of smog have this effect remain to be discovered. Smog is sometimes described as *photochemical* air pollution; that is, the gases and other particulate matter in the atmosphere are altered by the presence of sunlight. This also is a subject for more research.

As cities increase in size, new industries develop and new products are created, the chances are that the problem of air pollution will get worse instead of better in the next generations unless it is vigorously attacked now. Since air pollution, despite its predilection for cities, follows no political boundaries, the over-all attack on it must be organized cooperatively and on a comparatively broad basis. Certainly in the United States there is a role for the federal government.

Practical Attacks on Air Pollution

Some complex research problems must precede the application of new techniques to the control of air pollution. We must, for example, have more knowledge of the interreactions of pollutants in the atmosphere; we must know more about their synergistic (heightened) effect on physical and biological systems; we need better instruments—automatic instrumentation —to find out these other things.

In addition to research efforts, though including them, the present attack on air pollution should embrace the following steps:

¶We must more accurately and completely *appraise* present and potential air-pollution levels in specific localities. This would be mapping the problem and showing the danger points.

¶Local communities must be encouraged and stimulated to participate in *air-pollution abatement.* This may require administrative or legal action, such as industrial zoning, enforcement of nuisance ordinances, or even planning to limit the number of people in some geographic areas.

¶We must *improve methods* and instruments for continuous recording of air pollutants in the more heavily affected geographic localities.

¶We must make more complete and accurate *analyses of weather* conditions on a large scale and correlate them with data on air pollution in specific areas.

¶We must find ways to promote *interjurisdictional agreements* on the control of air pollution, so that touching or distant communities can get together in the solution of the problems that affect all, but that none can solve alone.

In the United States the federal government entered the field of air pollution relatively recently. The first legislation empowering the U.S. Public Health Service to deal with the field as a single entity, in focus, dates back only to 1955. Since then it has been more readily recognized, and translated into laws and appropriations, that air is a national resource we cannot squander.

"Let's Clear the Air": A National Conference. A national conference on air pollution under the title, "Let's Clear The Air," was held in Washington, D.C., in December 1962, under the auspices of the U.S. Public Health Service. On this occasion, Luther L. Terry, Surgeon General of the Public Health Service, said:

The filters in air-sampling devices throughout the country are still coming out black or gray. I am not discouraged, however, for we have reached agreement on a fundamental principle: that it is every man's right to breathe air which is not a hazard to his health or property and that this right must take precedence over a great number of lesser rights, real or imagined. . . .

While everyone cannot be expected to possess detailed knowledge of every aspect of air pollution, it is essential that virtually everyone have a basic understanding of the problem. This understanding is needed by the business man when he plans the design and location of a new factory, by the city council member when he is faced with the task of zoning a city or determining the flow of traffic, by the physician when he treats a patient with respiratory disease and by countless others.

An interesting observation on the variety and complexity of the problem was offered by S. Smith Griswold, control officer of the Air Pollution Control District of the County of Los Angeles, California (whom we have quoted before), as follows:

We have found that few communities have the same total air pollution problem. In Los Angeles 80% of our problem is motor vehicle emission; 20% comes from industry and other sources. In neighboring San Francisco, the problem is approximately 60% vehicular and 40% industrial. In Los Angeles we burn no coal and relatively little fuel oil; in Pittsburgh coal burning was once the major source of air pollution. In Los Angeles our air is very stable; we have light winds and low inversions. In Chicago and Cleveland the winds are brisk and inversions rarely a problem.

Despite the overall dissimilarity, the individual components of the problem are similar and the same correctives may be applied wherever those components are important. A steel furnace in Pittsburgh can be controlled in the same manner as a similar one in Los Angeles. A catalytic [petroleum] cracker in New Jersey can be controlled in the same degree as one in San Francisco.

Crankcase and Exhaust Devices for Automobiles. A statement by letter, from Edmund G. Brown, then governor of the state of California, called attention to the positive and pioneering efforts being made in this state, thus:

In 1959 the State department of public health adopted standards for the amounts of hydrocarbons and carbon monoxide which could be put into the air by the State's present car population. Our goal is to return air in California to 1940 quality. Following this the State legislature, through a special call in 1960, created the Motor Vehicle Pollution Control Board, a 13-man agency, serving without compensation, to test and certify emission control devices.

The board has, to date, certified 15 crankcase emission devices for factory installation. It has approved the principle of these devices for used cars. . . . More than a million cars in our State now have crankcase devices and when another 6 million car owners install them, we shall see a significant reduction in that source of pollution.

The governor's letter also indicated that progress was being made with exhaust control devices, a more complex engineering problem. These tailpipe or afterburner devices are aimed at eliminating 65% of all hydrocarbons and most of the carbon monoxide.

Wolfgang E. Meyer, chairman of a conference panel on "The Automobile, the Truck, and the Bus," confirmed the fact that the automotive engineers and industry had successfully resolved the crankcase emission problem. He pointed, however, to several other problems, among them, the diesel engine. He said:

The diesel engine differs from the gasoline engine in that it uses less volatile fuels, that it operates at higher air-fuel ratios, and that it employs different fuel supply and ignition means. These as well as other factors account for important differences in the combustion process and consequently in exhaust emissions. Diesel exhaust is lower in hydrocarbons and carbon monoxide than that of gasoline engines, but slightly higher in oxides of nitrogen. . . .

Diesel engines, however, present a more serious problem with regard to smoke and odor as compared to gasoline engines. Properly maintained and adjusted diesel engines emit, at their worst, only very faint smoke. The black diesel exhaust smoke that justly causes complaints and concern can be controlled by scrupulous maintenance and retention of the factory adjustment of the fuel system. The causes of diesel odor have not yet been identified conclusively and therefore control methods are still lacking.

Political Aspect to Air Pollution. Despite the generally favorable reception at the national conference to the idea of "clean air," it is fair to note that caution was expressed and even some objection to putting all the recommended practices into effect. A "go-slow" attitude may be expected from those to whom air pollution control will be costly or from those on whose political toes it will step. There is a political aspect to the application of air-pollution control measures.

In a layman's viewpoint on the national conference, Howard K. Smith, well-known radio and television news commentator, touched on the political aspects. He quoted a telegram from the American Medical Association which said in part: "Believing that air pollution can and should be controlled, the American Medical Association endorses the concept of local, State, and Federal joint enterprise." Mr. Smith said he found "great stress on the idea that local government has the primary responsibility for air pollution control." But he asked:

When it comes to air pollution, what is local? An airplane pilot, on the first day of your sessions, talked of seeing the smudge from many cities blending together in a cloud which covered parts of several states. "The wind bloweth where it listeth" and our jurisdictional lines traced on the surface of the earth have little relevance. . . .

Man has within his grasp the control of his environment. Sometimes haltingly, sometimes grudgingly he controls it for the benefit of the greatest number. You who are dealing with the most basic commodity of all are riding the crest of an irresistible wave. We are going to clear the air. Let's clear it now.[2]

Water

Water is essential to human existence; hence most civilizations have been founded where there was an adequate water supply. With increasing world population, increasing water supplies are necessary. The usual water sources are rivers, lakes, wells, dams, and the like. With modern sanitary engineering these have generally been kept as safe sources of water for human consumption. Another phase of environmental engineering has been given over to the sanitary disposal of human and other wastes, so that they do not contaminate the sources of drinking water. Great progress has been made in providing pure water supplies for most urban communities in the United States.

At the 1964 American Medical Association Congress on Environmental Health, Dr. Charles L. Wilbar, Jr., of Harrisburg, Pa., said:

In the minds of some people, including some legislators, it seems that public health aspects of water pollution are being overshadowed by the need to keep the water pure for recreational, industrial, and agricultural purposes. . . . It would seem to me that physicians need also be interested in these aspects of water pollution control while remembering the primary importance of keeping water clean for health purposes.

Since 1900 fresh-water use in the United States has jumped eightfold—from around 40 billion to 325 billion gallons a day. By 1980 it

[2]*National Conference on Air Pollution Proceedings,* (December 10–12, 1962), Public Health Service Publication 1022; Washington, D.C.: U.S. Department of Health, Education, and Welfare, 1963. (For sale by the Superintendent of Documents, U.S. Government Printing Office, Washington 25, D.C., $2.75, 436 pages.)

is estimated that water needs will increase to 600 billion gallons a day—almost equal to the total fresh-water supply in sight. Under these circumstances water will have to be treated for re-use and re-used liberally. Conversion of sea water to fresh, potable water may become a necessity.

The United States has been generally fortunate in its water resources. However, with the rapidly increasing American population and the increased need for water in normal industrial production practices, a new look at America's water reserves, and how she will handle them, is justified. In the 1960's the United States had about 325 billion gallons of water available a day. Through conservation measures it is anticipated that this can be built to 600 billion gallons a day by 1980. If water use doubles from 1980 to the year 2000, it is difficult to see where the extra gallonage is coming from.

As water re-use becomes increasingly necessary, the key factor is *water quality.* This means that pollution wastes will have to be treated at their sources so they do not pollute waters that must be re-used. Improved treatment methods are being tried, because the fact is that there is already a considerable amount of water that could be used over and over again if a means could be found to remove the small but important amount of dissolved materials remaining after subjection to currently available treatment.

An unprecedented population and economic growth in the United States is demanding more water. Industry, the largest user of water, will need twice as much as is presently used by 1980. Those who use it for irrigation, municipal water supplies, and recreation will also be demanding more water. The increasing discharge of pollutants diminishes suitable water supply and hence contributes to the increasing water demands.

The Water Pollution Problem. In the 1880's water pollution made headlines when typhoid and cholera epidemics struck some cities. These diseases were discovered to be carried by waterborne bacteria. It was further discovered, then, that the city's water supply could be rendered safe by purification techniques, such as filtration and chlorination.

For four generations, now, city-dwellers and their suburban friends have been taking pure, safe drinking water for granted. "Just turn on the tap." But the situation is changing. Polluted, dirty water is causing a new and still not completely defined peril to human health. Every glass of water from the faucet is not necessarily clean and potable. New and unusual contaminants are getting into the American water supply. Some are wastes; others are chemicals found in the new pesticides, herbicides, and detergents. These inevitably return to surface or underground waters after they have been washed off croplands, out of barns, or out of kitchens and laundries. Cumulatively they may be hazardous. Drinking water in many communities is beginning to have a definite, unpleasant taste. In the southwestern part of the United States there is the special case of public water supplies, as well as waterholes used by cattle and wildlife, becoming contaminated by salt brine.

These present problems in environmental health and medicine should not come as a complete surprise. After all, in the last 50 years, we have doubled the United States population, tucked two-thirds of it into cities, and raised our industrial production about 900%. In these same years hundreds of thousands of new chemicals have been manufactured and found their way into streams. In some crowded localities water intake has been located dangerously close to sewer outlets. A combination of forces, none of which are rapidly abating, are polluting the waters and bid fair to continue doing so unless remedial measures are adopted.

The three basic uses for water in the United States are (1) municipal, the smallest; (2) agricultural, for irrigation; and (3) industrial, by far the largest. In 1960, industry consumed about *half* the available water, about 160 billion gallons a day; irrigation, about 43%—141 billion gallons; and municipalities, a mere 7%, about 22 billion gallons. By 1980, according to some estimates, industry will be consuming about *two-thirds* of the 600 billion gallons a day then hope-

fully available, with 166 billion gallons going for irrigation (27%) and a mere 37 billion gallons for municipalities (6%).

The water challenge now before the nation is to complete, as rapidly as possible, engineering works which are necessary to capture 600 to 650 billon gallons of water a day, and furthermore to treat water in such a way that each gallon is usable at least twice. Water re-use is nothing new. The water of the Ohio River, for example, is used 3.7 times before it reaches the Mississippi. But water to be re-used must be of suitable quality. Unfortunately, water-pollution control programs have not developed as rapidly as the need for them. As a result, at least in the United States, pollution has become the Number 1 water resource problem.

What is Pollution? Since water pollution is a far-reaching and increasing problem in environmental health in the United States, it will be worthwhile to go into some detail concerning what is meant by pollution and what is specifically causing it, as well as recommendations in some cases of what can be done about it. "Pollution" may be defined as anything that degrades the quality of water. Water becomes polluted, unsuitable for re-use, when *over*burdened with any of the following things:

1. *Organic wastes,* which are contributed by domestic sewage and industrial wastes of plant and animal origin.

2. *Infectious, disease-producing agents,* also originating in domestic sewage and some kinds of industrial wastes.

3. *Plant nutrients,* which promote nusiance growths such as algae and water weeds.

4. *Synthetic-organic chemicals,* such as detergents and pesticides, potentially toxic, the result of new chemical technology.

5. *Inorganic chemicals* and mineral substances. These result from mining, manufacturing, and oil plant operations. They interfere with natural stream purification, destroy fish, cause "hard water," complicate water treatment processes.

6. *Sediments,* which damage hydroelectric operations, choke streams, destroy fish and spawn.

7. *Radioactive* pollution, from mining of radioactive ores and processing them; also from "fallout,"

8. *Temperature increases,* from power plants and water impounding. Increased temperature may have harmful effects on aquatic life, may reduce water's capacity to assimilate wastes.

Water pollution in the United States is no longer a local affair. Long stretches of streams are degraded. Conventional waste treatments are hard pressed to hold the line against the sheer mass of biological and chemical pollutants entering their intakes. Sewage construction has not matched our population growth and movement. Coastal waters in 23 states are increasingly subject to pollution from waste discharges of coastal cities, a situation adversely affecting shellfishery, finfishery, recreational and waterfront property values, and creating health hazards.

Groundwater pollution, also increasing, is still essentially a local affair, with different causes in different localities. Seawater is intruding to pollute groundwater in a number of coastal states, such as Maryland, New Jersey, Texas, and California. In the oilfields of the Midwest and Southwest brine disposal practices are causing salt pollution of groundwaters, particularly seepage from evaporation pits. In an increasing number of metropolitan suburban areas, where a large part of the population must rely on individual septic tanks for its waste disposal, this has resulted in serious pollution of groundwaters which must basically provide this same population with its water supply. Industrial waste-storage lagoons, improperly located in permeable soils, are also often responsible for local ground water pollution. One of the most hopeful steps on the part of industry, a move encouraged by experience with oil brine, is to look to deep *underground* strata for disposal of highly poisonous, untreatable, or radioactive wastes.

We have been discussing the specialized problems in the United States; but we should point out that most of the world's population uses water supplies that are unsafe and insufficient in quantity, disposes of excreta and waste dan-

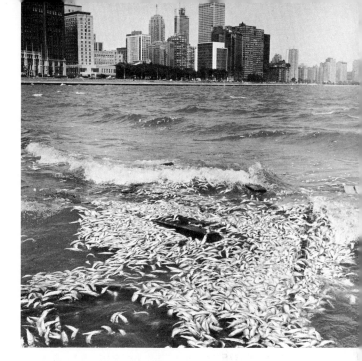

IN THE UNITED STATES pollution has become the major problem in water resources, a situation affecting fishing, recreational, and waterfront property values, and creating health hazards. These dead fish (alewives) are within full view of the magnificent skyline of Chicago. (Photograph by Hays-MONKMEYER)

gerously, and commits many other sanitary errors. The water pollution hazard is illustrated in a number of South American countries, where diarrheal diseases remain the leading cause of death for children from ages 1 to 4. We have an interesting example of the efforts made in one water-poor South American city of 350,000 (Arequipa, Peru) to improve the quantity and quality of the water supply—and thus reduce gastro-intestinal disease rates. An intelligent plan to pipe pure water to houses was set up, but it met resistance expressed in such phrases as: "Water is a gift from God. Why do we have to pay?" "We prefer river water; it is sweeter." "How can we wash if water is more expensive?"

How Much Water Pollution? Returning to the American scene, it will be worthwhile to investigate how much of what kind of water pollution we suffer and what the prospects are for reducing it. We can state the situation in terms of what we *have* accomplished and what remains to be done.

Municipal Wastes. In 1900 there were only 950

communities in the United States that had provided their citizens, numbering about 24.5 million people, with sewers. Since then the number of communities with sewers has increased to nearly 12,000 and the number of citizens served to about 125 million (60%). About two-thirds of these sewered municipalities have constructed sewage treatment works, serving perhaps 110 million people. At the same time the amount of municipal pollution has increased and is increasing because of more population, obsolescence of older sewage treatment plants, failure to construct needed new sewers, increased interception of industrial wastes by municipal sewers, and greater numbers of water-using devices in the home (automatic laundries, garbage grinders, etc.). Even if we build more sewers and sewage treatment plants at a greatly accelerated rate between now and 1980, we will still have as much municipal waste and pollution reaching the nation's streams as we do now!

Combined Sewer Systems. The discharge of mixed raw sewage and storm water into our streams from combined sewer systems overflows is one of the most harrassing water pollution problems a number of our cities face. Combined sewer systems are a product of mistaken, nineteenth-century engineering concepts. What happens in these old-fashioned combined systems is that a high percentage of raw sewage, sludge, and rainwater runs off directly into the receiving stream without going through the sewage treatment plant. Even occasional, "rainy season" overflows of raw sewage on receiving waters often create serious pollution problems, as exhibited in posting and closing beaches in New York City, Milwaukee, and other areas. There are still about 2000 American communities that depend wholly or partly on combined sewer systems.

Industrial Wastes. There are at least three classes of industrial wastes that rank as water pollutants: (1) organic industrial wastes, (2) inorganic industrial wastes, and (3) new chemical wastes. Some radioactive wastes and "heat pollution" will be considered under this heading.

Industry places a staggering demand on the nation's water resources. It uses water in scores of ways—as a solvent, a coolant, a washing agent, an ingredient, a means of transportation, etc. The amounts of water used sound fantastic. For example, it takes 200 gallons of water to produce a dollar's worth of paper; 1400 gallons to make a dollar's worth of steel. Talking in tons, it takes 320,000 gallons of water to produce a ton of aluminum; 600,000 gallons for a ton of synthetic rubber.

Organic industrial wastes are discarded substances of direct animal or vegetable origin which are originally taken into such industrial processes as fiber or food processing, textile manufacture, papermaking, or kindred industries. The U.S. Public Health Service estimated that in the 1960's the amount of organic industrial wastes, treated and untreated, going into the nation's watercourses was about *double* the total municipal waste load being dicharged! If production estimates are valid, the amount of industrial organic waste could double by 1980. It is not suprising under these circumstances that the U.S. Public Health Service also estimates that if industry is to do its fair share in keeping America's water clean, it will have to construct about 6000 first-class sewage treatment plants.

Inorganic industrial wastes originate from such processes as metal pickling, metal finishing, chrome tanning, mining, processing, and manufacturing a wide variety of metal and chemical products; and from mine-acid drainage. Something over 20,000 openings from abandoned or inactive mines account for more than half the total mine-acid discharge in the United States annually. This is estimated at 3.5 million tons of acid every year, disgorged into about 4000 miles of waterways. The acid kills fish, corrodes underwater structures, destroys the recreational value of streams, and makes necessary more extensive and expensive water purification processes for industry and municipalities. In the spring of 1964 the U.S. Public Health Service undertook two extensive projects in West Virginia to locate all mine openings and find effective ways of keeping drainage from entering streams.

Inorganic industrial wastes contain metals

such as iron, chromium, nickel, and copper; salts such as sodium, calcium, and magnesium; acids such as hydrochloric and sulfuric; and a host of other waste compounds. They degrade water quality by causing tastes, odors, and colors; excess saltiness and hardness; and corrosion. Some are toxic or potentially so.

New chemical wastes appear increasingly in our streams and water supplies. They are not removed by and are indeed resistant—and sometimes antagonistic—to present-day water and sewage treatment processes. The new synthetic wastes are present in low concentrations in most waters; but we have no idea what their long-range toxic effects on man and other living organisms may be. Some are known to be highly poisonous to fish and some forms of aquatic life. Others are known to cause persistent tastes and odors. It should be realized that at least half the thousands of new products now manufactured by the synthetic chemical industry were not in production, nor dreamed of, in 1940. With the rapid growth of the synthetic chemical industry a major new water pollution problem has emerged. Not only do the finished products become new chemical pollutants, the by-products in the manufacturing processes also contaminate streams.

Radioactive wastes are a relatively recent factor in the water-pollution problem. They are the result of the growth of our new nuclear technology. The sources of radioactive substances which may be responsible for water pollution are varied. They include mining and refining of radioactive minerals, such as uranium and thorium; escape of refined radioactive substances used in power reactors or for other industrial, medical, or research purposes; and nuclear weapons testing. In the mid-sixties the U.S. Public Health Service national water quality analytical network showed that the radioactivity in the country's lakes and streams was "well below the safe allowable concentration." However, there is always a potential hazard.

Heat pollution, so-called, is caused by the return to water courses from power plants and other industrial sources of relatively large quantities of water heated as the result of being used as a coolant in industrial processes. As water temperature goes up, the amount of oxygen it can hold in solution diminishes. Hence there is less oxygen to oxidize pollutants. Fish life in streams is also adversely affected. Unless effective controls are instituted, it is estimated that heat pollution will increase 100% between 1965 and 1975.

Other Sources of Pollution. *Land drainage wastes* include the silt, sediment, soils, mineral particles, agricultural pesticides, and fertilizers washed from the land by storms and floodwaters or drained off by rainwater. This may occur along an entire watershed. Sediment results from soil erosion, and this in turn is caused by denuding soil of its vegetative cover. Brush and forest fires may create this situation in some localities—giving the water of the nearby streams a "burnt" taste. More commonly land is denuded by bulldozers as the first step toward the erection of a housing development or the building of a new highway, which causes the same results.

Hard-surface runoff describes the waste material washed into streams by runoff of water from the hard-surfaced, chiefly urban areas—streets, highways, houses, industrial and other buildings, airports, etc. The urban runoff carries with it accumulated deposits, such as oils, organic matter, trash, soil, industrial dusts, other air pollutants, fertilizers, and pesticides used by weekend gardeners. The hard-surface runoff is nearly 100% of the rainfall, but a certain amount of this goes through sewer systems and water treatment plants.

Irrigation return flows are a major water pollution problem in 17 western states. As irrigation waters percolate through the soil, they dissolve significant amounts of minerals and other substances. Used over and over again, the concentration of mineral pollutants in these waters becomes damagingly high. Irrigation return flows often render streams unfit for further use, including irrigation, until their mineral content is diluted.

Agricultural pesticides and fertilizers have created perhaps the most important new land drainage problem involving water pollution. We shall discuss the pesticide and fertilizer problem later.

Recreation in and on the water—swimming, boating, water-skiing, etc.—can create measurable water pollution. Few recreational small crafts have proper waste disposal facilities, and they discharge galley and toilet wastes directly into the water. Motorboat and outboard motor exhaust wastes are becoming a serious problem in some areas. They leave in the waters significant concentrations of oil, lead, and combustion products, such as carbon monoxide, phenols, and benzpyrenes common to air pollution from automobile exhausts. Offshore drilling for oil has also contaminated once clear beaches, as at Santa Barbara, California in 1969.

Navigation is an old and still active source of water pollution in estuaries, harbors, and some coastal waters. With the opening of the St. Lawrence Seaway, which has opened the Great Lakes to 90% of the world's commercial vessels, the problem of water pollution in the Great Lakes has been greaty magnified. Many communities draw their drinking water from these lakes and there are many recreational beaches along them.

Few ships afloat today have any facilities for collection, treatment, or disposal of shipboard wastes. Ship pollution consists of bilge waters, sanitary sewage, garbage, spoiled cargo, oils, and anything else that can be thrown overboard. Theoretically bilge should be pumped outside a ten-mile harbor limit; but this regulation is not always honored. Stricter enforcement of sanitary regulations on the Great Lakes will be necessary as its cargo tonnage continues to increase.

How Can We Control Water Pollution? Unless the United States takes positive steps to control its increasing water pollution problem, it may find itself running out of safe, high-quality water for essential needs—personal, agricultural, industrial. The attack on the water-pollution problem must be threefold: (1) construction of more first-class water and sewage treatment facilities; (2) enforcement of laws against practices that create pollution; and (3) development of research procedures that will find ways to remove the new pollutants and better ways to get rid of the old contaminants.

The best modern sewage treatment plants provide a *primary* treatment, in which solids are given a chance to settle out; and a *secondary* treatment that depends on bacteriological action. This treatment removes only 75% to 90% of organic wastes, a smaller fraction of dissolved mineral solids, very little of the chemically new wastes. The U.S. Public Health Service is therefore encouraging *advanced waste treatment research*, through which it is hoped the conversion of waste water to fresh water may be genuinely achieved. In 1964 the Manufacturing Chemists Association undertook a research project to determine the behavior of organic chemicals in streams, lakes, and rivers. Among the new techniques for water purification under study, some of which may turn out to offer practical solutions to the water pollution problem, are absorption by carbon or other absorptive filter, distillation, foaming, freezing, ion exchange, solvent extraction, electrodialysis, and even electrolysis.

The individual can do relatively little, outside of obeying the laws against water pollution, to reduce this hazard of which he himself may fall a victim. He can as a *citizen*, however, raise a loud voice to encourage industry, voluntary agencies, and government agencies at all levels to do their jobs in controlling water pollution.

Measuring Water Quality. Realizing the need for continuing measures of water quality management through state, interstate, and other agencies, the U.S. Public Health Service in 1957 established a "National Water Quality Network." By 1962 more than one-third of the planned 300 sampling stations were in operation. Detailed analysis of samples is helpful in determining long-range water quality trends, in selecting sites for water use, and in developing comprehensive water resource programs. Another indicator of water pollution introduced by the U.S. Public Health Service is its annual "fish-kill" count, running into the millions (7.8 million in 1963). The U.S. Public Health Service has also undertaken a Pesticide Control Project to determine the presence of herbicides and insecticides in surface streams and ground waters so that their damage, if any, can be accurately assayed.

Water pollution control programs are now being developed for seven major river basins: Arkansas-Red, Colorado, Columbia, Great-Lakes-Illinois, Delaware, Chesapeake Bay, and Southeastern. As the nation grows, more and more developments in making pure water available will have to be undertaken. Industry will have to become more conscious of its responsibilities for water control and seek to provide clean, fresh water for economic as well as public health reasons. Water is now big business.

Food Contamination

The food a person eats is as much a part of his environment as the water he drinks or the air he breathes. Altogether air, water, and food provide the physical substance, the chemical elements, out of which living organisms, including man, are compounded. Just as population expansion and technological progress in civilization have created new problems of water and air pollution, they have also introduced new hazards of food contamination. True enough, the advances in microbiology and public health in the past century have happily eliminated some of the old hazards of unclean, impure food—for example, botulism and typhoid fever—but new risks have arisen.

The following statement from the *Report of the Committee on Environmental Health Problems to the Surgeon General* highlights the predicament of the 1970's:

The traditional food sanitation programs of [local] health departments generally speaking [cannot keep up] with the new responsibilities resulting from advances in food technology, changing eating habits, and population growth. So many new problems have arisen that many departments are no longer capable of providing adequate food protection. There is urgent need to reverse this trend toward obsolescence.

The food supply for metropolitan centers presents an increasing number and variety of public health problems, based on the potential hazards associated with technological changes, the continuing wide-spread occurrence of foodborne illnesses, rapidly changing economics and pattern of distribution, and the influence foods may have on man's response to environmental stresses. . . . Food protection is the keystone of environmental health.

The magnitude of the new problems faced by the official agencies responsible for food safety of the America public, that is, local and state health departments, the U.S. Public Health Service, and the Federal Food and Drug Administration (FDA) can be illuminated by the following fact: The American public spends $80 billion a year in retail stores for *food*. It spends another $35 billion for *meals* in restaurants, grills, hamburger stands, "drive-ins," etc. The American food industry devotes more than 1% of its income, a sum close to $1 billion a year, to research designed to develop *new* food products. In terms of budget alone the health agencies cannot keep up with the industry. New and unresolved problems are constantly arising as new foods are introduced. The food-protection service budgets of the Federal Food and Drug Administration and the U.S. Public Health Service operate in the low tens of millions of dollars.

The demand of the American public for foods of greater convenience, variety, and quality, and in ever-increasing quantity, is at the root of new problems in food safety. This human demand is certainly understandable. Man's relationship to his environment (including food supply) during his long evolutionary period was not unlike that of other animal species. The human race multiplied at a rate which was on the whole in excess of its food supply and accepted the marginal existence implicit in that multiplication. It is only today, and then only in a few countries like the United States, that people enjoy the possibility of having enough of the right kind of food to eat. Success in this direction has brought new kinds of problems of food contamination, and it has not eliminated all the old ones. It will be most illustrative to look at this in historical perspective.

Foods in America: An Historical Perspective. In general stores such as Abraham Lincoln kept when he was a young man fewer than a hundred

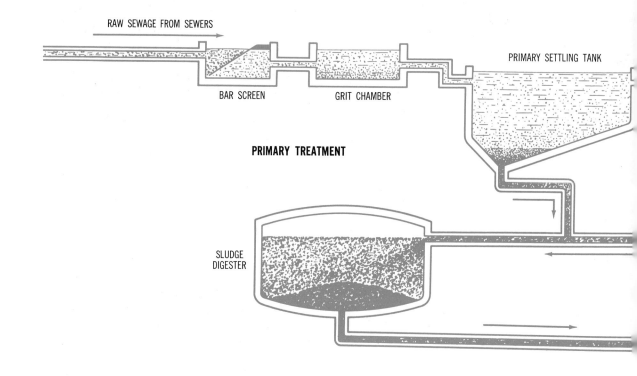

RAW SEWAGE FROM SEWERS

PRIMARY SETTLING TANK

BAR SCREEN   GRIT CHAMBER

PRIMARY TREATMENT

SLUDGE
DIGESTER

SEWAGE TREATMENT, MODERN STYLE, is one of the important functions of environmental sanitation designed and executed behind the scenes (and underground) by the professional public health workers and sanitary engineers whose efforts make possible healthier living in modern communities. The modern sewage treatment plant diagrammed above provides for both primary and secondary sewage treatment. *Primary treatment* removes about 35 percent of the polluting materials, such as body wastes, which are carried into the treatment plant by dirty sewage waters. *Secondary treatment,* which is considerably more expensive, removes nearly 85 percent of the pollution and permits the discharge of clean water from the plant into a stream or other natural waterway. Primary treatment is largely a matter of screening and permitting sewage water to stand for a considerable time in a settling tank, where waste matter settles to the

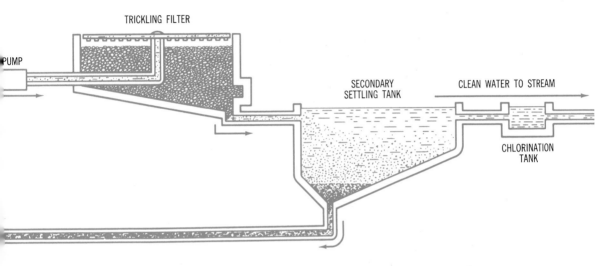

TRICKLING FILTER

PUMP

SECONDARY
SETTLING TANK

CLEAN WATER TO STREAM

CHLORINATION
TANK

SECONDARY TREATMENT

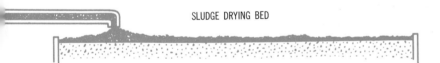

SLUDGE DRYING BED

bottom as "sludge" or rises to the top as "scum." The water between these two layers is then drained off. Secondary treatment depends on the action of bacteria to remove dissolved organic matter from the water. This takes place in a trickling filter, a bed of coarse stones, about six feet deep, on which bacteria grow. The water then goes through a secondary settling tank and finally a chlorination tank before being discharged. The sewage treatment plant does one other important job. Waste matter removed from the water is made useful by passing it through a sludge digestion tank and into sludge drying beds. It may then be used as land fill or for fertilizer. (The diagram shown here is from *The Living Waters*, U.S. Public Health Service Publication No. 382, revised 1961) food items were sold. These were mostly dried staples and produce from nearby farms. Perishable foods were consumed promptly or home-processed to preserve them a little longer. Milk was made into butter and cheese. Meat was salted down. The common preservative agents were salt, sugar, and vinegar. The causes of food-borne diseases and food spoilage were basically unknown.

Scientific advances in the second half of the nineteenth century led to remarkable progress in the production, manufacture, distribution, and service of food. Microbiology and epidemiology demonstrated the role of food (and milk) in spreading infectious diseases such as typhoid fever, tuberculosis, dysentery, and septic sore throat. Sanitation programs were set up, involving pasteurization of milk, inspection of dairy products, veterinary examination of food and dairy animals, inspection of restaurants, and education of food-handlers in hygienic practices. Adequate heat-processing of canned foods was insisted upon to destroy spore-forming bacteria which, without air, it was discovered, produced the highly virulent poison of botulism.

At about the turn of the twentieth century the traditional patterns of food marketing and consumption also began to change radically. Part of this was based on early urbanization; part on technological advances, such as the development of farm machinery, long-range railroad transportation, mechanical refrigeration in storage warehouses, and the commercial food industry. By 1900 food processing, chiefly canning, was moving rapidly from home kitchens to large factories and processing plants.

Then came shocking revelations of contamination and adulteration of commercially processed food. Housewives were terrified by public disclosure of filthy, fraudulent, and dangerous foods—foods doused with large amounts of dangerous chemical preservatives such as formaldehyde, salicylic acid, and boric acid; and candy colored with poisonous dyes. Such conditions led Congress to pass the original "Pure Food and Drug Law" of 1906. Appointed to enforce it was Dr. Harvey W. Wiley, the man whose 20-year fight against food contamination did most to show its need. Wiley conducted a dramatic "poison squad" experiment in 1903. In this sensational scientific experiment he fed a dozen young men measured amounts of chemical food preservatives and observed the harmful effects. Laws protecting food safety and purity have been strengthened many times since 1906.

Food production in the United States has advanced steadily in the twentieth century. Thanks to power-driven machinery, selection and hybridization of seed plants and animal sires, and agricultural chemicals, the American farmer now produces ten times as much food per acre as his Indian or African counterpart. But it is the agricultural chemicals, constantly being "improved," that have introduced new problems of food contamination. Agricultural chemicals include fertilizers, weed killers, feed supplements, fungicides, insecticides and pesticides. There are tens of thousands of them. Some are suspected of being carcinogenic (cancer-causing). Not all of them have been adequately tested. The pesticides in particular appear to offer the greatest risks, and a special amendment (1954) to the federal food and drug laws empowered the Food and Drug Administration to set safe limits or "tolerances" for residues of pesticides on fresh fruits and vegetables when shipped. We shall discuss the problem of pesticide contamination, which is an international problem, in great detail in the following chapter.

The technology of food processing, packaging, and distribution was changed radically after World War II. There came a still greater demand for complex, convenient, precooked foods, processed by increasingly complex machinery. Among the new foods were dried, precooked, and frozen products—which were not always sterile. New hazards were introduced—the risks of improper storage and the breakdown of refrigeration. Oldtime canning always included a step of heat sterilization. However, with use of some of the new packaging materials, foods are only partially sterilized—in the expectation that they will be preserved by unbroken refrigeration until consumed. This does not always happen.

Today, in contrast to Lincoln's day, you can buy 8000 different food items at America's supermarkets. Two dozen new ones are offered every day. The safety risks multiply, augmented by new modes of food service. Automatic vending machines now deliver both hot and cold foods and even complete meals. This business, presently around $300 million a year, is expected to increase. The American food industry in all its aspects probably does around $115 billion worth of business a year at retail prices. It is estimated that there are at least 450,000 establishments in the United States that manufacture, distribute, store, or sell food, in addition to 375,000 public eating places. The magnitude of the problems of inspection and surveillance is obvious!

And there is another mid-twentieth-century contaminant to which foodstuffs are liable: man-made radioactivity.

Three Basic Contaminants: Microbes, Chemicals, Radioactivity. The foodstuffs sold and served in America today run risk of contamination from three sources: (1) microbes, owing to faulty processing or handling; (2) chemicals, commonly known as "food additives," deliberately or indirectly added to food-stuffs; and (3) radioactivity, arising from controlled weapons testing, industrial, and accidental sources.

Not counting the occasional gastro-intestinal upsets that almost everyone experiences, it is estimated that a minimum of 1 million cases of definite food poisoning occur in the United States every year. The infective agents usually reported are the staphylococcal and salmonella or shigella organisms. In rare cases, such as the 1964 typhoid epidemic in Aberdeen, Scotland—traced to South American corned beef that had been prepared under less than the best sanitary precautions and had been kept in storage for many years—food infection and poisoning may be traced to other organisms.

There is another facet to this "poisoning" problem; namely, the long-range effect on health of chemicals directly or indirectly added to food. Studies of the results of cumulative effects of small amounts of food contaminants—chemical, microbial, and radiological—have just begun. The total risks are still undetermined.

Microbial Contamination of Food. Control of severe food-borne diseases, such as botulism and typhoid fever, in the past half-century has been so successful on the whole that it has left the impression that technical knowledge in this field is completely adequate. But current sanitation practices of the past decade and a half have failed to reduce a high incidence of food-borne infections. It is now believed that hitherto unsuspected fungi, bacteria, viruses, rickettsiae, and protozoa may be at least partly responsible for a number of these infections. For example, an outbreak of infectious hepatitis was traced to polluted shellfish, first in Sweden, then in the United States.

A local public health officer, William A. Dorsey, chief of the Richmond (Va.) Public Health Laboratories, pointed out in June, 1964, that there were significant changes in the way *Salmonella* food poisoning was attacking its victims. Formerly, the food poisoning occured as an epidemic and it was easy to trace the source of contamination. "Today," said Dr. Dorsey, "the poisoning is coming up as individual cases that are never concentrated in one particular area. In the Richmond area alone there are several hundred food plants putting out several thousand products. It's impossible to check them all. We're groping in the dark."

The situation described in Richmond is reflected nationwide. A survey of 63 frozen food plants conducted in 18 states in the mid-60's by the Food and Drug Administration revealed the same hazardous and unsanitary situation. After examining 3000 food samples, the Food and Drug Administration concluded: "Sanitary and operating practices in the plants were considerably below the levels desired."

The legal actions initiated by the Food and Drug Administration in recent years is *a priori* proof that strong steps, beyond a continuing program of persuasion and education, remain necessary to safeguard the food offered the American public from bacterial and chemical contamination. Approximately 3500 legal actions, that is, seizures, citations, prosecutions, and injunctions, are now instituted every year against food and drug manufacturers, wholesalers, retailers, and others who are apparently in violation of the laws. Approximately 7500 detentions of imported drugs and foodstuffs are recorded annually.

It is another interesting fact that industry often takes *voluntary* corrective actions as a result of Federal Food and Drug Administration inspections, which reveal batches of food to be adulterated or contaminated. In the first three years of the 1960's approximately 3500 members of the food industry voluntarily destroyed (or converted to feed, if allowable) nearly 60 million pounds of adulterated foods.

Chemical Additives; Radionuclides. Under the present operation of our scientific agriculture and highly technological food processing industry, it would be impossible to keep foreign chemicals—food additives—completely out of our foodstuffs and still feed the American people. It has been promulgated, for example, that if agricultural chemicals (principally fertilizers) were eliminated, the yield of American farms would drop by 10% to 90%. Among the food additives now commonly used in American foodstuffs are the following:

Nutrient supplements (e.g., vitamins, iodized salt); sugar substitutes (e.g., saccharin); preservatives (e.g., antioxidants, mold inhibitors, fungicides, sequestrants, citric acid, benzoic acid, salt, and vinegar); emulsifiers (e.g., lecithin, monoglycerides); stabilizers and thickeners (e.g., agar, gelatin); acids, alkalis, buffers, neutralizing agents (e.g., ammonium bicarbonate, calcium carbonate); flavoring agents (e.g., amyl acetate, methyl salicylate); bleaching agents, bread improvers (e.g., benzoyl peroxide, chlorine dioxide, chlorine); leavening agents; hardening agents; drying agents; chill-proofing agents; antifoaming agents; color additives (e.g., coal-tar colors); and livestock feed additives which leave a residue in milk, meat, eggs, and other human food.

A Food Additives Amendment became Federal law in 1958, and in 1960 the law was ex-tended to bring all food colors under the same type of control. The Food and Drug Administration now receives animal feeding tests on proposed new food additives before they are marketed. If satisfied that the additive is safe, the Food and Drug Administration issues an order permitting its use and establishes its tolerance (the amount which may be used). This is a great improvement over previous practice, but it is not perfect.

As the Food and Drug Administration itself has said: "The danger [is] not theoretical—it [is] real, as shown by a number of instances of chemicals having been found injurious only after they had been in use for a considerable period of time, including a chemical used for flour aging and an ingredient of imitation vanilla extract. Both had to be removed from the market after years of presumed safety." The Food and Drug Administration has also pointed out that some of the coal-tar colors which it originally listed as "harmless" under provisions of the 1938 law were later found to produce injury when fed to animals in large amounts and had to be removed from the list of certified colors.

In all questions about the risks of food additives, one must bear in mind that fundamental axiom of pharmacology and clinical medicine: "The dose makes the poison." (*"Dosa venum facit."*)

Finally, we must briefly mention radionuclide contamination of milk and other foods by fallout from nuclear explosions, by-products of atomic reactors, and residues of radioactive waste. About five-sixths of the strontium 90 that gets into the human body comes through the food chain, especially dairy products (where strontium replaces calcium). A great deal of study remains to be done on radionuclide contamination through the food chain. We shall say no more about the subject here because we have included a detailed discussion on the radiation hazards faced by twentieth-century man in the following chapter. This too is an international subject of concern. In terms of the hazards it faces, the world is shrinking.

SUMMARY

We have presented in this chapter the impact of the new pollutions that men of the twentieth century, and particularly those of the most technically developed countries, face. We have discussed air pollution, water pollution, and food contamination. The astonishing thing about these new hazards to human welfare is that they have arisen out of the scientific and technical progress which is also responsible for the population explosion and increasing urbanization of mankind—topics we shall touch on in the next chapter. In other terminology we can say that air, water, and food pollution, as well as the hazards of pesticides and radiation (also discussed in the following chapter), are to a large extent the outcome of the indifferent *social environment* in which we live. In every one of these five major areas of pollution and contamination, which are making a damaging impact on the physical and mental health of human beings, we have apparently less the will than the ways to bring them under control.

SUMMARY REVIEW QUESTIONS

1. What three essentials to life may be polluted or contaminated? What amount, on the average, of each of these three essentials are required daily by an adult?
2. What are some of the substances (name at least four) that may pollute the air we breathe? What might be some of the results of breathing this polluted air? In what areas is air pollution most likely to be a serious problem?
3. What are some of the methods by which the problem of air pollution can be abated? What is the relationship of the motor car to the problem of air pollution?
4. Are American water reserves adequate for the present? For the future? What is the key factor in providing water supplies for its many users? In addition to water necessary for daily human consumption, what other uses of water are essential to the American economy?
5. What are the principal water pollutants (name at least six) with which the United States must now contend? What are some of the sources (or reasons) of these old and new pollutants? How can water pollution be controlled? Whose responsibility is it?
6. What important steps have been taken in the United States since the middle of the nineteenth century to make food safer for human consumption? What new developments have taken place in the middle of the twentieth century to increase the risks of food contamination?
7. What are some of the principal "food additives" (name at least five) now used in the commercial processing of food sold to and consumed by the American public? What protection against dangerous food additives does the American public now have?
8. What in general would you say are the reasons for the new pollutions of air, water, and food which United States citizens of the middle twentieth century are facing?
9. Are the following statements sense or nonsense? Why? *Industry is the largest consumer of the American water supply. . . . All this talk about air, water, and food contamination is nonsense. . . . Ignorance and apathy are the real limitations upon the control of air pollution. . . . The causes of food-borne diseases and food spoilage are still basically unknown. . . . The dose makes the poison.*
10. What do the following terms mean to you: Salmonella, hard-surface runoff, pasteurization, smog, exhaust devices, organic wastes, "National Water Quality Network," agricultural chemicals, ciliary action, strontium 90?

Worth Looking Into: *A Study of Pollution—Air,* a staff report to the Committee on Public Works, U.S. Senate (88th Congress, 1st session). *A Study of Pollution—Water,* a staff report to the committee on Public Works, U.S. Senate. *What Consumers Should Know About Food Additives* (pamphlet), Federal Food and Drug Administration. *Environmental Health Problems,* report of a committee to the Surgeon General of the U.S. Public Health Service. For more complete references, see Appendix E.

6 Youths Bid Elders Clean Lakes

William M. Blair
Special to The New York Times

Washington, March 4—

The younger generation questioned today the right of the older generation to hand down contaminated lakes and rivers that upset the balance of the human environment.

With the aplomb of seasoned witnesses, six high school seniors from the Cleveland metropolitan area told Congress of watching the slow death of Lake Erie from pollution, the strangulation of the fishing industry and the closing of swimming beaches.

They demanded more stringent controls over pollution, more research, and "crash" programs to save Lake Erie and other water resources. They denounced "big business" as the greatest offender of public property and local governments for allegedly favoring private profit over public interest.

Water Loses Oxygen

Lake Erie is afflicted with an advanced case of "chemical aging" because of a long infusion of sewage and industrial wastes. This infusion has sapped the water of oxygen, exterminated the higher fish species and caused a runaway growth of obnoxious plants.

The four boys and two girls appeared before the House Public Works Committee in favor of water quality bills that would put new restraints on pollution and polluters.

They rattled off, under questioning, the amounts of nitrates and phosphates finding their way into lakes and streams and talked of "eutrophication," a word that many committee members still find hard to pronounce (it means the process of becoming rich in dissolved nutrients).

They won praise from Fred Schwengel, Republican of Iowa, a former high school teacher, for exercising the right of petition. He also praised them for showing the public an example of a "majority" of today's youth in contrast to restless young demonstrators who he said were "doing the wrong things at the right time." His view was echoed by other committee members.

"I am not an expert on pollution, but anyone can see and smell the flagrant abuse of the biosphere," Virginia Robinson, 17 years old, of the Hathaway Brown School, a private girls' school, told the committee. "Perhaps pollution should be as important as the defense budget, or the space program or highway construction."

Sees 'Lack of Conscience'

She suggested that if Congress provided Federal funds to match Cleveland's recent $100-million anti-pollution bond issue on a 9-to-1 ratio, as in highway construction, "the Lake Erie problem could be coped with meaningfully."

Mary Helston, 17, of the Laurel School, also a private school, found "a general lack of conscience about destructive waste removal."

"Is it your right to hand down to us contaminated lakes and rivers that are obviously detrimental to the ecological balance of our environment?" she asked.

George Scott Langer, 17, of the Cleveland Heights High School, said that the students' testimony was intended "not to convey facts, but rather to motivate your concern for water pollution." The "minimum life ex-

SOURCE. Reprinted with permission of *New York Times*. This article appeared on March 5, 1969.

pectancy" of Lake Erie is five years at the present rate of pollution, he said.

John Coventry, 18, of the University School, presented a petition with 13,000 signatures urging Congress to start a "crash" program to save Lake Erie. The signatures, he said, were collected in a week and more are on the way.

Attack On Business

Ronald H. Traub, 17, of the Shaker Heights High School, said, "Big business, one of the greatest offenders in water pollution, fails to understand one basic concept—that water courses are public property. Local government shirks its responsibility when it decides in favor of private profit to the disadvantage of the public."

Jeffrey T. Kline, 17, of the Hawken School, spoke of the "mounting international problem of pollution" and "too much delay" in pollution control.

The youths were brought to Washington by Representative Charles A. Vanik, Democrat of Ohio, after he learned of their interest and work in various areas of pollution control.

Answers to Special Exercise, pages 402, 403, and 404.

1. Doctors Carry Disease
   Completely correct. This is an excerpt from Oliver Wendell Holmes' famous and classical essay on the "Contagiousness of Puerperal Fever," read before the Boston Society for Medical Improvement in 1843 and published in the shortly defunct *New England Quarterly Journal for Medicine and Surgery.*

2. Ocean Gives Up Secret
   Complete nonsense. How would you pronounce "Foni Gey"?

3. New Triumph for Medicine?
   An utter fabrication. Note the dateline on the story.

4. Controlled Sleep Found Effective in Peptic Ulcer.
   Quite legitimate. A news story from *Scope* (medical weekly) for June 18, 1958. The report is perfectly reasonable, even though other physicians might disagree with it or even later disprove it. Full responsibility is pinned upon the World Congress of Gastroenterology and the investigator from Warsaw, Poland.

5. Be Beautiful (advertisement)
   You would have to be pretty naive to believe this completely *fake advertisement.* There is no such brand name as "BEE BEAUTIFUL."

6. In Acne (advertisement)
   Perfectly legitimate medical advertisement which appeared in a number of reputable medical journals. It is reprinted here with the permission of the advertiser, Winthrop Laboratories, New York.

7. Why Take Chances with Your Health?
   This is another completely *fake* advertisement, written in the presumptuous news-story form that charlatans often adopt. Note the parade of normal human reactions, such as fatigue after a hard day's work, put forward as symptoms of vitamin deficiency. Observe the high-sounding titles "International Vitamin and Minerals Institute of America" and "Vitamin Subscription Bureau." If the fakery of this advertisement does not otherwise strike you, note the *number* of vitamins and minerals claimed to be included in the theoretical formula of "Vitaboos" (which do not exist) and the "degree," after the name of the mythical character, Dr. John Hitzmuller-Smythe. This one shouldn't fool you—but it illustrates many of the advertising techniques by which quacks and charlatans operate to hoodwink their victims. Finally, note the high price for seaweed!

8. 2 Sunscreen Preparations that may be recommended with confidence (Bronztan).
   A completely legitimate and forthright advertisement that appeared in respectable medical journals and cites specific references to publication in another reputable medical journal to back up its modest and specific claims. This is believable, legitimate advertising. It is reprinted with permission of the advertiser, Shulton, Inc., Clifton, N.J.

23

ENVIRONMENTAL HEALTH
AND WORLD HEALTH

THE PHYSICAL GEOGRAPHY OF THE GLOBE has remained basically fixed since long before the existence of man. Despite some minor evolutionary changes, the flora and fauna of the world have not altered within the memory of man. The fundamental physical and biological environments—background, framework, if you will—within which the human race has been set down on Earth have not changed. What has changed, easily within the memory of even young men, is the social environment of the globe. Much of this is the result of the improvement in the concepts and practices of environmental health that have occurred, at an increasingly rapid pace, within the last century. The gross outcome is what is today called "the population explosion."

The newly governing factor in today's world is its population, and the distribution of this population. Man is more a product and victim today of his social environment (with overtones of his ideological environment) than ever before in his history. Understanding of today's world, including its health problems, depends on appreciating the signficance of its population distribution—by continents, countries, and big cities (see tables on next page).

There are factors abroad in the world which will tend to push populations up—selectively by countries and continents. There are other factors which may starkly limit population growths. In this chapter we shall discuss both kinds of factors, for example, the question of the use of pesticides and insecticides, and activities of the World Health Organization.

Populations of the World's Largest Cities

The populations of some foreign cities cannot be exactly compared with others or with large U.S. cities because of different administrative practices employed in tabulating or calculating populations. The Tokyo metropolitan area, for example, include 10 cities. The New York–Northeastern New Jersey standard consolidated area population is 15 million; Chicago–Northwestern Indiana, 6.8 million. Greater Paris population (15 mile radius) is 8.6 million; Greater Moscow, 7 million; Metropolitan Calcutta, 5.5 million. Minimum populations for the mid-1960's, by latest standard enumerations and estimates, are:

POPULATION OF THE WORLD—CONTINENTS*

	Estimated population	Land area (sq. km.†)
Asia	1,780,000,000	26,940,000
Europe	434,000,000	4,955,000
North America	276,000,000	24,248,000
Africa	269,000,000	30,366,000
South America	153,000,000	17,793,000
Oceania	17,000,000	8,558,000
U.S.S.R. (excluded from totals for Asia and Europe)	221,000,000	22,402,000
TOTALS	3,150,000,000	135,262,000

*From the Statistical Office of the United Nations, Mid-year, 1962.

†One sq. km. (square kilometer) is the equivalent of 0.386 sq. mi.

TEN LARGEST NATIONS

	Population in millions
1. China	697
2. India	441
3. U.S.S.R. (Soviet Union)	221
4. U. S. (United States)	200
5. Japan	96
6. Indonesia	96
7. Pakistan	96
8. Brazil	75
9. West Germany	57
10. United Kingdom	53
British Commonwealth of Nations (including India, Pakistan and the United Kingdom)	738

POPULATION OF WORLD'S LARGEST CITIES

Tokyo, Japan	11,027,000
New York City, U.S.A.	10,694,000
London, England	7,881,000
Shanghai, China	6,900,000
Mexico City, Mexico	6,815,000
Moscow, U.S.S.R.	6,507,000
Chicago, U.S.A.	6,220,000
Bombay, India	4,785,000
Cairo, Egypt	4,197,000
Sao Paulo, Brazil	4,098,000
Peiping, China	4,010,000
Rio de Janiero, Brazil	3,909,000
Hong Kong, China	3,739,000
Leningrad, U.S.S.R.	3,341,000
Tientsin, China	3,220,000
Manila, Philippine Islands	3,100,000
Buenos Aires, Argentina	2,967,000
Jakarta, Indonesia	2,907,000
Paris, France	2,811,000
Berlin, Germany	2,190,000

Pesticides: Boon or Bane?

One of the major reasons for the present high population of the globe has been the discovery, control, and now hopefully eradication of insect-borne diseases. Until the turn of the twentieth century the population growth of every continent

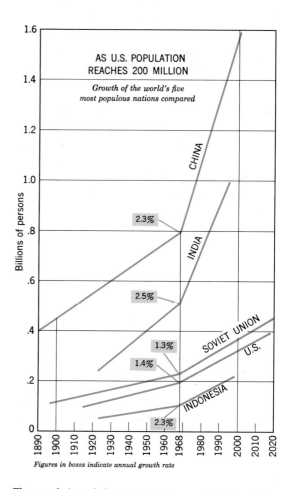

AS U.S. POPULATION REACHES 200 MILLION

Growth of the world's five most populous nations compared

Figures in boxes indicate annual growth rate

The population of the United States reached 200 million people in November, 1967. It took 53 years for the nation's population to double. At present growth rates, it will double again in another 50 years. The chart shows that populations in China, India, and Indonesia will double at a still more rapid rate, whereas Russia's population growth curve will be much more like that of the United States. For each country, the graph begins at the date when its population was half what it was in 1967 and ends at the year where it will double again.

was dampened by death from insect-borne diseases.

The pressing questions about pesticides and insecticides—whether or not to use them, which ones to use if any, how to use them, what limitations to place upon their use—are still subject to debate, investigation, and research. They are unquestionably the leading environmental health questions on the stage of world health. Populations will undoubtedly rise or fall depending on how correctly these questions are answered. These new synthetic chemicals, of which the prototype is DDT, introduced in 1942, have stamped on insect-borne diseases in every country in the world. Before coming to the issue of the "great debate"—briefly, are pesticides going to do more harm than good?—it will be illuminating to present the history that leads up to it.

Insect-Borne Diseases

The opening of the Panama Canal in 1914 was a cogent triumph for Pasteur's germ theory of disease and a marked victory over insect-borne diseases. The isthmus of Panama had long had the reputation of being the "hellhole of the Pacific"; specifically, it was a hotbed of yellow fever. The French had attempted to build a canal across the isthmus between 1881 and 1888; but all the engineering genius of Ferdinand de Lesseps, who had previously built the Suez Canal, could not prevail against the country's sanitary conditions. It is estimated that the French lost through disease one-third of all their employees.

In 1902 President Theodore Roosevelt sent Colonel William C. Gorgas to Panama as chief sanitary officer. He knew what to do before the civil engineers could safely go to work—primarily, get rid of the mosquitoes. Behind this crucial knowledge, which made the building of the canal more a triumph of sanitary than civil engineering, stood the genius and heroism of the men who in the previous half a century had made epidemiology an eminently practical science.

The *proof* that communicable disease could be insect-borne, and the elaborate and peculiar ways in which this actually occurred, was a momentous step in the discovery of the common means of transmission of communicable disease. It had been vaguely and uncritically suspected for centuries. But it was the scientific work during the last quarter of the nineteenth century that made this crude suspicion a certainty and opened the way to practical public-health measures for the control of all insect-borne diseases.

The Itch Mite. Probably the first insect unquestionably indicted as a cause of disease was the itch mite, although in this case the tiny insect buried in the skin was itself the disease, called scabies or "the itch." It is claimed that an old woman proved this fact to the grave and learned physicians of the eighteenth century, who finally accepted her facts and proceeded to write scholarly books about it. Even in the nineteenth century it was folk wisdom that provided the hunch for the first definite, large-scale scientific proof that insects transmit the germs of disease.

The Tick. The American meat industry was menaced by attacks of "Texas fever" in northern cattle. The cowboys said it was caused by ticks; most scientists laughed at them. But not all. In 1889 the U.S. Department of Agriculture sent young Theobald Smith to investigage the cause of Texas fever. By ingenious and critical experiment he proved beyond a doubt that the cowboys were right. The ticks carried the microorganisms of the cattle infection. If the cattle were dipped to kill the ticks, Texas fever disappeared. Actually, as Smith had found out, baby ticks not blood-gorged adults transmitted the disease. In 1893 he published a classic paper on the subject. But since it dealt with an animal disease, it attracted relatively little public attention.

The Flea and the Rat. The following year there was an outbreak in Hong Kong of that most dreaded human disease, plague. Yersin, from Pasteur's laboratory, and Kitasato, a Japanese physician who was an assistant to the great Robert Koch, went to China to investigate it. They not only found the microorganism of the human disease, the plague bacillus; they also found it in rats and in the fleas that infested rats. This immediately suggested the chain of transmission of plague and the practical means of controlling epidemics. Get rid of the rats! Rat-proofing and deratization, especially of ships, have since become standard public-health procedures. The flea was now added to the list of vectors of disease, and the business of indicting other insects was in full swing.

The Tsetse Fly. Theobald Smith's paper on the insect transmission of cattle fever made a great impression on Dr. David Bruce, a disease-hunter in the employ of the British Army Medical Service. Bruce had already made a reputation for himself by discovering the microorganism of undulant fever in goats and goats' milk on the island of Malta. In 1895 Bruce went to South Africa to investigate *nagana,* a disease of horses. He had guessed that an insect might transmit the disease. He found that insect—the tsetse fly.

Later investigation by Bruce and others proved that African sleeping sickness, a disease of man, was also transmitted by the tsetse flies. And the tsetse flies, it was further proved, got it from the wild animals of the African jungles which were a reservoir of the microbe fatal to man.

Malaria Control. *The Mosquito.* The most dramatic tale in the quest for the insect vectors of disease is that of the mosquito. This insect was demonstrated by Ronald Ross and others to transmit malaria and by Walter Reed and others to carry yellow fever also.

Ross, like Bruce, was a member of the British Army Medical Service; he was also an accomplished mathematician and poet. Stationed in India, he desperately pursued proof of the opinion earlier vocied by Nott, King, and Manson that the mosquito did transmit malaria. On the hot evening of August 20, 1897, Ross peered through his microscope to discover one form of the malarial parasite in the minute, dissected stomach wall of a mosquito. He celebrated this discovery in verse. "I have found thy secret deeds,/Oh, million-murdering death," he wrote.

Within a year he had traced the parasites to the salivary gland of the mosquito. From this position they had free exit through the mosquito's stylet ("stinger"). These were the crucial facts in the proof that the *bite* of a mosquito infected with malarial parasites actually carried the disease to man.

A great deal of work remained to be done to find out exactly what kind of mosquitoes could convey the malarial parasites; they turned out to be females of the genus *Anopheles.*

Still more investigation was required into the life cycle of the mosquito and into the conditions under which these dangerous pests could be most effectively destroyed. The Italian scientist, Battista Grassi, shared the 1902 Nobel Prize with Ross for his discoveries in this direction. Mosquito control was thus shown to be the key to malaria control.

Contrary to some popular belief, mosquitoes do not travel far from their birthplace. Practically speaking, malaria control boils down to keeping mosquitoes from biting individuals who already have malarial parasites in their blood. The newer insecticides, of which DDT is a prime example, have revolutionized the techniques of mosquito control. They have not wiped out malaria yet—but they have made malaria eradication a reasonable and early possibility.

Yellow-Fever Control. The suspicion that the mosquito was associated with yellow fever had been advanced by Josiah Knott and most emphatically, in 1881, by Dr. Carlos Finlay, of Havana, Cuba. After the Spanish-American War, Cuba became for a time a United States responsibility. In 1900 Major Walter Reed, Dr. James Carroll, Dr. A. Agramonte, and Dr. Jesse W. Lazear were sent to Havana as a commission to study yellow fever, there rampant.

Lazear died of yellow fever early in the course of the investigation. A true martyr of science, he had permitted himself to be bitten by a mosquito suspected of carrying the disease. At Camp Lazear, named in his honor, Reed continued the essential experiments.

They required human volunteers who would permit themselves to be bitten by mosquitoes; others who would expose themselves to the contaminated bed clothing and other excretions of yellow-fever victims. Among those who offered themselves for the experiment were John R. Kissinger and John J. Moran. They refused any monetary compensation for running the risk of death. In an immortal phrase, Kissinger said that they had volunteered "solely in the interest of humanity and for the cause of science."

"Gentlemen," said Major Reed, rising and touching his cap, "I salute you."

With the help of his courageous volunteers, Reed indisputably proved that only persons bitten by mosquitoes who had previously bitten other persons with yellow fever could carry the disease. The offending mosquito, *Aëdes aegypti,* was a different brand from that which carried malaria. Mosquito control promptly controlled yellow fever in Havana, Panama, and wherever else it could be effectively applied. However, the disease remains endemic in Africa and is still found in monkeys in the South American jungles.

The New Insecticides

Insect control and destruction programs, based on available knowledge and materials, followed rapidly upon the momentous discoveries of the nature of the insect-borne diseases. The big break-through came during World War II with the introduction of DDT and other synthetic chemicals that came to be called insecticides and later pesticides. Scores of diseases have been conquered by them.

Epidemic typhus has plagued man for centuries. This "traditional" rickettsial disease, transmitted by the body louse, accompanies disasters. It has been known as war fever, famine fever, jail fever, ship fever, and camp fever. In World War II, specifically in 1943, typhus was again breaking out. When American troops arrived in Naples in December 1943, typhus was present. However, a vigorous campaign against it was immediately instituted, primarily with the insecticide, DDT. Freely blown into clothes with a dust gun, DDT quickly killed body lice and interrupted transmission of the disease. From this first blazing demonstration, DDT has gone on to control typhus wherever it lifts its head—even endemic (murine) typhus.

Insecticides have played a major role in the eradication of *Aëdes aegypti* and yellow fever from all of Central America and almost all of South America—probably also from Mexico—but the history is complicated because the eradication campaign has been going on for more than three decades and many things have changed. Earlier techniques called for sealing off and eliminating all possible breeding places. Later a perifocal, pinpoint method of applying DDT was developed, and this has provided a cheap and effective operational procedure.

Effective as campaigns against typhus and yellow fever have been, the greatest results of the use of insecticides have been against malaria. This disease has depopulated large areas, is accused of being responsible directly or indirectly for one-half of the world's mortality, and steals the "joy of living" from millions.

As noted, efforts to control malaria were made by other techniques (oil spraying) and other larvicides (e.g., Paris green) before DDT and other modern insecticides became available. It was hopeless to attack the anopheline mosquitoes in their enormous breeding areas, as in India, but another method proved effective. DDT is a contact poison which enters the mosquito through its feet. The mosquito was therefore eliminated by spraying indoor walls of homes with DDT—twice a year. When the mosquito, after eating, came to rest on the walls, it absorbed the poison. By this method the transmission of malaria was halted and the disease drained out of specific populations in less than three years. The effectiveness of the early campaigns encouraged the World Health Organization to undertake a malaria eradication campaign. DDT was generously used in the attack.

In 1968 World Health Organization revised its goals. It now believes that unless basic medical services in many countries become better developed in detection and treatment, total eradication of malaria is not attainable. Furthermore, the mosquito vectors have acquired resistance to many of the insecticides used in agriculture. However, by 1968, there were only 564 million people living under uncontrolled malarious conditions instead of the original 1420 million.

Another disease which has responded to DDT attack is onchoceriasis, often called river blindness. This disease is caused by a filarial nematode, which is transmitted by small black flies in Africa, South and Central America. Approximately 20 million people are infected. The microfilariae invade all the tissues of the skin, producing severe dermatitis with intense itching. It is worst in the eyes and may go on to produce total blindness. The vector flies of onchoceriasis breed in flowing water, mostly in small streams. Usually attached to stones, the larvae are highly susceptible to DDT. They can be killed by DDT applications as low as 0.1 p.p.m. (parts per million) applied for 15 minutes, although the chemical is usually applied at the rate of 0.05 p.p.m. for 30 minutes—which will not kill fish.

Another disabling disease of a large share of tropical mankind is bilharziasis, or schistosomiasis, commonly carried by snails in snail-infested waters. The infecting blood fluke (trematode) is spread in waters by urinary and fecal contamination. Its tiny larvae infect the snail. After a few weeks the snail liberates free-swimming cercariae, which penetrate the skin of people working, swimming, or wading in the stream. Like malaria, schistosomiasis causes a lifetime of disability. It is estimated that the disease is prevalent in 15 African and Middle Eastern countries. In Egypt possibly 26 million out of 107 million population are infected. The disease cannot be controlled by pesticides alone; other sanitary measures must also be employed.

"Pesticides Upset Balance of Nature." In 1962 there was a book published which rudely interrupted the success stories being piled up by the new insecticides and pesticides; and the "great debate" was on. The book was *Silent Spring* (Boston: Houghton Mifflin Co.); the author was Rachel Carson (d. 1964), a scientist, author, and brilliant observer of ecological cycles on the face of the globe. Miss Carson's book is a reasoned, well-documented, scientific, but impassioned plea against the indiscriminate use of pesticides, insecticides, herbicides, and other "agricultural chemicals" across the face of the globe. Her thesis is made clear in the following passage (quoted with permission):

The history of life on earth is a history of the interaction of living things and their surroundings. . . . It is only within the moment of time represented by the twentieth century that one species—man—has acquired significant power to alter the nature of his world, and it is only within the last twenty-five years that this power has achieved such a magnitude that it endangers the whole earth and its life. The most alarming of all man's assaults is the contamination of the air, earth, rivers, and seas with dangerous and even lethal materials. This pollution has rapidly become almost universal. . . .

It is widely known that radiation has done much to change the very nature of the world, the very nature of its life . . . [but] it is less widely known that many man-made chemicals act in much the same way as radiation; they lie long in the soil, and enter into living organisms, passing from one to another. Or they may travel mysteriously by underground streams, emerging to combine, through the alchemy of air and sunlight, into new forms, which kill vegetation, sicken cattle, and work unknown harm on those who drink from once pure wells. As Albert Schweitzer has said, "Man can hardly recognize the devils of his own creation."

The Statistical Evidence. The statistical evidence concerning pesticides gives some substance to Miss Carson's worry. Over 45,000 pesticide formulations are registered for sale with the U.S. Department of Agriculture! The new synthetics are rapidly replacing the older inorganic insecticides (arsenicals, copper, zinc sulfate, boron, sulfur). Each new pesticide brought on the market is usually more "powerful," that is to say, more toxic, than the one it is intended to supplant.

The quantities of pesticides, insecticides, and other "agricultural chemicals" now produced and used sounds almost fantastic. In the early 1960's this amounted to about 700 million pounds a year; and it was predicted that the output would be increased to 7 billion pounds a year by 1970. Most of these synthetic chemicals have been used by United States farmers. Primarily they have sprayed them one or more times a year on some 30 million acres of cultivated cropland. Some has gone for other purposes—application to pastures, highway right of ways, mesquite, and other nuisance plants. Many of these materials have a long residual toxicity in soil or water.

Most pesticides are removed only in part by ordinary water treatment. Water samples show them present in most major lakes and rivers. It can be assumed that they are washed in by normal land drainage processes. Some may be dropped or drift into the water. It is known that these water-borne pesticides are responsible for some large fishkills and that they wipe out certain chains of aquatic life. But the crucial question, hotly debated, remains unsettled: At what concentration will these pesticide residues become drinking water contaminants of serious toxicity? Opinions differ.

At the American Medical Association's 1964 Congress on Environmental Health Problems, Wayland Hayes, Jr., M.D., of the U.S. Public Health Service pointed out that pesticides kill about 200 people a year in the United States from accidental poisoning and that about 2000 cases of nonfatal pesticide poisoning occur. At the same meeting, Irma West, M.D., of Berkeley, California, declared vigorously: "There is no question that widespread, substantial contamination of the environment has arisen primarily from the massive use of the persistent chlorinated hydrocarbon pesticides. . . . Unforeseen, irrevocable, and undesirable side effects have risen on a sizable scale . . . because the chemicals involved were not checked out from all angles beforehand."

On the other hand another physician at the environmental health congress, Mitchell R. Zavon, M.D., of Cincinnati, Ohio, had a completely different opinion. He said: "The effect of pesticides on our general environment will probably require many years of research to evaluate. There is presently 'no evidence' . . . that the extremely small amounts of certain pesticides [e.g., dieldrin, lindane] which may be found in our food or in our general environment cause us any harm." He suggested that in some pesticide intoxications it may be the solvent which is the culprit.

The "great debate" on the hazard of pesticides appears in miniature in many scientific, technical, and popular journals. The following excerpts from an exchange of letters in *Science* (June 12, 1964, p. 1294) must stand as token for thousands more like it. A professor of biology writes:

"Thanks are due *Science* for the description of the Lower Mississippi fishkill by pesticides. . . . It is surprising that this was not first-page news all over the country. . . . In spite of repeated assurances that endrin and dieldrin were safe, obviously they are not safe. They have not been adequately tested. Have any of the new insecticides been adequately tested?"

A member of an Agricultural Experiment Station at a state university complains that the original *Science* report is "grossly unfair" because it condemns government regulation of pesticides as "weak and confused" and "piecemeal and inadequate" and "dissipated in political and bureaucratic bickering." The agriculturalist writes: "The use of pesticides is essential for the continued production of food and fiber crops, for the protection of human health through control of lice, flies, rats, and cockroaches. . . . Pesticides, when misused in high concentrations, can be dangerous. The public has a right to know. . . . However, in our worry about this problem let's not lose sight of the fact that we must have food and clothing from crops whose production would be impossible or much more expensive without pesticides."

The last word on pesticides (boon or bane?) will probably never be spoken. The latest words will depend on first-rate research. Some of the important research questions which must be taken up are: Do insecticides like DDT decompose in the soil or leach out? How are pesticides retained and released in various types of clays and other soils? What are the interactions between pesticides and soil microorganisms? Are pesticides retained by fish? Absorbed and accumulated by land and water plants? Some states have banned the use of DDT, and further research is going forward. Latest reports have asserted the risks of DDT and ask for substitutes for it.

Radiation Hazards

Mankind has been exposed to ionizing radiation ever since the very first stage of its evolutionary development. It worried no one, because no one knew about it. The first inkling of the existence of ionizing radiation and its production by what we now call atomic energy came in that "miracle decade" of modern science, 1895 to 1905. Then William Conrad Roentgen discovered X-rays, Henri Becquerel first observed natural radioactivity in the image of a key on a *wrapped-up* photographic plate inadvertently left in a drawer with a piece of uranium, and Pierre and Marie Curie isolated and discovered radium. Madame Curie correctly interpreted that its powerful radioactivity and gradual disintegration were being caused by an intra-atomic breakdown.

Atomic energy is produced when atoms break up. Among other things that happen under these circumstances is the emission of *gamma rays* from the site of the break-up. Gamma rays are electromagnetic waves, much like X-rays but of shorter wave length. Very powerful gamma rays and X-rays can penetrate several feet of lead. When atomic energy is kept under control, it is readily possible to protect against its hazards. When it is uncontrolled and reaches critically high levels, it may produce acute or delayed *radiation sickness,* which appears in many forms.

Human beings on Earth are being constantly bombarded by atomic energy from natural sources, such as cosmic rays and naturally occurring radium and other radioactive substances in the earth's crust. It is estimated that this amounts to about 3 *roentgens* (the standard measure of radiation) in 30 years.

Medical X-Ray Risks. Since 1900 the people of civilized countries have been exposed to a second major source of ionizing radiation—namely, medical and dental X-rays. The biological dangers of X-ray and radium were not appreciated at first by the early workers with these energy sources and a goodly number of physicians and scientists in the early 1900's died as "martyrs to radiation" used in examining and treating patients.

Medical necessity requires that X-ray pictures be taken to save life and limb and protect against ravages of disease. In fact more than 50 million diagnostic X-ray films or fluroscopic examina-

tions for medical purposes are now made annually in the United States. Dentists take twice as many, more than 100 million, X-ray pictures of teeth a year. The important thing is that all this X-raying be done with the highest possible safety standards.

It is now possible, however, to protect against a substantial part of the radiation hazards of medical and dental X-rays. This can be done, for example, by getting rid of all obsolete and badly working X-ray equipment, by using well-established protective devices such as lead shielding and new ones like aluminum filters and cone adaptors, by "faster" X-ray film, by periodic checking of all X-ray equipment, and by avoiding needless X-ray examinations and treatment. The National Tuberculosis Association and the U.S. Public Health Service have given up their past recommendations for mass or routine chest X-rays for screening populations for tuberculosis.

Particularly to be deplored and eliminated is the use of atomic energy by shoe clerks in shoe stores that employ fluoroscopes for fitting shoes. In some states, they have been banned.

Genetic-Mutation Risks. The individual risk from the medical use of X-rays must be evaluated against the potential seriousness of the conditions for which they are properly indicated. There is, however, another major danger from ionizing radiation—that of damaging the gonads (testes and ovaries) and creating harmful mutations of the genes that transmit hereditary characteristics. Geneticists strongly advise against provoking any gene mutations beyond those produced by natural background radiation.

While some geneticists would still argue the point, the present consensus is that the risk of any given individual having a child with inborn defects is not significantly increased above normal by submitting to the use of safely shielded X-rays for properly indicated medical or dental needs. The amount of theoretical harm done by correctly administered X-ray dosages is so small that it has never actually been detected or measured. Properly given dental X-rays involve such a limited area of the body that they contribute negligibly to whole body or gonadal radiation.

Nuclear Weapons—Atomic Fallout Risks. The third source of radiation hazards to which the human race is now exposed came into existence in 1945 with the first atomic bomb. Since then there has been great scientific, popular, and political furor over the legitimacy of testing or using such weapons. The explosion of an atomic weapon above the surface of the earth causes atomic fallout, which creates dangers that by their very nature are beyond the control of exposed persons.

A particular problem is posed by the long-lived isotope strontium 90, chemically similar to calcium. Blown into the atmosphere and later descending to earth, this isotope could be absorbed by plants and passed on to man in meat, milk, and other foods. In the human body it would tend, like calcium, to lodge in the bones and might therefore damage the blood-forming organs and produce leukemia, especially in children. The reality of this theoretical risk is constantly being evaluated. For example, the U.S. Public Health Service has expanded to every state its program of measuring the kinds and amounts of radioactivity in the meals of selected school children. These regular diet studies permit more accurate estimates of the daily intake of radioactive substances by children and young adults.

The Federal Radiation Council, in a report issued in May 1963, stated:

Iodine 131 doses from weapons testing conducted through 1962 have not caused undue risk to health.

Health risks from the present and anticipated levels of strontium 90 and from fallout due to testing through 1962 are too small to justify measures to limit the intake by modification of the diet or altering the normal distribution and use of food.

In May 1964, John D. Harley, of the U.S. Atomic Energy Commission pointed out that natural radioactive isotopes (background radiation) give Americans a bigger dose of radiation every year than arrives through radioactive fallout, although the dose from fallout is a "significant fraction" of the natural dose.

Committee Reports on Radiation Hazards. In 1956 the U.S. National Academy of Sciences published a study on atomic-radiation hazards. The study committees sought, among other things, to decide what amount of radiation the male and female sex organs could safely take without undue risk of producing gene changes that might be harmful to future generations.

They arrived at the tentative conclusion that exposure to man-made radiation, including diagnostic and therapeutic X-rays, should not exceed 10 roentgens during the first 30 years of life, counting from the date of *conception*. They said, however: "This is a reasonable quota (for a population) not a harmless one. It should most emphatically not be assumed that any exposure less than 10 roentgens is, so to speak, all right. The idea is to stay as far under the quota as possible. As geneticists we say, 'Keep the dose as low as you can.'"

The National Academy of Sciences report also estimated that the amount of man-made radiation resulting from A-bomb and H-bomb tests continued indefinitely at the 1950 to 1955 rate would add $\frac{1}{2}$ a roentgen in 30 years of exposure to the other radiation hazards to which human beings are exposed.

The report further recommended that every effort should be made "to reduce the radiation exposure from X-rays to the lowest limit consistent with medical necessity."

"Proper safeguards always [should] be taken to minimize the radiation dose to the reproductive cells," the report emphasized.

In 1958 a United Nations Scientific Committee studying the effects of atomic radiation issued a report which in general confirmed the earlier American one. The United Nations committee pointed out that there are still vast areas of ignorance about atomic-radiation hazards since so many "conclusions" about its effects in man are based upon extrapolations of effects observed in rats and mice. The committee unanimously agreed that fallout from nuclear-weapons tests presents a hazard to mankind. "Even the smallest amounts of radiation," it stated, "are liable to cause deleterious genetic and perhaps also somatic (whole-body) effects."

However, on the key question of stopping nuclear-weapons tests or adopting other measures to control radiation dangers, the majority of the United Nations committee sidestepped. It held that these matters "involve national and international decisions which lie outside the scope of its work." The whole question is still debatable.

Cumulative Hazards of Ionizing Radiation. For a gneration, ending in the middle 1960's, mankind can be said to have been living in the formative period of the nuclear age. Since World War II the problems of radiation have been magnified and dramatized. One of man's major problems for the seventies, and thereafter, is to control radiations from all sources, so that he can cope with the artificial environment created by the influence of the atomic industrial revolution. Even in the mid-sixties it was estimated that in the United States alone about half a million people were working on jobs in which radiation was an actual or potential danger.

In considering and planning against the hazards of radiological health, it must be admitted that there are major programs both in the United States and other nations specifically aimed at activities which could lead to exposure of large numbers of people. In these cases the health effects are weighed against considerations of national policy. Another major factor in the public health aspect of radiation is the difficulty in assessing the effects of ionizing radiation. The hazard to the individual is related to the cumulative total of radiation exposures continuously or intermittently received throughout life.

Many sources, old and new, as we have noted, contribute to the cumulative total of radiation which an individual receives through his lifetime. First, of course, there is the natural or "background" radiation, to which man has always been exposed. This includes cosmic rays from space and radiation from naturally radioactive materials present in all parts of the world. The average person in the latitude of the United States receives a total background dose of about 100 milliroentgens per year. Exposure to medical X-rays contributes roughly the same dosage level (when averaged out) as background radiation, especially in North America and Western Europe.

The greatest potential problem of radioactive contamination, if the problem goes uncontrolled, lies in the continuing development of atomic energy. A committee of the U.S. Public Health Service estimated that the accumulated volume of radioactive wastes will increase from about 1.5 million gallons in 1965 to 2 billion gallons in 1995!

The Division of Radiological Health of the U.S. Public Health Service has taken prime responsibility for protecting the American public against radiation dangers. The task, however, is an exceedingly complicated one in which other federal, state, and local government agencies must share. Since, except in rare accidents, acute radiation injury to individuals is rarely seen, the primarily objective of the Division of Radiological Health is the reduction of unnecessary radiation exposure, whatever its source and no matter how small the amount, in order to limit the possible long-term statistical effects upon large numbers of people.

How Much Radiation? A difficult question here has been whether there is such a thing as a safe threshold dose of radiation, below which adverse effects would not appear. Unfortunately, when calculated on a large scale, this does not seem to be the case. Accumulating evidence, particularly on the genetic effects of radiation, as noted, suggests that even small doses to the gonads prior to reproduction will be accompanied by an increase in genetic mutations, most of which will be deleterious.

Any dose chosen as "standard" must therefore be assumed to involve some risk of injury in exposed population groups. The setting of standards cannot therefore be an exclusively scientific task, since there is a need of balancing certain risks against acceptable standards. For use of United States government departments a radiation protection guide is established on the best judgment of the Federal Radiation Council (FRC). This council, incidentally, has estimated the harmful effects from the fallout of all nuclear tests through 1961 as astonishingly minor—

primarily affecting only about 110 people.

Once ionizing radiation is released into the environment, complex measures must be developed and applied to reduce its hazards. Though difficult, the task is not hopeless; and many hopeful experiments are under way. Some control of the radioactive iodine and strontium levels in milk, for example, can be achieved by altering the feeds of dairy cattle.

There can be no question but that in the last third of the twentieth-century mankind's *potential* risk from radiation hazards is bound to increase. However, with the ever-sharper attention and control measures, bulwarked by research directed to holding down or dissipating radiation effects, it is increasingly possible in a peaceful world for the operational hazards of ionizing radiation to be minimized. This is the goal for mankind to seek.

Atomic-Waste Disposal. The use of atomic energy for peaceful purposes also involves some radiation hazards, but up to 1960 these were not taken very seriously because so few (about a dozen) nuclear reactors were actually in operation. One risk is possible accident, but a far more pressing one is what to do with atomic wastes. We have no means of rendering atomic wastes harmless and they will continue to accumulate in the environment. You can't drop them into the ocean or scatter them to the winds. So far they have been buried in the ground, sometimes flushed down abandoned oil wells. The disposal of atomic wastes represents a real and only partially solved problem of environmental sanitation and public health.

Radiation Sickness. There appears to be a great public horror about the "mysterious" effects of radiation upon the human system. There is actually less mystery about this than popularly imagined.

The terms *radiation sickness, injury, or reaction* are used to describe the damage done to body tissues by exposure to radiation from X-rays, gamma rays, radium, radon, atomic energy, and other radioactive substances. The damge, of course, will depend both on the amount of exposure— the dose—and the individual's personal tolerance

for or resistance to radiation. The harmful effects may be acute or delayed.

Acute radiation sickness sometimes occurs in patients who are receiving X-ray treatment for conditions that cannot be expected to respond as adequately to other kinds of treatment, if available. The symptoms are loss of appetite, nausea, vomiting, and diarrhea. The treatment is symptomatic but the symptoms usually disappear in a day or two if no further exposure to X-ray radiation occurs.

Massive doses of radiation, as encountered in atomic explosions, can produce such severe reactions that death shortly ensues. The actual causes of death in these cases, however, can usually be attributed to severe *anemia*, since the blood-forming organs are exceptionally sensitive to radiation; to internal *bleeding*, since the capillary blood vessels are adversely affected; to secondary *infections*, since the white blood cells are knocked out; or to severe *burns*, with changes in the body-fluid balance, since any radiated energy is a form of heat.

In *delayed radiation sickness* the same mechanisms of body damage and possible death operate, but the severe symptoms develop more slowly and insidiously, sometimes over a course of many years. Early symptoms may include easy fatigue and lethargy and (in women) cessation of *menstruation*. Radiation injury in peace-time *can* be avoided by strict obedience to safety rules and regulations in establishments where possible radiation damage is a known hazard.

World Health Organization

Since the fourteenth century, when quarantine (40-day detention) was introduced at Italian seaports, it has been increasingly recognized that conditions affecting community health are not and cannot be contained within its political boundaries. Germs recognize no boundary lines, nor can ideas be kept in a bottle. Personal health and community health are interwoven with world health. What happens in Bangkok may have repercussions in Boston. Yellow fever in Guatemala can travel by plane to Georgia. Dis-

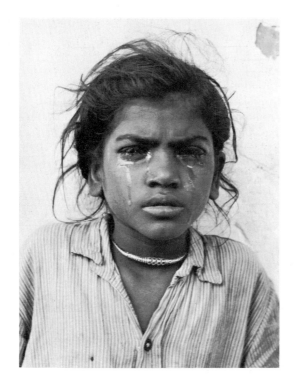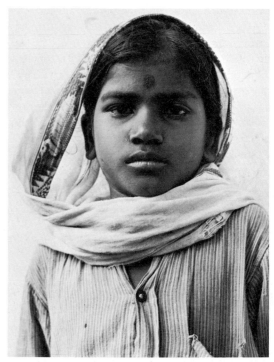

TRACHOMA: Nearly 400 million people suffer from trachoma. Although this eye infection does not kill, its victims often become blind. A World Health Organization assisted trachoma team in India is systematically working in village by village, where the infection rate is as high as 80–90 percent of the population. Aureomycin saves the eyesight of many like this child photographed before and after receiving treatment. The World Health Organization (WHO) is forging ahead on many fronts against many enemies, some of which are illustrated on the following pages. (Photographs courtesy of World Health Organization).

ease, like fire, is best fought at its source. The United States today has an inextricable stake in world health.

This responsibility is formally recognized in at least two ways: by United States membership in the World Health Organization—commonly abbreviated WHO—and by American participation in the World Medical Association, which is composed of over 50 national medical associations, including the American Medical Association. WMA now represents more than 700,000 physicians. The United States is the largest single national contributor to WHO.

WHO was organized in June 1946, in New York City, largely under United States leadership. It now includes over 130 member nations of the United Nations. Within the limitations of its small budget, WHO functions as an inter-national public health agency. It is concerned with raising standards of medical education, fortifying national health services, assisting in campaigns for the control of communicable diseases, and codifying and classifying medical information of international importance. It runs up warning flags of epidemics and endemics anywhere. In protection of the health of its own citizens at home and abroad, and in many other ways, the U.S. has been amply repaid for its investment in WHO.

WHO is the latest in a hundred-year series of international conferences, conventions, and organizations devoted to safeguarding international health. The first international sanitary conference was held in 1851. By 1909 this seed had become the International Office of Public Health (*L'Office International d'Hygiene Publique*) with staff headquarters in Paris. Meantime, in 1902, the Pan American Sanitary Bureau was established at a conference in Washington, D.C. In 1923 the Health Organization of the League of Nations was established with central offices in Geneva, Switzerland. It outlasted the League itself and pointed the way for WHO.

WHO is governed by a World Health Assembly, to which three official delegates may be appointed by each member nation. It has six regional offices, which hold annual regional meetings of their own. Its genuine decentralization of offices, almost unique in international affairs, has considerably strengthened WHO by making it more responsive to the health needs of its member countries.

Principal World Health Problems. The programs to which WHO has assigned priorities for attention reflect the major health problems of the world at large. Its first three priorities were malaria, tuberculosis, and venereal disease. Other "priority" areas that WHO has spearheaded include maternal and child health programs, environmental sanitation, and campaigns against plague, cholera, yellow fever, smallpox, and typhus.

Some of WHO's most successful efforts have been in international disease reporting, in building corps of trained health workers in many countries, and in stimulating nations to the control of communicable diseases with modern techniques. For example, WHO sent six malaria experts to a demonstration area in Greece. With DDT, spraying equipment, and local cooperation, the farm production of this area increased by about 25% in one year! One of the knottiest problems WHO faces is nutrition, since this is related to the world food supply.

Its fundamental approach has been to help people of different nations to help themselves to healthier living. Under its impetus, for example, a midwife in Ceylon can be found conducting classes for mothers in a thatched health center built by the people of the little village where it stands. Continuing and intelligent health education is necessary to get people to adopt the health services by which they will profit.

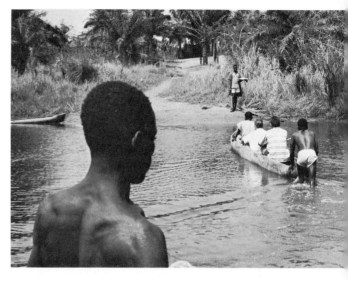

MALARIA: Fighting malaria in Africa is uphill work. In addition to financial, political, and administrative difficulties, the population is generally scattered and often mobile. The very construction of dwellings raises problems. Mosquitos may be resistant to insecticides, and the climate itself may shorten the effect. In this illustration, a spraying team prepared to spray houses in a remote village.

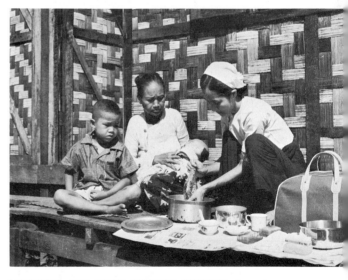

MATERNAL AND CHILD WELFARE SERVICES: Burma's infant mortality rate was estimated several years ago at nearly 300 out of every 1000 live births in many towns. With the guidance of experts furnished by World Health Organization, the United Nations Children's Fund is helping the government to establish 500 maternal and child welfare centers. As a part of the program, trained midwives visit mothers to demonstrate to them proper techniques of child care.

Environmental Health and World Health   **495**

In 1968 WHO celebrated its twentieth anniversary. Its accomplishments in the ten preceding years were considerable. It assisted 72 member states in establishing or improving health services; 16 of these projects were in Africa. Conferences on housing and urban development were held in Mexico, Madrid, Pittsburgh, and Stockholm. In 1968, 169 water supply projects were taking place in 83 countries. The membership of 131 nations at the 21st Assembly adopted a budget of $60,747,800 for 1969. It has established an international center at Delft, Netherlands for the purpose of coordinating research and acting as a clearinghouse of information.

"Little Dictionary of Infectious Diseases." In 1962 WHO issued a "Little Dictionary of Infectious Diseases" listing some of the more or less tropical ills it was fighting and telling how well it was doing against them. The following quotations are from the "Little Dictionary:"[1]

Bilharziasis. Disease caused by parasite that lives part of its life in freshwater snails. This disease hits young people and reduces working capacity. Irrigation often helps to spread. . . . Prevention is by sanitation, clearing water courses of aquatic plants and treating snail-breeding places with molluscicides. Synonym: snail fever, schistosomiasis.

Cholera. Intestinal disease caused by bacteria that contaminate water and food. The patient becomes dehydrated and can die in less than an hour. . . . With a vaccination jet-gun (useful in epidemics), injections can be given twenty times more rapidly than with usual syringe. Main areas of infection (1961): India and Pakistan. Prevention by clean water supplies.

Goiter. A disease caused by diet deficiencies. The remedy has been known for a century. Add iodine to kitchen salt. Still goiter affects 200 million people.

Leprosy. Ten million sufferers throughout the world, of whom only 20% receive treatment of

any kind. Less infectious than tuberculosis. If detected in time, can be completely cured by sulfone drugs.

Malaria. Transmitted by mosquitoes. Fought with insecticides (to kill the mosquitoes) and drugs (to kill the parasites in the bloodstream of sufferers). 140 million cases estimated 1962. Difficulty: some mosquitos have developed resistance to certain insecticides.

Onchoceriasis (river blindness). Caused by minute worm transmitted to man by black flies. 200 to 300 million people are believed to be infected. Control measure: insecticides to reduce fly population.

Plague. Transmitted to man by fleas carried by rats. Natural reservoir of infection: wild rodents, including squirrels. Dread scourge of man for many centuries. In India alone an annual average of over 500,000 deaths was reported between 1898–1908. [In 1967, 5619 cases were reported from South Vietnam, where the disease is endemic. However, great success in patient care. Prevention through rat control.]

Smallpox. Today, 150 years after the discovery of smallpox vaccine, this disease is an anachronism. It could be entirely eliminated if 80% of the world's population were vaccinated. Difficulties: fake certificates of vaccination, speed and volume of modern travel, lack of health workers. Countries most heavily infected: India, Pakistan, Central Africa. Revaccination necessary. [In 1967, about 120,000 cases were reported throughout the world.]

Trachoma. A virus disease that can lead to blindness. According to WHO, a sixth of the world's population (500 million people) is infected. In areas where practically the whole population has it, 1% of adults are totally blind and 4% are economically blind. Control through antibiotics.

Tuberculosis. 309 million persons were tuberculin-tested and 117 million vaccinated with BCG between 1941 and 1960 in 41 countries with a total population of 800 million. With modern drugs, particularly isoniazid, patients can be treated at home.

Typhus. Transmitted by lice. Killed hundreds

[1] "Little Dictionary of Infectious Diseases," *World Health*, The Magazine of the World Health Organization, 15: 4, 5–8 (July–August 1962).

of millions of people in the past. Control through DDT powder on body and clothes in order to destroy lice.

Yaws. A widespread, disfiguring, treponemal disease, causing deepseated infirmity if untreated. Can be cured by a single injection of long-acting penicillin (10 to 15 cents per treatment). 280 million people examined and 35 million treated between 1950 and 1960.

Yellow Fever. Transmitted to man by virus-carrying mosquito. Practically eliminated from the Americas. A few centers of infection remain in Africa. Not present in Asia. Forest reservoir of infection: mainly monkeys.

Zoonoses. Diseases transmitted from animal to man include psittacosis (parrot), Q-fever (goats, cattle), anthrax (cattle, horses), brucellosis (cattle, sheep, goats, etc.), and trichinosis (swine).

WHO alone cannot take credit for all the improvements in the world health that have occurred since World War II. But it has certainly taken some of the giant steps in that direction.

Other international organizations that contribute to world health include the Food and Agriculture Organization (FAO) of the United Nations and UNICEF (United Nations International Children's Emergency Fund).

The United States State Department, under a program known as AID, supports and conducts many health programs throughout the world. In 1967, for example, the agency expended around $50 million on health projects.

A Healthier World. The world *is* getting healthier. Expectation of life at birth has increased appreciably, sometimes dramatically, throughout the world. In Puerto Rico it increased by 22 years in 15 calendar years (1941 to 1955)! In Ceylon it increased by 17 years! The lowest life expectancy is still in India (32 years at birth), the highest in the Netherlands (72.5), Sweden, Norway, Israel, England, New Zealnd, the United States, and Canada. In the Soviet Union the average length of life was 64 years in 1955—the figure at which the United States stood a decade earlier. Females outlive males in every country of the world except Guatemala,

Ceylon, and India, where the males win by a fraction of a year.

Coupled with generally increased birth and marriage rates, the lowered death rates have added about 900 million people to the face of the earth since World War II. World population now stands over 3 billion! Asia claims more than half—over 1.75 billion. China, the largest nation, claims to have about 700 million people; India, next largest, 440 million. The United States, the wealthiest nation, has passed 200 million.

If the world's so-called population explosion continued at the rates of the early 1960's, it is estimated that the world population would reach 4 billion by 1980, 6 billion by 2000. This is unlikely, for the possible checks on population, as pointed out by Thomas Malthus back in 1798, will probably come into operation. The world cannot contain more people than it can feed.

The Space Age and Aerospace Medicine. We are living in what is called the "space age." If it must be dated by a specific event, it may be conceded to have begun on October 4, 1957, when the Russians launched the first artificial earth satellite, Sputnik I. We are also, however, living in the "atomic age" or "nuclear age," which may be dated back to December 2, 1942, when scientists working underneath the football stadium at the University of Chicago initiated and controlled the first self-sustaining, man-made, nuclear chain reaction. It is further asserted that we are now living in the "tranquillizer age" and the "aspirin age." Still we cannot claim that we have outlived the "electrical age," the "stream age" and the "iron age," all of much more ancient vintage.

The space age is interesting and characteristic in that it exhibits mankind's proclivity for exploring problems beyond his immediate ken long before he has resolved problems at home. We have put men on the moon before we have eliminated malaria, number one killer of mankind on earth. Practically speaking, the problem of surviving space travel affects the lives of only a few dozen earth dwellers, specially selected American astronauts and Russian cosmonauts. However, the intense research in aerospace medicine, the "human engineering," and particularly the development of new medical instrumentation and protective devices on their behalf may improve the health and welfare of millions of people who never get off the ground. Aerospace medicine, a step beyond global epidemiology, is a relatively new and fruitful medical and research specialty; but fascinating as it may be, it does not yet touch the lives of anywhere near so many people as such older and more mundane specialties as surgery and sanitary engineering.

Aerospace medicine is primarily concerned with the reactions of human beings under special kinds of *stress* (see page 151); for example, long and boring confinement in small capsules, wherein the normal cycles of day and night are lost; ability to withstand thrusts of pressure (acceleration) up to eighteen times the force of gravity (*g*); weightlessness; extreme heat; disorientation; tumbling; exposure to noise and vibration; and breathing an atmosphere ten times as loaded with carbon dioxide as the normal atmosphere on earth. Astronauts must also be protected against excess solar and radiant energy in space. The "ideal" build for the spaceman—stocky; short, sturdy neck; no heavy muscular development—is not necessarily the preferred physique for men who will spend their whole lives operating only against the perpetual pull of earth's gravity. (See page 459.)

Man in His Social Environment: The Present Situation

It would be difficult to conclude this text more eloquently than in the words spoken by the great Canadian psychiatrist and humanitarian, first director of the World Health Organization, Dr. Brock Chisholm, at the 1962 International Conference on Health and Health Education in Philadelphia, as follows:

As is true for all other forms of life, man's environment has always been a very important, even determining factor in his physical, mental, and social development. His basic equipment of muscle, eye, ear, tactile sense, erect posture, op-

posable thumb, and his brain, plus a long gestation period, long period of defenselessness of his young, omnivorous digestive system, gregarious tendency, and other specific qualities, have determined or allowed the methods he has used of surviving and developing his social and cultural patterns.

Man's particular superiority over all other known forms of life seems to lie largely in the degree of development of his brain, his ability to think, to imagine, to plan for the future, and to base his decisions on a very wide range of information and experience. Man's ability to communicate, and thus to acquire experience from others, has been of immense importance to his rapid development, over the last few thousand years, of ability to manipulate or control his environment. His power of adjustment to wide variations of environment and of adaptation of the environment to his own requirements have increased very greatly even in this century.

At the present time it seems that man's most important and dangerous lag is in relation to the human part of his environment, in his social relationships. For the first time man is now capable of destroying mankind. His technical skills have now produced a new situation, totally unknown to any previous generation, in which this generation holds a veto power over continuing human evolution and even existence.

There is no precedent for this situation and no established patterns of adjustment to it or methods of dealing with it. Perhaps still worse, there is no tradition of concern in any culture for this kind of problem. The environment in which man now finds himself is, for the first time, dangerous to all mankind, and it appears that man's social organization and habitual behavior patterns are quite inadequate for dealing effectively with the new relationships involved in this new situation. Because our power to destroy life has become absolute, our ancient and universal method of survival, by competition to the death between survival groups, has become suicidal on a racial scale. . . .

If these observations are valid, as I believe they

are, it is clear that a widespread reorientation is necessary, involving our own reeducation of ourselves into patterns of thinking and social behavior designed for survival in this new kind of world in which we, precariously, exist. No challenge of this degree of importance has ever before faced any human generation, but also no previous generation possessed the advantages we have of psychological and sociological understanding and of facility of communication.

Whether we will use those abilities effectively is still to be decided; that depends on our mental and social health. At the present time a large part of the responsibility for what will happen to the human race rests, inescapably, with the health professions. The very least that should be expected from the health professions is a demonstration of concern about man's ability to react appropriately and effectively to new and dangerous situations, with some appreciation of the factors in individual development which tend to facilitate or to obstruct progress toward a level of mental and social health necessary for human survival.

SUMMARY

As the world's population, white, black, yellow, and brown, increases—thanks largely to application of the principles of environmental health—the social and ideological environments surrounding each of us are altered. How perceptibly, how radically time alone can tell. Meanwhile we must contend with new hazards in our biological and physical environments—for example, pesticides (boon or bane?) and the effects of ionizing radiation from space, radioactive minerals in the earth's crust, medical and dental X-rays, atomic power plants and wastes, and nuclear fallout from weapons.

By and large, medicine and mankind have triumphed over the insect-borne diseases that once decimated large populations. Despite the present incidence of malaria, yellow fever, river blindness, and other communicable diseases noted by the valiantly working World Health Organization (WHO), the outlook for their eventual eradication is favorable. We know what to do about them—which previous generations did not. This long-lived generation's greatest risk, as Dr. Brock Chisholm points out, could be, and probably is, the threat of the misuse of nuclear energy, which could leave dominion over the face of the globe to the cockroach and other radioresistant insects.

The physical health and survival of the human race is inextricably interwoven with its mental health and moral vision.

SUMMARY REVIEW QUESTIONS

1. What is the "population explosion"? What has brought it about? What is its principal significance? How, eventually, is it likely to be checked?
2. In terms of population, what are the three largest continents, the four largest nations, and the five largest cities in the world?
3. What are some of the most important insect-borne diseases (name at least four)? What roles in the conquest of insect-borne diseases did the following men play: William C. Gorgas, Theobald Smith, David Bruce, Ronald Ross, Walter Reed?
4. When, where, and how was DDT, the first of the well-known modern insecticides, first spectacularly used and thus established as an important means for the control of insect-borne diseases? How does DDT function in the control of malaria and yellow fever? What are some of the other tropical diseases against which DDT and other new insecticides offer a primary method of control?

5. What are pesticides? What are the risks arising from their indiscriminate use? How and where are they primarily used today? What are the arguments for the use of pesticides?

6. What are the present sources of ionizing radiation to which human beings in different countries are exposed? In what countries are the risks probably greatest—and why?

7. Exactly what are the risks of ionizing radiation in the United States? What measures are being taken to minimize these risks?

8. What is the World Health Organization (WHO)? How was it organized? What are its chief functions? What are some of the important world health problems it has tackled?

9. What are some of the infectious diseases (name four) which are still worldwide problems? In what ways, if any, has progress been made in controlling these diseases? How serious a problem on an international scale is blindness? Why?

10. What changes, if any, do you think must be made in the ideational environment of mankind to assure the survival of the human race?

11. Are the following statements sense or nonsense? Why? *This generation holds veto power over continuing human evolution and even its existence. . . . Pesticides are a boon. . . . The World Health Organization has failed in its basic purposes. . . . The population explosion of the twentieth century is one of the best things that has ever happened to the human race. . . . The risks of ionizing radiation are now completely under control. . . . Man can hardly recognize the devils of his own creation.*

12. What do the following terms mean to you: radiation sickness, ecology, WMA, genetic mutation, plague, *Anopheles,* zoonoses, trachoma, Thomas Malthus, social environment?

Recommended For Further Reading: *Silent Spring* by Rachel Carson. *An Essay on the Principle of Population* by Thomas Malthus (1798). *Plague on Us* by Geddes Smith. *Doctors to the World* by Murray Morgan. *The Next Million Years* by Sir Charles Galton Darwin. For more complete references, see Appendix E.

A Selected Reading

Resources in America: The Coming Crisis

John P. Milton

Those of us who live in North America are on the brink of a fundamental revolution in our understanding of environment. We are finally coming to realize that the resources of our continent are limited and that they are bound together by a delicate web of complex interrelationships. In his recent book, *Science and Survival*, biologist Dr. Barry Commoner suggested that "The age of innocent faith in science and technology may be over." When we examine the past for the unforeseen effects of applied new technology, the conclusion that we have unknowingly promoted serious forms of environmental degradation seems inescapable. In looking to the future, it seems equally clear that the impact of technology upon our environment is accelerating, and that the size and permanence of many changes are going to be on a scale entirely new to man.

For many years the assumption that man was capable of adapting indefinitely to a changing environment dominated our approach to the two greatest environmental forces of our age: population growth and technological change. We are

only now beginning to question this basic assumption for our own country. And when we consider the history of population growth and technological change abroad, a clearer picture begins to emerge of man's basic limitations.

The Indian Example

There are today over half a billion people in India. Before the end of the century the same country will probably contain over a billion individuals. In the past, most Indians lived in rural villages, but now the villages are full and huge numbers of people are overflowing into large urban centers where there is little food and housing to sustain them. According to the *New York Times*, some 100,000 Indians are homeless and over a million are living in shanties that lack even the bare minimum of sanitary facilities. The specter of famine lies ahead for many of these people.

As India's population grows, the need to increase her agricultural production is becoming critical. The surplus granaries of the highly-developed nations are almost empty, and despite

worldwide efforts to stimulate agricultural production, population growth has consistently outstripped the ability of farm technology to keep up with it. Here we see one of the greatest miscarriages of technology. Through the well-intentioned introduction of medical technology alone, India's death rate was cut drastically while little effort was made to cut birth rates to a level that would keep her population in balance with her available resources. Now much of the world is aware of this problem, yet many experts remain pessimistic about our ability to invoke technology either to increase food production adequately or reduce birth rates quickly enough to solve India's problem.

The staggering difficulties that beset India hold true in varying degrees for over two-thirds of the world's population—a human tide in excess of two billion individuals now living in the "developing" regions of Asia, Africa, and Latin America. These regions have about half the world's total agricultural land resources, yet by the end of this century these same limited land resources—barring

SOURCE. John P. Milton is the director of the Office of International Affairs for the Conservation Foundation in Washington, D.C. The article presented here was released by the Population Reference Bureau on May 13, 1968; it has been somewhat abridged.

some spectacular breakthrough in food as from plankton or artificial photosynthesis—will have to feed nearly five billion people. Sir Julian Huxley, the famous British biologist, has said: "The problem of population is the problem of our age."

. . . At this point one may ask what direct effect this problem has on the United States. One may also ask whether we can ever isolate our continent from the dislocations, social and economic, of the less-developed world.

The U.S. Is Not An Island

Few of us realize how dependent our relatively affluent society is upon the rest of the planet. At present, our 200 million people consume about 40 percent of the total raw material resource output of the free world. And our rate of consumption of these raw materials has been rising steadily. We are growing more, not less, dependent upon the rest of the world. But as the developing countries accelerate their own industrial development—which they now see as their only hope—we can expect their demands for the world's natural resource output to grow rapidly. Within a short period of time we can expect to face much more active competition for this limited supply of raw materials.

Our future, then, is intimately linked with the future of the developing nations. And until they undertake to halt their population explosion as a primary step in successful development planning, we can only expect increasing social turbulence among over two-thirds of the world's people. As a world power, the United States is apt to become embroiled in revolutionary upheavals not of our own making—upheavals which will affect us politically and materially no matter what our official response may be. Thus, our best internal planning cannot succeed in the long run without global responsibility in the field of population growth.

Within the United States also, the size and distribution of our own population will have a major effect on the quality of our nation's environment. In 1967 the U.S. population rose above 200 million. Fifty years ago there were only 103 million Americans. By the end of another fifty years if present trends continue, our population will soar to some number between 324 million and 482 million.

What will a nation of 400 to 500 million Americans be like? At the 200-million level the problems of urban environment already seem insurmountable. But in the years ahead we will face the continuing concentration of more and more people in our already crowded urban clusters, and we will see the emergence of megalopolises. Together these vast super-cities may contain nearly one-half our country's population, including the majority of the scientifically-advanced, intellectual, and creative elements. But they may also contain sizeable extensions of the urban porverty now so familiar to us all.

Our Dwindling Resources

How will we deal with such massive urban environments? Every year the spread of U.S. cities consumes a million and half acres of open space—and much of this has been prime agricultural land. In California alone by the year 2000, I estimate that at least half the best crop land will have gone into urban industrial or residential use. Will we come to regret the loss of such fertile regions in the age of enormous populations and scarcer food that lies ahead?

As our population, urbanization, and the scope of our technology increase, the demands upon our nation's water resources will also accelerate rapidly. In a recent Water Resources Report, the National Academy of Science and the National Research Council estimated that we will be withdrawing 600 billion gallons per day in 1980 and 900 billion gallons per day in the year 2000— against an average run-off of just 1200 billion gallons. The report went on to say:

"At the present time, the limited pure-water resources of the arid west are almost at an end. Several states, such as Arizona which draws 60% of its water supply from over-pumped wells, have real cause for concern at this point. Some states in the manufacturing belt of the east are beginning to find themselves faced with the possibility of deterioration of their fresh-water resources."

To view the problem another way, for every addition of 1,000 people, we will need 36.5 million more gallons of water each year, as well as more sewers and treatment plants to deal with another yearly 62,000 pounds of organic water pollutants.

There will not only be a

problem of water distribution in coming years, but also a major crisis in water quality. The seriousness of this situation comes into focus when we remember that the watersheds most available to urban centers are also those most likely to be affected by pollution. In 1966 the Senate Public Works Committee recommended six billion dollars for the next five years to stimulate local construction of sewage treatment plants. The Committee went on to say that "the (total) cost of pollution control could well exceed $100 billion." Clearly we are only beginning to calculate the true costs incurred by rapid industrial development and the intemperate application of technology.

There are other, less obvious effects of the pollution of our environment. Despite the warnings voiced by Rachel Carson, Robert Rudd and others, we continue to shower increasing amounts of pesticides—largely for agricultural purposes—on our soil. These poisons are leached out and carried into rivers, where they contribute to lowered fish productivity, then reach the ocean, to be concentrated by diatoms. Dr. Lloyd Berkner has pointed out that "our supply of atmospheric oxygen comes largely from these diatoms—they replenish all of the atmospheric oxygen as it is used up. But if our pesticides should be reducing the supply of diatoms, or forcing evolution of less productive mutants, we might find ourselves running out of atmospheric oxygen."

The Knowledge Gap

So it is, then, that the rapid growth of modern technology is shaping the human habitat of tomorrow in ways we may not adequately foresee. Perhaps the most difficult aspect of the technological revolution is that we have consistently failed to understand the environmental risk involved in each application of new technology. We have already subjected our bodies to DDT, tetraethyl lead, and other potential poisons without knowing how close we have come to committing suicide; exposed our lungs to smog; suffered an increasing incidence of chronic respiratory disease; risked the long-term genetic and physiological effects of radioactive fallout; filled our rivers with chemical and organic pollutants; and committed great masses of people to a new, highly-stressful life in congested megalopolises —all without really knowing if the supposed short-term benefits would be worth it when measured against the long-term costs.

How many of these environmental changes induced by new technology are irreversible? How can we reduce the long-term environmental risks in such situations? I have mentioned the potential depletion of the world's free supply of oxygen. Another long-term atmospheric change that may profoundly alter human life is directly related to our use of fossil fuels. By burning the stored-up reserves of coal, oil, and natural gas, we have raised the carbon dioxide content of the atmosphere about ten percent over the past 100 years. Due to carbon dioxide's "greenhouse effect," which allows sunlight to pass through it but which reduces re-radiation of heat into space, the earth's temperature is liable to rise—if we continue utilizing fossil fuels. It has been estimated by the President's Science Advisory Committee that this increase in retained heat could lead to a slow melting of the polar ice caps— eventually raising the sea level 400 feet and inundating vast land areas and all of the world's present major ports.

How are we to prevent such a catastrophe? Nuclear power has been hailed as one solution. Certainly, the dangers of an increasing concentration of atmospheric carbon dioxide and the respiratory effects of rising air pollution would be effectively reduced. But how will we safely dispose of the massive amounts of radioactive wastes? A number of countries are already dumping toxic by-products from atomic energy plants into the sea. The United States has stored them in concrete blocks and buried them in the ocean, in caves, salt domes and deep wells. What are the risks from this process of groundwater contamination, especially in earthquake zones where vertical shearing of strata may take place? What happens to radioactive materials released into the oceans, either directly or perhaps indirectly through container decomposition?

I have mentioned only a few of the key factors that will affect the future environment of America: the growth of world population in relation to our nation's heavy dependence on raw materials abroad; the growth and changes in distribution of population within the United States; the emergence of huge megalopolises; the increased demands upon limited internal resources, such as water; and the impact of technology-caused pollution on the environment.

If we impose no conscious restraints in our power to "conquer" nature, our material and population growth will either stabilize at the point where shortages of food, water, breathable air, raw materials, energy resources, and space exert their own tyranny, or where epidemic disease and warfare become the primary controls of human numbers.

A

COMMON HUMAN AILMENTS
A Short Reference Catalogue*

This brief, alphabetical catalogue of common, adult human ailments brings together in one convenient place for ready reference the pertinent facts about prevalent chronic and "minor" illnesses always of interest to students of health. It is questionable, of course, whether there is such a thing as a "minor" illness. Any one of them might be the forerunner of or develop into a major illness or even a surgical emergency. For example, a common cold may be the forerunner of pneumonia.

What patients call "illnesses" or "diseases" are often what doctors view only as signs, symptoms, or complaints of disease. Furthermore, the person who is suffering from a "minor illness" doesn't usually consider it "minor." His pain is real and immediate.

The aim of this catalogue is not to make bad doctors but rather good patients out of willing students. This information should be especially useful in later life. The chronic diseases are problems largely because their causes remain obscure and the treatment for them is still only partially effective.

Included in this catalogue are the well-advertised diseases—mostly neurological disorders—for the control of which many voluntary health agencies have been established. Omitted from this catalogue are those disease conditions which are elsewhere discussed in this text. These conditions are, however, listed here with a cross reference to the text.

abdominal pain. One of the greatest indictments against laxatives is the rush to use them in the presence of abdominal pain. Categorically, *don't do it*! In the presence of abdominal pain lasting more than an hour, not only don't take a laxative but don't take anything to eat or drink until you have consulted a physician—this should be done promptly. There are a number of serious medical emergencies heralded by sharp abdominal pain. Among them is appendicitis, or inflammation of the useless appendage to the human digestive tract described as the vermiform appendix. With one very important exception—cancer—most gastrointestinal disorders express themselves through pain in the abdomen. Persistent abdominal pain demands medical care.

The cause of some cases of abdominal distress is obvious: overindulgence in food or drink. This pain can be relieved by vomiting, or by lying down quietly with the knees drawn up. Among other possible causes of abdominal pain are food allergy, food poisoning (gastrointestinal infection), and psychological stress—

*See also "Little Dictionary of Infectious Diseases," page 496.

often a factor in "nervous stomach," colitis, and peptic ulcer, a breach or erosion of the inner wall of the stomach or duodenum.

acne See page 171.

alcoholism See page 67.

allergy An allergy is an excessive and peculiar sensitivity to offending substances, called allergens, which do not adversely affect most people. Common allergens are food (see food allergy, page 508), pollens (see hayfever, page 509), dusts and hair. The symptoms of allergy—allergic reactions—may be expressed on the skin as hives and rashes, in the mucous membranes—as a stuffed nose or bronchial asthma—and in the digestive tract. Desensitization to some allergens is possible, but avoidance of them is usually indicated.

angina pectoris Angina pectoris literally means pain or strangling in the chest. Probably 95% of all instances occur in patients with heart disease, specifically, with disease of the coronary arteries. (See heart

505

disease, page 325). A common remedy for anginal pain is nitroglycerin. A small pellet placed under the tongue is rapidly absorbed and, by relaxing the blood vessels, soon relieves the chest pain.

appendicitis Appendicitis is an infectious inflammation of the worm-shaped (vermiform) appendix, a projection or pouch, some 1 to 6 inches long, that protrudes from the part of the large bowel called the cecum. The condition is fairly common in the late teens and middle age. An attack of appendicitis often comes on suddenly with a sharp *abdominal pain* (see abdominal pain). Treatment is surgical—the removal of the appendix. However, with sulfa drugs and antibiotics, it is now possible to reduce infection and the risk of a bursting appendix before operating, Before modern chemotherapy, emergency surgery was frequently required. Deaths from appendicitis are now at a low figure.

asthma Asthma is a symptom, not a disease. It describes the type of wheezing, labored breathing, that occurs with many forms of *allergy* (see allergy). Bronchial asthma is the most severe, and most often fatal, of allergic diseases. Such attacks may last for minutes, hours, or days. The patient wheezes and coughs; his breathing becomes difficult—almost as if something were crushing his chest. The severity of the attack is owing to the narrowing of bronchial tubes by spasmodic contraction and to the excess secretion of mucus. Relief of attacks is usually obtained by the administration of adrenalin. Long-term treatment involves discovery of the offending allergen and desensitization to it, if possible. Antihistamine drugs are also employed to relieve or abort asthmatic symptoms or attacks.

arthritis See rheumatism, page 511.

apoplexy See stroke, page 331.

athlete's foot See page 171.

boils Boils are more or less painful but usually limited infections. They generally begin in hair follicles and are principally caused by staphylococcus organisms. A simple boil, or furuncle, has a single core and may be no more than a pimple. More serious are a mass of boils, close together and with several cores, called a carbuncle.

Boils generally occur where the skin and hair roots are chafed or irritated, as on the back of the neck, in the armpits and on the buttocks of rowers and riders.

Boils should not be indiscriminately pinched or squeezed—especially those on the face or in the ear.

The walled-off infection may thus be induced to spread dangerously.

Small, simple boils can be treated by protecting them from irritation with a small adhesive tape and gauze bandage until the boil comes to a head in about a week, breaks, and evacuates its small core of pus. The bandage should be continued until healing is complete.

Large or painful boils should not be tampered with. See a physician. He may have to lance the boil to let out pus. He may also administer an antibiotic.

cancer See page 331.

cerebral palsy (CP) Cerebral palsy (CP) describes a group of disorders, all stemming from brain damage before, during, or shortly after birth and remaining more or less fixed. The common and classical symptom of cerebral palsy is inability to control body movements. In the spastic type of the disease, the body twitches, the muscles move without control, the face makes strange grimaces. In the athetoid type, the muscles tighten up, become rigid, often go into tremor (shaking). Unfortunately the handicaps of cerebral palsy are not limited to the muscle spasms. Among the 550,000 cerebral-palsied infants, children, and adults in the United States, half to three-quarters also suffer from speech defects, half are mentally retarded, half have eye defects, and one-quarter have impaired hearing.

cirrhosis of the liver Cirrhosis, or hardening, of the liver has crept up to be among the principal causes of death in the United States. In cirrhosis a vast number of the normally functioning cells of the liver are replaced by hardened, leathery cells, something like scar tissue. In a "hobnailed liver" the hardening process has gone so far that the outer surface of the liver appears covered with small nail-like projections.

Cirrhosis of the liver is most commonly associated with chronic alcoholism, and is one of the most unpleasant and fatal results. The death rate in cirrhosis is high, ranging around 20% to 25% of the cases. It is now generally considered that the cases of cirrhosis associated with alcohol are actually the result of the nutritional deficiency, particularly the lack of B vitamins, to which the chronic alcoholic is frequently subject.

There are other less common but definite causes of cirrhosis; notably obstruction to flow of bile from the liver, as from gallstones, and certain chronic infections, such as syphilis and malaria. The treatment of cirrhosis is chiefly nutritional (high-vitamin, high-protein diet) and palliative—to relieve such untoward symptoms as bleeding from the esophagus.

common cold See page 362.

constipation Constipation, or costiveness, means retention of feces from any cause. When it appears unexpectedly and acutely, it must be regarded as a *symptom* of some underlying disorder, and medical treatment must be directed at the cause. The kind of chronic constipation that many people worry about, however, is usually a delusion or a neurosis. Quite often it is caused by the very remedy—a laxative—which the victim has prescribed for himself to relieve himself of an imaginary ailment.

An unbelievably great number of people in the United States falsely believe themselves to be constipated and treat themselves accordingly. Generous advertising of laxative remedies has contributed to this illusion "Be regular, be regular, be regular," drum the advertisements. This is hokum. There is no law of nature or hygiene which decrees that a human being must move his bowels regularly once a day or suffer ill health. Regularity in evacuation of feces is a highly individual matter; it makes no difference whether it be three times a day or once in three days.

Definitely misguided is the zeal to "get regular" by the use of laxatives, cathartics, or purgatives of any description. Physicians have come to prescribe these evacuant drugs less and less frequently.

The laxative habit—and it should be noted that many laxative drugs are habit-forming—is to be deplored and avoided. It is expensive too. The American public spends as much as $50 million a year on needless laxatives.

The ill effects of constipation are greatly exaggerated. The symptoms which failure to move the bowels every day are said to produce—weariness, headache, sluggishness and malaise—are not caused by constipation. They are more likely to be symptoms of some localized or systemic fault, often psychic in origin, of which the constipation is just another symptom. Investigators have found that these symptoms can be reproduced simply by stuffing cotton into the rectum. The false popular opinion, however, is that these symptoms result from self-poisoning (auto-intoxication!) with products that are elaborated in the lower intestine because unevacuated feces are allowed to stand there. This so-called explanation of auto-intoxication is pure bosh. The feces have an unpleasant odor, but they are not very toxic.

The enema habit is as bad as the laxative habit. The bowels will function most effectively if they are left alone.

Constipation can be prevented, so far as it needs to be, by an intelligent mental attitude, a properly selected diet with a normal amount of roughage, adequate fluid intake and reasonable daily exercise. Normal peristalsis pushes the mass of feces accumulated in the lower intestines into the rectum, whence nerve endings telegraph a call for defecation. If the "call of nature" is not heeded, the fecal mass retreats back into the sigmoid. The physiological signal for emptying the bowels should be heeded when it occurs. If it is not sounded for several days at a time, that is still no occasion for needless worry and certainly no command to visit the drugstore or medicine cabinet for a purge.

Improper toilet training in early childhood is at the root of many people's foolish fear of being constipated. Too many mothers praise small children when they move their bowels on schedule and scold them when they don't. This forgotten, repressed childhood experience often induces in adult life a haunting sense of guilt or anxiety when bowels fail to move. It is foolish, of course, but sometimes the cure for constipation, as for colitis, diarrhea, and other disorders of the digestive tract, lies in psychotherapy.

dental caries See page 189.

diabetes Diabetes mellitus is a chronic, metabolic disease. About 40% of the 4.2 million people in the United States who have it don't yet know it.

The body organ primarily at fault in diabetes is the pancreas. It fails, for obscure reasons, to secrete from its islet cells sufficient insulin to permit complete oxidation of carbohydrates in the body tissues. This is a metabolic failure. The unoxidized carbohydrates then circulate uselessly in the bloodstream as "blood sugar" or pass off in the urine, which is sweet. The victims of untreated diabetes are subject to diabetic coma and gangrene. Treated according to the best modern methods, in which his lifelong and whole-hearted cooperation is obtained, the diabetic today can hope for a practically normal span of life.

The treatment of diabetes is a careful regimen of diet, in which carbohydrates are restricted but not eliminated; exercise; cleanliness, to prevent gangrene; and if necessary, the administration of insulin by injection or tolbutamide—a new drug—by mouth.

Diabetes appears to run in families and is associated with overweight in middle age. It is diagnosed by the presence of sugar in the blood and urine. The symptoms of the disease, through which its presence may be suspected, include: excessive thirst, frequent urination, weakness and drowsiness, loss of weight in spite of great appetite, and boils. Diabetes is one serious disease for which scientific medical care can usually supply a nearly complete method of control for known cases. Nevertheless, some arterial changes take place in spite of "adequate" control.

epilepsy Epilepsy describes a group of nervous disorders characterized by convulsive seizures ("fits") and generally involving loss of consciousness. Violent attacks are described as "grand mal"; mild attacks, lasting a few seconds, as "petit mal." Contrary to popular misconception, the epileptic is more of a danger to himself than to other people. When a fit is on him, he must be protected so that he does not hurt himself.

Epilepsy was known to the ancient Greeks, who called it "the sacred disease." The disease is now known to be associated with abnormal electrical disturbances in the brain ("brain waves"), which can be detected by electroencephalography. It can now be kept under control with new anti-convulsant drugs, notably dilantin. Of the estimated 1,500,000 epileptics in the United States, a very high proporiton can now hold jobs and get along as safely and well as other people. Much antiquated superstition and legislation still restricts job and other opportunities for epileptics.

food allergy Allergies or allergic diseases are in a sense the opposite of deficiency diseases. In allergy the body responds, sometimes violently, not to the lack of some food or other essential but to the presence or even minute excess of some specifically offending substance. In a way allergies are poisonings.

It is common experience that some foods agree with us better than others. There is an old proverb, "One man's meat is another man's poison." One test of disagreeable foods is that they stay with you for a long time and can be tasted long after they have been eaten. It is better to avoid or eat most sparingly of the foods that—as the saying goes—"repeat on you." For some people, however, there are foods that do far worse than "repeat." They cause a variety of unpleasant symptoms both in the digestive tract itself and in other parts of the body. The typical example is "strawberry rash." An individual who is sensitive or allergic to strawberries may find his skin breaking out in an itchy rash when he eats them. Hives are among the most common symptoms of food allergies, but many more are possible, including the asthma and nasal congestion that are the familiar symptoms of pollen allergy (hay fever). The gastrointestinal tract displays its own opposition to offending foods with such symptoms as indigestion, nausea, vomiting, and diarrhea.

The exact mechanism of food or other allergy is not understood. The unpleasant symptoms are relieved by avoiding the offending allergens, or sometimes by desensitization to them. The discovery of an allergen is often a piece of medical detective work. The elimination diet, in which groups of food are omitted regularly from the diet according to plan until the offending food is found, is one of the tools for dealing with food allergies. Quite often, but not necessarily, the offending allergen turns out to be a specific protein, such as that of milk, eggs, wheat, chocolate, or seafood. However, any food on any menu may sometimes prove to be allergenic to some individuals. It is im-portant to note that people sometimes outgrow their food allergies, especially the allergies of childhood.

food poisoning Food poisoning is really a severe intestinal infection, which breaks out into uncomfortable symptoms—abdominal pain, vomiting, diarrhea, cold sweat, and headache—anywhere from a few hours to a day and a half after the contaminated food was eaten. The offending microorganism is usually one of the group described as *Salmonella,* though other microbes can be responsible. The most dangerous, fortunately, is the rarest—the organism which causes botulism, a severe, sometimes fatal form of food poisoning which reaches the central nervous system. Prompt medical attention should be obtained if and when symptoms of food poisoning occur.

Actually food posioning is a rare rather than a common occurrence on the American scene. It is not so rare in countries without high standards of sanitation and public health.

Food poisoning is commonly the result of failure to store food properly, especially in summer. If food smells or tastes peculiar, you should avoid it.

glaucoma Glaucoma is a serious disease whose locale is within the eye itself; probably 1 in every 8 or 9 cases of blindness results from this disease. In glaucoma the pressure of the fluids within the eyeball unaccountably rises. This intraocular tension makes the eyeball hard, and the pressure, if unrelieved, destroys fibers from the optic nerve to the retina. The disease can be treated with considerable success, if it is discovered in time.

Glaucoma usually strikes in and after middle age. In a small portion of the cases, the disease comes on suddenly (acute glaucoma). Its earliest symptom is clouded vision, with or without pain around the eyes. Most commonly, glaucoma creeps up insidiously, offering only intermittent symptoms. You should, however, be checked for this dangerous, blinding disease, if warning symptoms occur. The doctor does this with an instrument, called the tonometer, that measures fluid pressure inside the eyeball.

A check-up is indicated if you are regularly or occasionally plagued by any of the following symptoms: blurred or foggy vision, loss of side vision, rainbow-colored rings around lights, inability to adjust vision to darkened rooms (as when entering a motion picture theatre), need to change glasses frequently without any new pair being really satisfactory.

gonorrhea See page 361.

halitosis Halitosis or bad breath is a symptom rather than a disease. The usual cause is infected teeth or gums; but it may also occur as a result of nose and throat infections, some lung disorders (notably bronchiectasis), diabetes (in which case the breath has a sweetish, vinegary odor), indigestion, and the eating of odorous foods, like garlic. Bad breath cannot be rinsed away; it will continue to recur until the underlying cause is corrected.

hayfever The discomforts of hayfever follow a seasonal pattern and afflict the upper respiratory system, chiefly the nose. Hayfever is an *allergy*—extreme sensitivity—to various plant pollens, especially ragweed. It is related, therefore, to such other allergic reactions as hives, "strawberry rash," bronchial asthma, and food allergy.

Hayfever can be quite mild or so severe as to cause loss of sleep and weight. The disease occurs most commonly in late summer and fall, but sometimes also in spring and early summer, when it may be called "rose fever."

Some of America's estimated 4 million hayfever patients are relieved by antihistamic drugs; others by desensitizing injections of the pollen to which they are sensitive (after this has been determined by skin tests). Still others go to resorts more or less free of irritating pollens, or try to stay in air-conditioned rooms during their hayfever season. No single treatment relieves all victims.

headache Headache is probably the commonest complaint a doctor hears. The possible underlying causes are staggeringly numerous. One *simple* medical classification lists 200! No one should attempt to diagnose the cause of his own headache.

Running to a doctor with every little headache sometimes indicates a morbid anxiety about one's health (hypochondria). But medical attention should be sought with reasonable promptness if headaches are frequent, severe enough to interfere with sleep, or accompanied by other symptoms, particularly changes in vision. A severe headache is usually accompanied by a feeling of nausea, often by vomiting. Headaches run the gamut from mild to severe.

Numerous headache remedies are on the market sold in drugstores without medical prescription. Some fizz; some do not. The fizz is no therapeutic advantage. Few, if any, of these remedies are more effective than plain aspirin; they just cost more. Their active ingredient is usually the same as that in aspirin, a form of salicylic acid. Caffeine, the active drug in coffee and tea, is sometimes added. Some so-called headache remedies contain sedative drugs, like salts of bromine (bromides), whose continued use can be harmful.

heart disease See page 325.

hemorrhoids Hemorrhoids, sometimes called piles, are a special case of varicose veins. They are swollen veins located just inside, just outside, or across the walls of the anus. Two out of three adults have, or have had, them. They are associated with sedentary occupations.

The mere presence of hemorrhoids means little. The problem is to keep them from becoming annoying or seriously infected. Safe, though somewhat delicate, surgery can usually provide permanent relief for chronic, truly bothersome cases, but it is not always necessary.

Even "bleeding hemorrhoids" are not necessarily dangerous. There is some risk of infection, but the bleeding often provides a natural cure for the piles. It fills them with little blood clots, which causes them to shrivel up and disappear. When bleeding arises from scratching or irritation of *external piles,* situated outside the anus, there is little to worry about. The bleeding from *internal piles* may appear more alarming.

The problem is to be sure that the cause of the bleeding is hemorrhoids and not any other more serious condition of the lower bowel, such as an early signal of cancer. For this reason medical examination at an early date is advisable.

Itching is the chief complaint associated with hemorrhoids. It is usually brought on by misguided efforts to relieve it; namely, violent scratching, overtreatment with salves and ointments, and intemperate use of cathartics or laxatives to self-treat constipation. Itching is often the result of secondary infections superimposed on the varicose veins, particularly fungus infections similar to those found in athlete's foot.

hepatitis See page 365.

indigestion Indigestion is not a disease but a symptom, often the first of the symptoms, which foretells the possible advent of the more serious disorders of the gastrointestinal tract—cancer, ulcer, food allergy, food poisoning or food infection. Because of its role as a warning signal, it should not be treated lightly—with a quick dose of bicarbonate of soda—or neglected. If indigestion persists, it should be investigated. There are some simple forms of indigestion (or dyspepsia) which have obvious causes and do not betoken serious disease. Air-swallowing, for example, will form gas on the stomach, lead to belching and discomfort. These symptoms disappear when the air-swallowing stops. "Heartburn," which has nothing to do with the heart, describes the slight regurgitation of acid secretions from the stomach into the esophagus.

influenza Influenza, the clinical and statistical companion of pneumonia, is essentially a virus invasion of the lungs. Many types of virus have been indicted and efforts to provide effective immunization attempted—but only with partial success. It is sometimes difficult for doctors to distinguish clinically between influenza and pneumonia. The virus disease is debilitating but rarely itself fatal. It "softens up" the lungs for the later, more dangerous bacterial attack. Death rates from pneumonia go up when influenza epidemics are around. (See pneumonia, below.)

infectious mononucleosis See "student's disease," page 512.

leukemia Leukemia, sometimes referred to as cancer of the blood, is a serious disease characterized by wild overgrowth of the tissues that manufacture white blood cells (leukocytes). The overgrowth of cells may occur in the lymph tissue or the bone marrow. In any case there appear more white blood cells, mature and immature, than the body can handle. The disease may progress slowly (chronic leukemia) or rapidly (acute leukemia). Treatment calls for irradiation of bone marrow, bleeding, and drugs. In the mid-1960's leukemia was the form of cancer for which greatest promise of successful treatment by drugs (chemotherapy) could be held out. There was some suspicion, then, that leukemia was, or was related to, a virus disease.

mental illness See page 53.

multiple sclerosis (MS) Multiple sclerosis (MS) is a progressive disease characterized by loss and destruction of the fatty myelin sheaths that act essentially as insulation for the nerves. Scar tissue forms in the damaged areas and nerve messages are "short-circuited," distorted, or eventually blocked.

The symptoms of multiple sclerosis are therefore many and varied, including paralysis and numbness of different parts of the body, double vision, dragging of one or both feet, loss of bladder and bowel control, and slurred speech. Multiple sclerosis is primarily a disease of young adults. Together with other demyelinating diseases it tragically afflicts, with occasional remissions, about 500,000 Americans.

muscular dystrophy Muscular dystrophy is a progressive, inexorably fatal disease primarily of the *voluntary muscles,* which gradually weaken and waste away over a period of years. The weakened patient often succumbs in the meantime to a minor illness, like the common cold. More than half of the estimated 200,000 victims of muscular dystrophy in the United States are children between the ages of 3 and 13. Few will reach adolescence, almost none maturity—unless intensive research turns up some new clue or cure.

narcotic addiction See page 80.

nervous breakdown See page 57.

Parkinson's disease Parkinson's disease, or shaking palsy, is a degenerative disease in which something

goes wrong with the nerve ganglia at the base of the brain. The outstanding symptoms are tremor (shaking), which usually begins in the hands, and rigidity of body muscles. The victim hates to move. His posture slumps, and in extreme cases he loses height. Speech is often impaired.

New drugs, largely antispasmodics which relieve muscle tension, physical therapy, psychotherapy, and sometimes surgery can help greatly to relieve the risk of disability. Most of the 1,500,000 victims of Parkinson's disease in the United States are older people who need more encouragement than they usually get from their families and friends.

peptic ulcer Peptic ulcer, also called stomach ulcer, is a chronic, often recurrent disease that seems to have an affinity for high-pressure executives, self-drivers, and highly emotional, tense, nervous people. Peptic ulcer is a psychosomatic disease. In susceptible individuals anxiety and emotional stress tend to bring on ulcers and bring them back.

The disease itself is a breach or erosion in the inner lining, or more rarely in the entire wall of the stomach or duodenum. A true stomach ulcer is a gastric ulcer. The others are properly called duodenal ulcers, and they are about ten times as frequent as gastric ulcers. From the standpoint of symptoms and treatment, however, both are pretty much alike.

An excess of hydrochloric acid from the stomach always accompanies a true peptic ulcer. It is this acid which eats away at the site of the ulcer, causing pain and complications (such as bleeding).

The classical symptom of peptic ulcer is hunger pain, which comes on before and between meals and can be relieved by taking food or alkalis. Most people with ulcers must eat frequently and avoid irritating foods as well as emotional stress. Adequate and continuing medical care is necessary.

Peptic ulcer is an exceedingly common affliction in the American population, much more so among men than women. The condition usually begins in early adulthood, disappears after adequate treatment, then recurs more or less frequently. About 1 patient in 6 or 7 may eventually require surgery.

pneumonia Pneumonia is an acute, infectious, communicable disease of the respiratory system. It strikes suddenly and abruptly. Most frequently it follows in the wake of a neglected cold or other upper-respiratory infection, such as influenza ("flu"). The symptoms that herald pneumonia include chills and fever; a rapidly rising temperature; rapid or difficult breathing; coughing; expectoration of sticky, rust-colored sputum; pain in the side, chest, or shoulder, which becomes worse with attempts at deeper breathing; and a marked feeling of illness. These symptoms should prompt anyone to seek medical help immediately. The diagnosis may not be pneumonia, but this is not a disease to take chances with; prompt treatment must be instituted.

Pneumonia, together with the closely allied condition *influenza,* still ranks first among *infectious diseases* as a cause of death in the United States. It kills about 60,000 people a year. However, it is no longer quite the dread disease it was before modern sulfa drugs and antibiotics. Pneumonia used to kill 1 in every 3 or 4 people it attacked. Now 19 out of 20 people recover.

No one is immune from pneumonia, for the microbes that cause it are commonly present in the nose and throat. However, it is most dangerous at the extremes of life, in infancy and old age, and among alcoholics or people debilitated by other disease. Terminal pneumonia has been called the "friend of the aged," because it often carries off elderly, suffering patients quickly and with little pain. However, pneumonia is the foe of newborn and young children, often dealing death at the termination of some other disease. Males contract pneumonia more often than females.

Essentially pneumonia is an inflammation in the lungs, caused by one of a large variety of infective agents. Most commonly, however, the invading organism is the pneumococcus, of which there are at least 32 different types. The air sacs in the lungs become filled with fluids—pus and serum—and the usual absorption of oxygen and disgorgement of carbon dioxide is inhibited in some or all parts of one or both lungs. If a person dies of pneumonia, he has in effect "drowned" in his own body fluids. When an area of the lung is completely congested by the by-products of infection, it is said to be consolidated.

Two general types of pneumonia are recognized: lobar pneumonia, which is the type just described, and bronchopneumonia. In this second type, small areas of infection occur at the ends of the bronchi and are usually scattered over both lungs. The bronchopneumonias are more variable in their form and course than the lobar pneumonias.

They occur, for example, as hypostatic pneumonia in elderly patients who have long been bedridden and whose lungs have become congested as a result of lying flat on their backs. Bronchopneumonias also appear in the form of atypical virus pneumonia, a condition which has become widely recognized in recent years.

There is no practical method of specific immunization against pneumonia. The great hope of prevention lies in obtaining prompt treatment of the less serious upper-respiratory infections—like the cold, sinusitis, bronchitis, and middle-ear infection—which are sometimes followed by pneumonia. Fatigue, chilling, poor nutrition, alcoholism, physical exhaustion, and anything else that lowers bodily resistance should be avoided. Cold weather, or, more exactly, changes in

the weather from warm to cold, seem to be environmental factors favoring the development of pneumonia. In the United States, the statistics show that there are definite "pneumonia months," January, February, and March, when the death rate may be four to eight times as high as in the summer months. (See influenza, page 509.)

polio Poliomyelitis—more exactly, acute anterior poliomyelitis; and more popularly, infantile paralysis—once best advertised and most feared summer and childhood disease has joined the ranks of conquered health hazards. In 1952, 54,000 cases were reported in the United States. In 1964, fewer than 150 cases occurred! This happy result was brought about by the development of successful vaccines against the disease; first the Salk killed-virus injectable vaccine, later the Sabin live-virus oral vaccine.

Polio is an acute infection with a chronic aftermath. The infecting agent is any one of three known types of polio virus. For reasons still unknown—despite success in preventing the disease—this virus, multiplying in the intestines and circulating in the blood, sometimes (once in perhaps 200 cases) crosses the blood-brain barrier, invades the motor nerves of the central nervous system, and causes paralysis of arms, legs, trunk, or diaphragm. These cases are called "respiratory polio," since breathing is seriously impaired. A so-called iron lung or equivalent treatment is required for them.

Both the Salk and Sabin vaccines are used for protection against polio. There has been an increasing tendency to use the oral vaccine because of its ease of administration—simply a drop of vaccine on a lump of sugar to be swallowed by the person being immunized. Three administrations are required, one for each of the three types of polio virus. All infants should be immunized against polio during the first year of life and routinely reimmunized when they enter school, says the U.S. Public Health Service.

There are, however, in the United States approximately 300,000 people who were crippled by paralytic polio before the Salk vaccine was introduced in 1955. Perhaps one-third of them still require or would benefit by additional treatment.

radiation sickness See page 493.

rheumatism and arthritis Rheumatism is a fairly old-fashioned word that describes a variety of aches and pains in the muscles, bones and joints. Probably 11 million Americans are afflicted at any one time. *Arthritis,* which literally means inflammation in a joint, is the modern term for the majority of rheumatic ailments. Among the others are *fibrositis,* or inflammation of muscle sheaths; *sciatica,* pain in the thigh and leg along the course of the sciatic nerve; *lumbago,* pain in the lower back; and *wryneck.*

Improved medical diagnoses have made it possible to pinpoint many of the vague conditions formerly blanketed under the term rheumatism. More specific and effective treatment can therefore be offered.

All rheumatic ailments are characterized by inflammation or other changes in connective tissue. They usually come and go over the years. If untreated, they usually progress. Most forms of rheumatism are made worse by emotional stress, too much exercise, overfatigue, and exposure to inclement weather. The rheumatic patient who claims he can feel it in his bones when bad weather is approaching is often right.

Arthritis arises from many causes, some well identified, others still obscure. There are many forms of treatment for it. Certainly there is no specific diet to cure it. The arthritic patient needs only a well-balanced diet. The two principal forms of arthritis are (1) rheumatoid and (2) degenerative.

Rheumatoid arthritis is a disease not only of the joints but of the whole body system—particularly the connective tissue. This tissue reacts sensitively to infection, to endocrine disturbances, and to emotional stress. The condition may appear gradually or suddenly, often beginning in the hands and progressing until the patient is confined to a wheel-chair or hospital bed. Women are afflicted three times as often as men—and the disease sometimes disappears during pregnancy. The treatment for rheumatoid arthritis includes drugs—particularly the new ones of the cortisone family and the old standby, aspirin—rest, heat, physical therapy, and even orthopedic surgery.

Degenerative arthritis is a chronic joint disease of old age. It rarely occurs before age 40, and is not crippling or deforming. It represents the normal aging of joint tissues, a gradual wearing out from day-to-day use. Probably 80% of the people who reach their fiftieth birthday have some degenerative changes in their joints, but only 5 to 10% are troubled by them.

Weight-bearing, obesity, hard physical labor, minor injuries, and anything else that adds wear and tear on the joints contribute to this disease. The weight-bearing joints—ankles, knees, hips and spinal vertebrae—are most commonly affected. The early symptoms are usually mild stiffness and aching in the joint, relieved by using the joint. Degenerative changes cannot be reversed, but the painful symptoms can be relieved.

Rheumatic diseases are a happy hunting ground for peddlers of aspirin at high prices and promoters of foolish nostrums. They should be avoided in favor of adequate medical diagnosis and treatment.

sinus trouble Sinus trouble follows the path, pattern, and seasons of colds and other respiratory infections. The nasal sinuses are part of the respiratory system. The discomfort of sinus trouble originates principally from the inflammation and swelling of the mucous membranes lining the sinuses. This, in turn, is a response to acute or long-standing infection. The first problems in sinusitis, therefore, is to get rid of the underlying infection. Antibiotic and sulfa drugs given by mouth are often prescribed.

The shrinking of the mucous membranes of the nose and sinuses can often be accomplished by the application of drugs like adrenalin, amphetamine, and ephedrine. Occasionally these drugs are given by inhalation. The inhaler frequently used by people with colds and sinus trouble, if used too frequently, may do more harm than good. It will give immediate temporary relief, but, by irritating the mucous membranes, leave the inflammatory condition worse than it was before.

The prevention of sinus trouble is of first importance to about 1,400,000 people in the United States who suffer from it. People seriously subject to this condition should avoid swimming, diving, and overtaxing outdoor exercise. When the weather is cold, they should *sleep with the windows closed.* Cold air irritates and overstimulates the mucous membranes of the sinuses, especially during the period of lowered metabolism characteristic of sleep.

sore throat A sore throat can be a case of pharyngitis, laryngitis, or tonsillitis. There is, however, usually some infection and inflammation in all parts of the throat. The infecting organism is commonly called the streptococcus; hence the expression, "strep throat." Medicated gargles are of doubtful value in treating a sore throat; but the application of heat, by gargling five minutes with hot water, generally brings symptomatic relief. Except in the most minor cases a sore throat should be a signal for a visit to your doctor. The sore throat may be the beginning of something more serious. On the other hand it may be quickly cured by administration of the proper antibiotic.

stomach-ache See abdominal pain, page 505.

stroke See page 331.

"student's disease" Some college-health-service physicians believe that a disease which appears far more commonly among college students than is generally realized is *infectious mononucleosis.* It is otherwise known as glandular fever or "student's disease"—exactly because it occurs so commonly in student populations. The symptoms include fever, headache, malaise, fatigue, sore throat, and swelling in lymph glands or tissues, such as those in the arm-pits. Laboratory examinations reveal the presence of an unusual (mononuclear) type of white blood cell.

The disease is a rather vague one. It usually lasts

for 1 to 3 weeks and has no aftereffects. Treatment is entirely symptomatic—including bed rest during the acute fever.

stye A stye is a boil-like infection of the eyelashes. See boils, page 506.

syphilis See page 358.

tuberculosis Tuberculosis is classified as an infectious, communicable, and usually chronic disease. The infecting agent is the tubercle bacillus (*Mycobacterium tuberculosis*).

Once the tubercle bacillus enters the body, it can settle in any part—bones and joints, bladder, kidneys, and adrenal glands, for example. But in 90% of the cases, the affected organs are the lungs, so that the serious disease problem is *pulmonary tuberculosis.*

The nineteenth-century picture of tuberculosis was that of a pale but bright-eyed young lady, like Dumas' Camille, spitting into a blood-stained handkerchief and wasting away with "galloping consumption." Today tuberculosis is largely a disease of old men, and if its characteristic patient were to be painted, he could reasonably be a shuffling old panhandler from Skid Row. Over half the deaths from tuberculosis in the United States now occur in men over 40.

New drugs have revolutionized the treatment of tuberculosis. The antibiotic streptomycin was the first that gave promise of usefulness. In the 1950's isoniazid and drugs like it were introduced. These drugs render the tuberculosis patient non-infectious to others and thus make it possible to treat the disease safely at home. This has sharply reduced the need for beds in special tuberculosis hospitals and sanatoriums.

There are some patients, of course, for whom the full panoply of hospital care is essential—including bed rest, good food, special drugs, and surgery. Ailing lungs must sometimes be put at rest and this is accomplished by "splinting" the lung, as it were, through various surgical operations.

While tuberculosis remains a threat of great magnitude in many other parts of the world, in the United States it has certainly lost its title of "Captain of the Men of Death." In 1900 tuberculosis was the biggest killer in the country. Its death rate ran around 200 deaths per 100,000 population. This rate has fallen steadily since. By 1961, the death rate was under 6 and only about 10,000 people a year were dying from tuberculosis. The world picture is much blacker; about 3 million people a year are still dying of tuberculosis.

The chief obstacle to eliminating the disease entirely from the American scene is the existence of an estimated 400,000 active cases—of which about 150,000 are unknown to the people who have the disease. It is also estimated that there are 800,000 people with inactive or arrested cases. The big control problem is to find the still undiscovered cases and bring them under proper treatment. There is a high concentration of the disease in non-white groups, Negroes, Indians, and Orientals, among whom special efforts to control the disease are warranted.

varicose veins Varicose veins are simply swollen or dilated veins, slightly overloaded with bluish venous blood. They often can be seen through the skin as blue lines or purple patches. Leg veins are most commonly affected. (See also hemorrhoids.)

virus diseases See page 363.

B

FIRST AID
Condensed* and Illustrated

First aid intelligently employed can save lives and reduce disabilities. Probably the most important axioms of first aid are: (1) "Never do anything that may harm the injured person," and (2) "Call a doctor as soon as possible." However prompt action is required in many cases, as noted in a number of the alphabetically arranged entries on this and following pages.

animal bites Wash wounds freely with water. Hold under running tap for several minutes if possible. Apply sterile gauze dressing (or compress) and always see your doctor immediately. (Obtain name and address of owner of animal, so it may be held in quarantine.)

bandages Necessary to hold dressings in place and for other purposes, three types of bandages are illustrated here: (1) Triangular bandage for hand or foot. With triangle spread out, place hand or foot in the middle of it, as shown. Pull forward peak of triangle over the injured hand or foot. Cross the two other points of the triangle well above the wrist or ankle. Tie the loose ends and tuck them under.

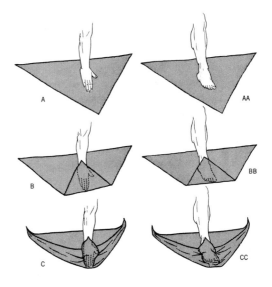

*All entries except the illustrated ones are by courtesy of Associated Hospital Service (Blue Cross) and United Medical Service (Blue Shield) of New York City.

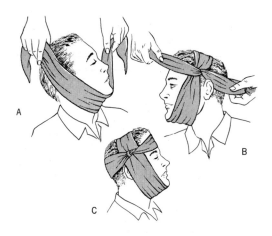

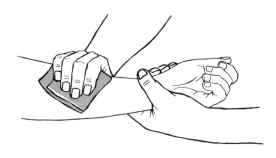

(2) Cravat bandage for ear or check. Place the middle of a wide cravat bandage over the dressing or compress on the cheek or ear. (A) Carry one end of the bandage over the top of the head and the other under the chin. (B) Cross the ends at the opposite side. (C) Carry one end (the short one) around the forehead and the other end around the back of the head. Tie the two ends over the dressing.

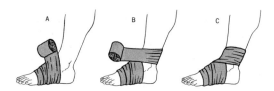

(3) Roller bandage: figure-of-eight bandage for ankle. (A) Anchor the bandage firmly with several turns around the instep and foot. (B) Bring the bandage diagonally upward across the front of the foot and then around the ankle. (C) Use several extra turns around the ankle, if necessary. Finally, carry the bandage diagonally downward across the front of the foot and around the instep (B again). Make several of these figure-of-eight turns, overlapping the previous turn by about two-thirds of the width of the bandage.

bleeding Apply direct pressure over the wound, preferably with a sterile gauze dressing, as shown above. Act promptly, however, with whatever is at hand. Have the patient lie down. If bleeding from arm or leg is severe, it may be advisable to put finger pressure on either the right or left brachial or femoral artery. The brachial artery can be located midway between the armpit and the elbow. The femoral artery emerges just below the groin on the front inner half of the thigh.

breathing stopped Artificial respiration should be started as soon as possible. Experts agree that the mouth-to mouth (or mouth-to-nose) is the most practical technique for emergency ventilation of the lungs. Wipe or remove any foreign matter from victim's mouth. Tilt his head back so his jaw is jutting out. Take a deep breath. Open your mouth wide and place it tightly over the victim's mouth. Simultaneously pinch the victim's nostrils shut with your thumb and forefinger, as shown below (A), or close the nostrils by pressure of your cheek, (B) below. Blow into the

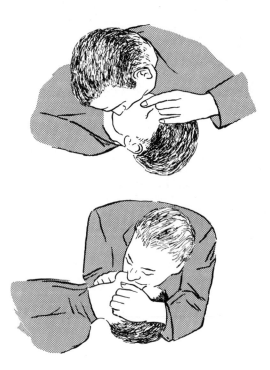

victim's mouth. Remove your mouth for the sound of air being exhaled. Repeat your blowing effort 12 times a minute for adults, 20 times for children. You may place a cloth, e.g., a handkerchief, between your mouth and the victim's.

bruises Apply ice bag or cold cloths for 25 minutes. If skin is broken, treat the same as minor cuts.

carrying or moving injured persons Transportation of the injured or wounded is often a serious problem which can sometimes be conveniently solved by the simple chair carry, pictured here. There are many other litters and carriers in use.

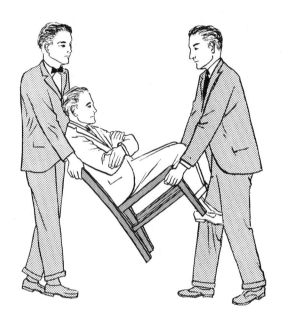

eyes *Foreign Bodies*—Remove by gently touching with point of clean handkerchief or by washing eye with clean tap water. If failure results after one or two attempts, consult a physician. *Never rub the eye. Chemicals*—If any chemical spatters into eyes, wash eye with clean tap water and consult physician at once.

fainting Keep in lying position, with head slightly lowered. Loosen any tight clothing about the neck. Pass smelling salts or aromatic spirits of ammonia gently a few inches benearh nose (not too close to nose). Sprinkle face lightly with cold water. If person does not respond within a short time, summon physician at once and keep person warm with blankets until physician arrives.

foreign bodies *Slivers*—Apply skin antiseptic such as mild tincture of iodine to injured part. Sterilize needle point by passing it through a flame and use it to "tease out" sliver. Again apply antiseptic; let dry and cover with suitable bandage.

frostbite *Symptoms*—Pain followed by appearance of grayish-white color in exposed part. *Treatment*—Gently cover a frozen part with the hand or expose to cool air or place in cold water, so that thawing will occur gradually. *Do not rub; do not expose to stove or fire; do not put in hot water;* such procedures may cause serious permanent damage.

fractures Deformity of injured part usually means a fracture. If fracture is suspected, *do not attempt to move injured person;* summon a doctor at once.

headache Look for causes—Constipation, eyes, nerves. Headache may occasionally be relieved by one or two aspirin tablets swallowed with water. If headaches are frequent, always consult your doctor.

heat cramps Caused by exposure to heat. *Symptoms*—Cramps in muscles of abdomen and extremities. Heat exhaustion may also be present. *Treatment*—Same as for heat exhaustion.

heat exhaustion Caused by exposure to heat—either sun or indoors. *Symptoms*—Face pale, skin wet and clammy, pulse weak, temperature subnormal. Usually conscious. *Treatment*—Keep in lying position with head low. Wrap in blanket. Give salt water to drink (teaspoonful of salt to pint of water) in small amounts at frequent intervals. Give a cup of strong coffee or tea or one teaspoonful of aromatic spirits of ammonia, well diluted, as a stimulant. Call physician immediately.

insect bites Remove "stinger" if present. Apply paste of baking soda and water. If swelling is pronounced, apply ice bag or cold cloths over the paste.

minor burns & scalds Apply white vaseline to burned area and bandage lightly with sterile gauze. If burn is deep or extensive, always consult physician.

minor cuts Apply pressure with sterile gauze until bleeding stops; then apply mild tincture of iodine. Allow to dry and bandage with sterile gauze.

minor scrapes *If dirty,* sponge off gently with wet gauze, blot dry and cover scraped area with a simple bandage. *If* scrape is *deep* and *dirty,* see your doctor.

poison ivy Wash exposed part immediately with soap lather five or six times but do not use brush or other rough material. If area involved is extensive or seems to be spreading, consult physician.

puncture wounds If puncture wound extends deeper than the skin surface, always consult a doctor. Serious infection can rise unless such wounds are properly treated.

sprains Elevate injured part and *apply ice bag* or cold cloths for 25 minutes immediately after injury. If swelling is pronounced do not attempt to use injured part until seen by physician.

sunstroke Caused by exposure to heat—usually sun's rays. *Symptoms*—Headache, skin hot and dry, red face, high fever, strong pulse. Usually unconscious. *Treatment*—Keep in lying position with head elevated. Apply cold cloths to body to cool. Call physician immediately.

toothache If cavity is present, moisten small piece of cotton with oil of cloves and apply to cavity. If no cavity is present apply ice bag or hot water bottle to cheek for comfort. For any toothache always consult your dentist.

unconsciousness Never attempt to give anything by mouth. Put in flat lying position, turn head slightly to one side, loosen any tight clothing about neck. Always summon a physician in every case unless you are sure it is a simple fainting spell.

C

CALORIE COUNTER OF COMMON FOODS

This convenient calorie counter is an adjunct to Chapter 10, Nutrition, Diet, and Weight Control. It can be used to formulate good, mixed diets necessary to health. For measurement of sizes of "servings" or portions use the following scale: 1 cup equals 8 ounces; 3 teaspoons equal 1 tablespoon; 4 tablespoons equal ¼ cup.

It should be noted and acknowledged that calorie counts of foodstuffs in portions commonly served will show some variations in different tables and compilations. The reasons for these discrepancies are obvious. The "portions" or "servings" of food differ in quantity. The exact descriptions of the foods do not tally. There are differences in the quality, time of harvest, and methods of preparation of foods which carry the same name and general description. Nevertheless, there is general agreement on the calorie counts set forth here.

FOOD	MEASURES	CALORIES
Almonds	12–15	100
Apple butter	1 tablespoon	40
Apples, baked	1 large and 2 tablespoons sugar	200
fresh	1 large	100
Applesauce, sweetened	½ cup	100
Apricots		
canned in sirup	3 large halves and 2 tablespoons juice	100
dried	10 halves	100
Asparagus, fresh or		
canned	5 stalks 5 inches long	15
Avocado	½ pear 4 inches long	265
Bacon	2–3 long slices cooked	100
Bacon fat	1 tablespoon	100
Banana	1 medium 6 inches long	90
Beans		
canned with pork	½ cup	175
dried	½ cup cooked	135
lima, fresh or canned	½ cup	100
snap, fresh or canned	½ cup	25
Beef (cooked)		
corned	1 slice 4 inches by 1½ by 1	100
dried	2 ounces	100
hamburger	1 patty (3 ounces)	300
round, lean	1 medium slice (2 ounces)	125
sirloin, lean	1 average slice (3 ounces)	250
tongue	2 ounces	125
Beets, fresh or canned	2 beets 2 inches in diameter	50
Biscuit, baking powder	2 inches in diameter	100
Blackberries, fresh	1 cup	100
Blueberries, fresh	1 cup	90
Bologna	1 slice 2 inches by ½ thick	100

FOOD	MEASURES	CALORIES

Breads

Boston brown	1 slice 3 inches in diameter, ¾ thick	90
corn (1 egg)	1 2-inch square	120
cracked wheat	1 slice average	80
dark rye	1 slice ½ inch thick	70
light rye	1 slice ½ inch thick	75
white, enriched	1 slice average	75
white, enriched	1 slice thin	55
whole wheat, 60%	1 slice average	70
whole wheat, 100%	1 slice average	75
Broccoli	3 stalks 5½ inches long	100
Brownies	1 piece 2 inches by 2 by ¾	140
Brussels sprouts	6 sprouts 1½ inches in diameter	50
Butter	1 tablespoon	95

Cabbage, cooked	½ cup	40
raw	1 cup	25

Cake

angel	⅒ of a large cake	155
chocolate or vanilla, no icing	1 piece 2 inches by 2 by 2	200
chocolate or vanilla, with icing	1 piece 2 inches by 1½ by 2	200
cup cake with chocolate icing	1 medium	250
Cantaloupe	½ of a 5½ inch melon	50
Carrots	1 carrot 4 inches long	25
Cashew nuts	4–5	100
Cauliflower	¼ of a head 4½ inches in diameter	25
Caviar	1 tablespoon	25
Celery	2 stalks	15

Cheese

American cheddar	1 cube 1⅛ inches square or three tablespoons grated	110
cottage	5 tablespoons	100
cream	2 tablespoons	100
Cherries, sweet	15 large	75

Chicken

broiled	½ medium broiler	270
roast	1 slice 4 inches by 2½ by ¼	100

Chocolate

fudge	1 piece 1 inch square by ¾ thick	100
malted milk	fountain size	460
milk, with almonds, sweetened	1 ounce	150
milk, unsweetened	1 ounce	140
mints	1 mint 1½ inches in diameter	100
sirup	¼ cup	200
unsweetened	1 square	160
Cider, sweet	1 cup	100
Clams	6 round	100
Cocoa, half milk, half water	1 cup	150
Coconut	½ cup fresh	175

FOOD	MEASURES	CALORIES
Cod liver oil	1 tablespoon	100
Cod steak	1 piece 3½ inches by 2 by 1	100
Cola soft drinks	6-ounce bottle	75
Collards	½ cup cooked	50
Cooking fats, vegetable	1 tablespoon	100
Corn	½ cup	70
Corn sirup	1 tablespoon	75
Cornflakes	1 cup	80
Cornmeal	1 tablespoon uncooked	35
Cornstarch pudding	½ cup	200
Crackers		
graham	1 square	35
peanut butter-cheese sandwich	1 cracker	45
round snack-type	1 cracker 2 inches in diameter	15
rye wafers	1 wafer	25
saltines	1 cracker 2 inches square	15
Cranberry sauce	¼ cup	100
Cream		
heavy	2 tablespoons	120
light	2 tablespoons	65
whipped	3 tablespoons	100
Cream-puff shells	1 shell	85
Cucumber	½ medium	10
Custard, boiled or baked	½ cup	130
Dates	4	100
Egg	1 medium size	75
Eggplant	3 slices 4 inches in diameter ½-inch thick, raw	50
Endive	average serving	10
Escarole	average serving	10
Figs, dried	3 small	100
Flour, white or whole grain	1 tablespoon unsifted	35
Frankfurter	1 sausage	125
Gelatin, fruit flavored		
dry	3-ounce package	330
ready to serve	½ cup	85
Ginger ale	1 cup	85
Gingerbread, hot water	2 inches by 2 by 2	200
Grape juice	½ cup	80
Grapefruit juice, unsweetened	1 cup	100
Grapes		
American or Tokay	1 bunch—22 average	75
seedless	1 bunch—30 average	75
Griddle cakes	1 cake 4 inches in diameter	75

FOOD	MEASURES	CALORIES
Halibut	1 piece 3 inches by $1\frac{3}{8}$ by 1	100
Ham, lean	1 slice $4\frac{1}{4}$ inches by 4 by $\frac{1}{2}$	265
Hard sauce	1 tablespoon	100
Hickory nuts	12–15	100
Hominy grits	$\frac{3}{4}$ cup cooked	100
Honey	1 tablespoon	100
Ice cream	$\frac{1}{2}$ cup	200
Ice cream soda	fountain size	325
Jellies and jams	1 rounded tablespoon	100
Kale	$\frac{1}{2}$ cup cooked	50
Lamb, roast	1 slice $3\frac{1}{2}$ inches by $4\frac{1}{2}$ by $\frac{1}{8}$	100
Lard	1 tablespoon	100
Lemon juice	1 tablespoon	5
Lettuce	2 large leaves	5
Liver	1 slice 3 inches by 3 by $\frac{1}{2}$	100
Liverwurst	2 ounces	130
Lobster meat	1 cup	150
Macaroni	$\frac{3}{4}$ cup cooked	100
Maple sirup	1 tablespoon	70
Margarine	1 tablespoon	100
Marshmallows	1	20
Milk		
buttermilk	1 cup	85
condensed	$1\frac{1}{2}$ tablespoons	100
evaporated	$\frac{1}{2}$ cup (1 cup diluted)	160
skim milk, dried	$2\frac{1}{2}$ tablespoons	100
skim milk, fresh	1 cup	85
whole milk	1 cup	170
yogurt, plain	1 cup	120–160
Mints, cream	$\frac{1}{2}$-inch cube	5
Molasses	1 tablespoon	70
Muffins		
bran	1 medium	90
1-egg	1 medium	130
Mushrooms	10 large	10
Noodles	$\frac{3}{4}$ cup cooked	75
Oatmeal	$\frac{3}{4}$ cup cooked	110
Oil (corn, cottonseed, olive, and peanut)	1 tablespoon	100
Okra	10–15 pods	50
Olives		
green	6 medium	50
ripe	4–5 medium	50
Onions	3–4 medium	100
Orange	1 medium	80
juice	1 cup	125
Oysters	5 medium	100

FOOD	MEASURES	CALORIES
Parsnips	1 parsnip 7 inches long	100
Peaches		
canned in sirup	2 large halves and 3 tablespoons juice	100
dried	4 medium halves	100
fresh	1 medium	50
Peanut butter	1 tablespoon	100
Peanuts	10	50
Pears		
canned in sirup	3 halves and 3 tablespoons juice	100
fresh	1 medium	50
Peas		
canned	½ cup	65
fresh, shelled	¾ cup	100
Pecans	6	100
Pepper, green	1 medium	20
Pickles, cucumber		
sour and dill	10 slices 2 inches in diameter	10
sweet	1 small	10
Pies	(sectors from 9-inch pies)	
apple	3-inch sector	200
lemon merigue	3-inch sector	300
mincemeat	3-inch sector	300
pumpkin	3-inch sector	250
Pineapple		
canned,		
unsweetened	1 slice ½ inch thick and 1 tablespoon juice	50
fresh	1 slice ¾ inch thick	50
juice, unsweetened	1 cup	135
Plums		
canned	2 medium and 1 tablespoon juice	75
fresh	2 medium	50
Popcorn	1½ cups popped	100
Popovers	1 popover	100
Pork chops, lean	1 medium	200
Potato chips	8–10 large	100
Potato salad with		
mayonnaise	½ cup	200
Potatoes		
mashed	½ cup	100
sweet	½ medium	100
white	1 medium	100
Prune juice	½ cup	100
Prunes, dried	4 medium	100
Pumpkin	½ cup	50
Radishes	5	10
Raisins	¼ cup	90
Raspberries, fresh	1 cup	90
Rhubarb, stewed		
and sweetened	½ cup	100
Rice	¾ cup cooked	100
Roll, Parker House	1 medium	100
Rutabagas	½ cup	30

FOOD	MEASURES	CALORIES
Salad dressing		
boiled	1 tablespoon	25
French	1 tablespoon	90
mayonnaise	1 tablespoon	100
Salmon, canned	½ cup	100
Sardines, drained	5 fish 3 inches long	100
Sauerkraut	½ cup	15
Sherbet	½ cup	120
Soup, condensed	11-ounce can	
bouillon		25
mushroom		360
noodle		290
tomato		230
vegetable		200
Spaghetti	¾ cup cooked	100
Spinach	½ cup cooked	20
Squash		
summer	½ cup cooked	20
winter	½ cup cooked	50
Strawberries, fresh	1 cup	90
Sugar		
brown	1 tablespoon	50
granulated	1 tablespoon	50
powdered	1 tablespoon	40
Sweetbreads	1 pair medium-sized	200
Swiss chard	½ cup leaves and stems	30
Tangerines	1 medium	60
Tapioca, uncooked	1 tablespoon	50
Tomato juice	1 cup	60
Tomatoes, canned	½ cup	25
fresh	1 medium	30
Tuna fish, canned	¼ cup drained	100
Turkey, lean	1 slice 4 inches by 2½ by ¼	100
Turnip	1 turnip 1¾ inches in diameter	25
Veal, roast	1 slice 3 inches by 3¾ by ¼	120
Waffles	1 waffle 6 inches in diameter	250
Walnuts	8	100
Watermelon	1 slice 6 inches in diameter 1½ inches thick	190
Wheat		
flakes	¾ cup	100
germ	1 tablespoon	25
shredded	1 biscuit	100

Alcoholic Beverages

Beer	8 ounces	120
Gin	1½ ounces	120
Rum	1½ ounces	150
Whiskey	1½ ounces	150

FOOD	MEASURES	CALORIES
Wines		
champagne	4 ounces	120
port	1 ounce	50
sherry	1 ounce	40
table, red or white	4 ounces	95

—Metropolitan Life Insurance Company

D

GLOSSARY AND SELECTIVE DICTIONARY
OF COMMON MEDICAL TERMS

abdomen. Body cavity bounded above by the diaphragm and below by the pelvis. It contains the stomach, intestines, and other internal organs.

abnormal. Outside the range of the normal, irregular.

abortion. The detachment and expulsion from the uterus of the embryo or fetus before it has become capable of living. It can occur spontaneously or be artificially induced.

abrasion. Rubbing or scraping off of skin or mucous membrane.

abstinence. The act of completely giving up something, such as liquor, sexual intercourse, narcotics.

accommodation. Power of the eyes to focus.

Achilles tendon. The tendon that binds the muscles in the calf of the leg to the heel bone.

acid. A chemical substance that, in solution, releases hydrogen ions. Acids taste sour, turn blue litmus paper red, unite with bases to form salts, and in general have chemical properties opposed to those of *alkalis* (or bases).

acidosis. A higher than normal acid content of the blood. It occurs, for example, in an advanced condition of diabetes.

acne. A skin disorder caused by an inflammation of the sebaceous glands of the skin.

ACTH. A hormone manufactured in the pituitary gland which stimulates the adrenal gland to release the hormone cortisone.

acute illness. Severe, usually critical, often dangerous illness.

addiction. The state of being completely in the grip of some habit. Drug addiction is characterized by an overwhelming compulsion, desire, or need to continue use of a drug, and producing psychological and physical dependencies on it.

Addison's disease. "Bronze skin" disease, named after Thomas Addison (1803–1860), a British physician. It results from underactivity of the adrenal glands.

adhesions. The sticking together of body tissues not normally joined. Distressing adhesions sometimes follow surgery.

adrenals. Endrocrine glands, above the kidneys, that secrete adrenalin and other hormones.

aerosol. A solution atomized into a fine mist, either a drug for inhalation or a substance for spraying in a room.

afterbirth. Placenta and membranes expelled from the womb a few minutes after the birth of a child.

aggression. A forceful, attacking action or feeling usually directed toward another person, and generally having a great emotional content.

airsickness. A form of motion sickness resulting from unaccustomed rapid motion.

alarm reaction. The first reaction to stress placed upon a person or any part of his mind or body.

albinism. Congenital absence of pigment in the skin, hair, and eyes; hence usually white in color.

alcoholism. An illness resulting from the prolonged and repeated use of alcoholic beverages frequently as a compensation for deep-seated personality problems.

alkali. The opposite of an acid; chemically a basic substance that turns red litmus paper blue.

allergy. An oversensitivity and overreaction to something in the internal or external environment. Examples of allergic reactions (or diseases) are hay fever and "strawberry rash."

alopecia. A condition in which the hair falls out; baldness.

altitude sickness. A condition that sometimes occurs at high altitudes, as on mountain tops or in airplanes, caused by lack of oxygen in the blood and brain.

alveolus. Air sac of the lungs; also socket of the teeth.

amblyopia. Dim or poor vision.

ameba. A microscopic, one-celled animal.

amino acid. Any one of some 30 or more chemical compounds, all containing nitrogen, that are the building blocks of body protein.

amnesia. Loss of memory; especially inability to remember past experiences.

amniotic sac. So-called "bag of waters"; an "elastic bottle" in which a growing infant floats during its life in the mother's womb.

amphetamine. A drug used to stimulate the central nervous system, increase blood pressure, reduce both appetite and nasal congestion. A common ingredient in "pep pills."

analgesia. The relief of pain without loss of consciousness.

anemia. A blood disease, of which there are many types; most commonly result from the failure of the blood-forming system in the bone marrow to manufacture enough or the right kind of red blood cells.

anesthesia. Loss of feeling or sensation.

aneurysm. The bulging out of the wall of an artery or vein.

angina. A spasmodic or suffocating pain, or the disease that causes it. *Angina pectoris* is pain in the chest, a form of heart disease.

anopheles. The kind of mosquito that carries malaria.

antibiotics. A group of drugs that kill or stop the growth of harmful microorganisms in the body. Most antibiotics (such as penicillin) are derived from cultures of molds or bacteria.

antibody. A substance produced in and by the body that protects against specific disease infections.

antidote. Anything that counteracts a poison.

antigen. Anything, usually a chemical substance, that prompts the body to manufacture antibodies.

antihistamine. A drug that counteracts the effect of histamine in the body; commonly used in treating allergy.

antitoxin. A substance in the blood that particularly fights a specific toxin (poison); for example, diphtheria antitoxin.

anxiety. A state of uneasiness, or apprehension arising in the unconscious mind, related to a fear which is nonspecific (i.e., a vague danger).

aphrodisiac. Anything that stimulates sexual desire or appetite.

apoplexy. A stroke resulting from a damaged blood vessel in the brain.

appendicitis. Inflammation of the useless, worm-shaped appendix, a small pocket or projection, one to six inches long, that protrudes from a part of the large bowel.

arteriosclerosis. The thickening and hardening of the arteries.

artery. Any of the blood vessels leading away from the heart.

arthritis. Literally, inflammation of a joint. It is one of the number of diseases and disorders called rheumatism.

asthma. A wheezing type of breathing and shortness of breath often resulting from an allergy.

astigmatism. A structural defect of the shape of the cornea or crystalline lens of the eye which distorts vision.

ataraxics. Class of tranquillizing drugs, used to calm the mind without depression of mental faculties.

atherosclerosis. A serious form of hardening of the arteries which arises from deposits of fat on the inner lining of the blood vessels.

"athlete's foot." Slang for ringworm of the feet.

atrophy. Wasting away of flesh, tissue, cell, or organ. For example, tonsils atrophy with increasing age.

anorexia. Extreme loss of appetite for food.

autonomic. Self-governing, as the autonomic nervous system.

autopsy. Examination of a body after death (post mortem) to determine exact cause of death.

avitaminosis. Mild or severe disease state caused by lack of vitamins.

axon. A nerve cell process which conducts nerve impulses away from the central cell body.

bacillus. A microbe, a germ; specifically a rod-shaped bacterium.

bacteria. Germs or microbes, more exactly, one-celled plants; they can be seen only under a microscope. "Pathogenic" bacteria cause disease, but not all bacteria are pathogenic.

barbiturates. A class of narcotic drugs; chemical compounds of many varieties and names, commonly used as sleeping pills, sedatives, and hypnotics.

basal metabolism. The minimum amount of energy required by the body at rest to keep up its normal functions such as food digestion, blood circulation, and maintenance of body temperature.

"bends." An occupational disease of "sand-hogs," deep sea divers, or others who work in an atmosphere of compressed air. Unless slowly decompressed, nitrogen bubbles form in the victim's blood stream, producing terrific pain.

benign. Harmless, not malignant; usually refers to tumors, new growths of body tissue.

beriberi. A deficiency disease due to lack of vitamin B (thiamine); characterized by inflammatory changes in the nerves.

bile. A complex body fluid that dissolves fat. It is manufactured in the liver, stored in the gall bladder. Bile backing up into the blood stream produces *jaundice*, a yellowing of the skin.

biopsy. The removal and microscopic examination of living tissue from the body. It is important in the diagnosis of cancer.

bisexual. Having both male and female sexual interests or characteristics.

"bleeder's disease." *See* **hemophilia.**

blood count. A laboratory test useful in the diagnosis of disease. A small sample of blood is dropped on a square-ruled glass slide, which is examined under a microscope in order to count the number of red blood cells, white blood cells, and other blood elements per square millimeter.

blood pressure. The force exerted by the blood beating against the artery walls.

blood test. Any laboratory test performed with a blood sample.

blood vessels. Elastic tubes of various sizes that carry blood throughout the body to and from the heart.

Blue Cross. Hospital insurance; specifically the symbol for prepaid, voluntary group plans which pay hospital bills. It may protect not only the subscriber but also his dependents.

Blue Shield. Medical insurance; specifically, the symbol for certain voluntary, prepaid health insurance plans which pay surgical and medical bills.

botulism. An extremely dangerous type of food poisoning arising from food comtaminated with *botulinum*, which is sometimes found in improperly canned or preserved foods.

brain stem. All of the brain except the cerebrum and cerebellum. It includes the motor and sensory nerve tracts, and the nuclei of the cranial nerves.

bronchi. The two main branches of the wind-pipe going into the lungs.

bursitis. Inflammation of a *bursa,* the small sac of heavy fluid found in various joints, such as the knee and elbow.

Caesarean section. Delivery of an infant through an incision in the mother's abdominal wall and the uterus.

caffeine. A stimulating drug present in coffee, tea, cocoa, and some cola drinks. It stimulates the heart, nervous system, and kidneys.

calorie. A unit of heat. The large calorie is the amount of heat needed to raise one kilogram of water one degree Centigrade. Commonly used as the measure of energy (heat) yielded by different foods.

cancer. A group of diseases characterized by abnormal and uncontrolled growth of body cells.

canker sore. A small ulcer, chiefly of the mouth and lips.

cannabis. The dried flowering tops of hemp plants, *Cannabis sativa,* known as marihauna, hashish and bhang.

capillaries. The smallest of the blood vessels in the circulatory system.

carbohydrate. An organic chemical compound; one of the chief classes of foodstuffs, represented by starches, sugars, dextrins, and other energy foods.

carbon dioxide. A gas (CO_2). It is normally formed in the human body through oxidation of foodstuffs. It is also the gas used to give the "fizz" to carbonated beverages.

carbon monoxide. A highly poisonous gas (CO) formed by incomplete burning (combustion) of carbon. It is a regular byproduct of automobile exhaust gases.

carcinoma. A malignant new growth (cancer) arising in epithelial cells (skin or glands). The condition may respond to treatment or may spread (metastasize).

cardiac. Relating to the heart.

cardiovascular system. The entire system of heart and blood vessels.

caries, dental. Tooth decay.

castration. Commonly refers to removal of a male's sexual organs (usually testicles, but sometimes penis also). Castration of the female means removal of both ovaries.

cataract. Clouding of the crystalline lens of the eye; it usually occurs in later life.

cementum. The bony material covering the root of a tooth, located underneath the tooth enamel.

cerebellum. The part of the brain behind and below the cerebrum.

cerebral palsy. Primarily a lack of muscular control caused by brain damage before, during, or soon after birth.

cerebrum. The large, main, upper "thinking" part of the brain, divided into two hemispheres.

cervix. A neck or narrow part; most commonly, the neck (or forward part) of the uterus.

chancre. The first open sign of syphilis. It is a small, painless sore or ulcer that appears at the site where the infecting spirochete of syphilis entered the body.

chancroid. Soft chancre; an uncommon venereal disease.

chemotherapy. The treatment of disease with chemical substances (drugs).

chiropodist. Podiatrist; an individual who diagnoses and treats disorders of the feet.

cholesterol. A fatlike substance found in all animal fats and oils, and in many other tissues of the human body.

chromosomes. Colored bodies, thread or rod-like in shape, which can be seen under a microscope when a "mother cell" is dividing into two "daughter cells." Genes, which control heredity, are located at specific positions along the chromosome threads.

chronic illness. A persistent, prolonged, and recurring illness.

chyme. The semifluid, homogeneous, creamy material produced in the stomach by gastric digestion of food.

ciliary muscles. Small muscles of the eye that help control its focus.

circumcision. The cutting away of the foreskin or some part of it.

cirrhosis. Hardening of a bodily organ as the result of inflammation or other disease process. Cirrhosis of the liver means destruction of its important functioning cells. This condition is usually brought on by chronic alcoholism.

claustrophobia. The abnormal fear of being shut up in a closed space.

cleft palate. An opening or fissure in the roof of the mouth; usually accompanied by harelip. Both of these conditions are first discovered at birth. No cause is known.

climacteric. "Change of life." The syndrome of endocrine, somatic, and psychological changes taking place at the ending of the reproductive period in the female (menopause), or accompanying the normal lessening of sexual activity in the male.

coagulate. To clot, as blood; to curdle, as milk solids becoming cheese.

cocaine. A narcotic drug obtained from coca leaves; addictive. Cocaine salts are sometimes used as local anesthetics.

cochlea. Snail-shaped bony structure of the inner ear, about the size of a pea. It carries end-organ receptors of the hearing process.

codeine. A narcotic drug derived from opium and related to morphine.

coitus. Sexual intercourse.

colitis. Inflammation of the bowels.

communicable disease. A disease which is capable of being transmitted from one person to another; sometimes through a chain of carriers (vectors). For example, malaria is carried by the mosquito.

compulsion. The act of being irresistibly driven to perform some action, often irrational.

conception. The fertilization of the ovum by the sperm; the beginning of pregnancy.

congenital. Conveyed from mother to child during intrauterine life, such as congenital syphilis; not inherited in the genes.

conjunctivitis. Inflammation of the conjunctiva, the tissue lining the outer surface of the eyeball and the inner surface of the eyelid.

contact lenses. Small lenses, made of glass or plastic, that fit directly over the cornea of the eye and under the eyelid.

contraception. Birth control; the prevention of conception by any means.

convulsion. A "fit" or seizure; usually uncontrollable by the afflicted person. Convulsions are a symptom of brain irritation; hence they occur as a result of such conditions as brain inflammation, brain tumor, skull fracture, or epilepsy.

cornea. Transparent outer surface of eyeball.

coronary. Usually refers to the "crown" of small blood vessels (arteries) that supply the nourishment of the heart itself.

coronary occlusion. Anything that stops the flow of blood through the coronary arteries of the heart. This is the form of heart disease usually called a "heart attack."

coronary thrombosis. A blood clot in the coronary arteries causing coronary occlusion.

cortisone. A hormone normally produced in the cortex of the adrenal glands. It is now manufactured as a drug and is useful in treating many diseases; for example, arthritis and some eye and skin ailments.

cretin. A dwarfed, misshapen, mentally retarded individual whose condition was caused by a prenatal lack of thyroxin, owing to lack of iodine in his mother's diet.

cryptorchidism. Undescended testes; the failure of the testes to descend normally into scrotal sac.

cutaneous. Relating to the skin.

cyanosis. Blue skin resulting from lack of oxygen in the blood.

cyst. A membranous sac enclosing a thin or heavy fluid. Cysts in the ovary are quite common.

cystitis. Inflammation of the bladder.

DDT. A powerful, common, cheap, and potentially hazardous pesticide. Its full name is dichloro-diphenyl-trichloro-ethane.

deficiency disease. Disease caused by lack of foodstuffs (or medication) containing elements, such as vitamins and minerals, essential to life and health.

degenerative diseases. A class of diseases (in contrast to infectious or psychogenic diseases) which are characterized by deterioration of tissues. Examples are rheumatism, heart attack, and cancer.

dehydration. A condition occurring when excessive or abnormal amounts of water are removed from the body, as by profuse sweating or frequent urination.

delirium. A state of restlessness, excitement, and wild talk, that sometimes follows a high fever, head injury, or disease.

delirium tremens (D.T.'s). An acute mental disturbance characterized by delirium with trembling and great excitement, accompanied by anxiety, sweating, some hallucinations. It is one of the symptoms of alcoholic psychosis, also seen in addiction to opium.

delusion. A false belief or irrational idea that is clung to despite logical proof to the contrary. Delusions of persecution or grandeur sometimes occur in mental illness.

dementia. Loss of mind; mental deterioration.

depilatory. Substance or method for removing unwanted hair from the surface of the skin.

depression. "The blues," a melancholy and downcast mood. If extreme or prolonged, it can be considered as a form of mental illness.

dermatitis. Inflammation of the skin from any cause.

dermis. Inner layers of the skin.

diabetes mellitus. A metabolic disorder in which the body is unable to burn its intake of sugar, starches, and other carbohydrates because of faulty activity of the pancreas.

diagnosis. The doctor's (or clinics') best judgment as to what is specifically wrong with a patient. This is the core of the art of medicine. Rational treatment depends on correct diagnosis.

diaphragm. The sheet of muscle that separates the chest cavity from the abdominal cavity. Moving up and down, it supplies most of the muscle power for breathing. A *vaginal diaphragm* is a fitted rubber or plastic cap that covers the mouth of the womb to prevent entrance of semen during sexual intercourse. It is one of the means of achieving birth control.

diarrhea. Frequent or excessive bowel movements.

diastole. The resting stage of the heart between beats (systole). Diastolic blood pressure is the pressure recorded at this in-between time.

digestion. The conversion of food into materials to be assimilated by the body cells.

digestive system (alimentary system). Comprises a 24 to 36 foot long flexible tube, beginning at the mouth and ending in the anus. It transforms food taken into the mouth into nutrient substances that can be assimilated by the cells of the body.

dipsomania. Severe addiction to alcohol.

disorientation. The loss of proper bearings; a state of mental confusion as to time, place, or identity.

diuretic. Anything that promotes excretion of urine.

DNA (deoxyribonucleic acid). One of the exceptionally long spiral molecules that are in fact the *genes* on the chromosomal chains. They determine the genetic constitution of living matter. DNA forms the genetic pattern; RNA, sometimes called "messenger RNA" carries it to the new cells where it will be adapted.

dorsal. The backside of any organism, as contrasted with the ventral (front or belly) side.

ductless gland. Endocrine gland which pours its secretions (hormones) directly into the blood stream without passing through any specific duct.

dysentery. A bowel disorder, characterized by pain in the abdomen, diarrhea, cramps, and sometimes bloody stools.

dysmenorrhea. Difficult and painful menstruation.

dyspnea. Difficult breathing; shortness of breath.

ecology. The study of organisms (including man) as they relate to each other in a stable or changing environment.

-ectomy. A word ending that means that something has been cut out or removed; for example, *tonsillectomy,* or removal of tonsils.

ectopic. Out of place.

ectopic pregnancy. A pregnancy in which the fertilized ovum attaches itself and begins to grow somewhere in a uterine tube instead of the womb.

eczema. A skin disease of uncertain origin. The skin is rough and red and has patches of rashes.

edema. Swelling of body tissues as a result of being waterlogged with fluid.

ego. That portion of the unconscious mind which possesses consciousness, maintains its identity, and recognizes and tests reality.

electrocardiogram. Often abbreviated EKG or ECG, it is a wavy, graphic, "picture" on a tape that records the electrical action of the heart muscle. EKG's are used in diagnosing, treating, and managing heart diseases.

electroencephalogram (EEG). A graphic picture of the electrical impulses of the brain on a moving tape; "brain waves."

electrolysis. A method or removing unwanted hair.

emasculation. Castration of the male; removal of testes or testes and penis.

embolus. Anything carried along in the blood stream that causes sudden blockage of a vein or artery. Often the embolus results from a thrombus (a clot of blood broken off from the spot where it was formed).

embryo. Unborn, developing infant-to-be during first few months of intrauterine growth.

embryology. The science and study of life before birth; notably conception and intrauterine life.

empathy. Recognizing and entering in to the feelings of another person or set of circumstances. Empathy thus goes beyond sympathy, which is feeling for, but not acting out of feelings and impulses.

emphysema. A lung disease, most common in older people, in which the air sacs of the lungs have been stretched too thin and broken down.

empyema. A collection of pus within a body cavity, usually the chest.

encephalitis. An inflammation of the brain.

endemic disease. Disease confined to a particular group of people or locality.

endocrine glands. The ductless glands whose secretions (hormones) regulate and control most bodily functions. The seven important endocrine glands, from the head downward are: pituitary, thyroid, parathyroid, thymus (?), adrenals, islet cells of the pancreas, and gonads (testes or ovaries).

endogamy. Marriage within the tribe, caste, or social group.

endometrium. Inner lining of the uterus. Part of it is shed during menstruation.

enuresis. Bed-wetting; involuntary discharge of urine.

enzymes. Organic substances, mostly proteins, capable of entering into and bringing about chemical reactions in living organisms. Enzymes act as chemical catalysts.

epidemiology. The study of disease as it spreads and involves large groups of people.

epidermis. Outer layers of the skin.

epidermophytosis. Fungus infection of skin, notably "athlete's foot."

epilepsy. A disease characterized by seizures ("fits") with impairment or loss of consciousness.

epithelial. A type of body cells that make up the skin, mucous membranes lining body organs, and glands.

erythema. Reddening of the skin from various attacks upon it.

erythrocyte. Red blood cell.

etiology. The causes of disease.

eugenics. The effort to improve the human race by attention to mating and breeding.

euphoria. A sense of extreme well-being; sometimes exaggerated and unwarranted.

eustachian tube. Auditory tube; narrow passageway from the middle ear to the back of the throat (pharynx). It was named after the Italian anatomist, Bartolommeo Eustachia (1520–1574) who first described it.

exhibitionism. The display of one's body for the purpose, conscious or unconscious, of indirectly satisfying sexual urges.

exogamy. Marriage outside of the same kinship group or clan.

extrovert. A personality type whose interest is turned outward toward external values. The extrovert is frequently trying to escape his own inner thoughts and emotional conflicts. He is restless.

fainting. Temporary loss of consciousness as a result of diminished supply of blood to the brain.

fallopian tubes. Tubes from the ovaries to the womb; oviducts. Named after Gabriello Fallopius (1523–1562), Italian anatomist who first described them.

fantasy. A psychological mechanism by which a harsh reality is converted into an imaginary experience to satisfy the individual's subjective demands.

fatigue. "That tired feeling," "loss of pep," can be one of the most important symptoms of disease. Fatigue may be physical, resulting from physical labor, or emotional, the result of conflicts in the unconscious mind.

feeblemindedness. Old name for mental retardation of varying degrees.

fertility. The ability to sire, conceive, or bear offspring.

fetishist. A person who gets sexual gratification from an object (such as a lock of hair) regarded with unreasoning devotion.

fetus. The developing infant-to-be in the uterus after the first eight weeks of pregnancy; before eight weeks, called an embryo.

fibroid. Generally describes a type of harmless or benign tumor or new growth inside the uterus.

fibrositis. A form of muscular rheumatism.

filariasis. The name for several tropical diseases, caused by threadlike worms, which block the lymph channels. This causes enormous swellings of arms, legs, and scrotum.

flatus. Gas or air on the stomach or in the intestines; sometimes expelled from the mouth as a belch or from the anus as "passing wind."

fluoridation. Addition of fluorides to (public) water supply to aid in preventing tooth decay.

fluoroscope. A machine used to examine, not photograph, the interior of the body by means of roentgen rays shining on a fluorescent screen.

follicle (of hair). The hair roots from which the hair grows. (*See also* **graafian follicle.**)

foot-candle. A standard unit in measurement of intensity of illumination from a source of light; the amount of light projected at one foot from the flame of a standard candle.

fracture. Broken bone.

frigidity. A woman's lack of normal interest in, sometimes an aversion to, sexual intercourse.

frustration. A condition of increased emotional tension resulting from failure to achieve sought gratifications.

functional. A word used to describe many disease conditions in which no visible or laboratory evidence can be found to explain the patient's complaints. The opposite state is "organic," in which something definitely wrong with the body can be found.

fungicide. Anything that kills a fungus.

fungus. A low form of plant life; most commonly a microscopically small vegetable organism. Some fungi (plural of fungus) can cause annoying and sometimes dangerous infections. Most fungus infections are on the skin. Athlete's foot is typical.

galactosemia. A hereditary disorder of carbohydrate metabolism in early infancy; characterized by vomiting, diarrhea, jaundice, poor weight gain, and malnutrition.

gallstones. Concretions of elements that make up bile; for example, cholesterol. These have backed up and accumulated in the gallbladder.

gamma globulin. A fraction of the blood plasma which carries antibodies.

ganglion. A knotlike mass of nerve-cell bodies located outside the central nervous system. May also refer to a form of cystic tumor on a tendon, as in the wrist.

gangrene. Death of body tissue over an area large enough to be visible; caused by damage to the circulation of blood.

gastric. Relating to the stomach; as, for example, gastric juice.

gene. The biological unit of heredity; self-reproducing and located in a definite position on a particular chromosome. Genes are *molecules* of the nucleic acids, DNA or RNA.

genetics. The study of heredity as determined by the genes.

genitalia. The reproductive apparatus (organs).

genotype. The genetic make-up of an organism; its fundamental hereditary constitution, as determined by its genes.

geriatrics. That branch of medicine that is concerned with the diseases and disabilities of older people.

german measles. *Rubella;* a mild virus disease. Hazardous in early months of pregnancy, it may cause malformation of fetus.

germicide. Anything that kills germs.

germs. Disease-producing microorganisms. The concept of the germ theory of diseases was established in the late 19th century by Pasteur and Koch.

gingivitis. Inflammation of the gums.

glands. Body organs that manufacture some fluid that they secrete from their cells. Thus we have glands, like the sweat glands and mammary glands (breasts), that secrete their "product" through definitely defined ducts, and also ductless glands, such as the endocrine glands (pituitary, thyroid, etc.) that secrete their hormones directly into the blood stream.

glaucoma. A serious disease of the eye, marked by hardness of the eyeball, causing vision impairment or blindness.

globulin. A fraction of blood serum, that can be separated out of it.

glucose. Sugar in the form in which it usually appears in the blood stream (blood sugar).

gluteal. Related to the buttocks, which are made up of the large *gluteus maximus* muscles.

glycogen. Animal starch formed by and stored in the liver, where it is reformed into glucose (blood sugar).

goiter. Enlargement of the thyroid glands in the neck.

gonads. Essential sexual glands; testes in the male, ovaries in the female.

gonorrhea. The most common and most curable veneral disease; caused by the *gonoccocus* microorganism; effectively treated with penicillin and other antibiotics.

gout. A metabolic disease in which the body fails to get rid of uric acid. The typical picture of gout is that of a middle-aged man with an exquisitively sensitive and swollen big toe.

graafian follicle. "Pocket" in the ovary in which an individual ovum matures (one each month) and from which it is released when ripened.

group therapy. A group discussion or other activity with a therapeutic purpose, generally consisting of a therapist and several clients or patients.

gynecologist. Specialist in diseases of women.

habituation. The condition resulting from the repeated use of a drug, with a compulsion to continue its use. There may be psychic but *not physical* dependence on the drug, which is the distinction between habituation and addiction.

halitosis. Bad breath.

hallucination. Hearing, seeing, or feeling things that do not actually exist; a mental mirage.

hardening of the arteries. A condition marked by thickening, hardening, and loss of elasticity in the walls of the arteries. Deposits of sodium salts and hardening take place chiefly in the middle layer of the arteries.

harelip. A notch in the upper lip, giving it the appearance of a rabbit's (hare's) lip. This congenital malformation is usually accompanied by cleft palate.

hay fever. A catarrhal inflammation of the nose and eyes, caused by allergy to various plant pollens, especially ragweed.

heartburn. A burning sensation in the food tube (esophagus), which passes near the heart on the way to the stomach. Heartburn has nothing to do with the heart.

hemiplegia. Paralysis of one side of the body.

hemoglobin. The red coloring matter of the blood which carries the oxygen.

hemophilia ("bleeder's disease"). A hereditary disease in which the blood lacks the elements necessary for clotting.

hemorrhage. Bleeding.

hemorrhoids (piles). Swollen or distended varicose veins situated just outside, inside, or across the walls of the anus.

hepatitis. Inflammation of the liver. *Infectious hepatitis* is caused by a virus. *Serum hepatitis* is transmitted by way of blood, as in use of inadequately sterilized needles.

heredity. The genetic transmission of a quality or trait from parent to child; for example, the tendency for red-haired parents to have red-haired children (and grandchildren).

hermaphrodites. Individuals of doubtful or obscure sex, since they usually have sex organs of both sexes.

hernia. The protrusion of a loop or part of some internal organ of the body through an abnormal hole or slit. In *inguinal hernia* a loop of bowel protrudes into the scrotum.

heroin. A narcotic drug; probably the most dangerous.

herpes. A virus infection, in which blisters develop on the skin and mucous membranes.

heteroxesual love. Love for a person of the opposite sex.

Hippocratic oath. The physician's oath, dating back to the great Greek physician, Hippocrates (460–377? B.C.). It promises among other ethical promises, that the physician will guard his life and art (medicine) in "purity and holiness."

histamine. A chemical substance occurring in all animal and vegetable tissues. When the human body becomes oversensitive to its quantity of histamine, an allergy may result.

hives. *See* **urticara.**

Hodgkin's disease. A malignant disease first described by the British physician, Hodgkin, in 1852. It brings about the swelling of the lymph glands in many parts of the body.

homeostatis. The tendency of the internal environment of the body to return to normal whenever it is disturbed or assaulted.

homicide. Murder; sometimes justifiable.

homosexuality. The sexual attraction toward those of the same sex. Lesbianism is female homosexuality.

hormones. Chemical substances, produced in the body by the endocrine glands and having specific effects on the activities of certain other organs and of each other.

hydrophobia. Literally means fear of water. It is a common name for the virus disease, *rabies,* as it appears in human beings.

hydrotherapy. Any treatment with water; commonly hot-and-cold baths.

hymen (maidenhead). A thin, perforated, mucous membrane that stretches across the opening of the vagina. The hymen is usually broken by first sexual intercourse, but it may be broken in other ways.

hyper-. A prefix meaning too much, above normal.

hyperkinetic. Abnormally increased body movements.

hyperopia. Farsightedness.

hypertension. Consistent elevation of the pressure of blood above a normal range. Generally called "high blood pressure."

hyperthyroidism. Excessive secretion from the thyroid gland, usually causing goiter.

hypnosis. An artificially induced passive state (trance) in which there is responsiveness to suggestions and commands if these do not conflict seriously with the subject's own conscious or unconscious wishes.

hypo-. A prefix to medical terms which indicates too little, not enough, or below normal. Also used with reference to a hypodermic syringe for giving injections under the skin.

hypochondriac. One who has a morbid anxiety about his health; a person who "enjoys" poor health.

hypodermic. Under the skin; the same as subcutaneous. Also refers to a hypodermic syringe for giving injections ("shots") under the skin.

hypokinetic. Abnormally decreased movements.

hypotension. Low blood pressure.

hysterectomy. Surgical removal of the uterus.

hysteria. A psychoneurosis, the emotional conflicts of which are often converted into physical symptoms. Some characteristics are: lack of control over acts and emotions, morbid self-consciousness, anxiety, and simulating various physical disorders (hysterical blindness, deafness, paralysis, etc.).

iatrogenic. Caused by the doctor. Originally applied to disorders caused by autosuggestion based on physician's remarks at examination of the patient.

id. The prime mover of the unconscious mind, out of which develop the ego and superego.

idealization. Unconscious habit of looking up to other people, usually parents.

illusion. A false or misinterpreted sensory impression; that is, seeing, hearing, or otherwise sensing something that is not really there.

immunity. The power of an individual to resist an infection to which he might be susceptible. Immunity can be *active* or *passive.*

immunization. Vaccination (the two words now mean practically the same thing); providing immunity against some specific diseases by injections (or "shots"). Infants are routinely immunized against such diseases as whooping cough, tetanus, diphtheria, polio, mumps, and measles.

impacted. Usually refers to wisdom teeth so firmly imbedded in the jaw that they do not normally erupt above the gum line.

impetigo. A highly contagious infection of the skin, principally found among newborn babies and young children.

impotence. Inability of the male to have an erection of the penis so that he can have sexual intercourse.

incest. Sexual intercourse between individuals whose relationship is too close to permit a legal marriage.

incontinence. Inability to hold back urine or bowel movements.

incubation period. The time between contact with a source of infection and the outbreak of symptoms.

infection. The entry, presence, and multiplication of disease-producing microorganisms in the body, and the reaction of the tissues to their presence and to the toxins generated by them.

influenza. A virus-caused disease that may attack the respiratory, nervous, or gastrointestinal system.

infrared. The range of electromagnetic waves beyond red in the visible spectrum of light. Infrared rays provide intensive heat for careful, dry heat treatment.

injection. A "shot"; anything forced into the body through a hollow needle with a syringe and plunger behind it.

ink-blot test. *See* **Rorschach test.**

insemination. Fertilization of an ovum by a sperm; conception.

insomnia. The inability to sleep.

instinct. A native or hereditary factor in behaviour which leads to a goal natural to a species.

insulin. A hormone formed by the islet cells of the pancreas and secreted into the blood, where it regulates the metabolism of sugar. Used in treating diabetes.

intern. A medical school graduate who is working (and often living) in a hospital to get at least a year of practical training before being licensed to practice medicine.

intravenous. Inside a vein.

introvert. An individual whose interest is focused within himself.

I. Q. Intelligence quotient; the numerical result of a test which attempts to measure intelligence.

irradiation. Treatment with any form of radiant energy: heat, light (sunlight), x-ray, radium emanations, or radioisotopes.

islet cells. Part of the pancreas, they secrete insulin necessary for carbohydrate digestion.

isometric exercise. The practice of performing muscular contractions to maximum ability for brief periods of time (seconds) to increase muscle strength.

isoniazid. A group of drugs, given by mouth, which are highly effective in the treatment of tuberculosis.

isotonic exercise. Ordinary exercise in which the body or limbs move as a result of making contractions and extensions of the muscles.

-itis. A suffix denoting inflammation and usually disease of a body part, for example; tonsill*itis.*

jaundice. A disease symptom that causes the skin and the whites of the eyes to turn yellow.

keratin. The hard protein substance, containing sulfur, that is the chief component of hard body tissues, such as hair, nails, horns (in animals), and the outer layer of the skin.

ketosis. "Vinegar breath"; a disturbance of normal acid-base relationships in the body. It is sometimes a complication of diabetes.

kinesiology. The study and science that deals with human motion and locomotion.

kinesthesia. The combination of sense perceptions and judgment by which a human being "feels" muscle tension and thus judges in himself and in others muscular motion, weight, and position.

kleptomania. An uncontrollable compulsion to steal; a form of mental illness.

laceration. A tear; any wound or injury in which skin, muscle, or other tissue is torn.

lactation. The act and time of giving milk from the breasts.

lactic acid. A thick, almost colorless, liquid that sours milk, disinfects wounds, and accumulates in the muscles as they become fatigued.

lanolin. Wool fat; used in some cosmetics.

laryngitis. Inflammation of the larynx; sore throat.

laughing gas. The popular name for nitrous oxide, sometimes used for inhalation anesthesia.

leprosy. An ancient, serious and chronic disease caused by infection with a specific microorganism (*Hansen's bacillus*). One form of leprosy particularly affects the skin; another, the nerves.

lesbianism. Homosexuality between women.

lesion. An injury to any part of the body from any cause that results in damage to the part.

leukemia. A serious disease of the blood-forming organs, which then produce too many white blood cells. Leukemia is sometimes called cancer of the blood.

leukocyte. White blood cell.

libido. The psychic energy of the unconscious mind; sometimes refers to sexual desire and drive.

ligament. A tough band of tissues that connects bones or supports body organs.

liver extract. Processed from the livers of meat animals, it is used in the treatment of pernicious anemia.

lobotomy. A cutting into a lobe of the brain to sever fibers as a treatment for certain types of mental illness. Now rarely used.

lockjaw. Tetanus; an acute, infectious disease. Its major symptom is the tightening of the jaw muscles, called trismus.

lues. Another name for syphilis; the adjective is "luetic."

lymph. The fluid, outside the blood vessels, in which the cells and tissues of the body are constantly bathed.

lymphatic system. The channels and small vessels that collect tissue fluid (lymph) and transport it back to the veins so that it re-enters the circulating blood stream.

maidenhead. *See* **hymen.**

malaise. A generally sick feeling, often accompanied by nausea and vomiting.

malaria. A mosquito (*anopheles*)-borne disease, characterized by intermittent attacks of chills, fever, and sweating.

malignant. Refers primarily to cancer. A truly cancerous growth or tumor is called malignant. The phrase "malignant hypertension," a rapidly increasing high blood pressure, is also used.

malnourishment. Failure to receive adequate nourishment for any reason. The usual cause is a diet inadequate in vitamins, minerals, and other nutritional substances.

malocclusion. Failure of teeth in upper and lower jaws to come together properly.

malpighian cells. Second (from the top) layer of skin whose growing cells contain skin pigment (melanin) that largely determines human skin color.

malpractice. Failure of a physician to treat a patient with the skill and attention that could reasonably be expected of him.

mammary. Relating to breasts.

mania. Frenzy or madness, a sign of mental illness. It may be characterized by violence of behavior, overtalkativeness, wild ideas, or undue excitement.

manic-depressive psychosis. A mental illness characterized by mood swings in the direction of excitement (manic phase) or extreme fatigue and despondency (depressive phase). It may be cyclic or periodic.

Mantoux text. A skin test for tuberculosis.

marihuana. A drug produced from the tops and leaves of the female *cannabis* plant; it is considered a hallucinogen, not a narcotic, but it produces a psychological dependency.

masochism. The psychological tendency to take pleasure in receiving pain; in its extreme form, a sexual perversion.

mastication. The act of chewing food.

mastoiditis. Inflammation in the mastoid bone, on the side of the head near the ear.

matriarchy. A pattern of social organization in which the mother is the dominant figure, descent is traced in the female line, and all children belong to the mother's family line.

M. D. Doctor of Medicine.

megalomania. Irrational belief in one's own greatness; delusions of grandeur.

melancholia. The deeply melancholy state of mind and body in which fear, anxiety, pessimism, indecision, and unwillingness to act dominate the mental outlook.

melanin. A dark pigment found in the skin, hair, and other body parts.

menarche. Onset of menstruation.

Mendelian laws. Patterns of heredity, in terms of dominant and recessive characteristics, first evolved by the Austrian abbot, Gregor Mendel (1822–1884).

meningitis. Inflammation of the meninges, the membranes that envelop the brain and spinal cord.

menopause. "Change of life"; the time when menstruation stops, marking the end of the child-bearing period.

menorrhagia. Profuse menstrual bleeding.

menstruation. The periodic discharge of blood from the vagina, usually about every 28 days. This blood and other tissue come from the inner lining of the uterus. The function of this lining is to receive a fertilized ovum. If none appears, the lining is again shed, with some bleeding.

mental illness. The exaggeration of personal behavior to the point where it strikes other people as queer, odd, abnormal, or dangerous. The bulk of so-called mental illness is really emotional maladjustment. The most common of the severe mental illnesses is schizophrenia.

mental mechanisms. The defenses adopted by the ego for the relief of painful conflicts in the unconscious mind. These defenses include: regression, projection, rationalization, and fantasy.

mental retardation. A condition characterized by faulty development of intelligence, which damages an individual's ability to learn and to adapt to the demands of society.

meprobomate. A chemical substance used as a tranquilizer.

metabolism. All of the physical and chemical processes that take place in the living body; the building up (anabolism) and breaking down (catabolism) processes that release energy for the use of the body.

metastasis. The spread of disease within the body, usually by way of the blood stream or lymph channels. Metastasis is particularly used to describe the migration of cancer cells from the site of their original growth to other parts of the body.

metatarsal. Any one of the five more or less parallel bones of each foot that reach from the ankle joint to the toes. They form the metatarsal arches of the feet.

metazoa. Comparatively large wormlike organisms that cause disease; for example, tapeworm, hookworm.

microbe. A tiny living organism, a microorganism, that can be seen only under a microscope. The smallest of these organisms are viruses and can be seen only with an electron microscope. Microbes are also germs; but only relatively few of them cause illness in man.

microbiology. The science which is concerned with the study of microorganisms; synonymous with bacteriology.

microorganism. A minute living organism, visible through a microscope. (*See* **microbe.**)

migraine. A type of headache usually confined to one side of the head, and often preceded by warning signals, such as flashes of light before the eyes.

miscarriage. A spontaneous abortion; premature expulsion of contents of the pregnant uterus.

mitosis. The common method of cell division into two "daughter cells" from one "mother cell."

mongolism. A condition of severe mental and physical retardation, characterized by an oblique slant of the eyes and a short flat-bridged nose.

monogamy. Marriage with one person at a time.

mononuclueosis, infectious. An acute, infectious disease characterized by fever and swelling of the lymph nodes in the neck. It is sometimes called the "kissing disease" or the "student's disease."

mons veneris ("mount of Venus"). The pad of rounded fatty tissue just above the female sex organs.

morbidity. Sickness.

moron. A person of low intelligence, whose mental age is between eight and twelve years.

morphine. A narcotic drug derived from opium.

motion sickness. Dizziness, headache, nausea, and vomiting produced by unaccustomed motions of vehicles of transportation. The seat of the illness is in the semicircular canals of the ears, where the sense of balance resides.

motor nerves. The nerves leading from the central nervous system out to the nerve endings in different parts of the body. These parts are put into action by the nerve impulse.

mucus. The thick, slippery fluid excreted by the mucous membranes of the body; for example, by the lips.

multiple sclerosis. A crippling disease of the central nervous system and nerve pathways; usually attacking young adults. The insulating tissue that covers the nerve fibers (the myelin sheath) degenerates in patches and is replaced by scar tissue. Hence messages from the brain to the muscles and organs are "short-circuited."

muscle tone. Describes the state of a muscle when it is partially and firmly contracted and is on the alert to contract more.

muscular dystrophy. A progressive disease whose principal characteristic is the wasting away of the striped, voluntary muscles of the body. It begins in early childhood.

myocardium. Heart muscle.

myopia. Nearsightedness.

myxedema. An endocrine disorder caused by thyroid deficiency. It is a disease of middle life; far more common in women than in men. Puffy face and hands, low body temperature, are some of its symptoms.

narcissism. Self-love. Narcissus, in Greek mythology, fell in love with his own image as reflected in a pool.

narcolepsy. A condition in which there is uncontrollable desire to fall asleep at any time of the day or night.

narcotics. Any drugs that produce sleep and stupor and at the same time relieve pain. Most narcotics are derivatives of opium, for example, morphine and heroin.

nausea. Tendency to vomit; sick at the stomach.

necropsy. Autopsy; postmortem examination of a body.

necrosis. Death or destruction of body tissue (or cells) while still in place and surrounded by living tissue. Gangrene and bedsores are examples.

neisserian infection. Another name for gonorrhea.

neoplasm. Any new growth or tumor. Malignant neoplasm means cancer.

nephritis. Inflammation of the kidneys.

nervous breakdown. A popular term for any kind of mental illness which is serious and prolonged.

neuralgia. Pain in a nerve, arising from a specific nerve and running along its course in the body. Examples: migraine headache, toothache.

neurasthenia. Nervous weakness or exhaustion; a mild form of mental illness characterized by extreme fatigue and loss of energy.

neuritis. Inflammation of a nerve. The body areas served by these nerves are usually tender and painful.

neurologist. A medical specialist concerned primarily with disorders of the nervous system.

neuron. A nerve cell.

neurosis. (Also called psychoneurosis.) A disturbance in an individual's psychic constitution. It is a milder form of mental illness, less severe than a psychosis. The disease is produced by conflicts in the unconscious mind, often too severe to be relieved without psychiatric treatment.

niacin. Nicotinic acid; the pellagra-preventive factor of the vitamin B complex.

nicotine. The principal active substance (alkaloid) in tobacco. Pure nicotine, even in small doses, is a dangerous poison.

nucleic acids. Acids formed in the nucleus of a cell. The two important ones are DNA (deoxynucleic acid) and RNA (ribonucleic acid), which provide the genes (molecules) that govern heredity.

nucleus (of cell). The cell's core, center, and reproductive system. It contains the thread-like chromosomes that separate into two chains when one cell breaks down into two cells.

nullipara. A woman who has never borne a child.

nutrient. Nourishing; any substance that supplies food to the body.

nutrition. The essential body process of assimilating food. Failure of nutrition may result from a faulty, limited diet or from the body's failure to absorb food.

nymphomania. Extreme, abnormal sexual desire in the female; comparable to satyriasis in the male.

obesity. Fat and overweight.

obstetrics. The medical speciality that deals with the events of pregnancy and childbirth.

occlusion. The condition of being closed. The closure of the small arteries of the heart brings on coronary occlusion. In dentistry, occlusion describes the fit of the teeth of the upper and lower jaws when the mouth is closed.

occupational diseases. Those arising out of the course of one's work or occupation, unless adequate safety or preventive measures are taken. Examples: lead poisoning in painters, black lung in coal miners.

occupational therapy. Part of the process of total rehabilitation. It means providing the patient (in or out of a hospital) with interesting opportunities to exercise those muscles and talents that can be strengthened and lead toward a life as normal as possible. Included in occupational therapy projects are such things as weaving, painting, carpentry, dance, and many other hobby-crafts.

oculist. Eye specialist; an older term for ophthalmologist.

Oedipus complex. A construct in Freudian psychoanalysis. The name derives from Oedipus Rex who, in Greek mythology, was destined by the gods to kill his father and marry his mother. The Freudian theory contends that there is a normal stage in the psychological development of a male child, usually around the ages of five to seven when he wants to replace his father in the affections of his mother.

olfactory. Related to the sense of smell.

ophthalmia. Inflammation of the eyes; conjunctivitis. The gonococcus germ often threatens the sight of the newborn if the mother herself has gonorrhea. To prevent damage to the eyes of the newborn (*gonococcal ophthalmia*) the physician is required by law to instill in all newborn babies' eyes some drug or antibiotic which will kill the gonococcus.

ophthamologist. Eye specialist; physician; also called oculist.

opiate. Any painkiller or narcotic, particularly one derived from the opium poppy.

opium. The crude product of the resins derived from the flowering tops of the female poppy plant (*papaver somniferum*).

optician. A technician who grinds the lenses of eye glasses and adjusts their frames.

optometrist. A person licensed to give limited eye care; to examine the eyes for the purpose of prescribing eye glasses and recommending specific eye exercises.

organism. Any living thing, from a polio virus to a whale.

orgasm. The climax; the moment of the highest pitch of sexual excitation.

orthodontics. A speciality of dentistry which deals with straightening and realigning the teeth to achieve proper occlusion of the upper and lower teeth.

orthopedics. The medical specialty that deals primarily with the results of disease or accident to the bones, joints, and muscles.

osmosis. The passage of fluid solutions through membranes that ostensibly separate them. For example, the nutrient-carrying blood plasma seeps through capillary blood vessels to bring needed nourishment.

osteopath. Abbreviated to D. O. for Doctor of Osteopathy; a medical practitioner who has been trained in and accepts the teachings of osteopathy. Some D. O.'s are also M. D.'s.

otitis. Inflammation of the inner, middle, or outer ear.

otologist. Ear specialist.

otosclerosis. A form of progressive deafness caused by formation of spongy bone around the tiny inner bones of the ear.

oviducts. The tubes, one on each side of the body, through which the ova descend from the ovary to the womb. (Also called uterine tubes or fallopian tubes.)

ovulation. The time when a mature ovum is released from the ovary; approximately the midpoint of the menstrual cycle.

ovum. Egg; the human ovum is the female reproductive cell, a sphere approximately $\frac{1}{20}$ of an inch in diameter.

palliative. A drug or treatment which relieves or alleviates pain but has little or no affect on its underlying cause.

palpation. Examination by hand; feeling with the fingers or whole hand for signs of disease.

palpitation. Rapid heartbeat of which a person is acutely aware.

palsy. Paralysis.

pancreas gland. A large, long internal organ, located behind the lower part of the stomach. It is an important part both of the digestive system and endocrine system. Scattered through it are islet cells which secrete insulin necessary for proper digestion of sugars and starches (carbohydrates).

"Pap test." Laboratory examination for detection of possible uterine cancer. Named after originator, Dr. George Papanicolaou.

"paramedical" specialties. A growing list of minor specialties, whose work complements that performed by the physician. Thus, for example, we have physical and occupational therapists, x-ray technicians, and more recently "physician's aides."

paranoia. A chronic form of mental illness in which the patient suffers from delusions of persecution or illusions of grandeur.

paraplegia. Paralysis of both legs and lower part of the body. It results from accident to or disease of the spinal cord.

parasite. A plant (for example, a fungus) or an animal (protozoa) that lives and feeds on another plant or animal, presumably to the detriment of its host. A virus is a type of parasite in a cell.

parathyroid glands. Endocrine glands, four small ones, attached to each of the two thyroid glands in the neck.

paresthesia. Abnormal feeling, heightened sensibility, such as burning, pricking, or crawling sensation on the skin.

parietal. Refers to walls of any body cavity, usually the skull.

Parkinson's disease. A degenerative disease in which some unknown process takes place at the clusters of nerve cells at the base of the brain. The disease is named after the English physician, James Parkinson (1755–1824) who first described it.

parotid glands. The saliva-producing glands in the back of the mouth, near the ears.

pasteurization. A method of "sterilizing" milk, wine, and other fluids without boiling or destroying their intrinsic flavors. Named after the French chemist, Louis Pasteur (1822–1895).

pathogenic. Anything that causes disease, whether a microorganism or any other material.

pathological. A diseased condition.

pediatrics. The medical specialty relating to the care of children.

pediculosis. Lousiness; infestation with lice.

pellagra. A vitamin deficiency disease, once common in the South. The vitamin lacking in this condition is niacin, a part of the vitamin B complex. The symptoms of pellagra include sore tongue and mouth, skin eruptions, digestive disturbances (diarrhea), mental depression, backache, and general weakness.

penicillin. An antibiotic derived from the mold, *Penicillium notatum*. Effective against a wide range of microbes, including those that cause syphilis, gonorrhea, pneumonia, and sore throat.

perfectionist. An individual who, to avoid criticism, sets his goals so high that he cannot be reasonably criticized for failure to reach such impossible goals.

periodontal disease. Inflammation, infection, or other disorder of the periodontal membranes; commonly called *pyorrhea.*

periodontal membrane. Soft tissue surrounding teeth.

periosteum. The elastic lining around the bones; consisting of two layers of fibrous tissue.

periphereal nervous system. The nerves that reach the outer surfaces of the body and return sensations, felt on their end-organs (sensory nerves), to the central nervous system which immediately dispatches "orders" to the part by way of the motor nerves.

peristalsis. The wavelike motion, brought about by alternating contraction and relaxation of the smooth muscle tissues of the gastrointestinal tract. This motion carries food and gastic juices along from the stomach to the rectum.

peritoneum. The strong membrane that lines the abdomen.

peritonitis. Inflammation in or of the peritoneum.

pertussis. Whooping cough.

pesticides. A wide range of chemical substances, starting in the 1940's with DDT, which are applied to dwellings or field crops to kill undesirable insect pests; for example, the *anopheles* mosquito which carries malaria.

peyote. A hallucinating drug obtained from Mexican cactus.

phagocyte. A white blood cell that engulfs and destroys microbes that infect the body.

phallus. The male organ; the penis and representations of it, as found in phallic worship rites.

pharmacist. Druggist, apothecary, licensed to fill physicians' prescriptions.

pharmacology. The science that deals with drugs; in particular the formulation and testing of new drugs.

pharmacopoeia. An authoritative and official treatise or book that describes drugs and tells in exact detail how to make and use them. Many countries have an official pharmacopoeia.

pharyngitis. Sore throat.

phenotype. The individual organism resulting from the reactions between its genotype (the purely hereditary factors) and its environment.

phlebitis. Inflammation of the walls of a vein.

phlegm. Thick mucus, coughed up or spit out of the mouth.

phobia. Abnormal, morbid fear; for example, claustrophobia; fear of enclosed places.

physical therapy. The treatment of disease by physical methods. Among these are the use of heat, cold, water (hydrotherapy), ultraviolet light, massage, and exercise.

physiology. The science and study of the functions or actions of living organisms in their gross or minute structures.

piles. *See* **hemorrhoids.**

pink eye. *See* **conjunctivitis.**

pituitary gland. An endocrine gland located at the base of the brain; sometimes called the "master gland."

placebo. A sugar pill or other "make-believe" medicine, given merely to satisfy the patient's desire for drug treatment; or used as a control in a scientific medical experiment.

placenta. The pancake-shaped tissue attached to the wall of the uterus during pregnancy. Through it the fetus is nourished from its mother's blood. The placenta is normally expelled from the uterus five to ten minutes after birth.

plasma (blood). The fluid part of the blood in which the various blood cells are suspended.

plastic surgery. The reconstruction of facial and other skin and soft tissues to relieve disfigurements, deformities, and other visible blemishes.

plexus. A knot or tangle of tissues, usually applied to nerves or veins. The *solar plexus* is a large network of nerves located on the outside of the stomach.

pneumonia. A serious, infectious disease of one or more lobes of the lungs; caused by invasion of the pneumococcus germ.

podiatrist. Chiropodist; nonmedical specialist in the care of the feet.

poliomyelitis. Polio; acute virus disease characterized by fever, sore throat, headache, and vomiting, frequently with stiffness of the neck and back. It may be minor or major, with possible crippling or fatal effects. Since vaccines for the prevention of polio were introduced in the United States in the midfifties, the incidence of the disease has fallen to fewer than 100 cases a year.

polyandry. The union of one woman to several husbands at the same time.

polygamy. Multiple or plural marriage; sometimes construed as the exclusive right of one man to several wives at the same time.

polygyny. The right of one man to several women, concubines as well as wives, concurrently.

polyps. New growths of body tissue; overgrowths of the mucous membranes that line many body cavities.

postmortem. After death. Usually refers to a postmortem examination of the body; an autopsy.

postnasal drip. A collection of mucus at the back of the nose from where it drips down to the throat.

postnatal. Following childbirth.

premature. Too soon, before expected; usually applied to an infant born before the full nine months of pregnancy.

prenatal. Before birth.

presbyopia. Old-sightedness; a type of farsightedness that comes with advancing years.

procaine. A local or topical anesthetic.

proctology. The medical specialty dealing with diseases and disorders of the rectum and anus.

progesterone. A female sex hormone.

prognosis. The physician's opinion, based on past experience, of the probable outcome of a specific disease or injury.

projection. The mental mechanism in which people project the blame for their own shortcomings on other people or things.

prophylaxis. The prevention of disease; frequently refers to the means of preventing venereal disease through the use of a condom.

proprietary. Any drug that can be sold without a doctor's prescription, including "patent medicines."

prostate gland. A gland in the male located just below the bladder and encircling the urethra. Enlargement of the prostate (usually in older men) causes difficulties in urination.

prosthesis. Any artificial replacement or substitute for a part of the body that has been lost or is missing. For example; a false tooth, a glass eye, a wooden leg, a plastic arm, or an artificial heart.

protein. The "meat" of a body; the prime component of the flesh of any living organism from the one-celled ameba to the blue whale. Some form of protein, or its "building blocks," the amino acids, are essential to a life-sustaining diet.

protoplasm. Living matter.

protozoa. One-celled "animals" of a variety of shapes and sizes; usually larger than bacteria. Typical example is the plasmodium which causes malaria.

pruritis. Itching.

pseudocyesis. False pregnancy. A woman believes herself to be pregnant and displays some of the early signs of pregnancy, for example, morning sickness and enlarged abdomen.

psittacosis. "Parrot fever"; transmitted to man by parrots, parakeets, and domestic fowl. It is a virus disease, causing an atypical pneumonia.

psoriasis. A chronic recurring skin disorder of unknown cause.

psyche. Mind; taken from the Greek word for soul, it is now used to describe the processes that arise in the conscious and unconscious mind.

psychiatry. The medical specialty dealing with mental illness and the restoration and maintenance of mental health.

"psycho." Slang expression for an individual currently or in the past afflicted with mental illness.

psychoanalysis. It has three meanings: (1) a method of treatment for some of the milder forms of mental illness (notably neuroses); (2) a method of research throwing light on mental illness and the nature of man's mind, both conscious and unconscious; and (3) a theory on how the human mind operates.

psychogenic. Caused by mental or emotional factors.

psychologist. An individual trained in the science of psychology; that is, the scientific study of the mind and the whole range of human and animal behavior. A well-trained clinical psychologist who treats emotional disorders usually has a Ph.D. degree.

psychoneurosis. *See* **neurosis.**

psychosis. The term now used to describe the more severe forms of mental illness; notably, schizophrenia, manic-depressive psychosis, and alcoholic psychosis.

psychosomatic. An illness or disorder in which the mental component seems to have a great or direct bearing; for example, hysterical paralysis and stomach ulcers.

psychotherapy. A planned and organized pattern of action, chiefly conversation between doctor and patient, designed to cure or alleviate mental illness. It is designed to give a patient greater insight into the nature of his illness.

ptomaine poisoning. Old fashioned and incorrect name for serious food poisoning. Ptomaines are a class of substances formed in the decay of flesh.

puberty. The years during which sexual maturity occurs. In the female it is marked by the onset of menstruation.

public health. Attention to the health of the community at large. The health officer and his staff take the steps necessary to achieve a healthy environment; for example, sanitation, epidemic control, and recording of vital statistics. Public health departments are tax-supported and have police power over situations within their realm of protective and preventive services.

pudenda. External sex organs, male or female.

puerperal. Related to childbirth and the days immediately following.

pulmonary. Related to the lungs.

pulmonary embolism. The blocking or closure of the pulmonary artery by a blood clot (an embolus); a frequent cause of sudden death.

purgative. A strong laxative.

pus. The fluid that accumulates around an inflammation. It contains dead cells and many white blood cells.

pyelitis. Infection of the kidney, usually its inner core.

pyorrhea. Literally, a flow of pus. The term is usually used to describe infection of the gums and the membranes that cover the roots of the teeth below the gum line.

quackery. False pretense to medical skills and achievements; charlatan is another name for a quack doctor.

quarantine. Means legal and, if necessary, forceable restriction of people from entering and especially from leaving countries or premises where communicable or contagious disease exists (or may be presumed to exist). The American astronauts who first set foot upon the moon were held in quarantine for two weeks after splashdown, to avoid the possiblity that they were carriers of unknown and potentially dangerous microorganisms from the moon.

quinine. Bark of the cinchona tree; a specific drug for treating all forms of malaria.

rabies. Called *hydrophobia* when it occurs in man; a virus disease, fatal if not treated with rabies vaccine. The disease is transmitted by the bite of rabid animals.

radiation. Emission of radiant energy, electromagnetic waves; as evident in x-ray beams, radium emanations, and atomic explosions.

radiation sickness. Injury or bodily damage occurring as the result of overdoses of radiant energy. Many survivors of Hiroshima suffered from delayed radiation sickness.

radiology. Sometimes called roentgenology; the medical specialty that deals with the use of radiant energy (for instance, x-rays) for the diagnosis and treatment of disease.

radioisotope. Any isotope of a chemical element or its compounds that has been made radioactive by treatment in an atomic energy pile. For example, radiocobalt is now used in the treatment of cancer.

rash. An abnormal, reddish coloration, or blotch on some part of the skin. The causes are many, including irritation, infection, and allergy.

rationalization. A common mechanism of the unconscious mind, through which an individual finds acceptable reasons for doing or thinking things that his superego does not approve.

rauwolfia. A drug derived from the Indian snakeroot plant(*Rauwolfia serpentina*) which grows in southeast Asia. In purified forms, which became available in the 1950's, it has proved an exceptionally valuable drug for the treatment of high blood pressure and an effective tranquilizer for use in treatment of mild to severe mental illness.

receptor. A nerve ending in a sense organ that responds to particular stimuli; thus the eye is stimulated by light, the ear by sound.

red blood cells. The cells that give blood its color. These cells contain iron in the form of hemoglobin. They transport oxygen to all cells of the body (via the blood stream) and bring back for exclusion (via the lungs) the waste product of cell metabolism, carbon dioxide.

reflexes. Involuntary acts performed in response to some stimulus from the nervous system. For example, the eyes blink when a light is flashed upon them.

refraction. (1) The deviation of light rays when they pass from one transparent medium to another (as from air to glass lenses). (2) The testing of eyesight for errors of refraction of the crystalline lens of the eye and prescribing lenses to correct these errors.

regression. The unconsciously motivated psychological mechanism in which a person reverts to earlier, childish types of behavior.

rehabilitation (medical). The restoration of a disabled person toward self-sufficiency or gainful employment at his highest possible skill as rapidly as possible.

renal. Related to the kidneys.

repression. A fundamental mental mechanism by which disagreeable, unpleasant, or painful thoughts and feelings are submerged into the unconscious mind.

reserpine. A drug, related to *rauwolfia*, for the treatment of heart disease and high blood pressure.

resident. A graduate physician, licensed to practice, who remains in the hospital framework to further his education in a medical specialty.

respiratory system. Includes the lungs and other parts of the body that have to do with the mechanism of breathing.

resuscitation. Artificial respiration; various kinds of maneuvers to restore breathing when it has been stopped by such events as drowning or electric shock.

rheumatic fever. An infectious disease that is most damaging when it scars the heart muscle or valves of the heart and thus produces rheumatic heart disease.

rheumatism. The popular term for *arthritis*. It describes a multitude of aches and pains in muscles, bones, and joints.

Rh factor. A substance included in red blood cells; important for typing blood for transfusions and in obstetrics. It is an hereditary characteristic.

rhinitis. Inflammation, usually with some swelling, of the inner lining of the nose.

rhythm method. A "safe-period" system of contraception based on knowledge of the fertility cycle.

rickets. A deficiency disease; specifically the lack of vitamin D in infancy and childhood. Lack of vitamin D causes brittleness and softness of the bones.

rickettsia. A class of microbes, larger than viruses but usually smaller than bacteria. It is named for Howard Taylor Ricketts (1871–1910), an American scientist. Among the diseases caused by rickettsia are typhus fever and Q fever.

RNA (ribonucleic acid). An exceptionally long spiral molecule that carries the genetic pattern from its model, DNA, to the cells newly being formed. *See* **DNA.**

roentgen. The roentgen or *r* is a measure of the amount of radiation exposure that will produce a certain amount of ionization in a specific volume of air. This unit is named after the German physicist, Wilhelm Conrad Roentgen (1845–1923), who first discovered x-rays (also called roentgen rays).

Rohrschach. A test in which the subject is shown a standard series of ink blots and asked to describe what he sees; used to determine aspects of personality.

rubella. *See* **German measles.**

rubeola. Measles.

rupture. The popular term for hernia. *See* **hernia.**

sacroiliac. The lower part of the back; the joints between the sacrum and ilium (hipbone) and the ligaments that join them. A common site of backache.

sadism. Deliberate cruelty, usually for the satisfaction of open or disguised sexual impulses.

salicylates. A large class of drugs that have the same general effects as aspirin, which is one of them.

salmonella. A genus of bacteria frequently responsible for food poisoning.

sarcoma. Cancer arising from connective tissues, such as the bones.

satyriasis. Abnormal and excessive sexual desire in the male. In the female this condition is called nymphomania.

scabies. "The itch"; a skin disorder caused by the boring of the itch mite beneath the surface of the skin.

schistosomiasis. A tropical disease caused by infestation of a particular kind of parasite (*schistosome*). These parasites are dependent on snails for one part of their life cycle.

schizophrenia. A term for dementia praecox (early madness) which is interpreted as a "split" in the mental functions. In general terms, it implies withdrawal from the real world into a fantastic (but sometimes logically fantastic) world of one's own. Schizophrenia is the most serious form of psychosis.

sclerosis. Hardening. It is used in such terms as arteriosclerosis; hardening of the arteries.

scurvy. A vitamin C deficiency disease.

sebaceous glands. Small glands near the surface of the skin and adjacent to hair follicles. These glands secrete sebum, an oily substance, which helps keep skin soft.

seborrhea. Excessive secretion of oily substance, sebum, from the sebaceous glands of the skin; an important factor in the development of adolescent *acne*.

"second sight." Better vision for reading and seeing in the later years of life. This improved vision is a result of the thickening of the lens of the eye.

However, this is usually a forerunner of cataracts of the eyes.

sedative. Any drug that reduces activity and allays excitement or overt anxiety.

semen. The white, slightly sticky, fluid produced by the male sex organs and ejaculated from them; the vehicle for sperm.

sensory nerves. A system of nerve endings that pick up sensations (for example, heat or bad smells) and convey them back to the central nervous system.

sepsis. Poisoning by microbes or their by-products in the living organism. It is the root of the words *asepsis* and *antiseptic.*

septicemia. Blood poisoning.

serology. The branch of science that deals with the study of antigens and antibodies in blood serum. Blood tests like the Wassermann and other similar tests for syphilis, are actually serologic tests.

shingles. A virus disease, caused perhaps by the same virus that brings on chicken pox. The first symptoms are a crop of small blisters on the skin.

shock. In medicine it usually means the rapid and sometimes fatal fall in blood pressure following injury (for example, a blow on the head), operation, or administration of anesthesia. The term shock is also used to designate *electric shock* given in some cases of mental illness. *Psychic shock* refers to emotional reaction to a sudden, shocking event.

"shots." Popular term for injections.

sign. Any objective evidence of a disease condition. Signs, in contrast to *symptoms,* can be seen, heard, felt, or even smelled by the examiner.

silicosis. An occupational disease of the lung caused by long-time inhalation of stone or sand dust.

sinusitis. Inflammation of a sinus; generally refers to the sinuses of the nose.

sleeping pills. Usually barbiturate drugs. Overdoses can be fatal.

sleeping sickness. Occurs as the result of some damage or disorder in the brain. Most commonly refers to African sleeping sickness, transmitted from domestic and wild animals to man through the bite of the *tsetse fly* and similar insects.

smog. A fog made heavier, darker, and irritating to the eyes by the smoke emitted from a city's smoke stacks and also by exhaust fumes from motor vehicles.

socialized medicine. A system of medical practice in which all physicians are employed by the state and all people in the state have the right to medical help without direct payment of a fee for service.

soma. Taken from the Greek word meaning "body" and used in contrast to *psyche,* or mind.

somnambulist. Sleep-walker.

spastic. Marked by muscle spasms; involuntary, repeated contractions of any set of muscles. A spastic child or adult is usually one whose rigid, stiff muscles or awkward muscular movements reflect some brain damage.

specimen. A sample for further study or medical laboratory examination; frequently refers to small sample of urine.

sperm. The fully developed male sex cell formed in the testes and capable of fertilizing the female ovum.

spirochete. A cork-screw shaped microorganism; such as the pale spirochete (*Treponema pallida*) that causes syphilis.

staphyloccus. Often abbreviated to "staph," this is the general name for a particular group of round, ball-shaped bacteria that grow in bunches like a cluster of grapes.

sterility. Barrenness; inability to bear or sire children. May be relative, not absolute.

sterilization. (1) The process of making surgical instruments and dressings completely free of germs by autoclaving under steam. (2) It also means making an individual incapable of further reproduction, often by simple surgical procedure.

stethoscope. An instrument that enables the physician to hear better what is taking place inside the body, by conducting sound.

stimulant. A drug that excites or stimulates some organ or part of the body to greater function or activity. Amphetamines and caffeine, for example, stimulate the central nervous system.

strabismus. Squint; cross-eye or wall-eye.

streptoccocus. Often abbreviated to "strep," this is the name for a class of dangerous microbes associated with several serious illnesses; for example, sore throat and rheumatic fever.

streptomycin. An antibiotic isolated from a soil mold.

stress. Pressure, physical or mental, usually persistent, that leads to the development of the stress syndrome.

stroke. Any sudden, severe attack of illness; usually an apopletic stroke, or apoplexy. This condition is caused by the breaking or clogging of a blood vessel in the brain.

"student's disease." *See* **infectious mononucleosis.**

subcutaneous. Under the skin.

sublimation. The directing, channelizing, and converting of basic drives and instincts into personally satisfying, socially acceptable, and useful activities.

sulfa drugs. A great number of powerful germ-fighting drugs, all of which (such as sulfanilamide) contain in some combination the chemical group called a sulfonamide radical which includes sulfur.

superego. Roughly, the conscience; in particular, the unconscious censor of an individual's thought, feeling, and action. It partially controls the ego.

suture. (1) Threadlike material, such as catgut, wire, silk, or cotton thread, for sewing up a wound. (2) Suture also describes the lines where the bones of the skull join together.

symptom. Subjective evidence of disease; something the patient feels but the doctor cannot see; for example, a headache.

synapse. The "spark" by which nerve impulses jump from one neuron to another.

syndrome. A set of signs and symptoms which, taken together, often point to the diagnosis of a specific illness.

syphilis. A contagious venereal disease, caused by a microorganism (*Treponema pallidum*), almost always transmitted by sexual intercourse. It leads to many structural and skin lesions if unchecked; but is curable with massive doses of antibiotics.

syphilophobia. Exaggerated and abnormal fear of syphilis.

systole. The short period of time when the heart muscle contracts to force blood through the arteries. This is the moment when blood pressure is at its highest in all the arteries in the body. Readings of blood pressure at these moments are also at their highest. When the heart is not in systole (working) it is in *diastole* (at rest).

taboo. Forbidden.

tachycardia. Rapid heart beat; usually over 100 beats per minute.

tampon. A plug of cotton or other absorbent material introduced into a body cavity to stop bleeding or soak up secretions. Tampons are safely and comfortably inserted into the vagina to absorb menstrual flow.

tendons. The glistening white connective tissues in which muscle fibers end and which attach the muscles to bones or other body organs. The *Achilles tendon* runs from the calf muscle of the leg to the heelbone.

testes. The male sex organs suspended in the sac of the scrotum at the groin outside the abdominal cavity.

testosterone. Male sex hormone.

tetanus. *See* **lockjaw.**

tetany. A disease state, marked by muscular twitching, tremors, spasms, and cramps. It can be traced to a fall in the amount of calcium in the blood stream. *Not* the same as tetanus.

thalamus. A part of the brain, situated at its base; the main relay station for sensory nerve impulses to the higher centers of the cerebrum.

thalidomide. A drug once commonly used in Europe as a tranquilizer or sedative. It was later discovered to produce fetal damage (deformed infants) if taken by a pregnant woman.

therapy. A technical word for treatment by any means.

thiamine. Part of the vitamin B complex.

thorax. The chest cavity, reaching from the neck to the abdomen.

thrombosis. Means the clogging of a blood vessel as a result of the formation of a blood clot within the vessel itself. When a thrombus breaks off from the site where it was formed and enters the blood stream, it is called an *embolus.*

thymus gland. An accessory gland, in the chest, whose function is not really known. It is sometimes considered an endocrine gland, but it wastes away during childhood.

thyroid glands. The two endocrine glands in the neck that secrete the hormone, thyroxin. When they are enlarged, they produce the condition called goiter.

thyroxin. The hormone secreted by the thyroid gland. It partially controls body metabolism.

tic. A twitching of muscles, especially of the face, constantly repeated.

"tired blood." Anemia.

tissue. A collection of body cells of the same kind in sufficient quantity to form a definable part of the anatomy; for example, skin tissue.

tolbutamide. Oral drug for treatment of mild forms of diabetes.

tolerance. The ability of the human body or other living organisms, notably microbes, to resist successfully the anticipated effects of drugs, poisons, or other stress.

tonometer. Instrument for determining the pressure inside the eyeball; useful in detecting early glaucoma.

tonsillectomy. Surgical removal of tonsils by snare, knife or electrocoagulation; the most common surgical operation.

torticollis. Wry-neck; head twisted on shoulders.

toxemia. Poisoning by way of the blood stream, usually from toxins (poisons) released by microbes. Toxemia also occurs in pregnancy, for reasons still uncertain.

toxicology. The scientific study of poisons and their antidotes.

toxin. A poison.

trachoma. A serious eye disease; a form of conjunctivitis.

traction. Pulling, drawing, or stretching action. It often refers to methods for setting broken bones.

tranquilizer. A drug which acts on the emotional state to calm without affecting clarity of consciousness.

trauma. An injury or wound to living tissue. *Birth trauma* means injury in the process of being born. In psychiatry, this may imply that being born is in itself a traumatic experience. *Psychic trauma* is an emotional shock that makes a lasting impression on the conscious or unconscious mind.

tremor. Involuntary shaking, trembling, or quivering of any part of the body or of the body as a whole.

"trench mouth." Vincent's infection; inflammation of the gums with ulcerations that may also extend to the tonsils.

trichinosis. A disease caused by infestation with a hairlike parasite, *Trichinella spiralis.* The infestation is transmitted from pigs to man by the eating of insufficiently cooked pork or pork products.

trypanosome. A protozoan (comparatively large) microorganism which infects the blood stream to cause a disease such as sleeping sickness.

tsetse fly. The insect carrier of African sleeping sickness.

tubercle. A nodule or small rounded mass sometimes found on the skin, bones, or in the lungs; especially the characteristic little nodule found in the lungs in the presence of tuberculosis.

tuberculosis. An infectious disease caused by the presence of the tubercle bacillus in the lungs (and sometimes other parts of the body).

tumor. New growth in the body of useless cells, benign or malignant (cancerous).

typanic membrane. Ear drum.

typhoid fever. A serious communicable disease caused by infection with a specific microbe (*Salmonella typhosa*). The disease, sometimes called an intestinal fever, is spread through the excretion of the microbe in feces (bowel movements).

typhus. Describes a large class of diseases (fevers) caused by microbes called *rickettsia.* They are all transmitted from man to man or from animal to man by insects (ticks).

ulcer, peptic. Open lesions in the stomach or duodenum.

ultraviolet rays. They are the electromagnetic radiations that occur beyond the violet end of the visible spectrum (rainbow) of light.

unconscious mind. The hidden, buried, and temporarily forgotten part of the human mind. Here occur the conflicts between its three parts (or constructs); the id (instincts), the ego (self) and the superego (conscience). This theoretical construct of the unconscious mind is central to *psychoanalysis.*

undulant fever. Also called Malta fever and brucellosis; perhaps the most common animal disease transmitted to man.

urea. The nitrogen-containing chemical substance which is the chief end-product of the decomposition of protein foodstuffs in the human or animal body. It is present in blood, lymph, and especially urine.

uremia. Poisoning by accumulation in the blood stream of waste products like *urea* that should normally be passed off into the urine by the kidneys.

urinalysis. Examination of patient's urine as an aid in detecting and diagnosing disease.

urticaria. Hives; an allergic reaction of the skin characterized by elevated white, pink, or red patches, which often itch.

uterus. Womb: the chief female sex organ.

vaccination. Immunization against specific diseases by inoculation, injection, or ingestion (oral vaccines) of any product of biologic origin designed to prevent or alleviate those diseases. Originally vaccination meant only inoculation with cowpox to prevent smallpox.

vaccine. Any biological material administered to protect against microbial invasion or damage. The vaccines are usually attenuated forms of the microbes against which they protect. They may confer brief or long-lasting immunity against the specific microbes which cause such diseases. There are about a dozen successful vaccines now available (polio, smallpox, diphtheria, yellow fever, measles, mumps, whooping cough, lockjaw, cholera, typhoid, paratyphoid fever, and rabies).

vagina. The birth canal and female organ of sexual intercourse.

valve. Usually refers to the structures of the heart and veins which keep blood from flowing the wrong way.

varicose veins. Dilated or swollen veins. The veins of the legs are by far the most commonly affected.

vascular. Relating to the blood vessels.

"V. D." Venereal disease.

vector. Anything that carries and thus tends to spread a specific disease. For example, malaria is carried by the *Anopheles* mosquito.

vein. Any blood vessel leading to the heart.

venereal disease. Diseases spread primarily by sexual intercourse; notably syphilis, gonorrhea, and chancroid.

ventral. Bellyside or frontside; the opposite of *dorsal* or backside.

vertebrae. The odd shaped bones that, piled one on top of the other, make up the spinal column or backbone. The adult human has 26 vertebrae.

vertigo. Dizziness; the sensation that the environment is revolving around you.

vessel. In medicine it means blood vessel; vein or artery.

veterinary medicine. The diagnosis, treatment, and prevention of disease in animals.

virus. A tiny parasite living, growing, and reproducing its kind inside a host cell. Viruses are the smallest of microbes. When viruses damage or destroy the host cells they invade, they produce virus diseases; for example, polio, smallpox, and rabies.

viscera. Internal organs of the abdomen and chest.

vitamins. Organic chemical substances, widely distributed in natural foodstuffs, that are essential to normal metabolic function in man, lower animals, and birds. Vitamins, also called accessory food factors, are needed only in small amounts, but lack of this necessary amount results in a vitamin deficiency disease (avitaminosis). Examples are scurvy, rickets, beriberi, and pellagra.

voyeurism. Sexual satisfaction through merely seeing sexual organs or watching sex acts.

Wassermann test. A blood test for detecting the presence and severity of syphilitic infections.

WHO. World Health Organization.

x-rays. Electromagnetic waves of very short wavelength. They have the property of (1) penetrating solids to produce an image on sensitized film or screen, and (2) in large doses, inducing certain chemical changes in living tissue that are beneficial in the treatment of malignant diseases. Wilhelm Conrad Roentgen, their discover in 1895, named them "x-rays," although in his honor they are now frequently called roentgen rays.

yaws. A tropical disease caused by a spirochete (*Treponema pertenue*).

yellow fever. An acute virus disease carried by mosquitoes and marked by fever, albuminuria, and jaundice (which gives a yellow color to the skin of the victim).

zoonoses. Animal diseases that can be transmitted to man.

zygote. A fertilized ovum in its earliest stages.

APPENDIX

E

CHAPTER REFERENCES AND BIBLIOGRAPHY

Chapter 1. Introduction:
Health in the College Community

Beyrer, Mary K., Nolte, Anne E., and Solleder, Marian K., *A Directory of Selected References and Resources for Health Education,* Minneapolis: Burgess Publishing Co., 1966.

Blaine, G. B., Jr. and McArthur, C., eds., *Emotional Problems of Students,* New York: Appleton-Century-Crofts, 1961.

Chesterfield, Lord (Philip Dormer Stanhope), *Letters to His Son.*

Evans, Alfred S., M.D., and Warren, Jeffrey, B.S., "Common Problems of College Students," *AMA Archives of Environmental Health* (June 1962).

Farnsworth, Dana, M.D., *Mental Health in College and University,* Cambridge, Mass.: Harvard University Press, 1957.

A Forward Look in College Health Education (Conference Report), Washington, D. C.: American Association for Health, Physical Education and Recreation, 1956.

Galdston, Iago, M. D., ed., *The Epidemiology of Health,* New York: Health Education Council, 1953.

Gomez, Joan, *Dictionary of Symptoms,* Marvin Gersh, ed., New York: Stein & Day, 1968.

Guide Book Describing Pamphlets, Posters and Films on Health and Disease, Baltimore, Md.: Maryland State Department of Health, 1967.

Hanrahan, James S. and Bushnell, David, *Space Biology: The Human Factors in Space Flight,* New York: Science Editions, 1961.

Inglis, Bryan, *Emotional Stress and Your Health,* New York: Criterion Books, 1958.

Ives, Charlotte Yale, R.N., Ph.D., "Perceptions of Prospective Elementary Teachers Regarding Their Preparation in Health Education," *The Journal of School Health,* **32:** 6 (June 1962).

Jores and Freyberger, *Advances in Psychosomatic Medicine,* New York: Basic Books, 1961.

Kiell, Norman, *The Universal Experience of Adolescence,* New York: International Universities Press.

Lerner, Monroe and Anderson, Odin U., *Health Progress in the United States: 1900–1960,* Chicago: University of Chicago Press, 1964.

Levenson, Edgar, M.D. and Kohn, Martin, Ph.D., "A Demonstration Clinic for College Dropouts," *The Journal of The American College Health Association,* **12:** 4 (April 1964), pp. 382–391.

Riesman, David, *The Lonely Crowd,* New Haven, Conn.: Yale University Press, 1962.

Rosen, George, M.D., *A History of Public Health,* New York: MD Publications, 1958.

Sanford, Nevitt, ed., *The American College: a psychological and social interpretation of the higher learning,* New York: John Wiley & Sons, Inc., 1962.

Smith, W. G., Hansell, N., and English, J. T., "Psychiatric Disorder in a College Population," *Archives of General Psychiatry,* **9** (October 1963), pp. 351–361.

Teacher Health, Los Angeles, Calif.: Health Education and Service Branch of the Los Angeles, Calif., City School Districts.

Whyte, William H., Jr., *The Organization Man,* New York: Doubleday & Company, Inc. (Anchor Books), 1962.

Wright, John J., Ph.D., "Environmental Stress Evaluation in a Student Community," *The Journal of the American College Health Association,* **12:** 3 (February 1964), pp. 325–336.

Chapter 2. Mental Health: Mind and Body

Adler, Alfred, *Understanding Human Nature,* New York: Fawcett Publications (Premier Books Series), 1957.

Becker, E., *The Revolution in Psychiatry: The New Understanding of Man,* New York: Free Press of Glencoe, 1964.

Brown, James A. C., *Freud and the Post-Freudians,* Baltimore, Md.: Penguin Books, 1961.

Candland, Douglas K., *Emotion: Bodily Changes,* Princeton, N.J.: Van Nostrand, 1962.

Cannon, Walter B., *Bodily Changes in Pain, Hunger, Fear, and Rage,* New York: Appleton-Century, 1929.

Cannon, Walter B., *The Wisdom of the Body,* rev. ed., New York: Norton, 1939.

Clouzet, M. C., *Sigmund Freud: A New Appraisal,* New York: Philosophical Library, 1963.

Committee on Adolescence of the Group for the Advancement of Psychiatry, *Normal Adolescence,* New York: Charles Scribners and Sons, 1968.

Fitzgerald, Alice and Schifferes, Justus J., ed., *Ten Million and One: Neurological Disability as a National Problem,* New York: Hoeber-Harper, 1957.

Hall, Calvin S., ed., *A Primer of Freudian Psychology,* New York: New American Library (Mentor Books Series), 1955.

James, William, *Psychology: The Briefer Course,* Gordon Allport, ed., New York: Collier Books, 1962.

James, William, "What Is an Emotion?" *Mind,* 9 (1884), p. 188.

Joint Commission on Mental Illness and Health, *Action for Mental Health: Final Report,* 1961, New York: Basic Books, 1961.

Jung, C. G., *The Undiscovered Self,* New York: New American Library (Mentor Books Series), 1959.

Kleitman, Nathaniel, *Sleep and Wakefulness—As Alternating Phases in the Cycle of Existence,* rev. ed., Chicago: University of Chicago Press, 1963.

Koupernik, C., "Problems of Mental Hygiene," presented at International Conference on Health and Health Education, Philadelphia, June 30 to July 7, 1962.

Kraines, S. H. and Thetford, E. S., *Managing Your Mind,* New York: Macmillan, 1943.

Laird, Donald A. and Laird, Eleanor C., *Sound Ways to Sound Sleep,* New York: McGraw-Hill, 1959.

Luce, Gay Gaer, and Segal, Julius, *Sleep,* New York: Coward-McCann, Inc., 1966.

Menninger, Karl, M.D., *The Human Mind,* 2nd ed., New York: Knopf, 1942.

Merritt, Houston, M.D., *Textbook of Neurology,* 3rd ed., Philadelphia: Lea and Febiger, 1963.

Mooseheart Symposium, Martin L. Reymert, ed., *Feelings and Emotions,* New York: McGraw-Hill, 1950.

The Nervous System, illustrated by Frank Netter, M.D., Summit, N.J.: Ciba Company, 1 (1957).

Pavlov, Ivan, *Conditioned Reflexes* (unabridged trans.), New York: Dover Publications, 1960.

Ridenour, Nina, *Mental Health in the United States: A Fifty Year History,* Cambridge, Mass.: Harvard University Press, 1961.

Saul, Leon J., *Emotional Maturity: The Development and Dynamics of Personality,* 2nd ed., Philadelphia: Lippincott, 1960.

Sherrington, Charles, *The Integrative Action of the Nervous System,* New Haven: Yale University Press, 1961.

Strole, Leo, Langner, Thomas S., Michael, Stanley T., Opler, Marvin K., and Rennie, Thomas A. C., *Mental Health in the Metropolis: the Midtown Manhattan Study,* New York: McGraw-Hill, 1962.

A Student Committee on Mental Health, *Psychedelics and the College Student,* Princeton, N.J.: Princeton University Press, 1967.

Truex, R. C. and Carpenter, M. B., eds., *Strong and Elwyn's Human Neuroanatomy,* 5th ed., Baltimore, Md.: Williams and Wilkins, 1964.

Weiss and English, *Psychosomatic Medicine: A Clinical Study of Psychophysiological Reactions,* 3rd ed., Philadelphia: W. B. Saunders Company, 1957.

Whittington, H. G., *Psychiatry on the College Campus,* New York: International Universities Press, 1968.

Wyburn, *The Nervous System: An Outline of the Structure and Function of the Human Nervous System and Sense Organs,* New York: Academic Press, 1960.

Chapter 3. The Unconscious Mind—Anxiety

Alexander, *The Scope of Psychoanalysis,* New York: Basic Books, 1962.

The Basic Writings of Sigmund Freud (translated by A. A. Brill), New York: Modern Library, 1938.

Berne, Eric, *A Layman's Guide to Psychiatry and Psychoanalysis,* New York: Simon and Schuster, 1968.

Blanton, Smiley, M.D., *Love or Perish,* New York: Simon and Schuster, 1956.

Freud, Sigmund, *A General Introduction to Psychoanalysis,* Garden City, N.Y.: Doubleday, 1943.

Freud, Sigmund, *The Problem of Anxiety,* New York: Norton, 1936.

Freud, Sigmund, *The Psychopathology of Everyday Life* (translated by A. A. Brill), New York: New American Library (Mentor Book Series), 1951.

Galdston, Iago, ed., *Freud and Contemporary Culture,* New York: International Universities Press, 1957.

Galdston, Iago, ed., *Historic Derivations of Modern Psychiatry,* New York: McGraw-Hill, Blakiston Division, 1967.

Goldstein and Palmer, *The Experience of Anxiety: A Casebook,* New York: Oxford University Press, 1963.

Grinker, Roy R., Sr., M.D., Grinker, Roy R., Jr., M.D., and Timberlake, John, "Mentally Healthy Young Male College Students," *AMA Archives of General Psychiatry,* June 1962.

Guthrie, Edwin R., *The Psychology of Human Conflict: The Clash of Motives Within the Individual,* Boston: Beacon Press, 1962.

Hall, Bernard H., ed., *A Psychiatrist's World: The Selected Papers of Karl Menninger,* New York: Viking Press, 1959.

Herma, Hans, Ph.D. and Kurth, Gertrud M., Ph.D., eds., *Elements of Psychoanalysis,* Cleveland: World Publishing, 1952.

Horney, Karen, *New Ways in Psychoanalysis,* New York: Norton, 1939.

Horney, Karen, *Our Inner Conflicts,* rev. ed., New York: Norton, 1956.

Jung, C. G., *The Undiscovered Self,* New York: New American Library (Mentor Books Series), 1959.

Reusch, Jurgen, M.D. and Bateson, Gregory, *Communication: The Social Motive of Society,* New York: Norton, 1951.

Rickman, John, ed., *A General Selection from the Works of Sigmund Freud,* New York: Doubleday (Anchor Books Series), 1957.

Robinson, James Harvey, *The Mind in the Making,* New York: Harper, 1921.

Silverman, S. L. and M. G., *Theory of Relationships,* New York: Philosophical Library, 1963.

Steiner, Heiri and Gebser, Jean, *Anxiety: A Condition of Modern Man,* New York: Dell Publishing, 1962.

Strachey, James, ed., *Standard Edition of the Complete Psychological Works of Sigmund Freud,* New York: Macmillan.

Strecker, Edward A., M.D. and Appel, Kenneth, M.D. (in collaboration with John W. Appel), *Discovering Ourselves,* 3rd ed., New York: Macmillan, 1957.

Sullivan, Harry Stack, *The Interpersonal Theory of Psychiatry,* New York: Norton, 1953.

Thigpen, Corbett H. and Cleckley, Hervey M., *Three Faces of Eve,* New York: McGraw-Hill, 1957.

Thompson, Clara, *Psychoanalysis: Evolution and Development,* New York: Grove Press (Evergreen Books), 1950.

Waelder, Robert, *Basic Theory of Psychoanalysis,* New York: Schocken Books, 1964.

Chapter 4. Mental Illness

Battista, O. A., *Mental Drugs: Chemistry's Challenge to Psychiatry,* Philadelphia: Chilton, 1960.

Brussel, James A., *The Layman's Guide to Psychiatry,* New York: Barnes and Noble, 1961.

Center for Studies of Suicide Prevention, and National Clearing House for Mental Health Information, *Bulletin of Suicidology,* Washington, D.C.: U.S. Government Printing Office, 1968.

"Conditioning Therapies vs. Psychoanalysis" (highlights from Meeting at the University of Virginia School of Medicine, Charlottesville, Va., April 13–14, 1962), *Medical Science,* **11:** 10 (May 25, 1962).

Dublin, Louis I., Ph.D., *Suicide: a Sociological and Statistical Study,* New York: Ronald Press, 1963.

Felix, Robert H., *Mental Illness—Progress and Prospects,* New York: Columbia University Press, 1967.

"Fifteen Indices," Joint Information Service, American Psychiatric Association, Washington, D. C., 1963.

Fish, *Schizophrenia,* Baltimore: Williams and Wilkins, 1962.

Freeman, Lucy, *The Cry for Love: Understanding and Overcoming Human Depression,* New York: Macmillan, 1969.

Glasser, William, *Mental Health or Mental Illness?* Psychiatry for Practical Action, New York: Harper, 1960.

Gorman, Mike, *Every Other Bed,* Cleveland: World, 1956.

Lemkau, Paul, M.D., *Mental Hygiene in Public Health,* rev. ed., New York: McGraw-Hill, 1955.

Locke, Norman, *Group Psychoanalysis: Theory and Technique,* New York: New York University Press, 1961.

Masserman, Jules H., ed., *Current Psychiatric Therapies,* Vol. VII, New York: Grune and Stratton, 1967.

Masserman, Jules, M.D., *Principles of Dynamic Psychiatry,* 2nd ed., Philadelphia: Saunders, 1961.

Menninger, Karl, M.D., *Man Against Himself,* New York: Harcourt, Brace, 1938.

Noyes, Arthur P., M.D., and Kolb, Lawrence C., M.D., *Modern Clinical Psychiatry,* 6th ed., Philadelphia: Saunders, 1963.

Pearson, ed., *Strecker's Fundamentals of Psychiatry,* 6th ed., Philadelphia: Lippincott, 1963.

Rosen, George, *Madness in Society,* Chicago, Ill.: University of Chicago Press, 1968.

Solomon, Philip, *Psychiatric Drugs,* New York: Grune and Stratton, 1966.

Ubell, Earl, "Has Psycho-Probing Helped Anyone?" *The New York Herald Tribune,* June 3, 1962.

Uhr, Leonard and Miller, James G., *Drugs and Behavior,* New York: John Wiley & Sons, Inc., 1960.

Wolberg, Lewis R., *Psychotherapy and the Behavioral Sciences,* New York: Grune and Stratton, 1966.

Mental Retardation

Committee on Mental Retardation, *Mental Retardation: A Family Crisis,* New York: Group for the Advancement of Psychiatry, 1963.

Farber, Bernard, *Mental Retardation: Its Social Context and Social Consequences,* Boston: Houghton Mifflin, 1968.

Information Office, National Institute of Neurological Diseases and Blindness, National Institutes of Health, *Research Profile #5: Summary of Progress in Mental Retardation,* Washington, D.C.: U.S. Government Printing Office, 1963.

Mayo, Leonard W. (Chairman), "Report of the President's Panel on Mental Retardation," *New Directions in Health, Education and Welfare* (Office of Program Analysis of the U.S. Department of Health, Education and Welfare), Washington, D.C.: U.S. Government Printing Office, 1963.

A Modern Plan for Modern Services to the Mentally Retarded, Washington, D.C.: U.S. Government Printing Office, 1967.

Penrose, *Biology of Mental Defect,* 2nd ed., New York: Grune and Stratton, 1963.

Reed and Reed, *A Genetic Study of Mental Retardation,* Philadelphia: Saunders, 1964.

Stringman, Luther W., "Mental Retardation," *New Directions in Health, Education and Welfare* (Office of Program Analysis of the U.S. Department of Health, Education and Welfare), Washington D.C.: U.S. Government Printing Office, 1963.

Tredgold and Soddy, *A Textbook of Mental Deficiency,* 9th ed., Baltimore: Williams and Wilkins, 1956.

Chapter 5. Alcohol and Alcoholism

Alcoholic Foundation, *Alcoholics Anonymous* (P.O. Box 459, Grand Central Annex, New York, N.Y.).

Atkins, A. J. and Gwynn, J. Minor, *Teaching Alcohol Education in the Schools,* Philadelphia: Saunders, 1959.

Bacon, Margaret and Jones, Mary Brush, *Teen-Age Drinking,* New York: Crowell-Collier, 1968.

Boyington, Gregory ("Pappy"), *Baa Baa Black Sheep,* New York: Putnam, 1958.

Chafetz, Morris E. and Demone, Harold W., *Alcoholism and Society,* New York: Oxford University Press, 1962.

Cooperative Commission on the Study of Alcoholism, *Alcohol Problems. A Report to the Nation,* prepared by Thomas F. A. Plaut, New York: Oxford University Press, 1967.

"Epidemiologic Studies and Control Programs in Alcoholism" (symposium), *American Journal of Public Health,* **57:** 6 (June 1967).

Jackson, Charles, *The Lost Weekend,* New York: Pocket Books.

Joint Information Services of the American Psychiatric Association and the National Association for Mental Health, *Treatment of Alcoholism: A Study of Programs and Progress,* Washington, D.C.: American Psychiatric Association, 1967.

Lolli, Giorgio, *Social Drinking: How to Enjoy Drinking Without Being Hurt by It,* Cleveland: World Publishing, 1960.

Mann, Marty, *Marty Mann's New Primer on Alcoholism,* New York: Rinehart, 1958.

Menninger, Karl, *Man Against Himself,* New York: Harcourt-Brace, 1938.

National Center for Prevention and Control of Alcoholism, National Institute of Mental Health, *Alcohol and Alcoholism,* Washington, D.C.: U.S. Government Printing Office, 1967.

Pittman, David J. and Snyder, Charles R., *Society, Culture and Drinking Patterns,* New York: John Wiley and Sons, Inc., 1962.

Pfeffer, Arnold Z., M.D., *Alcoholism,* New York: Grune and Stratton, 1958.

Roth, Lillian, *I'll Cry Tomorrow,* New York: Frederick Fell, 1954.

Roueché, Berton, *The Neutral Spirit: A Portrait of Alcohol,* Boston: Little, Brown, 1960.

Strachan, J. George, *Alcoholism: Treatable Illness,* Vancouver, Canada: Mitchell Press, 1968.

Todd, Frances, *Teaching About Alcoholism,* New York: McGraw-Hill, 1964.

Chapter 6. Drug Use and Abuse

AMA Council on Mental Health, "Marijuana and Society," *Journal of the American Medical Association,* **204** (June 24, 1968), pp. 1181–1182.

Ausubel, David P., M.D., *Drug Addiction: Physiological, Psychological and Sociological Aspects,* New York: Random House, 1958.

Black, Perry, ed., *Drugs and the Brain: Papers on the Action, Use and Abuse of Psychotropic Drugs,* Baltimore, Md.: Johns Hopkins Press, 1968.

Bloomquist, E. R., *Marijuana,* New York: Collier Books, 1968.

Blum, Richard H. and Associates, *Society and Drugs* (Vol. 1), and *Students and Drugs* (Vol. 2), San Francisco: Jossy-Bass, Inc., 1969.

Brown, Wenzell, *Monkey on My Back,* New York: Greenberg, Publishers, 1953.

Carey, James J., *The College Drug Scene,* Englewood Cliffs, N.J.: Prentice Hall (Spectrum Books), 1968.

Chein, Isidor, Gerard, Donald L., Lee, Robert S., and Rosenfeld, Eva, *The Road to H: Narcotics, Delinquency and Social Policy,* New York: Basic Books, 1964.

DeQuincey, Thomas, *Confessions of an English Opium Eater,* originally published in *London Magazine,* 1821.

Epstein, Stanley, ed., *The International Journal of Addictions* (Vol. 4), New York: Marcel Dekker, Inc., 1969.

Fort, Joel, M.D., *The Pleasure Seekers: The Drug Crisis, Youth and Society,* Indianapolis: Bobbs-Merrill Co., 1969.

Hoffer, A. and Osmond, H., *The Hallucinogens,* New York: Academic Press, 1967.

A Joint Committee on Narcotic Drugs of the American Bar Association and the American Medical Association, *Drug Addiction: Crime or Disease?,* Bloomington, Ind.: University of Indiana Press, 1961.

Keniston, Kenneth, "Heads and Seekers: Drugs on Campus, Counter-Cultures, and American Society," *The American Scholar* (Winter 1968–69), pp. 97–122.

Kitzinger, Angela and Hill, Patricia J., *Drug Abuse: A Source Book and Guide for Teachers,* Sacramento, Calif.: California State Department of Health, 1967.

Kleber, Herbert D., "Student Use of Hallucinogens," *Journal of the American College Health Association* **14:** 2 (1965), pp. 109–117.

Kolb, Lawrence, M.D., *Drug Addiction: A Medical Problem,* Springfield, Ill.: Chas. C. Thomas, 1962.

Laurie, Peter, *Drugs,* Baltimore, Md.: Penguin Books, 1967.

Louria, Donald B., *Cool Talk About Hot Drugs,* Albany, N.Y.: New York State Narcotic Addiction Control Commission (reprinted from *The New York Times*), 1967.

Louria, Donald B., *The Drug Scene,* New York: McGraw-Hill, 1968.

Murphy, B. W., Leventhal, Allan M., and Balter, Mitchel B., "Drug Use on Campus: A Survey of University Health Services and Counseling Centers, *"The Journal of the American College Health Association,* **17:** 3 (June 1969).

"Napan Newsletter," New York: National Association for the Prevention of Addiction to Narcotics.

Nowlis, Helen H., *Drugs on the College Campus: a Guide for College Administrators,* Detroit: National Association of Student Personnel Administrators, 1967.

Oursler, Will, *Marijuana: The Facts—The Truth,* New York: Eriksson, 1968.

Pollock, Marion B., "The Drug Abuse Problem, Some Implications for Health Education," *The Journal of the American College Health Association,* **17:** 3 (June 1969).

Proceedings of the Institute on New Developments in the Rehabiliatation of the Narcotic Addict (Fort Worth, Texas, February 1966), *Rehabilitating the Narcotic Addict,* Washington, D.C.: U.S. Government Printing Office, 1967.

Public Information Branch, National Institute of Mental Health, *Narcotics, Some Questions and Answers* (Public Health Service Publication No. 1827); *LSD, Some Questions and Answers* (No. 1828); *Marijuana, Some Questions and Answers* (No. 1829); *The Up and Down Drugs* (No. 1830), Washington, D.C.: U.S. Government Printing Office, 1968.

"A Remarkable New Drug Suddenly Spells Danger—LSD," *Life* (March 25, 1966), pp. 28–33.

Smith, Kline, and French, in cooperation with American Association for Health, Physical Education and Recreation (National Education Association), *Drug Abuse: Escape to Nowhere, A Guide for Educators,* Philadelphia: Smith, Kline, and French, 1968.

Strack, Alvin E., "Drug Use and Abuse," *Journal of Health, Physical Education and Recreation,* **39:** 1 (January 1968).

Vermes, Jean C., *Pot is Rot,* New York: Association Press, 1969.

Chapter 7. Physical Fitness—Personal Fitness

American Association for Health, Physical Education and Recreation, *Contributions of Physical Activity to Human Well-Being:* a supplement to the May 1960 *Research Quarterly,* Washington, D.C.: National Education Association.

Berger, Andrew J., *Elementary Human Anatomy,* New York: John Wiley, 1964.

Bowerman, William J. and Harris, W. E., *Jogging, a Physical Fitness Program for All Ages,* New York: Grosset & Dunlap, 1967.

Brownell, Clifford L. and Hagman, Patricia, *Physical Education: Foundations and Principles,* New York: McGraw-Hill, 1951.

Committee of the American Association for Health, Physical Education and Recreation report, "The Role of Exercise in Physical Fitness," Washington, D. C., 1943. (Reaffirmed in "Exercise and Fitness" statement, 1964.)

Cooper, Kenneth H., *Aerobics,* New York: Bantam Books, 1968.

Exercise and Health, Chicago: American Medical Association, 1958.

Focus on Dance I: articles of interest in all fields of dance, 1960; *Focus on DanceII:* an interdisciplinary search for meaning in movement, 1962, Washington, D.C.: American Association for Health, Physical Education and Recreation.

Harris, W. E., with Shea, James M., *Jogging,* New York: Grosset and Dunlap, 1967.

Johnson, P. B., Updike, W. F., Stolberg, D. C., and Schaefer, M., *Physical Education: A Problem-Solving Approach to Health and Fitness,* New York: Holt, Rinehart and Winston, 1966.

Joint Committee of the American Medical Association and the American Association for Health, Physical Education and Recreation, "Exercise and Fitness," *Journal of Health, Physical Education and Recreation* (May 1964).

Kiphuth, Robert, *How To Be Fit* (with exercises for men and women), rev. ed., New Haven: Yale University Press, 1956.

Krusen, Frank, M.D. and others, *Concepts in Rehabilitation,* Philadelphia: Saunders, 1964.

Matthews, Donald K., Stacy, Ralph W., and Hoover, George N., *Physiology of Muscular Activity and Exercise,* New York: Ronald Press, 1964.

Osler, Sir William, *The Alabama Student,* Oxford, England: Clarendon Press, 1908.

Pendman, Kenneth A., *Physical Education for College Students: Programmed Instruction,* St. Louis: C. V. Mosby, 1964.

President's Council on Youth Fitness, *Policy Statement on School Health and Physical Fitness,* May 31, 1962.

President's Council on Youth Fitness. *Youth Physical Fitness: Suggested Elements of a School-Centered Program* (Parts 1, 2), Washington, D.C.: U.S. Government Printing Office, July 1961.

Rasch, Philip J. and Burke, Roger K., *Kinesiology and Applied Anatomy,* 2nd ed., Philadelphia,: Lea and Febiger, 1963.

Rathbone, Josephine L., *Corrective Physical Education,* 6th ed., Philadelphia: W. B. Saunders, 1959.

Royal Canadian Air Force, *Five Basic Exercises (BX),* Ottawa, Canada: The Queen's Printer, 1962.

Royal Canadian Air Force, *XBX Plan for Physical Fitness* (for women), Pamphlet 30/2, Ottawa, Canada: The Queen's Printer, 1962.

Rusk, Howard, M.D., *Rehabilitation Medicine,* St. Louis: C. V. Mosby, 1958.

Schifferes, Justus J., *Guide to Physical Fitness,* New York: Collier Books, 1962.

Slusher, Howard S., *Man, Sport and Existence, a Critical Analysis,* Philadelphia: Lea & Febiger, 1967.

Souder, Marjorie A. and Hill, Phyllis, J., *Basic Movement: Foundations of Physical Education,* New York: Ronald Press, 1963.

Wallis, Earl and Logan, Gene A., *Figure Improvement and Body Conditioning Through Exercise,* Englewood Cliffs, N. J.: Prentice-Hall, 1964.

Weston, Arthur, *The Making of American Physical Education,* New York: Appleton-Century, 1962.

Wilbur, E. A., "A Comparative Study of Physical Fitness Indices as Measured by Two Programs of Physical Education, The Sports Method and The Apparatus Method," *Research Quarterly* (October 1943).

Your Guide to Physical Fitness: Agility, Strength, Endurance, New York: American Football Coaches Association and the Tea Council of the U.S.A. (distributors), 1963.

Isometrics

Adamson, G. T., "Effects of Isometric and Isotonic Exercise on Elbow Flexor and Spine Extensor Muscle Groups," *Health and Fitness in the Modern World.*

Berger, Richard A., "Effects of Dynamic and Static Training on Vertical Jumping Ability," *Research Quarterly,* **34:** 4 (December 1963), pp. 419–424.

Clarke, W. Harrison, ed., Development of Volitional Muscle Strength as Related to Fitness," *Exercise and Fitness,* Chicago: The Athletic Institute, 1960.

Flint, M. Marilyn, "Selecting Exercises," *JOHPER,* **35:** 2 (February 1964), pp. 19–23.

Hettinger, Th. and Mueller, E. A., "Muscle-Testing and Muscle Training" (*Muskelleisting und Muskeltraining*), *Arbeitsphysiologie,* **15:** 2 (October 1953), p. 111.

"Isometric Exercises To Build Your Strength," *Your Guide to Physical Fitness,* New York: American Football Coaches Association and the Tea Council of the U.S.A. (distributors), 1963.

Lindeburg, F. A., Edwards, D. K., and Heath, W. D., "Effect

of Isometric Exercise on Standing Broad Jump Ability," *Research Quarterly,* **34:** 4 (December 1963), pp. 478–483.

Morehouse, Lawrence E., "Physiological Basis of Strength Development," *Exercise and Fitness,* W. Harrison Clarke, ed., Chicago: The Athletic Institute, 1960.

Pierson, W. R. and Rasch, P. J., "The Injurious Consequences of Maximal Isometric Arm Exercises," *Journal of the American Physical Therapy Association,* **45** (1963), pp. 582–583.

Spackman, Robert R., *Isometric Exercise for the Whole Body,* Dubuque, Iowa: Wm. C. Brown, 1963.

Chapter 8. The Human Body in Health and Disease

Asimov, Isaac, *The Bloodstream: River of Life,* New York: Collier Books, 1961.

Asimov, Isaac, *The Genetic Code,* New York: New American Library (Signet Books Series), 1963.

Basmajian, J. V., M.D., ed., *Primary Anatomy,* 5th ed., Baltimore: Williams and Wilkins, 1964.

Berger, Andrew J., *Elementary Human Anatomy,* New York: John Wiley & Sons, 1964.

Best, C. H. and Taylor, N. B., *The Human Body: Its Anatomy and Physiology,* 3rd ed., New York: Henry Holt (Holt, Rinehart and Winston), 1956.

Brock, Thomas, ed., *Milestones in Microbiology,* Englewood Cliffs, N.J.: Prentice-Hall, 1961.

Caplin, Irving, *The Allergic Asthmatic,* Springfield, Ill.: Chas. C. Thomas, 1968.

Clendenning, Logan, M.D., *The Human Body,* rev. ed., New York: Knopf, 1937.

Copenhaver, W. M., ed., *Bailey's Textbook of Histology,* 15th ed., Baltimore: William and Wilkins, 1964.

Editors of *Scientific American, The Physics and Chemistry of Life,* New York: Simon and Schuster, 1956.

Frohse, Franz, Brodel, Max, and Schlossberg, Leon, *Atlas of Human Anatomy,* 6th ed., New York: Barnes & Noble, 1961.

Gerard, R. W., *Unresting Cells,* New York: Harper and Row (Torchbook Series), 1961.

Goss, ed., *Gray's Anatomy,* 27th ed., Philadelphia: Lea and Febiger, 1959.

Lockhart, R. D. and others, *Anatomy of the Human Body,* Philadelphia: J. B. Lippincott, 1959.

McElroy, William D., *Cellular Physiology and Biochemistry,* Englewood Cliffs, N.J.: Prentice-Hall, 1961.

Mercer, E. H., *Cells: Their Structure and Function,* New York: Doubleday (Anchor Books Series), 1962.

Ross and Wilson, *Foundations of Anatomy and Physiology,* Baltimore: Williams and Wilkins, 1963.

Shure, Norman and Harris, M. Coleman, *All About Allergy,* Englewood Cliffs, N.J.: Prentice-Hall, 1969.

Sproul, Edith E., *The Science Book of the Human Body,* New York: Pocket Books (Cardinal Edition), 1955.

Stanley, Wendell M. and others, *Viruses and the Nature of Life,* New York: E. P. Dutton, 1961.

Tokay, Elbert, *Fundamentals of Physiology: The Human Body and How It Works,* rev. ed., New York: Barnes & Noble, 1967.

Vesalius, Andreas, *Anatomy of the Human Body.*

Endocrinology

Brown and Barker, *Basic Endocrinology for Students of Biology and Medicine,* Philadelphia: F. A. Davis, 1962.

Hoskins, R. G., *The Tides of Life—The Endocrine Glands in Bodily Adjustment,* New York: W. W. Norton, 1933.

Mason, A. Stuart, *Health and Hormones,* New York: Penguin Books, 1960.

Riedman, Sarah R., *Our Hormones and How They Work,* New York: Collier Books, 1962.

Stress, Stressors, and Disease

Bernard, Claude, *An Introduction to the Study of Experimental Medicine,* New York: Collier Books, 1961 (originally published 1865).

Cannon, Walter B., "Organization for Physiological Homeostasis," *Physiological Review,* **9:** 399 (July 1929).

Cannon, Walter B., "Stresses and Strains of Homeostasis," *Physiological Review,* **189:** 1 (January 1935).

Cannon, Walter B., *The Wisdom of the Body,* New York: W. W. Norton, 1932.

Galdston, Iago, M.D., ed., *Beyond The Germ Theory: The Roles of Deprivation and Stress in Health and Disease,* New York: Health Education Council, 1954.

Galdston, Iago, M.D., ed., *The Epidemiology of Health,* New York: Health Education Council, 1953.

Selye, Hans and others, "Adaptation Reaction to Stress," *Psychosomatic Medicine,* **12:** 3 (1950), 155.

Selye, Hans, "General Adaptation Syndrome and Diseases of Adaptation," *Journal of Clinical Endocrinology,* **6:** 117–230 (February 1946).

Selye, Hans, *The Physiology and Pathology of Exposure to Stress,* Montreal: Acta, Inc., 1950.

Selye, Hans, *The Stress of Life,* New York: McGraw-Hill, 1956.

Chapter 9. Sense Organs:
Eyes, Ears, Nose, Mouth, Skin

Adler, ed., *Gifford's Textbook of Ophthalmology,* 7th ed., Philadelphia: W. B. Saunders, 1962.

Boies, *Fundamentals of Otolaryngology,* 4th ed., Philadelphia: W. B. Saunders, 1964.

Brauer, Earle W., *Your Skin and Your Hair,* New York: Macmillan, 1969.

Goldsmith, Norman, M.D., *You and Your Skin,* Springfield, Ill.: Charles C. Thomas, 1953.

Lubowe, Irwin I., M.D., *New Hope for Your Hair: A Scientific Guide to Healthy Hair for Men, Women, and Children,* New York: Collier Book, 1961.

Mann, Ida and Pirie, Antoinette, *The Science of Seeing,* New York: Penguin Books, 1950.

Middleton, A. W., ed., *Cosmetic Science,* 1962 (proceedings of the Second Congress of the International Federation of Societies of Cosmetic Chemists, London, 1962), New York: Macmillan, 1963.

Raiford, *Contact Lens Management*, Boston: Little, Brown, 1962.

Rothman, *The Human Integument*, Washington, D.C.: American Association for the Advancement of Science, 1959.

Seeman, Bernard, *Your Sight: Folklore, Fact and Common Sense*, Boston: Little, Brown, 1968.

Sloane, *Manual of Refraction*, Boston: Little, Brown, 1961.

Southall, James, P. C., *Introduction to Physiological Optics*, New York: Dover Publications, 1961.

Stewart, ed., *Turner's Diseases of the Nose, Throat and Ear*, 6th ed., Baltimore: Williams and Wilkins, 1961.

Sulzberger, Wolf, and Witten, *Dermatology: Essentials of Diagnosis and Treatment*, 2nd ed., Chicago: Year Book Publishers, 1961.

Vail, Derrick, M.D., *The Truth about Your Eyes*, New York: Farrar, Straus and Cudahy, 1959.

Von Buddenbrook, Wolfgang, *The Senses*, Ann Arbor, Mich.: University of Michigan Press, 1958.

Chapter 10. Nutrition, Diet, and Weight Control

Beaumont, William, M.D., *Experiments and Observations on the Gastric Juice and the Physiology of Digestion*, New York: Dover Publications, 1959 (originally published 1833).

Bogert, L. Jean, *Nutrition and Physical Fitness*, 7th ed., Philadelphia: W. B. Saunders, 1960.

Brock, *Recent Advances in Human Nutrition*, Boston: Little, Brown, 1961.

Burton, Bejamin T., *The Heinz Handbook of Nutrition*, New York: McGraw-Hill, 1959.

Food and Nutrition Board of the National Academy of Science, National Research Council, *The Role of Dietary Fat in Human Health*, Washington, D.C.: National Research Council, 1958.

Jolliffe, Norman, M. C., ed., *Clinical Nutrition*, 2nd ed., New York: Harper and Row, 1962.

Krehl, W. A., M.D., Ph.D. and Hodges, Robert E., M.D., "Sixth International Congress of Nutrition in Retrospect (report)," *Borden's Review of Nutrition Research*, **24:** 4 (October–December 1963).

Lind, James, *Treatise on Scurvy*, London, 1753.

McHenry, E. W., *Basic Nutrition*, rev. ed., Philadelphia: J. B. Lippincott, 1963.

Meyer, Lillian Hoagland, *Food Chemistry*, New York: Reinhold Publishing, 1960.

Mitchell, Helen S., and others, *Nutrition in Health and Disease*, 15th ed., Philadelphia: J. B. Lippincott & Co., 1968.

Tatkon, M. Daniel, *The Great Vitamin Hoax*, New York: Macmillan, 1968.

von Haller, Albert, *The Vitamin Hunters* (trans. from German by Hella Freud Bernays), Philadelphia: Chilton, 1962.

Wilson, Eva D., and others, *Principles of Nutrition*, New York: John Wiley & Sons, 1959.

Wohl, Michael G., and Goodheart, Robert S., *Modern Nutrition in Health and Disease*, 4th ed., Philadelphia: 1968.

Teeth

American Dental Association, *Teeth, Health and Appearance*, 4th ed., Chicago: American Dental Association, 1957.

Haines, Helen S. and Thoburn, Robert, *75 Years of Dentistry*, Gainesville, Fla.: University of Florida Press, 1960.

McClure, Dr. F. J., ed., for U.S. Public Health Service's National Institute of Dental Research, *Fluoride Drinking Waters*, Washington, D.C.: U.S. Government Printing Office, 1962.

Schloat, G. Warren, *Your Wonderful Teeth*, New York: Scribners, 1954.

Scott, James H. and Symons, Norman B. B., *Introduction to Dental Anatomy*, 4th ed., Baltimore: Williams and Wilkins, 1964.

Staple, Peter B., ed., *Advances in Oral Biology*, Vol. 1, New York: Academic Press, 1964.

World Health Organization, *Periodontal Disease*, New York: Columbia University Press, 1961.

Diet and Weight Control

Agricultural Research Service, U.S. Department of Agriculture, *Essentials of an Adequate Diet: Facts for Nutrition Programs* (Home Economics Research Report No. 3), Washington, D.C.: U.S. Government Printing Office, 1957.

Antar, Mohamed A., "Changes in the Retail Market Food Supplies in the United States in the Last Seventy Years in Relation to the Incidence of Coronary Heart Disease, with Special Reference to Dietary Carbohydrates and Essential Fatty Acids," *American Journal of Clinical Nutrition*, **14:** 169 (March 1964).

Bruch, Hilde, *The Importance of Overweight*, New York: W. W. Norton, 1957.

Committee on Dietetics of the Mayo Clinic, *Mayo Clinic Diet Manual*, 3rd ed., Philadelphia: W. B. Saunders, 1961.

Council on Foods and Nutrition of the American Medical Association, "Formula Diets and Weight Control," *Journal of the American Medical Association*, **176:** 439 (May 6, 1961).

Dach, Elizabeth M., *Your Emotions and Overweight*, New York: Mental Health Materials Center, 1957.

Dietary Fat and Its Relation to Heart Attacks and Strokes, New York: American Heart Association, 1961.

Fleck, Henrietta, Ph.D. and Munves, Elizabeth, Ph.D., *Everybody's Book of Modern Diet and Nutrition*, New York: Dell Publishing, 1955.

Food and Your Weight, Washington, D.C.: U.S. Government Printing Office, 1967.

Iowa State Department of Health and Iowa Dietetic Association, *Simplified Diet Manual*, 2nd ed., Ames, Iowa: Iowa State University Press, 1961.

Jolliffe, Norman, M.D., *Reduce and Stay Reduced*, rev. ed., New York: Simon and Schuster, 1957.

Leverton, Ruth M., *Food Becomes You*, Ames, Iowa: Iowa State University Press, 1960.

Lowenberg, Miriam E., *Food and Man*, New York: John Wiley & Sons, Inc., 1968.

Mayer, Jean, *Overweight: Causes, Cost and Control,* Englewood Cliffs, N.J.: Prentice Hall (Spectrum Books), 1968.

McHenry, E. W., *Foods without Fads,* Philadelphia: J. B. Lippincott, 1960.

Planning Fat Controlled Meals for 1200 and 1800 Calories, New York: American Heart Association, 1962.

Recommended Dietary Allowances, 6th rev. ed., A Report of the Food and Nutrition Board of the National Academy of Sciences, National Research Council, Washington, D.C.: National Research Council, 1968.

Rose, W. C., "A Half Century of Amino Acid Investigations," *Chemical and Engineering News,* **30:** 23 (June 9, 1952), pp. 2385–2388.

Schacter, Stanley, "Obesity and Eating," *Science,* **161:** 3843 (August 23, 1968), p. 751.

Schifferes, Justus J., Ph.D., *What's Your Caloric Number?,* New York: Macmillan, 1966.

Shearman, *Diets Are For People,* New York: Appleton-Century, 1963.

Stillman, Irwin Maxwell and Baker, Samm Sinclair, *The Doctor's Quick Weight Loss Diet,* New York: Dell Books, 1968.

U.S. Department of Agriculture, *Food: The Yearbook of Agriculture, 1959,* Washington, D.C.: U.S. Government Printing Office, 1959.

White, Philip L., ed., *Let's Talk About Food: Answers to Your Questions About Foods and Nutrition,* Chicago: American Medical Association, 1967.

Chapter 11. Education for Family Living

Baruch, Dorothy W. and Miller, H., *Sex in Marriage: New Understandings,* New York: Harpers, 1962.

Blanding, Sarah Gibson, "Educators Educated," *Saturday Review,* May 31, 1958, p. 12.

Butterfield, Oliver M., *Sex Life in Marriage,* rev. ed., New York: Emerson Books, 1963.

Calderone, Mary S., and Goodman, Phyllis and Robert P., *Release from Sexual Tensions: Toward an Understanding of Their Causes and Effects in Marriage,* New York: Random House, 1960.

Cavan, Ruth Shonle, *American Marriage: A Way of Life,* New York: T. Y. Crowell, 1958.

Clendenning, Logan, M.D., *The Human Body,* New York: Knopf, 1943.

Commission on Education for Family Life, *Education for Family Life:* The 19th Yearbook of the American Association for School Administrators, Washington D.C.: National Education Association, 1941.

Davis, Maxine, *Sex and The Adolescent,* New York: Affiliated Publishers, 1960.

Duvall, Evelyn Millis, *Love and the Facts of Life,* New York: Association Press, 1963.

Duvall, Evelyn Millis and Duvall, Sylvanus Milne, *Sense and Nonsense About Sex,* New York: Association Press, 1962.

Ellis, Havelock, *The Psychology of Sex.*

Franzblau, Abraham, *The Road to Sexual Maturity,* New York: Simon and Schuster, 1954.

Hoeflin, Ruth M., *Essentials of Family Living,* New York: John Wiley, 1960.

Gravatt, Arthur E., "Proceedings of a Symposium on Sex Education of the College Student," *The Journal of the American College Health Association* (May 1967).

Hofman, Hans, *Sex Incorporated—A Positive View of the Sexual Revolution,* Boston: Beacon Press, 1967.

Hollingshead, A. B., *Elmtown's Youth: The Impact of Social Classes on Adolescents,* New York: John Wiley, 1949.

Johnson, W. R., *Human Sex and Education; Perspectives and Problems,* Philadelphia: Lea and Febiger, 1963.

LeMasters, E. E., *Modern Marriage and Courtship,* New York: Macmillan, 1957.

Kinsey, Alfred C., Pomeroy, Wardell B., and Martin, Clyde E., *Sexual Behavior in the Human Male,* Philadelphia: W. B. Saunders, 1948.

Kirkendall, Lester, *Premarital Intercourse and Interpersonal Relations,* New York: Julian Press, 1961.

Kirkendall, Lester, *Sex Adjustments of Young Men,* New York: Garden City, 1949.

Liebman, Samuel, M.D., ed., *Emotional Forces in the Family,* Philadelphia: Lippincott, 1959.

Mead, Margaret, *Male and Female,* New York: Morrow, 1949.

Menninger, Karl, M.D., *Love against Hate,* New York: Harcourt, Brace, 1942.

Rice, Thurman, M.D., *Sex, Marriage and Family,* Philadelphia: Lippincott, 1946.

Richardson, Henry B., M.D., *Patients Have Families,* New York: Commonwealth Fund, 1945.

Staff of the Institute for Sex Research: Alfred C. Kinsey, Wardell B. Pomeroy, Clyde E. Martin, Paul H. Gebhard et al., *Sexual Behavior in the Human Female,* Philadelphia: W. B. Saunders, 1953.

Taylor, Gordon Rattray, *Sex in History,* New York: Vanguard Press, 1969.

Chapter 12. Preparing for Marriage

Bauer, W. W. and Bauer, Florence M., *To Enjoy Marriage,* New York: Doubleday, 1967.

Blanck, Rubin and Blanck, Gertrude, *Marriage and Personal Development,* New York: Columbia University Press, 1968.

Bowman, Henry A., *Marriage for Moderns,* 5th ed., New York: McGraw-Hill, 1965.

Crawley, Lawrence, Q. Malfetti, James L., Stuart, Ernest I., and Vas Dias, Nini, *Reproduction, Sex, and Preparation for Marriage,* Englewood Cliffs, N.J.: Prentice-Hall, 1964.

de la Mare, Walter, *Love: A Garland of Prose and Poetry Woven Together,* New York: Morrow, 1946.

Despert, J. Louise, M.D., *Children of Divorce,* New York: Doubleday, 1953.

Duval, Evelyn Mills, *Why Wait Till Marriage?,* New York: Association Press, 1968.

Farber, Seymour M. and Wilson, Roger H. L., eds., *Sex Education and the Teenager,* Berkeley, Calif.: Diabolo Press, 1967.

Farber, Seymour M. and Wilson, Roger H. L., eds., *Teenage Marriage and Divorce,* Berkeley, Calif.: Diabolo Press, 1967.

Fishbein, Morris, M.D. and Burgess, Ernest W., Ph.D., eds., *Successful Marriage,* Garden City, N.Y.: Doubleday, 1948.

Frazer, Sir James George, *The Golden Bough* (originally published 1890).

Jacobson, Paul H., *American Marriage and Divorce,* New York: Rhinehart, 1959.

Kinsey, Alfred C. and others, *Sexual Behavior in the Human Male,* Philadelphia: Saunders, 1948.

Krich, A. M., ed., *The Anatomy of Love,* New York: Dell Publishing, 1960.

Krich, Aron, ed., *Facts of Love and Marriage for Young People,* New York: Dell Publishing, 1962.

Krich, Aron, ed., *Men: The Variety and Meaning of Their Sexual Experience,* New York: Dell Publishing, 1960.

Krich, Aron, ed., *Women: The Variety and Meaning of Their Sexual Experience,* New York: Dell Publishing, 1960.

Lantz, Herman R., Ph.D. and Snyder, Eloise C., Ph.D., *Marriage: An Examination of the Man-Woman Relationship,* New York: John Wiley, 1962.

Lee, Alfred M. and Lee, Elizabeth B., *Marriage and the Family,* New York: Barnes and Noble, 1961.

Malinowski, Bronislaw, *Sex and Repression in Savage Society,* Paterson, N.J.: Littlefield Adams, 1962.

Menninger, William C. and others, *How To Understand the Opposite Sex,* New York: Cornerstone Library, 1964.

Merrill, Francis E., Ph.D., *Courtship and Marriage,* New York: Henry Holt, 1959.

Moore, Marcene and Wyatt, Trevor, *Sex, Sex, Sex,* Philadelphia: Pilgrim Press, 1969.

Murdock, George, *Our Primitive Contemporaries,* New York: Macmillan, 1934.

National Center for Health Statistics and the U.S. Public Health Service, *Marriage Statistics Analysis, United States, 1963,* Washington, D.C.: U.S. Government Printing Office, 1968.

Rubin, Isadore and Kirkendall, Lester A., *Sex in Adolescent Years—New Directions in Guiding and Teaching Youth,* New York: Association Press, 1968.

Saul, Leon J., *Fidelity and Infidelity and What Makes or Breaks a Marriage,* Philadelphia: Lippincott, 1967.

Southard, Helen F., *Sex Before Twenty: New Answers for Youth,* New York: E. P. Dutton, 1967.

Stone, Hannah M. and Abraham, *Marriage Manual,* rev. ed., New York: Simon and Schuster, 1952.

Westermarck, Edward, *The History of Human Marriage,* New York: Allerton House, 1922.

Winch, Robert F., *Mate Selection,* New York: Harpers, 1959.

Wylie, Burdett, ed., *Sex and Marriage: A Guide To Marital Relations,* Cleveland: World Publishing, 1949.

Religious Sources

Gordon, Rabbi Albert I., *Bride and Groom, A Manual for Marriage,* New York: The United Synagogue of America (Conservative), 1947.

Hoenig, Rabbi Sidney E., *Jewish Family Life,* New York: Young Israel Organization.

Jewish Program for National Family Week, 1944–1951, New York: Synagogue Council of America.

Lambeth Conference, 1948, *Encyclical Letter on the Church's Discipline in Marriage,* London: Hazell, Watson, and Viney, 1948.

Levy, Felix A., Ph.D., *Judaism and Marriage,* New York: Commission on Information about Judaism, Union of American Hebrew Congregations (Liberal, Reform).

National Council of Churches of Christ, *Christian Marriage,* New York: National Council of Churches of Christ, 1952.

Piper, Otto A., *The Christian Interpretation of Sex,* New York: Scribner, 1949.

Pope Paul VI, *A Statement on Birth Control* (part of an address to Cardinals of the Roman Catholic Church, Rome, July 23, 1964), reported in full in American newspapers.

Pope Pius XI, *Casti Connubii: Encyclical Letter on Christian Marriage* (St. Peter's, Rome, December 31, 1930), New York: The Missionary Society of St. Paul the Apostle, 1941.

Pope Pius XII, *The Apostolate of the Midwife – Moral Questions Affecting Married Life* (address to delegates attending the Congress of the Italian Catholic Union of Midwives, Rome, October 29, 1951), reported in full in American newspapers.

Schmiedler, Edgar, O.S.B., Ph.D., *Marriage and the Family,* New York: McGraw-Hill, 1946.

Chapter 13. Heredity and the New Genetics

Asimov, Isaac, *The Genetic Code,* New York: New American Library (Signet Science Series), 1963.

Beadle, George, "Molecules, Viruses and Heredity," *Science and Resources,* Henry W. Jarrett, ed., Baltimore: Johns Hopkins Press, 1959.

"The Chromosomes of Man," *Lancet* (London), No. 7075 (April 4, 1959).

Dunn, L. C. and Dobzhansky, Theodore, *Heredity, Race and Society,* New York: New American Library (Mentor Books Series), 1952.

Fast, Julius, *Blueprint for Life: The Story of Modern Genetics,* New York: St. Martin's Press, 1964.

Galton, Francis, *Memories of My Life,* New York: Dutton, 1909.

Goldschmidt, Richard B., *Understanding Heredity: An Introduction to Genetics,* New York: John Wiley, 1952.

Goldstein, Philip, *Genetics is Easy,* New York: Viking Press (Explorer Books Series), 1961.

Hereditary Basis of Disease (a review of research grants supported by the National Heart Institute, 1949-1967), Washington, D.C.: U.S. Government Printing Office, 1968.

Lenz, *Medical Genetics,* Chicago: University of Chicago Press, 1963.

Mendel, Gregor, "Experiments in Plant Hybridization" (trans. by the Royal Horticultural Society of London), originally published in *Proceedings of the Natural History Society of Brunn,* Vol. 4, 1865.

Morgan, Thomas Hunt, *A Critique of the Theory of Education,* Princeton, N.J.: Princeton University Press, 1916.

Muller, Herman, *Studies in Genetics,* Bloomington, Ind.: University of Indiana Press, 1962.

Peters, James A., ed., *Classic Papers in Genetics,* Englewood Cliffs, N.J.: Prentice-Hall, 1959.

Scheinfeld, Amram, *The Basic Facts of Human Heredity,* New York: Washington Square Press, 1961.

Stevenson, A. C., ed., *Human Genetics,* London: British Council Medical Department, 1961.

Watson, James, *The Double Helix,* New York: Atheneum, 1968.

Winchester, A. M., *Heredity: An Introduction to Genetics,* New York: Barnes and Noble, 1961.

Chapter 14. Human Reproduction

Baruch, Dorothy and Miller, H., *Sex in Marriage,* New York: Hoeber-Harpers, 1962.

Davis, Maxine, *Facts About the Menopause,* New York: McGraw-Hill, 1951.

Dickinson, Robert Latou, *Atlas of Human Sex Anatomy,* 2nd ed., Baltimore: Williams and Wilkins, 1949.

Edsall, Florence S., *Change of Life,* New York: Woman's Press, 1949.

Fluhman, *The Managements of Menstrual Disorders,* Philadelphia: Saunders, 1956.

Greenhill, J. P., *Office Gynecology,* 7th ed., Chicago: Year Book Publishers, 1959.

Guttmacher, Alan F., M.D., *Birth Control and Love,* New York: Macmillan, 1969.

Guttmacher, Alan F., *Planning Your Family,* New York: Macmillan, 1969.

Knepp, Thomas H., *Human Reproduction:* Health and Hygiene, Carbondale, Ill.: Southern Illinois University Press, 1967.

Lincoln, Miriam, *You'll Live Through It,* New York: Hoeber-Harper, 1950.

Masters, William H., M.D. and Johnson, Virginia (Reproductive Biology Research Center, St. Louis, Mo.), *Human Sexual Response,* Boston: Little, Brown, 1966.

Portnoy, Louis, M.D. and Saltman, Jules, *Fertility in Marriage,* New York: Collier Books, 1962.

Scheinfeld, Amram, *Twins and Supertwins,* Philadelphia: J. B. Lippincott Co., 1967.

Velardo, *Essentials of Human Reproduction,* New York: Oxford University Press, 1958.

Chapter 15. Birth of a Baby

Allan, *Essentials of Human Embryology,* New York: Oxford University Press, 1960.

Calderone, Mary Steichen, ed., *Abortion in the United States,* New York: Hoeber-Harper, 1958.

DeLee, Sol T., *Safeguarding Motherhood,* 4th ed., Philadelphia: Lippincott, 1958.

Dr. X (as told to Lucy Freeman), *The Abortionist,* New York: Doubleday, 1962.

Eastman, Nicholas, *Expectant Motherhood,* rev. ed., Boston: Little, Brown, 1963.

Featheringill, Eve Stanton, *Primer for Pregnancy,* New York: Collier Books, 1962.

Fielding, Waldo L. and Benjamin, Lois, *The Childbirth Challenge,* New York: Viking Press, 1962.

Gebhard, Paul H., Pomeroy, Wardell B., Martin, Clyde E., and Christenson, Cornelia V., *Pregnancy, Birth and Abortion,* Philadelphia: W. B. Saunders, 1958.

Gilbert, Margaret Shea, *Biography of the Unborn,* Baltimore: Williams and Wilkins, 1963.

Greenhill, J. P., *Obstetrics,* 12th ed., Philadelphia: W. B. Saunders, 1960.

Guttmacher, Alan F., M.D., *Having A Baby,* New York: Signet Books, 1950.

Guttmacher, Alan F., M.D., *The Story of Human Birth,* New York: Penguin, 1948.

Hamilton, Boyd, and Mossman, *Human Embryology,* 3rd ed., Baltimore: Williams and Wilkins, 1962.

Levine, Milton I. and Seligman, Jean H., *A Baby Is Born,* New York: Simon and Schuster, 1949.

Mitchell, Robert M. and Klein, Ted, *Nine Months to Go,* Philadelphia: Lippincott, 1960.

Our Obstetric Heritage: The Story of Safe Childbirth, Hamden, Conn.: Shoe String Press, 1962.

Read, Grantly Dick, *Childbirth without Fear,* 2nd ed., New York: Harper, 1953.

Wilson, *Atlas of Obstetric Technic,* St. Louis: Mosby, 1961.

Chapter 16. The Big Killers:
Heart Disease and Cancer

Cardiovascular (Heart Disease)

Allen, E. V. and others, *Peripheral Vascular Disease,* 3rd ed., Philadelphia: W. B. Saunders, 1962.

Blakeslee, Alton and Stamler, Jeremiah, *Your Heart Has Nine Lives: Nine Steps to Heart Health,* Englewood Cliffs, N.J.: Prentice-Hall, 1963.

Burch, *A Primer of Cardiology,* Philadelphia: Lea and Febiger, 1963.

Giusti, George and Hoffman, Rudolf, *Heart: Anatomy, Function and Diseases,* New York: Dell Publishing, 1962.

A Handbook of Heart Terms, Washington, D.C.: U.S. Government Printing Office, 1964.

Marvin, H. M. and others, *You and Your Heart,* New York: New American Library, 1957.

Moses, *Atherosclerosis,* Philadelphia: Lea and Febiger, 1963.

Page, Irvine H. and others, *Strokes: How They Occur and What Can Be Done About Them,* New York: Dutton, 1961.

Paul, John R. and others, *The Epidemiology of Rheumatic Fever,* 3rd ed., New York: The American Heart Association, 1957.

Report of the Ad Hoc. Committee . . . of the American Heart Association, "Dietary Fat and Its Relation to Heart Attacks and Strokes," *Circulation,* **23** (January 1961).

Southwood, A. R., *Heart Disease: Some Ways to Prevent It,* Springfield, Ill.: Chas. C. Thomas, 1962.

Steincrohn, Peter B., *Common Sense Coronary Care and Prevention*, New York: Holt, Rinehart and Winston, 1963.

U.S. Public Health Service, *Strike Back at Stroke*, Washington, D.C.: U.S. Government Printing Office, 1958.

Cancer

American Cancer Society, "The Hopeful Side of Cancer" (pamphlet), 1960.

Cameron, Charles S., *The Truth About Cancer*, New York: Collier Books, 1967.

Chaklin, A. V., "Geographical Differences in the Distribution of Malignant Tumors," *Bulletin of the World Health Organization*, **27**: 337–358 (1962).

Field, *Cancer: Diagnosis and Treatment*, Boston: Little, Brown, 1959.

Glemser, Bernard, *Man Against Cancer*, New York: Funk & Wagnalls, 1969.

Harris, R. J. C., *Cancer*, Baltimore: Penguin Books, 1962.

National Cancer Institute, *Progress Against Cancer*, 1961, Washington, D. C.: U.S. Government Printing Office, 1962.

On Cancer and Hormones: Essays in Experimental Biology, Chicago: University of Chicago Press, 1963.

Viruses and Cancer: Progress Report XV, New York: Sloan-Kettering Institute for Cancer Research, 1963.

Tobacco

Berkson, J., "Smoking and Lung Cancer: Some Observations on Two Recent Reports," *Journal of the American Statistical Association*, **53**: 28 (1958).

Chester, Eustace, *When and How to Quit Smoking*, New York: Emerson Books, 1964.

Cohen, Jacob and Heimann, R. K., "Heavy Smokers with Low Mortality," *Industrial Medicine and Surgery*, **31**: 3 (March 1962).

McFarland, J. W. and Folkenberg, E. J., *How To Stop Smoking in Five Days*, Englewood Cliffs, N.J.: Prentice-Hall, 1964.

National Clearing House for Smoking and Health, *Bibliography on Smoking and Health*, 1967 Cumulation, Washington, D.C.: U.S. Government Printing Office, 1967.

Peters, J. M. and Ferris, B. G., Jr., "Smoking and Morbidity in a College Age Group, *American Review of Respiratory Diseases*, **95**: 783–789 (May 1967).

Rosenthal, G. and James T., eds., *Tobacco and Health*, Springfield, Ill.: Chas. C. Thomas, 1962.

Smoking and Health: Report of the Advisory Committee to the Surgeon General of the U.S. Public Health Service, Washington, D.C.: U.S. Government Printing Office, 1964.

Smoking and Health: A Report of the Royal College of Physicians (London), New York: Pitman Publishing, 1962.

U.S. Public Health Services, *The Health Consequences of Smoking*, Washington D.C.: U.S. Government Printing Office, 1967.

World Conference on Smoking & Health, September 11, 12, 13, 1967; Summary of the Proceedings, New York: American Cancer Society, 1969.

Chapter 17. Protecting Against Communicable Disease and other Health Hazards

"Acute Respiratory Diseases of Viral Etiology" (symposium), *American Journal of Public Health,* **52:** 6 (June 1962).

Adams, John M., *Viruses and Colds, The Modern Plague,* New York: American Elsevier Publishing Co., 1967.

Anderson, Gaylord W., M.D., Arnstein, Margaret G., R.N., M.P.H., and Lester, Mary R., R.N., M.P.H., *Communicable Disease Control,* 4th ed., New York: Macmillan, 1962.

"Bookshelf on Virology," *American Journal of Public Health* (April 1961).

Brock, Thomas, ed., *Milestones in Microbiology,* Englewood Cliffs, N.J.: Prentice-Hall, 1961.

Bryan, Arthus H. and Bryan, Charles G., *Bacteriology,* New York: Barnes and Noble (College Outline Series), 1962.

Burnet, *The Integrity of the Body: A Discussion of Modern Immunological Ideas,* Cambridge, Mass.: Harvard University Press, 1962.

Clark, Duncan and MacMahon, Brian, eds., *Preventive Medicine,* Boston: Little, Brown, 1967.

Clendenning, Logan, ed., *Source Book of Medical History,* New York: Dover, 1960.

The Control of Communicable Disease in Man: An Official Report, 9th ed., New York: The American Public Health Association, 1965.

de Kruif, Paul, *Microbe Hunters,* New York: Pocket Books, 1959.

Directory of Medical Specialists, Vol. 11, Chicago: A. N. Marquis Co., 1963.

Directory of Physicians, Chicago, Ill.: American Medical Association, published periodically.

Dobell, Clifford, ed., *Antony Van Leeuwenhoek and his "Little Animals,"* New York: Dover, 1960.

Doetsch, *Microbiology: Historical Contributions from 1776–1908,* New Brunswick, N.J.: Rutgers University Press, 1960.

Ehlers, Victor H. and Steel, Ernest W., *Municipal and Rural Sanitation,* 4th ed., New York: McGraw-Hill, 1951.

Fabricant, Noah D., M.D., *The Common Cold and How To Fight It,* New York: Ziff-Davis, 1945.

Gale, A. H., *Epidemic Diseases,* Baltimore: Penguin Books, 1959.

Garrison, Fielding H., *An Introduction to the History of Medicine,* 4th ed., Philadelphia: W. B. Saunders, 1960.

Hare, *An Outline of Bacteriology and Immunity,* 2nd ed., Boston: Little, Brown, 1963.

Hawker, Lilian E. and others, *An Introduction to the Biology of Micro-organisms,* New York: St. Martin's Press, 1960.

Hopkins and Schulze, *Practice of Sanitation,* 3rd ed., Baltimore: Williams and Wilkins, 1958.

Morton, R. S., *Venereal Disease,* Baltimore: Penguin Books, 1966.

Phelps, Earle B. and others, *Public Health Engineering, Vol. 1, A Textbook of the Principles of Environmental Sanitation,* New York: John Wiley, 1948.

Potter, William H., M.D., *You and Your Doctor,* New York: Bantam Books, 1962.

Proceedings of the International Infectious Mononucleosis Symposium, Evanston, Ill.: American College Health Association, 1967.

Public Health Service, *Health Statistics from the U.S. National Health Survey: Acute Conditions, seasonal variations, United States, July 1957–June 1961,* Washington, D.C.: U.S. Government Printing Office, June 1962.

Raffel, Sidney, *Immunity,* 2nd ed., New York: Appleton-Century-Crofts, 1961.

Rivers, Thomas M. and Horsfall, Frank Jr., eds., *Viral and Rickettsial Infections of Man,* 3rd ed., Philadelphia: Lippincott, 1959.

Roueché, Berton, *Annals of Epidemiology,* Boston: Little, Brown, 1967.

Saltman, Jules, *Immunization for All,* New York: Public Affairs Pamphlet No. 408, 1967.

Schifferes, Justus J., ed., *The Family Medical Encyclopedia,* Boston: Little, Brown, 1959.

Snow, John, M.D., *Snow on Cholera,* New York: The Commonwealth Fund, 1936.

Stamm, Donald, *Birds as Reservoirs of Virus Disease,* Ithaca, N.Y.: Report from 13th International Ornithological Congress at Cornell University, June 21, 1962.

Stanley, Wendell M. and Valens, Evans G., *Viruses and the Nature of Life,* New York: Dutton, 1961.

Stubbs, S. G. and Bligh, B. E. W., *Sixty Centuries of Health and Physic,* London: Sampson Low, Marston, 1932.

Syphilis, A Synopsis, Washington, D.C.: U.S. Government Printing Office, 1967.

Top, Franklin H., M.D., *Communicable and Infectious Diseases,* 5th ed., St. Louis: C. V. Mosby, 1964.

Vallery-Radot, René, *The Life of Pasteur,* New York: Dover, 1960.

Walker, Kenneth, *Patients and Doctors,* Baltimore: Penguin Books, 1957.

Winslow, C. E. A., M.D., *The Conquest of Epidemic Disease,* Princeton, N.J.: Princeton University Press, 1943.

Zinsser, Hans, *Rats, Lice and History,* New York: Bantam Books, 1960.

Chapter 18. Accident Prevention—Safety

Accident Facts, Chicago, Ill.: National Safety Council, published annually.

Accident Prevention Manual for Industrial Operations, 4th ed., Chicago, Ill.: National Safety Council, 1963.

Annual Safety Education Review—1968, Washington, D.C.: American Association for Health, Physical Education and Recreation, 1968.

Bacon, Selden D., ed., "Studies of Driving and Drinking," *Quarterly Journal of Studies on Alcohol,* No. 4, New Brunswick, N.J.: Center for Alcohol Studies, Rutgers University, 1968.

Editors of *Sports Illustrated, Sports Illustrated Book of Safe Driving,* Philadelphia: Lippincott, 1962.

First Aid Textbook; Life-Saving and Water Safety Manual; Accident Prevention, Washington, D.C.: The American National Red Cross.

Goldberg, Lawrence and Harvard, John D. J., *Road Safety Research: Alcohol and Drugs, A Report of the OECD Research Group,* Washington, D.C.: Office for Economic Cooperation and Development, 1968.

"Leading Causes of Fatal Accidents," *Statistical Bulletin* (Metropolitan Life Insurance Co.) (June 1964).

McInroy, Edward A., M.A., *The Collier Quick and Easy Guide to Driving.* New York: Collier Books, 1963.

"Motorcycle Accident Deaths Rising Rapidly," *Statistical Bulletin* (Metropolitan Life Insurance Co.), 48 (April 1967), pp. 2–4.

Nader, Ralph, *Unsafe at Any Speed,* New York: Grossman, 1965.

Schulzinger, Morris, M.D., *The Accident Syndrome,* Springfield, Ill.: Chas. C. Thomas, 1956.

Selzer, Marvin L., Gikas, Paul W., and Huelke, Donald F., *The Prevention of Highway Injury,* Ann Arbor, Mich.: Publications Division, The University of Michigan, 1968.

Strasser, M. K., Aron, J. E., Bohn, R. C., and Eales, J. R., *Fundamentals of Safety Education,* New York: Macmillan, 1964.

Suggested School Safety Policies, Washington, D.C.: American Association for Health, Physical Education and Recreation, 1964.

U.S. Public Health Service, *Types of Injuries: Incidence and Associated Disability, United States, July 1957–June 1961,* Washington, D.C.: U.S. Government Printing Office, 1964.

Chapter 19. Health Frauds

Cooley, Donald G., *The Science Book of Modern Medicines,* New York: Pocket Books, 1964.

Deutsch, Ronald M., *The Nuts Among the Berries,* New York: Ballantine Books, 1961.

Editors of Consumer Reports (A Consumer Union Publication), *The Medicine Show,* New York: Simon and Schuster, 1961.

Haggard, Howard W., M.D., *Devils, Drugs and Doctors,* New York: Harper, 1929.

Holbrook, Stewart H., *The Golden Age of Quackery,* New York: Macmillian, 1959.

Huff, Darrell, *How to Live with Statistics,* New York: Norton, 1954.

James, Don, *Folk and Modern Medicine,* Derby, Conn.: Monarch Books, 1961.

Krieg, Margaret, *Black Market Medicine,* Englewood Cliffs, N.J.: Prentice-Hall, 1967.

Krieg, Margaret B., *Green Medicine: The Search for Plants that Heal,* Chicago: Rand McNally, 1964.

Liston, Robert A., *What You Should Know About Pills,* New York: Pocket Books, 1968.

Milstead, K. L., Deputy Director Bureau of Enforcement, Food and Drug Administration, *The Food and Drug Administration's Program Against Quackery,* address delivered to

Yonkers (N.Y.) Academy of Medicine, May 16, 1962.

Proger, Samuel, ed., *The Medicated Society,* New York: Macmillan, 1968.

Rouché, Berton, *Curiosities of Medicine: An Assembly of Medical Diversions, 1552–1962,* New York: Berkley Publishing, 1964.

Seaver, Jacqueline, *Fads, Myths and Quacks and Your Health,* New York: Public Affairs Committee, 1968.

Sigerist, Henry, *Civilization and Disease,* Chicago, Ill.: University of Chicago Press, 1962.

Young, James Harvey, *The Medical Messiahs: A Social History of Health Quackery,* Princeton, N.J.: Princeton University Press, 1968.

Young, James Harvey, *The Toadstool Millionaires,* Princeton, N.J.: Princeton University Press, 1961.

Chapter 20. Community Health Organization and Costs

Background Material Concerning the Mission and Organization of the Health Activities of the Department of Health, Education, and Welfare, Washington, D.C.: U.S. Government Printing Office, 1966.

Bancroft, *Introduction to Biostatistics,* New York: Hoeber-Harper, 1957.

Beers, Clifford, *A Mind That Found Itself,* originally published 1906.

Blum, Richard H., *The Common Sense Guide to Doctors, Hospitals and Medical Care,* New York: Macmillan, 1964.

Carter, Richard, *The Gentle Legions,* Garden City, N.Y.: Doubleday, 1961.

Commission on Chronic Illness, *Chronic Illness in the United States,* Cambridge, Mass.: Harvard University Press, 1957.

Garland, Joseph and Stokes, Joseph A. III, ed., *The Choice of a Medical Career,* 2nd ed., Philadelphia: Lippincott, 1962.

Graunt, Capt. John and Peatty, Sir William, *Natural and Political Observations on the Bills of Mortality,* London, 1662.

Hill, *Principles of Medical Statistics,* 7th ed., New York: Oxford University Press, 1961.

Hilleboe, Herman and Larimore, Granville, *Preventive Medicine,* Philadelphia: Saunders, 1959.

Hobson, *The Theory and Practice of Public Health,* New York: Oxford University Press, 1961.

Kessler, Henry, *Rehabilitation of the Physically Handicapped,* 2nd ed., New York: Columbia University Press, 1953.

Kilander, H. Frederick, *School Health Education,* New York: Macmillan, 1962.

Krusen, Frank and others, *Concepts in Rehabilitation,* Philadelphia: Saunders, 1964.

Mustard, Harry and Stebbins, Ernest, *An Introduction to Public Health,* 4th ed., New York: Macmillan, 1959.

Office of Program Planning of the National Institutes of Health, *The Advancement of Knowledge for the Nation's Health* (report to the President on the Research Program of the National Institutes of Health), Washington, D.C.: Public Health Service, 1967.

Osborn, Barbara M., *Introduction to Community Health,* Boston: Allyn and Bacon, 1964.

Pearl, Raymond, *Introduction to Medical Biometry and Statistics,* 3rd ed., Philadelphia: Saunders, 1940.

Philadelphia (Pa.) Department of Public Health, *Annual Report 1961.*

Porterfield, J. D., ed., *Community Health: Its Needs and Resources,* New York: Basic Books, 1966.

Rosen, George, M.D., *A History of Public Health,* New York: MD Publications, 1958.

Rusk, Howard and Taylor, Eugene, *New Hope for the Handicapped,* New York: Hoeber-Harper, 1949.

Sills, David, *The Volunteers: Means and Ends in a National Organization,* Glencoe, Ill.: Free Press, 1958.

Vital Statistics of the United States, 1962, Washington, D.C.: U.S. Government Printing Office, 1964.

What Thirteen Local Health Departments Are Doing in Medical Care, Studies in Medical Care Administration, Washington, D.C.: U.S. Government Printing Office, 1967.

Wohl, *Long Term Illness: Management of the Chronically Ill Patient,* Philadelphia: Saunders, 1959.

Health Costs

Angell, *Health Insurance,* New York: Ronald Press, 1963.

Burrow, *AMA: Voice of American Medicine,* Baltimore: Johns Hopkins University Press, 1963.

Galdston, Iago, ed., *Voluntary Action and the State,* New York: International Universities Press, 1961.

Health Information Foundation, *An Inventory of Social and Economic Research in Health: 12th Edition,* Chicago: University of Chicago Press, 1963.

Lindsey, Almont, *Socialized Medicine in England and Wales: the National Health Service, 1948–1961,* Chapel Hill, N.C.: University of North Carolina Press, 1962.

A List of Current Health Insurance Books, 1968 Edition, New York: Health Insurance Institute.

Macleod, Kenneth I. E., M.D., M.P.H., "The British National Health Service and Its Meaning for Us," *Cincinnati Journal of Medicine,* **43:** 5 (May 1962).

Page, Sir Earle, *What Price Medical Cost?* Philadelphia: Lippincott, 1960.

Somers, Herman N. and Anne R., *Doctors, Patients and Health Insurance: The Organization and Financing of Medical Care in the United States,* Washington, D.C.: The Brookings Institution, 1961.

Source Book of Health Insurance Data, New York: Health Insurance Institute, available annually.

Weeks, Ashley, *Family Spending Patterns and Health Care,* Cambridge, Mass.: Harvard University Press, 1961.

Chapter 21. Environmental Health and Medicine

"Century of Progress Through Sanitation," Part II, *American Journal of Public Health,* **43:** 6 (June 1953).

Cohen, Jesse M., *Effects of Synthetic Detergents on Water Treatment and Quality on Water,* Cincinnati: Sanitary Engineering Center, 1959.

Congress on Environmental Health Problems, Sponsored by American Medical Association, Chicago, May 1–2, 1964.

The Control of Communicable Disease in Man: An Official Report of the American Public Health Association, 9th ed., 1965.

Environmental Engineering for the School, Washington, D.C.: U.S. Government Printing Office, 1961.

Environmental Health Planning Guide, Washington, D.C.: U.S. Government Printing Office, 1967.

Environmental Health Problems, Washington, D.C.: U.S. Government Printing Office, 1962.

Galdston, Iago, ed., The Epidemiology of Health, New York: Health Education Council, 1953.

"Man—His Environment and Health," American Journal of Public Health, Part II (January 1964).

Man in His Environment (proceedings of Fifth International Conference on Health and Health Education, Philadelphia, June 30–July 7, 1962, International Union for Health Education), International Journal of Health Education, 1963.

Middleton, F. M., Newer Chemical Contaminants Affecting Water Quality, Cincinnati: Sanitary Engineering Center, 1961.

Morris, Robert, "The City of the Future and Planning for Health," The American Journal of Public Health, 68, 1 (January 1968).

Odishaw, Hugh, ed., The Challenge of Space, Chicago: University of Chicago Press, 1962.

Phelps, Earl B. and others, Public Health Engineering: A Textbook of the Principles of Environmental Sanitation, Vol. 1, New York: John Wiley, 1948.

Rosen, George, M.D., A History of Public Health, New York: MD Publications, 1958.

The "Shattuck Report" — Report of the Sanitary Commission of Massachusetts: 1850, reprinted by American Public Health Association, 1950.

Spain, D. M., The Complications of Modern Medical Practice: A Treatise on Iatrogenic Diseases, New York: Grune and Stratton, 1963.

Chapter 22. Impact of the New Pollutions

Environmental Health Problems (report of a committee to the Surgeon General), Washington, D.C.: U.S. Government Printing Office, 1962.

Handbook on Programs of the U.S. Department of Health, Education and Welfare (10th Anniversary Edition), Washington, D.C.: U.S. Government Printing Office, 1963.

"Man — His Environment and Health," Part II, American Journal of Public Health (January 1964).

New Directions in Health, Education and Welfare (10th Anniversary Edition), Washington, D.C.: U.S. Government Printing Office, 1963.

Wilson, Billy Ray, ed., Environmental Problems: Pesticides, Thermal Pollution and Environmental Synergisms, Philadelphia: Lippincott, 1968.

Air Pollution

Air Pollution: Hearings Before a Subcommittee of the Committee on Interstate and Foreign Commerce (House of Representatives, 88th Congress, 1st Session), Washington, D.C.: U.S. Government Printing Office, 1963.

Environmental Health Problems (report of a committee to Surgeon General, pp. 65–96), Washington, D.C.: U.S. Government Printing Office, 1962.

Jaffe, Louis E., "The Biological Effects of Photochemical Air Pollutants (Smog) on Man and Animals," The American Journal of Public Health, 57: 8 (August 1967).

Mills, This Air We Breathe, New York: Christopher, 1962.

Stern, Arthur, ed., Air Pollution, Vols, 1 and 11, New York: Academic Press, 1962.

A Study of Pollution—Air, Washington, D.C.: U.S. Government Printing Office, September 1963.

U.S. Department of Health, Education and Welfare, National Conference on Air Pollution Proceedings, Washington, D.C.: U.S. Government Printing Office, 1963.

Water Pollution

Environmental Health Problems (report of Committee to Surgeon General, pp. 215–262), Washington, D.C.: U.S. Government Printing Office, 1962.

Harris, Robert R., "Dirty Water: A Problem in Economics, Conservation and Health," Journal of Health, Physical Education and Recreation (May–June 1962).

Milne, Lotus and Margery, Water and Life, New York: Atheneum, 1964.

A Study of Pollution—Water (staff report to Committee of Public Works, U.S. Senate), Washington, D.C.: U.S. Government Printing Office, June 1963.

Thorne, W., ed., Land and Water Use (symposium), Washington, D.C.: American Association for the Advancement of Science, 1963.

"Water and Environmental Sanitation" (including Bosch, Herbert M., "Adapting The Environment to Man," and Espinosa, Nilo, "Water—A Gift of God"), Man in His Physical Environment, Vol. 3, International Conference of Health and Health Education, published by International Journal of Health Education, 1963.

Food Contamination

Bicknell, Chemicals in Your Food and in Farm Products: Their Harmful Effects, New York: Emerson Books, 1961.

Environmental Health Problems (report to the Surgeon General, pp. 133–164), Washington, D.C.: U.S. Government Printing Office, 1962.

Food and Civilization, symposium at University of California, San Francisco Medical Center, May 15–17, 1964.

"Food Processing Methods May Be Cause of Food Poisoning," Health Bulletin (June 6, 1964).

Gunther, Residues of Pesticides and Other Foreign Chemicals in Foods and Feeds, Vol. 2, New York: Academic Press, 1963.

Maxcy, Kenneth, Preventive Medicine and Public Health, 8th ed., New York: Appleton-Century-Crofts, 1956.

Pesticides and Public Health (part of pesticide program of U.S. Public Health Service), Washington, D.C.: U.S. Government Printing Office, 1966.

Subcommittee on Pesticides of the Program Area Committee on Environmental Health, APHA, *Safe Use of Pesticides,* New York: American Public Health Association, 1967.

What Consumers Should Know About Food Additives; What Consumers Should Know About Food Standards: FDA: What It Is and Does (three pamphlets), Washington, D.C.: Federal Food and Drug Administration, 1963.

Chapter 23. Environmental Health and World Health

Chisholm, Brock, "Man in His Social Environment," *International Journal of Health Education,* **4** (1962).

Morgan, Murray, *Doctors to the World,* New York: Viking Press, 1958.

Simmons, James and others, *Global Epidemiology,* Vol. 1: India, the Far East and the Pacific Islands, 1944; Vol. 2: Africa and the Adjacent Islands, 1951; Vol. 3: The Near and Middle East, 1954. Philadelphia: Lippincott.

World Health Organization, *World Health* (magazine published 6 times a year).

Population

Brown, Harrison, S., *The Challenge of Man's Future,* New York: Viking Press, 1954.

Darwin, Sir Charles Galton, *The Next Million Years,* New York: Doubleday, 1952.

Editors of Fortune, *The Exploding Metropolis,* New York: Doubleday, 1958.

Erlich, Paul R., *The Population Bomb,* New York: Ballantine Books, 1968.

"Focus on World Population," *Intercom,* **6:** 1 (January-February 1964), published by Foreign Policy Association.

Hauser, P. M., ed., for the American Assembly, *The Population Dilemma,* Englewood Cliffs, N.J.: Prentice-Hall, 1963.

Higbee, Edward, *The Squeeze,* New York: Morrow, 1960.

Lenica, Jan and Sauvy, Alfred, *Population Explosion: Abundance or Famine?,* New York: Dell Publishing, 1962.

Malthus, Thomas, *An Essay on the Principle of Population,* London, 1798.

Osborn, Fairfield, ed., *Our Crowded Planet,* New York: Doubleday, 1962.

Petersen, William, *Population,* New York: Macmillan, 1961.

The Population Bomb, New York: Hugh Moore Fund.

U.S. Department of Commerce, *Historical Statistics of the United States, Colonial Times to 1957,* Washington, D.C.: U.S. Government Printing Office.

U.S. Department of Commerce, *Statistical Abstract of the United States 1963,* Washington, D.C.: U.S. Government Printing Office, 1963.

Vogt, William, *People! Challenge to Survival,* New York: William Sloane Associates, 1960.

Pesticides

"AMA Congress on Environmental Health (May 1964)," *AMA News* (May 11, 1964).

Carson, Rachel, *Silent Spring,* Boston: Houghton-Mifflin, 1962.

"Hazards of Pesticides," *Science,* **144** (June 12, 1964) p. 1294.

Kelly, Howard A., *Walter Reed and Yellow Fever,* Baltimore: Norman Remington, 1923.

Residue Reviews: Residues of Pesticides, and Other Foreign Chemicals in Foods and Feeds, New York: Academic Press, 1963.

Smith, Geddes, *Plague on Us,* New York: Commonwealth Fund, 1941.

Radiation Hazards

Becker, Barbara, "Radiation and Health," *The Journal of Health, Physical Education and Recreation* (February 1962).

Chadwick, Donald R., "Radiation and the Public Health," *Man—His Environment and Health,* Part II, *American Journal of Public Health* (January 1964).

Environmental Health Problems (Report of a Committee to the Surgeon General, pp. 205–215), Washington, D.C.: U.S. Government Printing Office, 1962.

Fallout Protection: What to Know and Do About Nuclear Attack. Washington, D.C.: Department of Defense, Office of Civil Defense, December 1961.

Oak Ridge Institute of Nuclear Studies, *Medical Division Research Report, 1963,* Washington, D.C.: Office of Technical Services, Department of Commerce, 1963.

Simon, Norman, "Radiation in the Diagnosis and Treatment of Disease," *Man—His Environment and Health,* Part II, *American Journal of Public Health* (January 1964).

O'Brien, R. D. and Wolfe, L. S., *Radiation, Radioactivity and Insects;* McLean, F. C. and Budy, A. M., *Radiation, Isotopes, and Bone;* Taliaferro, W. H. and L. C., and Jaraslow, B. N., *Radiation and the Immune Mechanisms,* part of a series of monographs on radiation biology, New York: Academic Press, 1964 *et seq.*

Williams, Smith, and Chalke, *Radiation and Health,* Boston: Little, Brown, 1962.

Your Radiologist, published by American College of Radiology (see especially Vol. 7, No. 2, Spring 1964 on safety factors).

APPENDIX

F

ACKNOWLEDGMENTS

Every book is the product of many minds and hands. I wish in this place to express sincerest thanks and make most grateful acknowledgment for assistance to the many individuals and organizations who have contributed in one way or another, mainly through critical reviews of material or by permission to quote them, to the completion of this book and its previous editions.

For critical reviews of material that appears in this book either in original or revised form, I want to thank:

Maurice Irvine, Ph.D., professor of English at Sarah Lawrence College, Bronxville, N. Y.*

Louis J. Peterson, Ph.D., San Jose State College, San Jose, Calif.

Ella Harris, M.D.; Sherwin Kaufman, M.D.: Rudolf Ekstein, Ph.D.; Marie Coleman; Richard G. Thurston, Ph.D.; Ralph Sikes, M.D.; Norman Goldsmith, M.D.*; David B. Kimmelman, M.D.; Ruth Frankel, Ph.D.; Clarence Frankel, D.D.S.; Perry Sandell* (American Dental Association); William J. Plunkert and Terence J. Boyle (National Council on Alcoholism); Laurence Wyatt and Henry Van Zyle Hyde, M.D. (Division of International Health, U.S. Public Health Service.

For introductions and forewords to this and previous editions:

William Hammond, M.D., Editor of the *New York State Journal of Medicine.*

John E. Sawhill, M.D., formerly University Physician, New York University.

Howard R. Craig, M.D., Director Emeritus of the New York Academy of Medicine.

For original artwork: Robert A. Jones; Louise Bush, Ph.D.

*Deceased.

For permission to use and quote specific material in the text, credit goes to the following organizations and individuals:

The American Association for Health, Physical Education and Recreation, for permission to quote from its committee report entitled "The Role of Exercise in Physical Fitness."

The American Medical Association, for permission to reprint quotations from the *Journal of the American Medical Association* and the *A.M.A. Archives of Neurology and Psychiatry;* and also the A.M.A. Communications Division, News Department, for specific information on physicians and hospitals and news releases on a variety of subjects.

The American Public Health Association for permission to reprint Tables 1 and 2 from "Acute Diseases of Viral Etiology: 1. Ecology of Respiratory Viruses—1961." (Jordan, *American Journal of Public Health,* June 1962, pages 898 and 899); copyright by the American Public Health Association, Inc., 1740 Broadway, New York 19, N.Y.

The Clarendon Press, for an extract from *The Alabama Student,* by Sir William Osler.

Harper and Brothers, for a selection from *The Mind in the Making* by James Harvey Robinson. Copyright 1921 by Harper and Brothers; copyright 1949 by Bankers Trust Company.

Houghton Mifflin Company, for permission to quote from *Silent Spring* by Rachel Carson.

Alfred A. Knopf, for extracts from *The Human Body* by Logan Clendenning.

J. P. Lippincott Company, for an extract from *Sex, Marriage and Family* by Thurman B. Rice.

Metropolitan Life Insurance Company for permission to use its height-weight tables, reprinted herein under caption "What Should You Weigh?"

Modern Medicine, for permission to adapt the chart that appeared in an article by Dr. Edward E. Gordon in the issue of December 15, 1957.

National Council of Churches of Christ in the United States of America, for extracts from *Christian Mar-*

563

riage, copyright, 1952, National Council of Churches; also from *Social Ideals of the Churches,* published by the Federal Council of Churches.

National Research Council, Food and Nutrition Board, for permission to reprint the "Table of Recommended Daily Dietary Allowances, Revised 1968.

Philadelphia Department of Public Health, for material from its Annual Report, 1961; notably illustrations of maps of the city.

Physicians News Service, Inc., for permission to reprint a news story that originally appeared in the June 18, 1958 issue of *Scope Weekly.*

The President's Council on Youth Fitness, for permission to reprint material from its publication, "Youth Physical Fitness," and particularly "A Presidential Message on the Physical Fitness of Youth" over the signature and under the presidential seal of former President John F. Kennedy.

Random House, for an extract from *Mind and Body: Psychosomatic Medicine* by H. Flanders Dunbar, copyright 1947.

Saturday Review, for permission to quote observations by Dr. Sarah Gibson Blanding from the issue of May 31, 1958. Permission also from Dr. Blanding, president of Vassar College.

W. B. Saunders Company, for extracts from *Sexual Behavior in the Human Male* by Alfred C. Kinsey, et al. (permission also from Dr. Kinsey and Dr. Paul C. Gebhard), and also from *Introduction to Medical Biometry and Statistics,* third edition, by Raymond Pearl.

The Science Press, for an extract from *The Foundations of Science,* authorized translation by George Bruce Halstead (Poincaré).

Shulton, Inc., for permission to reproduce their advertisement, "2 sunscreen preparations that may be recommended with confidence."

Union of American Hebrew Congregations, for excerpts from *Judaism and Marriage* by Rabbi Felix Levy; and from *Wife of Thy Youth,* by Rabbi Stanley R. Brav.

U.S. Department of Agriculture, Agricultural Research Service, in particular, Louise Page, Nutrition Analyst, Household Economics, for information and advice on the new "Essential 4" guide to an adequate diet. Also for the five charts on the "Essential 4" food groups, adapted from *Essentials of an Adequate Diet; Facts for Nutrition Programs,* Home Economics Research Report No. 3.

Winthrop Laboratories, for permission to reproduce their advertisement, "In Acne."

For illustrations, except original artwork, used in the text:

Wyeth Laboratories, Philadelphia, Pa., for permission to reproduce illustrations of Beaumont and St. Martin from original color painting by Dean Cornwell.

U.S. Department of Health, Education and Welfare, Public Health Service, National Institutes of Health for pictures from National Institutes: also for diagram on sewage treatment, pages 474 and 475, from "The Living Waters" (U.S. Public Health Service Publication No. 382, revised 1961); also for graph "The population of the United States," page 16.

Tea Council of the United States and the American Football Coaches Association, joint distributors of 16 page pamphlet, "Your Guide to Physical Fitness," from which the series of Isometric Exercises, appearing on pages 114 and 115, is adapted.

We wish to express our gratitude to the respondents to our surveys, whose helpful comments and suggestions have materially aided in shaping this book.

Justus J. Schifferes, PH.D.

INDEX

Abdominal pain, 12, 505

Abdominal strength and flexibility, test for, *ill*, 107

Abdominal swelling, 13

Aobrtion: definition, 319, 527; illegal, 234–235, 320; spontaneous, 320; therapeutic, 228, 320; legalization, 233; Roman Catholic viewpoint, 233

Accident proneness, 62; mental mechanisms of, 381; psychological sources, 374

Accidents: causes of, 373, 386; college, 384; factor in death, 325; home, 383–384; occupational, 384; outdoor, 384; philosophy of, 376–377: psychogenic origins, 8; rate, 441; statistics, 375–377. *See also* Automobile accidents

Acne, 169, 171, 527

Adler, Alfred, viii, 46–47, 58

Adolescents: adjustment problems, 243; causes of death, 325; dating behavior, 270; sex education, 24; sexual development, 229; sexual experience, 256

Adrenalin, 25, 148

Adrenals, 8, 146, 148–149, 527

Adrenocorticotropin (ACTH), 148, 152, 527

Adultery, 244, 257

Aerobics, viii, 111–112

Aerospace medicine, 441, 459, 497–498

Aerospace research, 459–460

Aggression, 527; eroticization of, 38

Agility, test for, *ill.* 107

Aging: exercise and, 110; fatigue and, 122; increased blood pressure, 141; loss of hearing, 165; normal physiological changes, 9–10; sperm production, 290

Air pollution, 448, 455, 457, 479; automotive causes, 466; carcinogens, 464; disasters, 461–462; geographical variations, 465–466; long-term effects, 463–465; Los Angeles, 453; Philadelphia, *ill.* 417; political aspects, 466–467; prevention, 465–467; problems of, 463–464; thermal inversion, 462. *See also* Environmental health; Environmental pollution

Alarm reaction, 8, 32, 527

Alcohol, 22; absorption into bloodstream, 179; addiction to, 62; automobile accidents, 379, 458; central nervous system effects, 81; customs surrounding, 78; complication of sleep, 34–35; depressant, 69; everyday use, 79; history, 81–82; impairment of driving ability, 68; lethal effect when combined with barbiturates, 35, 86, 93; levels of intoxication, 389–390; medicinal use, 72; physiological effects, 70–72; pre-

marital sex and, 222; prohibition laws, 75; religious attitudes, 77; similarity of effects to marihuana, 87–88; social functions of drinking, 77; student use of, 67; tolerance to, 68, 71–72. *See also* Alcoholism; Automobile accidents

Alcoholism, 22, 527; animistic explanation, 39; causes, 72–73, 77–78; central nervous system damage, 28, 54; chronic, 67, 69, 73; incidence, 69–70, 77; malnutrition, 73; prevention and control, 74–75; psychoses, 55; rationalizations, 70; risk of, 68; treatment 73, 75. *See also* Alcohol; Automobile accidents

Alibi artists, 45

Alimentary canal: embryonic development, 310; cancer, 333. *See also* Digestive system

Allergy, 505, 527; chronic alcoholism, 69; emergency medical identification, 386; food prejudices and, 177; skin manifestations, 171

Allport, Gordon, 46

Alopecia, 527

Ambition, 46

American Cancer Society, 420

American College Health Association, 4

American Diabetes Association, 420

American Heart Association, 420

American National Red Cross, 420

American Social Health Association, 420–422

Amino acids, 133, 137, 175–177, 182, 184, 528

Amnesia, 528; infantile, 41

Amniotic sac, 309, 317, 528

Amphetamines, 93, 96, 528; central nervous system effects, 86; characteristics, 84–85; complication of sleep, 34; fatigue and, 50; government regulation, 82; psychotherapeutic use, 59; psychological dependence on, 87; reasons for using, 99; signs of abuse, 90. *See also* Drugs

Anesthesia, 152, 528; in childbirth, 319

Anger, 8, 38; alcoholism, 73; displaced, 43; physiological effects, 26

Animal bites, first aid for, 515

Antabuse, 73

Anthrax, 497

Anthropology, 47

Antibiotics, 354, 441, 528

Antidepressants, 79. *See also* Drugs

Antihistamines, 35, 528

Anus, 143

Anxiety, 4, 39, 41, 47–49, 57, 152, 528; age of, 94; complication of sleep, 33; psychosomatic illness, 11, 14; relief, 51, 59; unconscious, 37, 44
Anxiety neuroses, 60
Appetite, 122
Aqueous fluid, 156
Arm and shoulder strength, test for, *ill.* 106
Arteries, 139–140, 528
Arteriosclerosis, 326–327, 341, 528
Arthritis, 120, 528
Ascorbic acid, 176–177, 185–186
Aspirin, 397–398
Asthma, 44, 506, 528
Astigmatism, 160, 528
Ataraxics, 58–59, 528
Atherosclerosis, 176, 326–329, 341, 528
Athlete's foot, 171, 528
Athletics, 128; psychotherapeutic value, 7, 117; red blood cells, 139; requirement of physical fitness, 109. *See also* Sports
Atomic energy, 499; waste disposal problems, 469, 492–493
Auditory nerve, 165
Automation, problems of, 444
Automobile accidents, 17, 386, *ill.* 378; alcohol, 74, 389–390; college dropouts, 6; cost of, 382; drugs, 86; environmental influences, 458; physical factors, 379; prevention, 377–380; psychogenic origins, 62, 380–382; rate, 73; vehicular defects, 375. *See also* Accidents
Automobiles, air pollution, 466
Automobile safety, 11
Autonomic nervous system, 26–27, 36, 132, 140, 179, 528
Axon, 29–30, 528

Bacteria, 354–355, 528; mouth, 190; resistance to, 169
Bacterial flora, colon, 182
Bacteriology, 352, 370
Bag of waters, *see* Amniotic sac
Balance, 31
Baldness, 171, 280. *See also* Alopecia
Bandages, first aid, *ill.* 515–516
Barbiturates, 86, 96, 528; addiction, 35; characteristics, 84–85; complication of sleep, 34; government regulation, 82; lethal effect when combined with alcohol, 35, 86, 93; psychotherapeutic use, 59; reasons for using, 99; signs of abuse, 90. *See also* Drugs
Bartholin's glands, 294
Basal metabolism, 127, 199, 528
Battle fatigue, 44, 57
Beaumont, William, 178, 208–210
Beer, 70
Behaviorism, 47
Benzedrine, 50, 59
Beriberi, 28, 185–186, 528
Bile, 179, 528
Biliary system, 132
"Biosocial" theory of personality development, 47
Biotin, 186
Birth control, viii, 234, 297–299; education, 304–305; problems, 301; Roman Catholic attitude, 259–260. *See also* Contraception
Birth rate, 216

Bleeding, first aid for, 516
Blindness: galactosemia, 63; iatrogenic, 441; incidence, 162; prevention, 161; trachoma, 494, 496
Blood clots, 327
Blood clotting, 151, 186–187
Blood, 139; composition, inherited, 280; iron, 188; loss, 152; Rh factor, 280
Blood-alcohol percentage, 69–70
Blood cells, 132
Blood-forming organs, 131; cancer, 333, 336
Blood pressure, 3, 139, 529; normal, 141
Bloodstream, elements of, 139
Blood types, 139
Blood vessels, 139–141, 529; surgery, 330
Blue Cross, 405, 428–430, 529
Blue Shield, 428–430, 529
Body types, 148, 197, 280
Bone marrow, 139
Bones: calcium requirement, 187; connective tissue, 132; foot, *ill.* 124; fractures, 152, first aid for, 517, knitting, 151; red blood cell manufacture, 118; vitamin D requirement, 187
Bone structure, 123
Brain, 26–28, 133; development, 310, 312; inflammation, 169; perception of reality, 155–157, 172; respiratory center, 143
Brain damage, 54–55, 63–64
Brain stem, 28, 529
Brain tumors, 28, 55. *See also* Cancer
Brain waves: abnormal, 177; sleep, 34–35
Bread-cereals group, "essential four," 195–196
Breast cancer, 333
Breathing failure, first aid for, 516–517
Bromides, 35
Bronchitis: air pollution, 462; tobacco smoking, 339
Brucellosis, 497
Bruises, first aid for, 517
Burns, 152; first aid for, 517

Caffeine, 50, 79, 529
Calcium, 187
Calisthenics, 110–111
Caloric balance, 198
Calories: allowances, 196; common foods, 519–525; definition, 126, 198, 529; expenditure rate, 126–127
Cancer, 12, 325, 341, 529; air pollution, 462, 464; chemotherapy, 334; "chimney-sweeper's," 450; college students, 8; common sites of, 333; contraceptive pills and, 302; curability, 331–332; detection, 335–336; fraudulent cures, 394; molecular attack on, 285; penile, 291; public health concern with, 412; role of heredity, 281; tobacco smoking, 338–340, 345
Cannon, Walter B., 25, 151
Capillaries, 139
Carbohydrates, 179, 191, 206, 529; dietary requirement, 177, 184; effect on cholesterol level, 176; relative caloric value, 199; sources, 184
Cardiovascular disease, 176, 460. *See also* Heart disease
Cardiovascularenal disease, 325. *See also* Heart disease
Cardiovascularenal system, 132, 146. *See also* Blood vessels; Circulatory system; Heart; Kidney; and Urinary system

Cytoplasm, 133

Dance, 104, 108, 111, 117
Danger signals of disease, twenty common: table, 12–13
Danger zone, automotive: table, 379
Dating, 222, 245, 263; changes in orientation, 266; courtship and, 265; feminine aggression, 270; personality types, 267; premarital sex, 237; source of satisfaction, 7
"Dating and rating," 265
Daydreams, *see* Fantasy
DDT (dichlorodiphenyltrichloroethane), 453, 485, 503, 530; malaria control, 486; onchoceriasis control, 487–488; restrictions on use, 489; typhus control, 487
Deafness, 166; causes, 165; hysterical, 44
Death: causes, college students, 8, 14, 17, 62, 375, variation with age, 325; rates, 15, 234
Degenerative diseases, 152, 530
Delinquent behavior, 62–63
Delirium tremens, 70, 72, 530
Dementia praecox, 56
Dendrite, *ill.* 29
Dendron, 30, *ill.* 29
Dental care, 430, 432
Dental caries, 189–191
Dentures, 190–191
Deoxyribonucleic acid (DNA), 135–136, 276, 283, 285–286, 531; composition, 137; model, *ill.* 284
Department of Health, Education, and Welfare, 418
Depressants: abuse, 83, signs of, 90; alcohol, 69; characteristics, 84–85; government regulation, 82
Depression, 11, 26, 98, 531
Dermatitis, 170, 531
Dermis, 168, 531
Detergents, 453
Diabetes insipidus, 147
Diabetes mellitus, 149, 183, 507, 531; association with obesity, 198; emergency medical identification, 385; inherited tendency toward, 280; mental retardation, 63; psychological effect, 457; public health concern with, 412; therapy, 11
Diaphragm, vaginal, 298, 531
Diarrhea, 13, 531
Diesel engines, air pollution, 466
Diet, 152; adequate, 10, 22; cholesterol content, 330; dental caries, 190; deficiencies, 11; fads, 205; fat-free, 185; food components, 206; neglect, 72; protective foods, 191; recommended daily allowances, table, 192–193; relation to cardiovascular disease, 176; weight reduction, 198
Digestion, 31, 531; chemistry of, 182–183; effect of adrenalin, 148; physiology of, early experiments, 208–210; regulation, 27–28
Digestive system, 132, 179–183, 206, 531, *ill.* 180–181; effect of alcohol, 72; fatigue, 122; normal condition, 196; oversensitive, 3. *See also* Alimentary canal
Dimethyltryptamine (DMT), 79, 89; characteristics, 84–85
Diphtheria, immunization, 14, 366
Disease: agents of, 150; classification, 152; insect-borne, 485–486; mistaken ascription to heredity, 281;

stress, 149–152; transmission, 355–358
Displacement, *see* Substitution
Divorce: rate among alcoholics, 73; religious attitudes, 256, 258, 263; statistics, 248; suggested reforms, 234
Dollard, John, 47
Douche, 299
Dreams, 33–34, 39
Drugs, 152; addiction and habituation, defined, 80–81; brain damage, 55; campus problem, 96; classes of users, 79–80; continuum, 96; degrees of use, 100; government regulation, 92; history, 81–83; medical uses, symptoms, and dependence potentials, chart, 84–85; mystique, 97–98; need for information, 100; orientation of society, 94; psychoactive, 79; psychotherapeutic use, 39, 59; rate of use, 79; reasons for using, 22, 80, 99; relief of anxiety, 49; role in identity search, 95; sleep, 35; testing, 394–395; treatment of alcoholism, 73
Drug abuse, vii–viii; behavioral signs, 89–90, 93; causes, 94; history, 92; traumatic, 97
Drug addiction, 62; attitudes toward, 82–83; crime, 82; environmental influences, 458; Negroes, 436; pressures to return to, 91; treatment, 91–93
Duodenum, 179
"Dynamic therapeutics," 113

Eardrum, 165
Ears, 172, *ill.* 164; wax, 165, 168. *See also* Inner ear; Middle ear; and Outer ear
Eating habits, 35, 196
Ecology, 441, 531
Education, role of family, 214
Ego, 39–42, 51, 531; fantasy, 44; functions, 22; sublimation, 45
Ego defenses, 40, 51; extreme, 54; rationalization, 43; unconscious conflicts, 41
Ego identity, drug use, 95, 99
Ehrlich, Paul, 354
Electric shock, 32
Electrocardiogram, 459, 531
Electroencephalogram, 459, 531
Electroshock therapy, 59
Embryo, 531; development, *ill.* 308; growth, 309–312, 320
Embryology, 307
Embryonic disc, 309
Emergency medical identification, 385–386
Emotional conflicts, 32, 240–241
Emotional deprivation, 32, 150
Emotional disturbances: college students, 6, 8; incidence, 14; menstrual cycle, 299; treatment, 9
Emotions, 25
Emphysema, 531, *ill.* 340; air pollution, 462; tobacco smoking, 339, 345
Employment, 46
Endocrine disorders, 146
Endocrine glands, 8, 32, 150, 220, 531
Endocrine secretions, 33, 139. *See also* Hormones
Endocrine system, 132, 146–149, 153, *ill.* 147; general adaptation syndrome, 152; mind-body mediation, 21–22, 25
Endogamy, 243, 532

Fractures, 532. *See also* Bones
Frascatoro, Girolamo, 350
Freckles, 170
Free fatty acids, 26
Freud, Sigmund, viii, 25, 58; concept of mental health, 21; Oedipus complex, 47; orthodox psychotherapy, 24; principles of mental health, 23; theory of personality development, 46; unconscious mind, 39
Fromm, Erich, 46–47
Frostbite, first aid for, 517
Frustration, 532; alcohol, 73; response to, 38; sublimation, 45; threat to health, 8; tolerance, 21
Fungi, 355, 532

Galactosemia, 532; hereditary, 285; mental retardation, 63
Gall bladder, 179
Galton, Francis, 275, 286
Gambling, 62, 73
Ganglion, 26–27, 29–30, 32, 533
Gastric juice, 179, 209, 533
Gastric secretion, 113
Gastritis, 9, 325
General adaptation syndrome, 151–152
Genes, 276, 282, 286, 533; chemical composition, 284; discovery, 278; dominant, 279; law of independent assortment, 279; number in human ovum, 284; protein synthesis, 135; recessive, 279; replication, 136; research, 285; sex-linked characteristics, 283
Genetic code, 137, 284, 286
Genetic laws, *ill.* 279
Genetic mutations, 490, 492
Genetics, 278–280, 285, 533
Genitourinary system, 132
Genotypes, 279, 533
German measles (rubella), 277, 533
Gestation, 312
GI Bill, 6, 251
Gingivitis, 191, 533
Glaucoma, 162–163, 508, 533
Glomerulus, 146
Glue sniffing, 90
Glycogen, 120, 122, 533
Goiter, 149, 496, 533
Golden Rule, 24
Goldstein, Kurt, 46
Golgi apparatus, 133, 135
Gonads, 533; development, 310–312
Gonorrhea, 361, 533
"Goof balls," *see* Barbiturates
Gossip, 45
Graafian follicle, 289, 297, 533
Grandmothers, 237
Gravity, 460
Group therapy, 58, 533
Growth, importance of thiamin, 186; rate, need for sleep, 33
Guilt, 39–41; alcohol, 73; sexual, 223, 235, 241; symbolic appeasement, 45

Hair, 171–172, 280
Halitosis, 508–509, 533

Hallucinations, 533; cocaine, 86; glue sniffing, 90; LSD, 88; schizophrenia, 56
Hallucinogens, 79, 87, 93; abuse, 83; characteristics, 84–85; college students, 89; dependence on, 96; government regulation, 82; history, 88; ill effects, 80; reasons for using, 99; signs of use, 91; traumatic effects, 98. *See also* Drugs; Marihuana; and Lysergic acid diethylamide
Happiness, narrow ideals of, 45
Hate, 38
Hayfever, 509, 533
Headache, 13, 41, 509; first aid for, 517
Head injuries, 55
Health: definitions, 3, 17, 445; misconceptions, xi
Health agencies, voluntary, 420–423, 432
Health cults, 14, 399, 401
Health education: ancient Greeks and Romans, 4; college dropouts, 5; philosophy of, viii; preparation for, 412; teacher's responsibility, 411; World Health Organization, xii
Health fads, 399, 401
"Health foods," 178
Health frauds, 393–397, 400
Health hazards, vii, 10; contraceptive pills, 302; direct causes, 11; environmental, 441; intrauterine contraceptive devices, 303; pollution, 479; self-protection against, 368, 370
Health insurance, 427–430, 433
Health personnel, 3
Health professions: career opportunities, 409–411; statistics, 406–407
Health programs, environmental, 448
Health resources, statistics, 408
Health services, inequities in, 424, 435–437
Health slogans, 5
Hearing: difficulties, 11; posture, 123
Hearing aids, 459, *ill.* 165–166
Heart, *ill.* 142; blood supply, 141; congenital defects, 328; development, 309–310, 312; jogging, 112; murmurs, 328; muscle, 132; palpitations, 32; stress from kidney infections, 146; stroke volume, 139; surgery, 326; transplantation, 326
Heart ailments, 462
Heart attack, 328–329; tobacco smoking, 340
Heart beat, fetal, 312
Heart disease, 11, 325, 341; college students, 8; death rate, 326; diet and, 175; fad diets, 205–206; molecular attack on, 285; obesity, 198; psychogenic origins, 44; public health concern with, 412; rheumatic, 328–330; tobacco smoking, 340, 345; types, 328–330
Heart failure, 329
Heart rate, 33, 141, 148
Heat cramps, first aid for, 517
Heat exhaustion, first aid for, 517
Hemoglobin, 139, 143, 188, 533
Hemophilia, 277, 280, 533; emergency medical identification, 385
Hemorrhage, 13, 533
Hemorrhoids, 509, 533
Hepatitis, viral, 365
Hereditary diseases, marriage and, 250
Hereditary, 533; cultural, 275–276, 286; definitions, 277;

Leukemia, 333, 336, 510, 535
Leukocytes, *see* White blood cells
Lewin, Kurt, 46
Libido, 37, 39, 535
Life expectancy, 9, 15; chart, 10; heart attack, 329; table, 11
Ligaments, 125, 535
Liver: bile production, 179; destruction of vitamin D, 177; development, 311–312; galactosemia, 63; portal circulation, 141
Longevity, 109, 280, 461
Love: being in, 25; capacity for, 21, 54; deprivation, 32; displaced, 43; homosexual, 38; idealistic, 38; imitative, 37; marital chastity, 236; marital fighting, 238; narcissistic, 37; need for, 23; oedipal, 37–38; romantic, 246–247, 263; sex and, 229, 232, 235, 240–241; stages, 37, 220
Loyalty, 38
Lungs, 112, 143; occupational hazards, 450–451. *See also* Cancer; Respiratory system; and Tobacco smoking
Lymphatic system, 132, 143, 535; cancer, 336
Lysergic acid diethylamide (LSD), 79, 93, 95; "casual" use, 96–97; characteristics, 84–85; government regulation, 82, 89; history, 88; nightmares, 94; psychotic reactions, 80, 97
Lysosomes, 135

Malaria, 442, 496, 499, 536; control, 486–487, *ill*. 495
Male reproductive system, 289–292, 299, *ill*. 291
Malnutrition, 176; alcoholism, 73; prevention, 191; role in disease, 150
Malpighian cells, 168, 536
Manic-depressive psychoses, 56, 536
Mann, Horace, 4
Marihuana, 79, 536; characteristics, 84–85; dependence on, 88, 96; government regulation, 82, 87; history, 81; physiological and psychological effects, 87, 98, 457; psychotic reactions, 80; reasons for using, 99; signs of use, 91; similarity of effects to alcohol, 87–88; social use, 96; thumbnail sketch of smoker, 97
Marriage, 263; ages at, 216, 249, 271–272; college students, 6, 248–249; courtship and dating, 245; early, 219; engagement, 245; fighting, 238; financial problems, 251, 255–256; forced by pregnancy, 222; functions of, 214; group, 217; improving patterns, 240; infidelity, 236; interracial, 250; interreligious, 258, 262; personality and, 251–253; religious viewpoints, 254–263; romantic monogamous, 218; sex, 241; sex education, 228; sex problems, 219; sexual fashions, 302; trial, 271; twenty questions for testing potential mate, 252–253; variations in rate, 249
Marriage brokers, *ill*. 247
Marriage contract, 257, 262
Marriage partner, selection, 249–251; taboos, 243–244
Masculinity, blurring of distinction from femininity, 231; stereotypes, 230, 233
Maslow, Abraham, 46
Mastication, 179, 536
Masturbation, 57, 222–224
Mating combinations, 217
Matriarchies, 213, 237, 536
Maturation, 220

Maturity, 23, 37
Measles, immunization toward, 14, 366, *ill*. 365
Meat group, "essential four," 195
Medicaid, 427, 431, 433
Medical advice, 398
Medical care, 430
Medical check-ups, 8, 370
Medical costs, 426–427, 432–433
Medical profession, attitude toward birth control, 234
Medical societies, 14
Medicare, 427, 431, 433
Medications, emergency medical identification, 386
Memory, 33, 39, 41
Menarche, 297, 536
Mendel, Gregor, 278–279, 286, 536
Meningitis, 55, 536
Menninger, Karl, 62
Menopause, 289, 297, 299, 536; atherosclerosis, 328
Menstrual cycle, *ill*. 296; emotional storms, 299; hormonal regulation, 148; ovulation, 297; "safe period," 298–299
Menstruation, 220, 289, 295–297, 299, 536; blood loss, 296; exercise, 113; painful, 296
Mental acuity, 4
Mental health, vii; Sigmund Freud, 21; improvement, 61; principles, 23–25, 36; public concern with, 412; signs of, 22; sublimation, 45–46
Mental hospitals, 57, 59–60
Mental illness, 22, 48, 65, 536; alcoholism, 69, 72; causes, 55; community services, 60; conditioning therapy, 59; degrees, 54; drug therapy, 39; environmental influences, 458; exhibitions of, 62–63; heredity, 281; incidence, 60; incipient, 6; nervous system, 39; precipitating factor, 55; prevention, 54, 61; treatment, 57–60; types, 55–57
Mental mechanisms, 22, 536; accident proneness, 381; ego defenses, 40–41; forms, 41–46, 51; health frauds and, 398–399
Mental retardation, 28, 65, 536; associated physical disability, 64; causes, 63; cretinism, 149; degrees, 64; incidence, 62–64; Negro children, 435–436; rehabilitation, 64, *ill*. 63
Meperidine, 80
Meprobamate (Miltown), 59, 73, 536
Mescaline, 79, 88; characteristics, 84–85
Metabolism, 536; food intake, 179; hormonal regulation, 146, 148; minerals, 187; muscles, 120–122; phosphorus, 188; sleep, 33–34, 143; thyroxin, 149; waste products, 122, 137–139
Metals, water pollution, 470
Metastasis, 333, 536
Methadone, 80, 84–85, 91–92
Metropolitan areas, 451, 464–465
Microbiology, 354, 370, 536
Microorganisms, 354, 370, 536, *ill*. 356, 357; classification, 355; discovery, 352, table, 353. *See also* Bacteria; Communicable diseases; and Fungi
Microscope, 132, 352
Midbrain, 32
Middle age: causes of death, 325; presbyopia, 160
Middle ear, 143, 163, 165
Milk group, "essential four," 194, *ill*. 195

Miller, Neal, 47
Minerals, 133, 175, 191, 206; dietary deficiency, 178; metabolism, 177; recommended daily dietary allowances, table, 192–193; regulation of metabolic processes, 187; relative caloric value, 199
Mitochondria, 135
Mitosis, 537. *See also* Cell division
Molecular biology, 136–137
Molecular disease, 285
Molecular reactions, 133
Money, 251
Mongolism, 282, 537
Monogamy, 217, 537; enforcement, 247; Jewish attitude, 261
Monosaccharides, 133. *See also* Sugars
Mons veneris, 295, 537
Montagu, Ashley, 49
Morality, "new," 95
Morphine, 80, 88, 92, 537; characteristics, 84–85; history, 81–82; signs of abuse, 90
Motherhood, 240
Motion sickness, 12, 163–165, 537
Motorcycle accidents, viii, 383
Mouth, 141, 172; cancer, 336; digestive function, 179
Multiple births, 289
Multiple sclerosis, 28, 510, 537
Mumps, 14
Murder, *see* Homicide
Murphy, Gardner, 47
Murray, Henry, 46
Muscles, *ill.* 121; metabolism, 120–122; tissue, 120, 132; tone, 33, 146, 537
Muscular contractions, 113
Muscular dystrophy, 28, 510, 537
Muscular Dystrophy Associations of America, Inc., 422
Muscular efficiency, 118
Muscular system, 131
Muscular tension, 122
Musculoskeletal system, 118–122, 128, 132
Muteness, hysterical, 44
Myelin sheath, 29
Myocardium, 141, 537
Myopia, 157, 537, *ill.* 158; correction, 159; inherited tendency, 280; progressive, 159

Nails, finger and toe, 172
Nalline, 92
Narcissism, 97–98, 537
Narcotics, 22, 92, 537; addiction, 82, 88; legal and medical definitions, 80
Nasopharynx, 141
National Association for Mental Health, 420–421
National Association for Retarded Children, 422
National Foundation, 420, 422
National Institutes of Health, 419, *ill.* 420
National Multiple Sclerosis Society, 421–422
National Tuberculosis Association, 420–422
Nearsightedness, *see* Myopia
Negativism, 24
Negroes: health problems, 435–446; patterns of family life, 237
Nephritis, 146, 537

Nerve cells, 133
Nerve impulses, 30
Nerve junctions, *ill.* 29
Nerves, 26
Nervous breakdown, 57, 537
Nervous reflexes, 30
Nervous stimuli, 31–32, 152
Nervous system, 132, *ill.* 27; alcohol, 72; cancer, 333; disorders, 28; electrical characteristics, 30; development, 309–310; functions, 36; general adaptation syndrome, 152; mediation of mind and body, 21–22; mental illness, 39; normal, 30; regulation of internal environment, 150. *See also* Autonomic nervous system; Central nervous system; and Peripheral nervous system
Neurasthenia, 57, 537
Neuroendocrine system, 132. *See also* Endocrine system; Nervous system
Neuron, 28, 36, 537, *ill.* 29; associative, 30–32
Neuroses, 55, 62, 537
Neurotic conflicts, alcoholism, 72–73
Neurotics, 44, 54
Niacin, 176, 185–186, 537
Nicotine, 79, 537. *See also* Tobacco smoking
Nicotinic acid, *see* Niacin
Night blindness, 161, 186
Nightingale, Florence, 351
Nightmares, 32, 94
Nocturnal emissions, 223, 290
Noise abatement, 448
Noise pollution, 416–417
Nondaters, 268
Nose, 141, 166–167, 172, *ill.* 145
Nosology, 152
Nucleic acids, 133, 537. *See also* Deoxyribonucleic acid; Ribonucleic acid
Nucleoli, 135
Nucleotides, 137, 284
Nucleus (of cell), 133–135, 283, 537
Nutrition: advances, 175, 277; children, 176; hormones, 146; nonsense, 205–206; pregnancy, 176; science, 178, 206; therapy, acne, 171
Nutritional deprivation, 32

Obesity, 73, 537; eating habits, 205; endocrine disorder, 148; psychogenic origins, 198; psychology, 204–205; relation to death rate, 197–198
Obstetric care, 304–305, 538
Obstetric shock, 152
Occupational diseases, 450, 538
Occupational hazards, 457
Occupational health, 448–451
Occupations, statistics, 449
Oculist, 157, 538
Odors, 166
Oedipus complex, 47, 538
Oil drilling, water pollution, 472
Old age, causes of death, 325
Oldsightedness, *see* Presbyopia
Olfactory cells, 166, 538
Onchoceriasis (river blindness), 496, 499; control, 487–488

ments, 183; International Congress of Nutrition, 176–177; recommended daily dietary allowances, 192–193; relation to atherosclerosis, 176; relative caloric value, 199; sources, 184; synthesis, 135; work capacity, 177

Protozoa, 355, 540
Psilocybin, 79, 88; characteristics, 84–85
Psittacosis, 497, 540
Psychasthenia, 57
Psychedelic drugs, 88, 96. *See also* Hallucinogens
Psychiatric complaints, 8, 9
Psychiatry, 58, 540; "interpersonal theory," 47; schools, 24
Psychoanalysis, 58, 540
Psychoanalytic theory, 39, 47
Psychological tests, 6
Psychopathic personality, 57
Psychopharmacology, 24
Psychoses, 54–55, 62, 541
Psychosomatic illness, 11, 14, 44, 152, 54
Psychotherapy, 541; acne, 171; alcoholism, 73; college students, 7; drugs, 59; types, 58
Puberty, 38, 541
Public health: definitions, 405, 541; code, Philadelphia, 417–418; departments, 432, functions, 412
Pulmonary circulation, 140
Puncture wounds, first aid for, 518
Punishment, 41, 46
Pyorrhea, 191, 541
Pyridoxine, 177, 186
Pyrimidines, 133

Q-fever, 497
Quackery, 10, 14, 205, 399, 401, 541
Quarantine, 454–455

Race, 237–238
Radiation, 455, 479, 541. *See also* X-rays
Radiation hazards, 487, 499; atomic wastes, 492–493; food contamination, 477–478; genetic, 490; medical, 490; nuclear fallout, 491
Radiation sickness, 493, 541
Radioactivity, 461
Radionuclides, regulation, 478
Rage, 25, 152
Rank, Otto, 58
Rape, 233–234
Rapid eye movements (REM), viii, 34
Rationalization, 43, 541; automobile accidents, 381
Reality principle, 40
Rebellion, 7, 95
Recommended daily dietary allowances, table, 192–193
Rectum, 143; cancer, 336
Red blood cells (erythrocytes), 118, 139
Reed, Walter, 486–487
Reflexes, 30–31, 541
Regression, 41–42, 381, 542
Reinforcement theory of learning, 47
Religion: fading importance, 95; marriage, 250, 253–263; observance, 7; training, 42, 46
Renal circulation, 140–141
Rennin, 179

Repression, 41, 381, 542
Reproduction, impulses toward, 287
Reproductive process, 287–289
Reproductive system, 132. *See also* Female reproductive system; Male reproductive system
Reserpine, 59, 542
Respiration, 31; daily air requirement, 461; mechanism, 143; oxygen requirement, 137; rate, 33; regulation, 27–28
Respiratory ailments: frequency, 9; air pollution, 462, 464
Respiratory system, 131, 153, 542, *ill.* 144; aerobics, 112; cancer, 333; development, 118; exercise, 110; lower, 143; oxygen circulation, 137; upper, 141–143
Rest, 22
Reticulo-endothelial system, 132
Retina, 26, *ill.* 27; astigmatism, 160; end-plates, 156; infection, 162; myopia and hyperopia, 159; rods and cones, 157; "visual purple," 186
Revenge, 38
Reward-punishment, 47
Rheumatic fever, 328–330, 542
Rheumatism, 511–512
Rh factor, 280, 542
"Rhythm" method of birth control, 298–299, 301–302, 542
Riboflavin, 186
Ribonucleic acid (RNA), 135–136, 276, 283, 285–286; composition, 137
Rickets, 185, 187, 542
Rickettsia, 355, 542
Rogers, Carl, 47
Royal Canadian Air Force, exercise program, 109–110

Saliva, 167, 179
Sanitation, 3, 368, 370, 469
Schistosomiasis (bilharziasis), 488, 496, 542
Schizophrenia, 56, 542; heredity, 281; serum factor, 56; treatment, 59
Scholarship resources, 5
Sclera, 156
Scrapes, first aid for, 517
Scrotum, 290
Scurvy, 11, 185–186, 197, 542
Seawater: desalinization, 454–455; evolution of life, 133
Sebaceous glands, 168, 542
Secondary sex characteristics, 220; female, 292; hair, 171; hormonal effects, 148–149, male, 290
Sedatives, 35, 59, 543
Self-esteem, 43
Self-medication, 10, 14, 50, 398
Self-mutilation, 62
Selye, Hans, 151
Semen, 288, 290, 543
Seminal vesicles, 290
Senile dementia, 56
Sense organs, 155–172
Sewage: disposal, 451–453; Lake Erie, 481; obsolete, 470; treatment, *ill.* 474–475; water pollution, 469–470
Sex: anxiety, 24; attitudes, 218–219, 227, 229–232, 239, 271–273; emotional conflicts, 241; legal regulation, 233–234; love and, 229, 232, 235, 240–241; marital,

Superstition, 48
Surgery, 152
Sweat glands, 143, 168
Swelling, 13
Swimming, 182
Symbolization, 45; automobile accidents, 381
Synapse, 30–31, 544
Syphilis: brain damage, 54–55; central nervous system damage, 28; congenital, 277; diagnosis, 360; Philadelphia, *ill.* 416; premarital examination, 250; stages, 360, transmission, 358–360
Systemic circulation, 140

Taste, 166
Teeth, 187–189, 206; embryonic development, 311–312
Tegumentary system, 131, 171–172
Television, 163
Temperature: circulatory system, 139; skin, 169; sleep, 33–34
Tendons, 544; foot, *ill.* 125
Tension, 111
Testes, 146, 288–290, 544; fetal descent, 312
Testosterone, 148, 290, 544; cancer chemotherapy, 335
Tetanus (lockjaw), immunization, 14, 366
Thermal inversion, 462
Thiamin, 185–187, 544
Thirst, abnormal, 183
Thorndike, Edward, 46
Throat, *ill.* 145
Thymus, 146, 149, 544
Thyroid, 146, 149, 544; disorders, 149; iodine requirement, 188
Thyroxin, 149, 544
Tobacco smoking, 341; addiction, 343, 345; campaigns against, 346; cancer risk, 338, 340; death and disease, table, 344; disease incidence, 339–340; pregnancy, 339; prevention, 345; statistics, 344
Tolbutamide, 11, 544
Tongue, 166–167
Toothache, first aid for, 518
Toothpaste, 191
Trachoma, 162, 496, 544, *ill.* 494
Tranquilizers, 22, 544; abuse, 83; complication of sleep, 34; everyday use, 79; psychotherapeutic use, 59; signs of abuse, 90; therapy, 48
Travel, 367–368, 453
Trichinosis, 497, 545
Tuberculosis, 442, 496, 513, 545; optical effects, 162; Philadelphia, *ill.* 416
Twins, 280, 289
Typhus, 487, 496, 545

Umbilical cord, 309, 318
Unconscious conflicts, 32, 40–41, 44
Unconscious mind, 39, 545; alcoholism, 73; anxiety, 37; behavior control, 37, 218; creativity, 33; fantasy, 44; mental mechanisms, 41; structure, 22, 39, 51; submergence of ego, 40
Unconscious reaction, 31
Unconsciousness, first aid for, 518
Undernourishment, 4
Underweight, 103

United Cerebral Palsy Associations, 422
United States Public Health Service, 418–420, 432, 447
Ureters, 132, 146
Urethra, 132, 146, 290
Urinary bladder, 132, 146
Urinary system, 132, 143–146; cancer, 333, 336
Urination, 13
Urine, 290
Uterine tubes, *see* Fallopian tubes
Uterus, 294, 299, 545; cancer, 333, 336; contraction, 318; embryonic development, 309; labor, 317; menstrual cycle, 297; position of fetus, 312; pregnant, *ill.* 313

Vagina, 294, 545
Vegetable-fruit group, "essential four," 195
Vegetarians, dietary protein sources, 184
Veins, 139; varicose, 513, 545
Venereal disease, 11, 358, 370, 442, 545; control, 361–362; effects on eyes, 162; effects on inner ear, 165; protection, 298; risk, 71; sixteenth century, 350. *See also* Communicable diseases; Gonorrhea; and Syphilis
Veterans Administration, 420
Virginity, 273, 295
Virology, 136
Virus diseases, 364
Viruses, 355, 545–546; cancer, 335; discovery, 352; research, 285
Vision: artificial light, 160–161; changes, 13; defects in focus, 157–160; faulty, detection, 155; postural effects, 123; normal, *ill.* 158; poor, 11
Vital statistics, 413–415
Vitamin A, 161, 186
Vitamin B, alcoholism, 72–73
Vitamin B_1, *see* Thiamin
Vitamin B_2 (G), *see* Riboflavin
Vitamin B_6, *see* Pyridoxine
Vitamin B_{12}, 186
Vitamin C, *see* Ascorbic acid
Vitamin D, 176–177, 185, 187
Vitamin deficiency diseases, 150, 152, 185–186
Vitamin E, 177
Vitamin K, 186
Vitamin pills, 178, 185
Vitamins, 133, 177, 179, 191, 206, 546; food additives, 478; overdoses, 187; recommended daily dietary allowances, 192–193; relative caloric value, 199
Vitreous fluid, 156
Voice change, 220
Vulva, 294

War, 44
Wassermann test, 360, 546
Water, 191, 206; dietary requirement, 183, 199; food component, 199; major uses, 468; rate of use, 467; relative caloric value, 199; safe sources, 467
Water pollution, 448, 455, 457, 461, 468–472, 503, 579; campaigns against, 481; chemical wastes, 471; control, 472–473; detergents, 453; fishkill, *ill.* 469; heat pollution, 471; industrial, 472; population explosion, 502; public responsibility, 482; radioactive wastes, 471; recreational wastes, 472